D1327787

WJ
141
12/06

10 FEB 09

OF01032

Books should be returned to the SDH Library on or before
the date stamped above unless a renewal has been arranged

Salisbury District Hospital Library
Telephone: Salisbury (01722) 336262 extn. 4432 / 33
Out of hours answer machine in operation

Urogenital Ultrasound

Urogenital Ultrasound

A Text Atlas

Second Edition

Dennis Ll Cochlin FRCR
Consultant Radiologist
Cardiff and Vale NHS Trust
University Hospital of Wales
Cardiff
UK

Paul A Dubbins MB BS BSc FRCR
Consultant Radiologist
Department of Medical Imaging
Derriford Hospital
Plymouth
UK

Barry B Goldberg MD
Professor of Radiology
Director, Division of Diagnostic Ultrasound
Thomas Jefferson University Hospital
Philadelphia, PA
USA

Ethan J Halpern MD
Professor of Radiology and Urology
Director, Jefferson Prostate Diagnostic Center
Thomas Jefferson University Hospital
Philadelphia, PA
USA

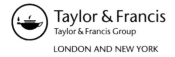

Taylor & Francis
Taylor & Francis Group

LONDON AND NEW YORK

© 1996, 2006 Taylor & Francis, an imprint of the Taylor & Francis Group
Taylor & Francis Group is the Academic Division of Informa plc

First published in the United Kingdom in 1996
by Martin Dunitz Ltd, an imprint of the Taylor & Francis Group

Second edition published in 2006
by Taylor & Francis, an imprint of the Taylor & Francis Group, 2 Park Square, Milton Park, Abingdon, Oxon OX14 4RN

Tel: +44 (0)20 7017 6000
Fax: +44 (0)20 7017 6699
E-mail: info.medicine@tandf.co.uk
Website: www.tandf.co.uk/medicine

All rights reserved. No part of this publication may be reproduced, stored in a retrieval system, or transmitted, in any form or by any means, electronic, mechanical, photocopying, recording, or otherwise, without the prior permission of the publisher or in accordance with the provisions of the Copyright, Designs and Patents Act 1988 or under the terms of any licence permitting limited copying issued by the Copyright Licensing Agency, 90 Tottenham Court Road, London W1P 0LP.

Although every effort has been made to ensure that all owners of copyright material have been acknowledged in this publication, we would be glad to acknowledge in subsequent reprints or editions any omissions brought to our attention.

Although every effort has been made to ensure that drug doses and other information are presented accurately in this publication, the ultimate responsibility rests with the prescribing physician. Neither the publishers nor the authors can be held responsible for errors or for any consequences arising from the use of information contained herein. For detailed prescribing information or instructions on the use of any product or procedure discussed herein, please consult the prescribing information or instructional material issued by the manufacturer.

A CIP record for this book is available from the British Library.

Library of Congress Cataloging-in-Publication Data

Data available on application

ISBN 1 84184 397 0
ISBN 978 1 84184 397 1

Distributed in North and South America by
Taylor & Francis
2000 NW Corporate Blvd
Boca Raton, FL 33431, USA

Within Continental USA
Tel: 800 272 7737; Fax: 800 374 3401
Outside Continental USA
Tel: 561 994 0555; Fax: 561 361 6018
E-mail: orders@crcpress.com

Distributed in the rest of the world by
Thomson Publishing Services
Cheriton House
North Way
Andover, Hampshire SP10 5BE, UK
Tel: +44 (0)1264 332424
E-mail: salesorder.tandf@thomsonpublishingservices.co.uk

Composition by Scribe Design Ltd, Ashford, Kent, UK
Printed and bound in Great Britain by CPI Bath

Contents

Contributors

Laurence Berman MRCP FRCR
School of Clinical Medicine
Department of Radiology
University of Cambridge
Cambridge
UK

Rosalie de Bruyn MB ChB DMRD FRCR
Consultant Paediatric Radiologist and Honorary Senior
Lecturer
Department of Radiology
Great Ormond Street Hospital for Children NHS Trust
London
UK

Lyn S Chitty PhD MRCOG
Senior Lecturer and Consultant in Genetics and Fetal
Medicine
Department of Clinical and Molecular Genetics
Institute of Child Health
London
UK

Dennis Ll Cochlin FRCR
Consultant Radiologist
Cardiff and Vale NHS Trust
University Hospital of Wales
Cardiff
UK

Paul Dubbins MB BS BSc FRCR
Consultant Radiologist
Department of Medical Imaging
Derriford Hospital
Plymouth
UK

Simon J Freeman MB BS MRCP FRCR
Consultant Radiologist
Imaging Directorate
Derriford Hospital
Plymouth
and
Visiting Lecturer
University of the West of England
Bristol
UK

Ethan Halpern MD
Professor of Radiology and Urology
Thomas Jefferson University Hospital
Philadelphia, PA
USA

Preface to the first edition

This book is a comprehensive study of genitourinary ultrasound. As ultrasound imaging is, by its very nature, a visual subject, the book takes the form of a text atlas. It is designed to be a reference work, but also to be easily read. To this end it is split into chapters which, while interrelated, are complete in themselves. The book is intended for radiologists, ultrasound technicians, urologists and all those involved with genitourinary ultrasound imaging.

Ultrasound imaging, while a well-established technique in the genitourinary system, is also a rapidly evolving modality. New imaging techniques are still being developed and new descriptions of the ultrasonic appearances of pathological conditions regularly appear in the literature. Against this background, this text provides a comprehensive account of state of the art ultrasound imaging and image interpretation.

Doppler studies are a relatively recent addition to genitourinary imaging, and they have an increasingly large place to play in various aspects of genitourinary studies, in some cases as a primary investigation, in others as an extension of the grey scale ultrasound examination. As Doppler studies are .essentially complementary to grey scale ultrasound studies, they are incorporated into the various chapters of the book, and not given a separate chapter.

Interventional ultrasound is, however, presented in a separate chapter. This is purely for convenience, as many of the techniques used in different anatomical sites and pathological conditions have much in common. The inclusion in a separate chapter should not imply that interventional ultrasound is, or should be, a separate discipline. Like Doppler, it should be regarded as a natural extension of the ultrasound examination. A chapter on paediatric ultrasound is included, as ultrasound is now the mainstay of paediatric genitourinary imaging. Many of the pathologies found in the paediatric age group are also found in adults. These are covered in the adult chapter. The paediatric chapter concentrates on those pathologies that differ in or are unique to the paediatric age group, and on the important differences in technique and interpretation that are essential to the practice and understanding of paediatric genitourinary ultrasound. Prenatal ultrasound is alluded to, as it affects investigation of the newborn, but the subject is not covered. This is properly the realm of obstetric ultrasound texts.

Unlike most ultrasound texts, no attempt have been made to include a chapter on the physics of ultrasound. Most practising ultrasonologists have been taught ultrasound physics and, for those that have not, there are excellent physics texts on the market that deal with the subject far more satisfactorily than could be done in a necessarily brief chapter. A chapter on the 'clinical' principles of Doppler is, however, included. Many ultrasonologists will have learned their skills before Doppler became generally used in the field. No serious attempt has been made to cover the physics of Doppler ultrasound. The Doppler chapter is firmly based on the clinical aspect – of what a sonologist needs to know in order to obtain and interpret diagnostic studies.

Chapters on renal dialysis and renal transplantation are included as they are an integral part of genitourinary medicine. The chapter on pancreatic transplantation is included as, at present, pancreatic transplants are nearly always combined with renal transplants in patients with diabetic nephropathy. Post-transplant studies of the pancreas are therefore usually combined with renal transplant studies and this task normally falls to the genitourinary imager.

Gynaecological ultrasound is not covered. Gynaecology is normally considered a separate discipline to genitourinary medicine, and there are many excellent texts devoted to this subject.

Why is a new book on this subject needed? This subject of genitourinary ultrasound is included in all general abdominal ultrasound texts as well as the few texts devoted purely to the subject. The many advances in genitourinary ultrasound have meant, however, that the subject is now too large to be adequately covered in general texts. While most of the monographs on the subject are some years old and thus do not include Doppler, the highly detailed studies made possible by high-resolution ultrasound equipment, and numerous advances in the ultrasonic interpretation of pathology and normal anatomy. There is therefore a need for a textbook of genitourinary ultrasound that is comprehensive and embraces all recent developments. This is such a book. It is an easily read, though comprehensive, text, generously illustrated for those studying the subject, and also a valuable reference work for those already established in the field.

Preface to the second edition

It is 10 years since the first edition was published. At the time we intended to produce a comprehensive study of genito-urinary ultrasound. The longevity of the first edition, we hope, bears witness to the fact that we have achieved a modicum of success in our aim. It also suggests, however, that the pace of change within ultrasound has been less rapid. Ultrasound remains central to the management of renal and urogenital disease process, but has retained a primary role in the initial investigation of the majority of conditions of the kidney while other technologies such as CT and MR may provide more specific diagnosis. This is particularly the case, for example, in the modern investigation or ureteric calculus disease. However, ultrasound retains a pre-eminent position in the investigation of the scrotum, of the renal transplant and of the urethra. Similarly, the advances that have taken place in prenatal diagnosis have influenced markedly the role of ultrasound in the neonate and young child. Consequently, the chapter on paediatric ultrasound reflects the close collaboration that is now necessary between pre- and postnatal imaging in offering the best continuity of care to patients with congenital disease or those diseases that manifest in the early neonatal period.

The sensitivity of Doppler and color Doppler has improved since the first edition, but the specificity of applying a particular diagnosis to processes involving neovascularity have not been fulfilled. Ultrasound remains subject to issues of body habitus and difficulties with bowel gas, as before. New technologies have resolved these difficulties only partly. Non-linear ultrasound, both applied to imaging and to Doppler, together with the development of contrast media of greater stability, have improved organ visualization in difficult patients, have contributed to characterization of certain pathologies and increased the ability to identify branch vessels and to afford their better interrogation.

The text book has been almost completely rewritten, partly to reflect the information available within the literature, but also to reflect the changing role of ultrasound in certain applications.

The majority of images have been replaced throughout the textbook and a number of images have been added, both to illustrate the new technology and to demonstrate the role of micro-bubble contrast agents. Inevitably, some images remain from the first edition, partly as a consequence of the rarity of some of the conditions that were illustrated and partly because we have been unable to improve on the original submissions.

We hope that our original intention that this should be an easy-to-read reference work has survived the extensive revision. Ultrasound is used by an ever-widening group of individuals as equipment becomes cheaper and more accessible. It is thus intended, not only to address the needs of radiologists, but also increasingly of urologists, renal physicians and sonographers.

Acknowledgments

We are pleased to acknowledge the contribution of Dr Rosalie de Bruyn and Lyn Chitty for the Pediatric and pre-natal urological ultrasound chapter; of Dr Simon Freeman for the chapter on The renal transplant; and of Dr Laurence Berman for the chapter on Ultrasound of the male anterior urethra.

The chapter on The bladder, while rewritten in part, is firmly based on the excellent chapter written by Dr Archie A Alexander in the first edition.

We are indebted to our wives and families for their encouragement and support during the writing of the book.

We acknowledge the help of our colleagues, sonographers and fellow radiologists who performed many of the studies that illustrate the book.

Finally, but not least, we thank Alan Burgess, Kelly Cornish and Caroline Milton at Taylor and Francis for their help in the preparation of the book.

1

The kidney

Paul Dubbins

GENERAL CONSIDERATIONS

Introduction

Ultrasound is established as the cornerstone of diagnosis in many conditions affecting the kidney. It is the investigation of first choice for renal failure, renal mass lesions, renal infections and diffuse parenchymal renal disease. Ultrasound is also of value in the investigation of renal colic, hematuria, abdominal trauma and congenital abnormalities, inherited cystic renal disease and renal vascular disease. Advances in computed tomography (CT) and magnetic resonance imaging (MRI) have altered the investigative pathway for renal disease, particularly, for example, in renal colic and in trauma management, but ultrasound remains a cost-effective primary investigation for a wide variety of disorders affecting the kidney.

Demonstration of sonographic anatomy requires that the ultrasound image be acquired with meticulous attention to technique, which will depend on an awareness of surface anatomy and anatomic relations.

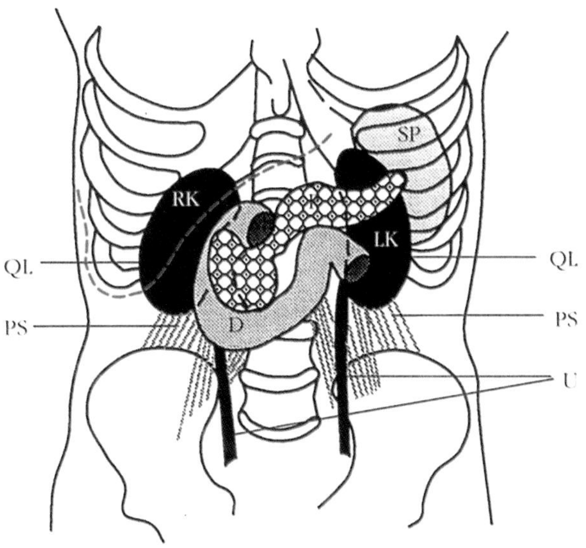

Figure 1.1
Anatomical relations of the kidneys. The dotted line indicates the normal position of the liver. RK = right kidney, LK = left kidney, SP = spleen, D = duodenum, QL = quadratus lumborum muscles, PS = psoas muscle, U = ureter.

Surface anatomy

The kidneys are oval structures which lie in a paraspinal location with their long axis approximately 20° to the vertical and their coronal axis approximately 10–20° from the true coronal. Thus, the upper pole of the kidney is situated more posteriorly and more medially than the lower pole. The hilum of the kidney usually lies just below the transpyloric plane, whereas the upper poles of both kidneys lie above the level of the costal margin. The lower poles usually extend well below the costal margin, although only the lowermost portion of either kidney extends below the 12th rib posteriorly (the two lowermost ribs are frequently resected at the time of nephrectomy). The course of the ureters usually follows the tips of the transverse processes to the pelvic brim, where they turn laterally and posteriorly, coursing over the surface of the pelvic wall muscles

before turning medially to enter the bladder at the trigone. The surface markings relative to the normal position of the kidney are shown in Figures 1.1 and 1.2.

Anatomical relations

The right kidney is related anteriorly and superiorly to the right lobe of the liver and the gallbladder and inferiorly to the hepatic flexure of the colon and to the small bowel (Figure 1.3). Posteriorly and posterolaterally, its relations are from above downwards to the ribs and intercostal muscles and the paraspinal muscles and quadratus lumborum. Laterally and inferiorly, the relations are the muscles of the

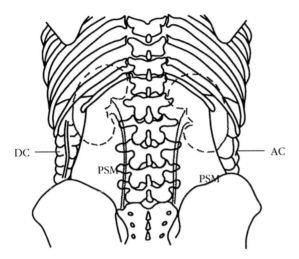

Figure 1.2
Surface anatomical markers for the kidneys from the posterior aspect. The normal axis of the kidneys is seen, their relationship to the lower ribs and to the paraspinal muscles (PSM). The relationship to the ascending colon (AC) and descending colon (DC) is also demonstrated. The relationship of the ureters to the tips of the transverse processes is shown.

abdominal wall. Medially, the kidneys are related to the psoas muscle and the transverse processes and bodies of the lumbar spine. Specifically on the right there is an anteromedial relationship to the adrenal gland, the pancreatic head and the second part of the duodenum and the inferior vena cava (Figure 1.4). On the left, the anterior superior relations are the spleen and tail of the pancreas, whereas medially lie the left adrenal gland, the third part of the duodenum and the aorta. The lower pole of the left kidney is anteriorly related to the splenic flexure of the colon and to the jejunum. For this reason a coronal approach to the left kidney yields the best images (Figure 1.5).

Gas within the colon and small bowel will frequently obscure the lower poles of both kidneys and, occasionally, rather more of the renal parenchyma. The ribs will obscure the upper pole of the kidney from an anterolateral approach and much of the kidney from a posterior approach. Much of ultrasound technique therefore is directed at utilizing available acoustic windows and optimizing points of access for renal imaging while taking into account the normal position and axis of the kidney (see Figures 1.1 and 1.2).

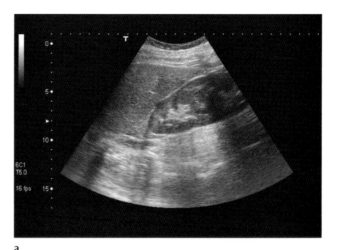

a

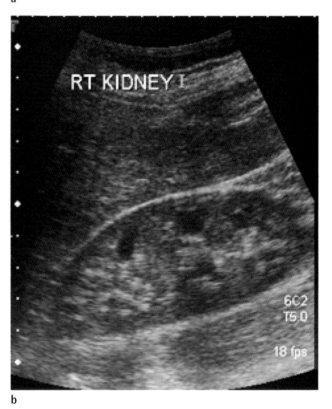

b

Figure 1.3
(a) Longitudinal scan through the right kidney, demonstrating the relationship to the right lobe of the liver anteriorly, the paraspinal muscles posteriorly and the adrenal bed superiorly. (b) Longitudinal section through the right kidney demonstrating the relationship between the right lobe of the liver, the psoas muscle and the perirenal fat.

Technique of examination

A flexible approach is required that acknowledges not only anatomical variation but also the physical principles which

contribute to the ultrasound information. Thus, to optimize the real-time grayscale image of renal anatomy, a scan plane perpendicular to the structure under study provides optimum information. By contrast, however, optimization

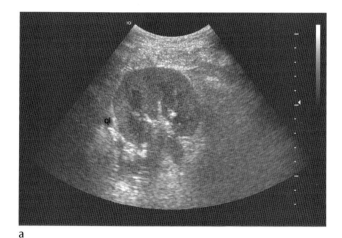

a

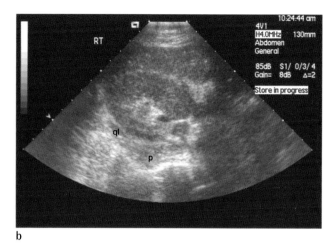

b

Figure 1.4
(a) Axial view of the right kidney demonstrating an approach from the flank. The quadratus lumborum (QL) is identified posterior to the kidney. The arrowhead identifies the renal hilum. **(b) Axial view of the right kidney, demonstrating the posterior relationship of the quadratus lumborum muscles (QL) and the postero-medial relationship of the psoas muscles (P).**

of a Doppler signal requires a vector of flow towards the transducer. In the investigation of renal vessels, therefore, the plane of scan which will best show the vascular anatomy is often at right angles to the plane which will afford optimal Doppler signal recording.

Probe selection

Probe selection depends upon body habitus, including weight, build, orientation of the ribs, presence of spinal deformity, etc. While a curved array will allow a wider field of view from near to far zone, a sector probe (tightly curved array or phased array) with its associated small footprint allows placement of the transducer in subcostal and intercostal location with minimal compromise of the fan of the scan plane. Linear-array transducers may be used in very slim patients where the advantage of a focus close to the transducer face is required. Most modern ultrasound probes have multiple frequencies/broadband capability which affords optimum visualization over the entire renal parenchyma.

Transducer frequencies are usually in the order of 3–7 MHz. The development of non-linear imaging (e.g. tissue harmonic imaging) has greatly improved visualization of the renal tract, particularly in those patients typically poorly visualized by ultrasound, the obese and the thick set. Furthermore, the use of non-linear imaging produces accentuation of sonographic artifacts such as acoustic enhancement and shadowing. It is possible, however, that given the slight reduction in dynamic range

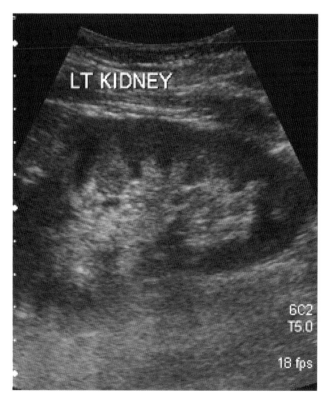

Figure 1.5
Coronal image of the left kidney. The upper pole is partially obscured because of difficult access through the ribs.

that occurs with tissue harmonic imaging, new observations will be required for the detection of renal calculi.

The kidneys

Little, if any, patient preparation is required. Patients presenting for upper abdominal ultrasound will frequently be fasted for 6 hours prior to the investigation, although this is largely to diminish bowel gas and afford distension of the gallbladder. However, if the kidneys are specifically to be examined, then many would recommend a fluid load in order to distend the calyces, thus allowing the separate identification of intrarenal vessels and also to increase urine flow and allow the regular demonstration of ureteric jets entering the bladder. Fasting the patient rarely improves the visualization of either kidney.

The supine position is the starting point for most abdominal ultrasound examinations and may be the only available approach in sick patients.

The right kidney can frequently be demonstrated in its entirety using the liver as an acoustic window with the patient supine.

Scans are performed in the sagittal and axial plane from the anterior approach using the liver or spleen as an acoustic window. Moving the probe to the costal margin and angling towards the feet may afford visualization of the lower pole where this is obscured by bowel gas.

Similarly, compression with the transducer face will often displace gas and allow visualization of the lower pole. A sequence of contiguous real-time images is created by gradual movement of the transducer from the midline to the flank, angling both subcostally and inferiorly in a slow rocking motion as the probe is moved across the abdomen. The axis of the scan plane is moved slightly off the sagittal between 10 and 20% to account for the normal axis of the kidney. Using this method the maximum length of the kidney can be measured from pole to pole and in the axial plane the anteroposterior (AP) and transverse diameter of the kidney can be measured at the hilum.

Sagittal and axial views of the kidney can also be demonstrated with the patient in the prone position. In this position the posterior ends of the ribs provides significant impediment to ultrasound imaging, particularly in the sagittal plane, although rather less so in the axial plane. This effect can be reduced by placing a pillow under the patient's midriff to reverse the lumbar lordosis and to widen the intercostal spaces.

The prone position is now used only infrequently, except for interventional procedures.

A modified coronal plane with the probe situated in the flank angling medially directing the axis towards the hilar region will allow the demonstration of the renal parenchyma and the renal sinus as well as the renal pelvis and the renal vessels as they course in to the hilum. The decubitus or partial decubitus position allows better coronal imaging of many patients. With the patient on the left or right side, the liver or spleen is displaced inferiorly, allowing more of the organ to be used as an acoustic

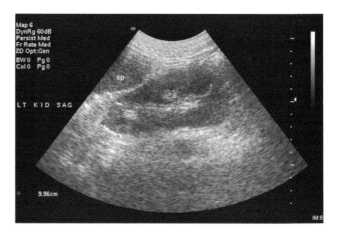

Figure 1.6
Coronal scan through the left kidney demonstrating the spleen and the kidney with a splenic hump consequent upon compression by the spleen. The lower pole of the kidney is partially obscured by adjacent shadowing from bowel gas.

window for the kidney. This position can be combined with an oblique intercostal scan with the probe axis aligned to the plane between the ribs which frequently corresponds to the anteroposterior plane of the longitudinal axis of the kidney (Figure 1.6).

Finally, the patient may be examined in the erect or sitting position. This occasionally displaces the liver or spleen further into the abdomen, when the lower pole of the kidney is difficult to demonstrate, but may also be necessary in a dyspneic person and also to demonstrate unusual renal mobility.

Our practice is generally to examine the kidneys in quiet respiration. This allows the use of respiratory excursion to increase the number of scan planes that are achieved for the same position of the probe (of particular importance where there is only a small acoustic window) but also demonstrates the normal motion of the kidney relative to the liver. Furthermore, it is important for the standardization of Doppler signals from the renal vessels. Occasionally it is necessary to perform a scan in suspended inspiration or expiration in order to better visualize one of the poles of the kidney.

Renal vessels

Renal vessels may be visualized in many patients from their origin at the aorta, through the renal hilum to the arcuate vessels.

With the patient supine it is frequently possible to examine the origin of the major renal vessels. The probe is placed

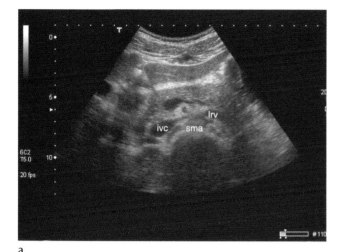

a

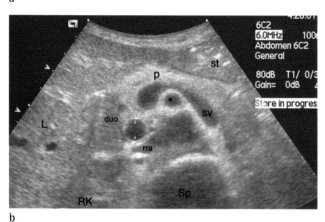

b

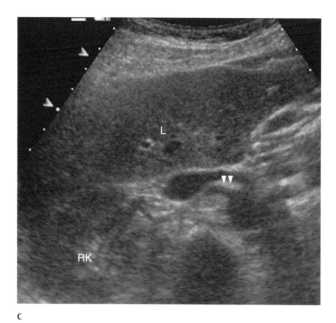

c

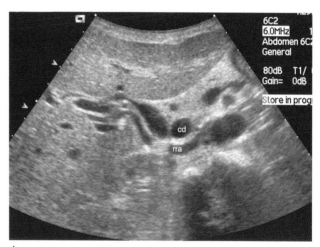

d

Figure 1.7

(a) Axial scan through the epigastrium demonstrating the inferior vena cava (IVC), the superior mesenteric artery (SMA) and the left renal vein (LRV). The SMA is situated immediately posterior to the splenic vein. **(b) Axial view through the epigastrium demonstrating the origin of the right renal artery (RRA) posterolaterally from the aorta.** The relationship of the renal vessels and of the right kidney to intra-abdominal structures is demonstrated. st = stomach, P = pancreas, SV = splenic vein, duo = duodenum, L = liver, Sp = spine. The superior mesenteric artery is identified by an asterisk. **(c) Axial view scanning through the right upper quadrant.** The origin of the right renal artery from the anterolateral margin of the aorta is demonstrated by the arrowheads as it courses posteriorly to the IVC. The liver (L) and right kidney (RK) are demonstrated. **(d) The right renal artery coursing posterior to the head of the pancreas towards the right kidney is demonstrated.** In this patient the common duct (CD) is dilated. Incidentally, there is mild intrahepatic bile duct dilatation. **(e) Transverse scan demonstrating the anterolateral origin of the right renal artery (RRA) and its course posterior to the IVC.** Cx = crus of the diaphragm, a = aorta, s = superior mesenteric artery, pv = portal venous confluence.

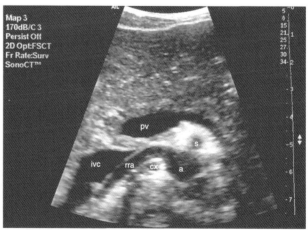

e

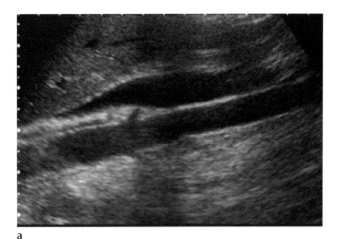

a

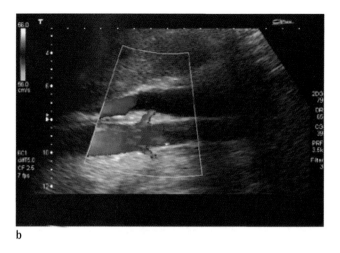

b

Figure 1.8
(a) Coronal view through the aorta, demonstrating the origin of the renal arteries. (b) Color flow Doppler of the coronal view of the aorta and IVC, demonstrating the origin of the renal artery.

midline in a transverse subxyphoid position. The aorta is visualized in the transverse plane. The probe is slid down the abdomen until the superior mesenteric artery is identified and the left renal vein is seen coursing between the aorta and the superior mesenteric artery on its journey from the left kidney to the inferior vena cava (Figure 1.7a,b). At this level the left renal artery can usually be demonstrated arising from the posterior aspect of the left side of the aorta and the right renal artery from the anterior aspect of the right side of the aorta (Figure 1.7c–e). The junction of the right renal vein with the inferior vena cava (IVC) can also be frequently demonstrated in this plane.

With the patient in the decubitus position (left side down), angling the probe towards the renal hilum allows visualization of the intrarenal branch vessels, the vessels at the hilum and, by further angulation, towards the IVC and aorta, the right renal artery and vein and frequently the left renal artery and vein. A scan plane slightly more posterior to this will demonstrate the IVC and renal veins (Figure 1.8).

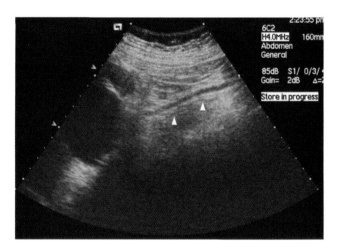

Figure 1.9
Mildly dilated ureter. The ureter is demonstrated adjacent to the psoas muscle by compression, with the transducer head in the left flank. The course of the ureter is demonstrated by arrowheads.

The ureter (see also Chapter 2)

The normal ureter can rarely be visualized for much of its intra-abdominal course. The pelviureteric junction can be demonstrated by axial and coronal views of the kidney but much of the ureter is obscured from the posterior approach by the transverse processes of the vertebrae and from the anterior approach by its small size and by multiple intervening loops of bowel (Figure 1.9). However, by scanning in the long axis over the transverse processes of the vertebrae and utilizing significant abdominal compres-

sion, or by flank compression with the patient in the decubitus position, the abnormal or dilated ureter can frequently be demonstrated for at least part of its course. In the pelvis the abnormal distal ureter can either be identified utilizing compression as it arcs over the iliac vessels or through a filled urinary bladder. By using scan planes slightly to the right and left of the midline obliqued to follow the long axis of the ureter, the pelvic course of the ureter can be seen in up to half of the patients, with at least one ureter being demonstrated in most patients (Figure 1.10). The scan plane is then changed to transverse, angling

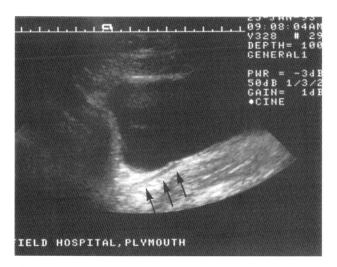

Figure 1.10
Oblique view of the distal ureter in the pelvis produced by angling the probe laterally from the midline with the plane of scan following the expected course of the ureter (arrows).

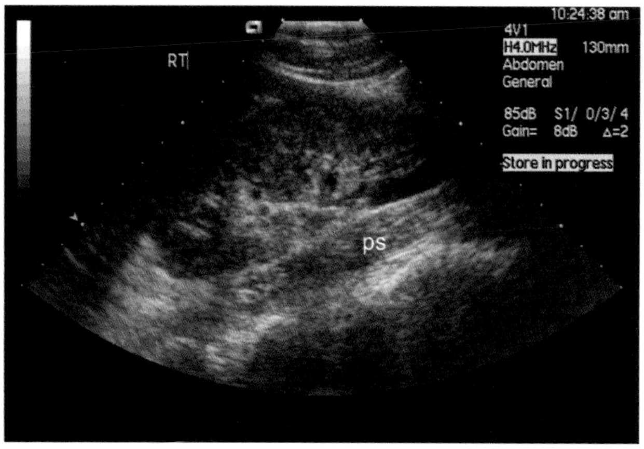

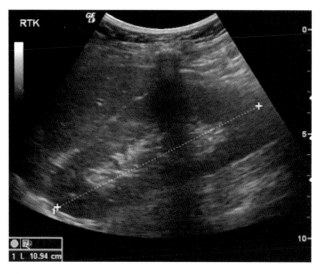

Figure 1.11
Coronal oblique view through the right kidney. This demonstrates the axis of the kidney. The lower pole of the kidney is displaced laterally and anteriorly by the increasing bulk of the psoas muscle (PS).

the probe downwards in order to demonstrate the bladder trigone and to detect ureteric jets.

Anatomical considerations

The kidney

The kidneys are bean-shaped organs between 9 and 13 cm in length situated in the deep paravertebral depression on the posterior wall of the abdomen. The paravertebral gutters slope slightly forwards and laterally as the psoas major muscles increase in bulk from above downwards. Consequently, the long axis of each kidney is not quite vertical but slopes laterally and slightly forwards from above downwards (Figure 1.11). The hilum of the kidney is the point at which the renal artery enters the kidney and the renal vein and the ureter leave it. The renal hilum is directed slightly anteriorly as well as medially. The kidneys are not quite symmetrical in position, the left being approximately 1.5 cm higher than the right, and being also therefore situated slightly more medially.

The sonographic appearances of the internal anatomy of the kidney depend upon the plane of scan. In the sagittal plane the features are those of an oval structure surrounded by a highly reflective (fibrous) capsule. In thin patients this renal capsule cannot be distinguished or separated from the capsule of the liver because of similar characteristics of reflectivity (Figure 1.12).

The cortex forms the more peripheral part of the kidney, covering the bases of the pyramids and also extending

Figure 1.12
Sagittal oblique scan through the right kidney with the cursors measuring the length of the kidney. The renal capsule is indistinguishable from the adjacent liver capsule. Incidental note is made of a rib shadow which passes through the center of the kidney.

down between the renal pyramids towards the sinus, forming the renal columns. Cortical thickness is usually between 1 and 1.5 cm. Renal cortical echogenicity is normally less than that of the liver and the spleen. However, this relationship changes with age. Younger patients, up to the age of 30 with normal renal function

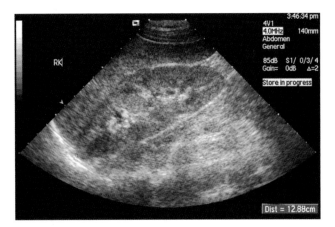

Figure 1.13
Sagittal image of the right kidney, demonstrating cortical echogenicity similar to that of the adjacent liver. The patient was clinically normal, with no evidence of renal disease.

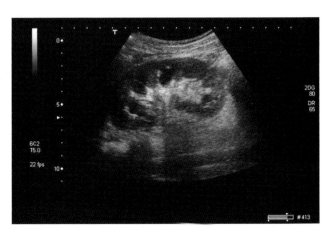

Figure 1.15
Coronal image of the left kidney demonstrating normal corticomedullary differentiation. The brightness of the renal sinus is demonstrated.

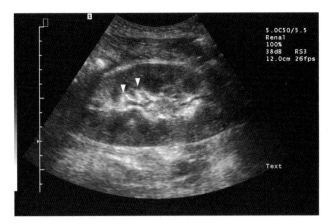

Figure 1.14
Sagittal scan through the left kidney. The normal relationship between the renal cortex and medulla is demonstrated. The renal sinus is seen centrally. Cupped calyces are identified at the upper pole (arrowheads).

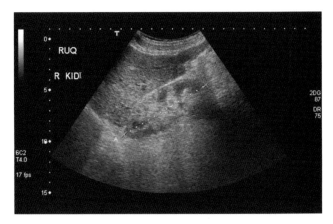

Figure 1.16
Sagittal image of the right kidney in an elderly patient demonstrating increase in cortical reflectivity. There was no evidence of diminished renal function.

may exhibit cortical reflectivity similar to that of the adjacent liver in as many as a third of the cases (Figure 1.13). This isoechoic appearance is also associated with prominence of the medullary pyramids. This appearance gradually decreases in frequency with advancing age, although in the elderly the overall renal echogenicity may increase without increase in prominence of the pyramids (Figures 1.14–1.16).

The medullary pyramids are a series of conical masses arranged with their bases directed towards the surface and their apices projecting into the minor calyces in the renal sinus, where they form the renal papillae. The renal cortex and columns are more highly reflective than the medullary pyramids but less so than the renal sinus. Renal pyramids may be differentiated from the cortex in approximately half of adult patients by differences in echogenicity. The ability

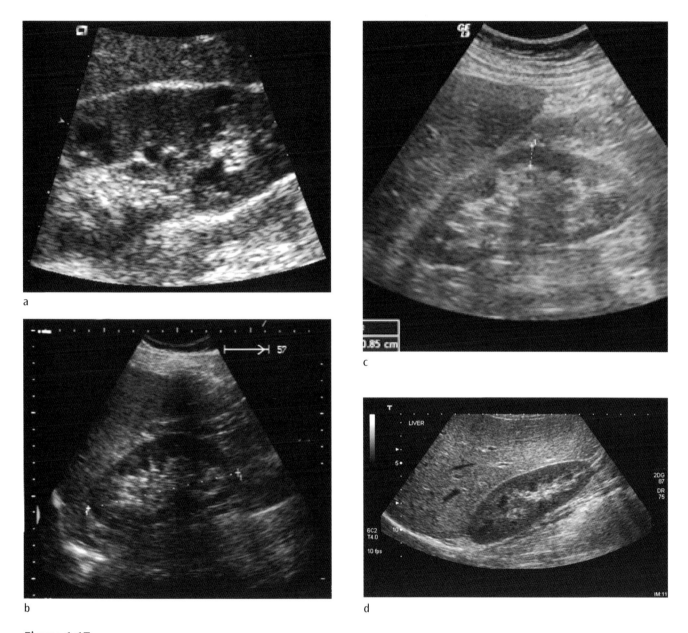

Figure 1.17
(a) **Normal reflectivity of the renal sinus.** (b) **Echogenicity of the renal sinus slightly less than in case (a), but the renal sinus is broader, implying greater fat content.** (c) **Marked fat content in an elderly patient.** This implies some renal parenchymal loss, although there was no evidence of abnormal renal function. (d) **The renal cortex is much less echogenic than the liver, although it remains normal.** The renal sinus contains little fat and contributes little to the overall renal volume.

to visualize the pyramids is dependent on patient age and also on body habitus. In the infant, the medullary pyramids are echo-poor in comparison to the cortex and in the first year of life are usually clearly distinguished from the cortex. In the adult, the difference in echogenicity reduces with increasing age.

Obesity influences the appearance of the kidney. Few obese patients exhibit cortical echogenicity equivalent to the liver because of increased hepatic reflectivity, few will

have easily demonstrable medullary pyramids and most will exhibit a broadened and bright renal sinus.

The renal sinus is the highly reflective central zone of the kidney, representing the confluence of the collecting system and sinus fat, vessels and nerves. As a general rule, the sinus is homogeneously echogenic, being of equivalent reflectivity to the renal capsule and perirenal fat (Figure 1.17). However, there are variations in the nature and distribution of renal sinus fat. Usually, broadening of the renal sinus

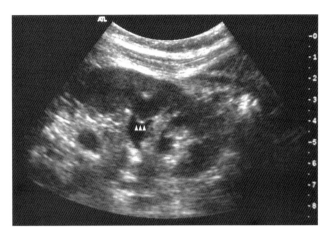

Figure 1.18
Coronal scan through the kidney demonstrating the difference in echogenicity between the cortex and medulla and also demonstrating the papilla of the pyramid extending into the calyx (arrowheads). The calyces were distended consequent upon a full bladder.

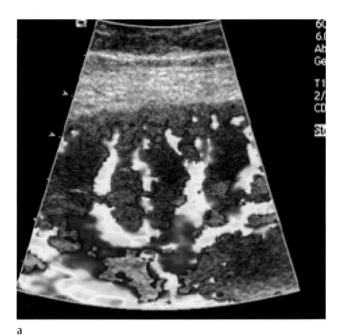

a

b

Figure 1.19
(a) Color flow Doppler, demonstrating vessels extending into the cortex. (b) Power Doppler, identifying striate vessels in the cortex.

secondary to fat produces a uniform appearance with bright echoes. However, in some patients the sinus fat may be inhomogeneous or, rarely, purely echo-poor.

Given a water load and a distended urinary bladder, some distension of the collecting system occurs in most patients sufficient to allow the demonstration of separation of the renal sinus echoes by echo-free fluid and the consequent demonstration of a split central renal sinus, thus also allowing the recognition of the renal sinus arteries and the papillae of the medullary pyramids (Figure 1.18). The peripheral branches of the renal vessels are well demonstrated in color and power Doppler modes (Figure 1.19).

Anatomical variations

As a general rule, the cortical surface of the kidney is smooth. In the fetus, however, the surface of the kidney is marked by a number of grooves that divide it into polygonal areas known as the lobes or renunculi, each one corresponding to a papilla, its pyramids and its surrounding cortex.

Persistent fetal lobation may be seen in childhood and is occasionally seen in the adult kidney. The features on ultrasound are represented by fine linear demarcation indenting the renal surface and consisting of a central pyramid and surrounding cortex.

There are other structural variations of renal anatomy that represent the persistence of the lobular structure, but these are subtler. Anatomical variations must be distinguished from significant pathology such as renal scarring. The echogenic triangle (Figure 1.20), or parenchymal junctional defect, parenchymal interjunctional line (Figure 1.21) and the intermediate cortical mass or hypertrophied column of Bertin may also represent persistent fetal lobation. However, the junctional line may represent simply a prolongation of the sinus fatty tissue towards the parenchyma and the column of Bertin

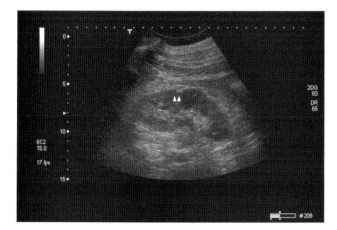

Figure 1.20
Coronal view of the left kidney. A junctional triangle is identified by the arrowheads.

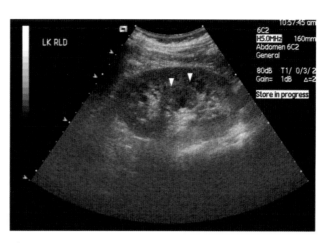

Figure 1.22
Column of Bertin. In this case the column of Bertin is clearly identified as a prolongation of the renal cortex into the renal sinus and containing a medullary pyramid (arrowheads).

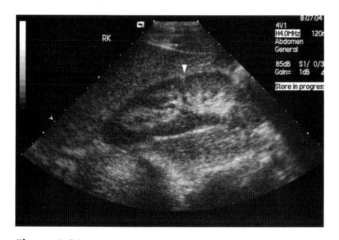

Figure 1.21
There is a line extending from the junctional triangle into the renal sinus, identified by the arrowhead.

represents true focal hypertrophy. The echogenic triangle, or parenchymal junctional defect, is a focal area usually present on the anterior surface of the kidney close to the upper pole and producing an apparent echogenic dimple in the kidney. The echogenic line, or parenchymal interjunctional line, is a linear brightly reflective structure crossing obliquely from the anterior surface of the kidney to the renal sinus, and is often associated with an echogenic triangle.

One or both of these features may be seen in 30% of normal adult kidneys and in 100% of adult kidneys where some form of ureteric duplication is present.

The echogenic triangle and echogenic line must be distinguished from renal scar tissue, which normally has a greater thickness, evidence of cortical thinning and abnormality of the adjacent calyces. This, of course, is not invariable in cases where the scar derives from a vascular abnormality rather than from renal infection/reflux.

The intermediate cortical mass, or hypertrophied column of Bertin, is a prolongation of the cortex between the medullary pyramids and into the renal sinus (Figure 1.22). This anatomical variant can produce a pseudomass effect. Differentiation from a pathologic mass is usually possible using ultrasound criteria. The reflectivity is usually equivalent to that of the normal renal cortex although some reports suggest that tubular abnormalities may be present which alter the echogenicity. Color flow or power Doppler have been used to document the normal distribution of renal vessels within the renal mass (Figure 1.23). More recently, administration of ultrasound contrast allows the demonstration of smoothly branching and ordered vessels. As a consequence of these features, it is now only rarely necessary to perform additional imaging studies such as CT or MRI (Figure 1.24).

The splenic or dromedary hump are minor adaptations of the surface of the kidney consequent upon pressure from adjacent organs, usually the spleen. The juxtaposition of the spleen to the pseudomass combined with normal echogenicity, and normal distribution of vessels on color flow Doppler will almost invariably allow recognition of this feature (Figure 1.25).

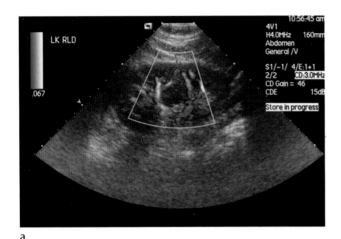

a

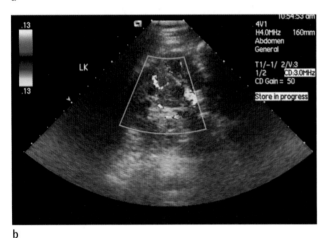

b

Figure 1.23
(a) Power Doppler demonstrates vessels displaced around the column of Bertin but with branches extending into the invaginated cortex. (b) Color flow Doppler again demonstrates displacement of vessels, but normal supply of the cortex.

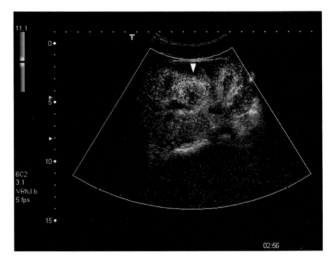

Figure 1.24
Contrast-enhanced imaging of the kidney. The arrowhead demonstrates normal cortical perfusion of the column of Bertin.

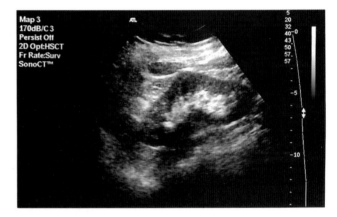

Figure 1.25
Left kidney, demonstrating a splenic hump.

Dilatation of the renal sinus with hydration

Without prehydration the renal sinus almost invariably shows no separation (less than 5% of individuals). But in over 50% of patients who have been prepared by hydration, there is a separation of the renal sinus with a range of between 2 and 14 mm, even in the absence of obstruction (Figure 1.26). Furthermore, if the hydrated patients are examined with a full bladder, the number of patients demonstrating distension of the renal sinus increases to over 90%.

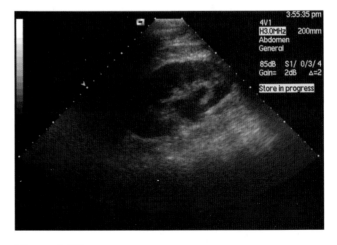

Figure 1.26
Separation of the renal sinus consequent upon a fluid load.

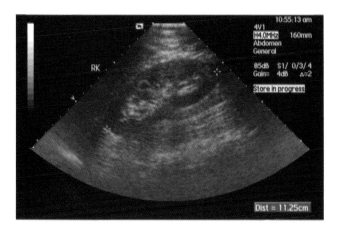

Figure 1.27
Long axis of the kidney. The kidney is measured at 11.25 cm. Taking care to ensure that the long axis is measured following the slightly oblique lie of the kidney is important.

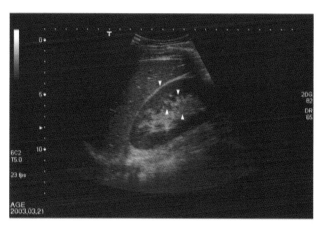

Figure 1.28
Comparison between the thickness of the parenchyma and renal sinus (arrowheads).

Renal length

Ultrasound is a reliable technique for evaluation of renal dimensions (Figure 1.27). Although it is possible to assess renal volume, the most commonly used measurement is renal length. Renal dimensions will be affected by the patient's age and hydration.

Male:
   Right kidney 11.3 ± 0.8 cm
   Left kidney 11.5 ± 0.9 cm
Female:
   Right kidney 10.8 ± 0.8 cm
   Left kidney 10.9 ± 1 cm

Renal volume is calculated by a modified prolate ellipsoid (length × width × depth)
   Male:
   Right kidney 147 ± 38 ml
   Left kidney 157 ± 37 ml
Female:
   Right kidney 118 ± 27 ml
   Left kidney 125 ± 26 ml
Renal volume is directly correlated with the weight, height and surface area of the patient. It is possible to derive a relative renal length by dividing the renal length by the height of the patient, but this has found limited clinical application.

Parenchymal thickness
Male:
   14.8 ± 0.17 mm (range 11–18 mm)
Female:
   13.6 ± 1 mm (range 11–16 mm)

The absolute and relative renal lengths diminish in the elderly, irrespective of renal function.

The ratio between the thickness of the parenchyma and the thickness of the sinus varies between 0.78 and 1.3 (Figure 1.28). This is important in determining renal parenchymal loss, where there are confounding features within the renal sinus. For example, increase in renal sinus fat may occur coincidentally with renal cortical loss, apparently maintaining renal length measurements. Similarly, the ratio is important in suspected hydronephrosis: for example, where the degree of calyceal distension in the hydrated patient is between 2 and 14 mm but the parenchymal sinus ratio is greater than 0.78, the likelihood of hydronephrosis is diminished.

Renal fascia and fat

The kidneys are closely related to the adrenal glands and both are enclosed within a weak fascia known as Gerota's fascia which is formed by the splitting of the fascial envelope of the abdomen into anterior and posterior layers. This encloses a variable amount of perirenal fat, which is usually of increased reflectivity compared with the renal cortex but may be of lesser reflectivity than the capsule and the renal sinus (Figure 1.29). The two layers of renal fascia fuse together a short distance above the adrenal gland and become continuous with the fascia on the undersurface of the diaphragm. Laterally, the two layers also fuse, but inferiorly and medially the fusion of the fascia is either incomplete or non-existent. This allows the mobility of the kidney inferiorly in renal ptosis and across the midline in

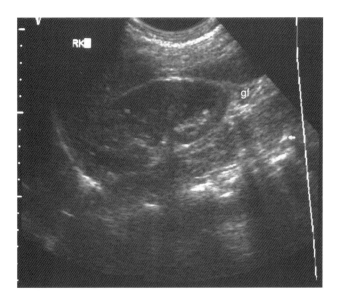

Figure 1.29
The relationship between Gerota's fascia (GF) and the lower pole of the kidney is demonstrated.

some patients with change in patient position (left posterior decubitus position, the right kidney crosses the midline) (Figure 1.30).

The main renal vessels

The renal arteries are lateral branches of the aorta that typically arise at the level of the second lumbar vertebra.

The right renal artery is an anterolateral branch of the aorta and can be visualized with the left renal artery (a lateral or posterolateral branch) using a coronal approach (Figure 1.31). The right renal artery then courses anteriorly for about 1 cm before descending obliquely posterior to the IVC (Figure 1.32) towards the right kidney. The left renal artery is a posterolateral branch of the aorta (Figure 1.33), and follows a posterolateral course behind the left renal vein to enter the renal hilum. The renal arteries divide into anterior and posterior divisions at the hilum, and subsequently into the segmental arteries.

The right renal vein has a short course and enters the inferior vena cava directly (Figure 1.34). On the left, the renal vein passes between the superior mesenteric artery and the aorta and is sometimes compressed between the two (the nutcracker effect). Occasionally, this compression coincides with loss of demonstration of the wall of the aorta, giving an apparent continuity between the vein and the artery (Figure 1.34b). In the past this has been mistaken for an aneurysm of the origin of the renal artery. Knowledge of this anatomical feature and the use of color flow and spectral Doppler will avoid this confusion.

The left renal vein usually receives the left gonadal vein, the left adrenal vein and the left lumbar veins.

Approximately 30% of patients with normally located kidneys will demonstrate anatomical variation of vascular supply. This is usually in the form of accessory renal arteries which arise usually close to the main renal artery but may arise anywhere along the aorta or the proximal iliac artery. Those that arise close to the renal artery may be visualized on ultrasound, although visualization is less reliable if the origin is distant from the main ostium.

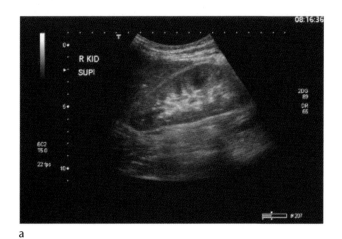

a

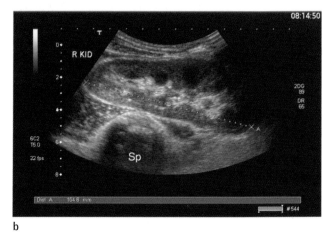

b

Figure 1.30
(a) Normal position of the right kidney. Patient in supine position. **(b) The patient in the decubitus position.** The kidney traverses the midline and lies transversely across the spine (SP).

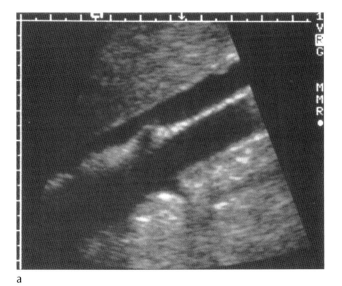

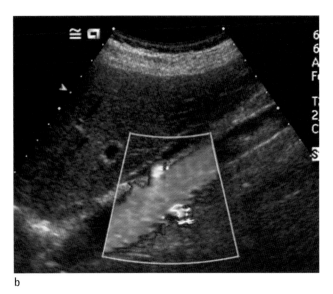

a   b

Figure 1.31

(a) **Coronal scan through the origin of both renal arteries demonstrating their relationship to the aorta and inferior vena cava.**
(b) **Color flow Doppler study of the origins of the renal arteries.** The right renal artery shows flow in red adjacent to the inferior
vena cava. Flow in the left renal artery demonstrates both blue and red features consistent with aliasing.

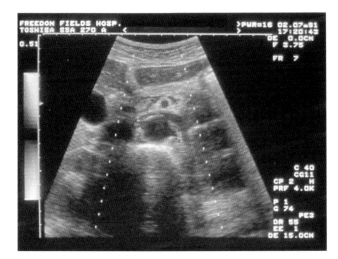

Figure 1.32

**Transverse color flow Doppler study demonstrating the
anatomical relations of the major renal vessels.** The splenic
superior mesenteric venous confluence configured in blue lies
immediately adjacent to the superior mesenteric artery in red.
Posterior to this, the left renal vein courses over the anterior
surface of the aorta, changing color flow configuration from
red to blue as the direction of flow changes. Posterior to this,
the right renal artery, which is an anterolateral branch of the
aorta, demonstrates blood flow towards the transducer in red,
whereas the left renal artery, a posterolateral branch of the
aorta, demonstrates blood flow in blue.

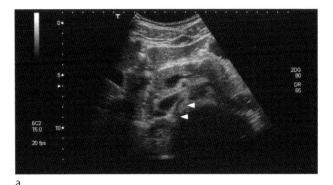

a

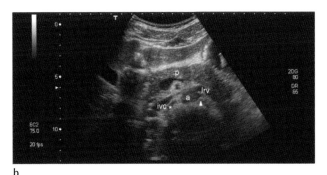

b

Figure 1.33

(a) **Transverse scan through the epigastrium demonstrating
the right renal artery (arrowheads) traversing posterior to
the inferior vena cava.** The head of the pancreas (p) is
identified anterior to the confluence of the splenic and
superior mesenteric veins. A = aorta. (b) **Transverse scan
through the epigastrium.** The right renal artery is identified (*)
and the left (^). The relationship of these vessels to the left
renal vein (lrv), the IVC, the pancreas (p) and the aorta (a) are
shown.

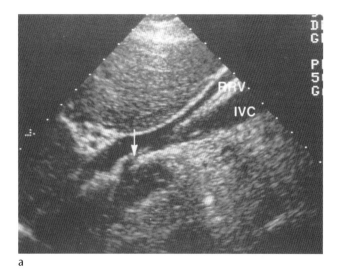

a

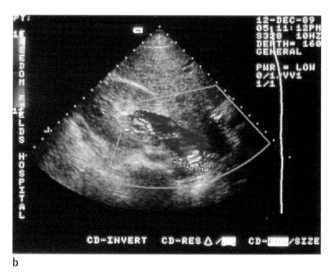

b

Figure 1.34
(a) Coronal oblique scan showing the origin of the right renal vein (RRV) from the IVC. The origin of the renal artery as it courses posterior to the inferior vena cava is identified by an arrow. **(b) Color flow Doppler study of the right renal vein.** The course of this vein is short and is subject to changes in intrathoracic and intra-abdominal pressure. The vein dilates, particularly with Valsalva maneuver.

Intrarenal vessels

There are usually five main segmental branches of the renal artery within the kidney. These divide into the interlobar arteries, which further branch into the arcuate arteries running along the base of the pyramids. In the normal kidney these do not anastomose and give rise to multiple fine striate or interlobular vessels which extend vertically into the renal cortex (Figure 1.35).

The segmental arteries can occasionally be demonstrated as a central sonolucent lumen in between parallel echogenic outer arterial walls. More peripherally, in the interlobar arteries, the vessels may be simply identified as pulsating echogenic linear structures or, in the case of the arcuate arteries, as pulsating echogenic 'dots' at the junction between cortex and medulla.

Doppler studies of the kidney and renal tract

Color and power Doppler

Color flow Doppler, power Doppler and spectral Doppler now allow the demonstration of global renal flow and flow within the major and branch renal arteries and allow the calculation of a number of indices which reflect intrarenal resistance and flow velocities. The techniques have poten-

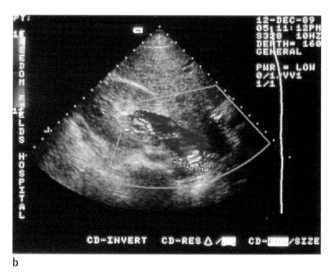

Figure 1.35
The left renal vein and left renal artery are demonstrated in color flow Doppler. The (blue) left renal artery arising from the (red) aorta is demonstrated by the arrowheads.

tial application in the evaluation of renovascular disease, renal infection, renal tumors and diffuse parenchymal renal disease. Color flow Doppler is used to identify the position of the major renal vessels and the intrarenal vessels. Variation in the size of the color flow box will allow the demonstration of flow to the entire kidney, or to a focal area of renal parenchyma if the size of the color box is reduced, when the sensitivity to flow and frame rate are

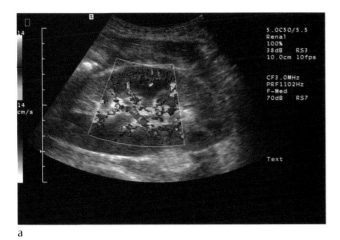 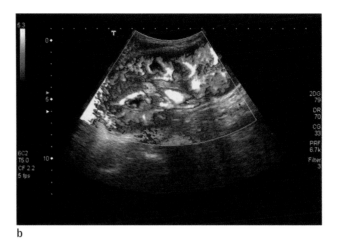

a   b

Figure 1.36
(a,b) Color flow and power Doppler images of the hilar, segmental, interlobular, arcuate and interlobar arteries.

increased. A combination of both techniques is used in the evaluation of flow to the renal parenchyma.

Color gain is increased until color noise is detected and then reduced until this just disappears.

Color flow suffers from similar technical limitations to all ultrasound, particularly beam attenuation with depth and angle dependence of detection of the Doppler signal. Although most machines also have an algorithm that diminishes motion artifact, this remains occasionally a problem in patients, for example, with dyspnea or as a consequence of prominent pulsation of a neighboring vessel such as the aorta. Power Doppler is less angle dependent and is better for demonstrating parenchymal flow, particularly at the poles of the kidney. It is important to ensure that, as far as is possible, in either technique, the angle that the ultrasound beam makes with the renal vasculature is optimized for best detection of flow. For the most part, this will involve a coronal approach for evaluation of the renal parenchyma and either a coronal approach or an axial approach angling to left and right with the probe in the midline for the main renal arteries (Figures 1.31–1.36).

Color sensitivities must be optimized to detect low flow within the parenchyma while also detecting higher flow velocities within the main branch vessels. Typical flow velocities within the main renal arteries will range from 40 to 120 cm/s, whereas in the branch vessels, particularly in the interlobular vessels, velocities may range from a few centimeters per second to 40 cm/s. Thus, pulse repetition frequency will need to be varied, dependent upon the

vessel being examined. High-frequency transducers will afford the resolution of a cortical color blush into individual interlobular vessels. However, this is only possible in slim patients. Patients who are obese, particularly those with significant peri- and pararenal fat, will only afford the use of lower-frequency transducers and, consequently, poor color sensitivity and spatial resolution. It is frequently possible in slim patients to demonstrate the vascular tree from the renal artery origin to the interlobular vessels. In the obese patient, it may be possible only to demonstrate vessels at the hilum and in the interlobar region.

Angle optimization is important for all Doppler assessment of the renal vasculature and, even when using power Doppler, sensitivities are improved if the Doppler angle is maintained at less than 60°. This is particularly important for the estimation of flow velocities which are angle dependent. Most Doppler transducers will use frequencies of the order of 2–5 MHz, with a sample volume of between 2 and 5 mm. A low-frequency wall filter is important to detect low flow velocities, particularly in smaller branch vessels. Pulse repetition frequency must be increased when evaluating vessels with high velocity flow, particularly where arterial stenosis is suspected.

Ultrasound contrast agents

Microbubble contrast agents are gradually gaining acceptance in the evaluation of intra-abdominal pathology. There is evidence that ultrasound contrast agents will improve

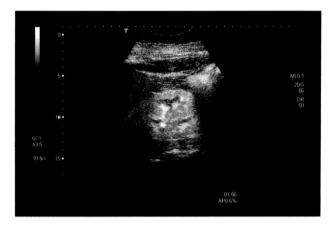

Figure 1.37
Parenchymal phase of contrast enhancement of the lower pole of the right kidney demonstrating high-intensity reflections from the central renal vessels and mid-range intensity from the perfusion of the renal cortex in contrast to the adjacent echo-poor medulla.

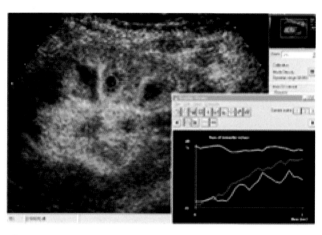

Figure 1.38
Time–velocity curves for perfusion of the renal sinus, the renal medulla and the renal cortex.

visualization of the renal vessels throughout their course and may be used where a renal artery stenosis is suspected to improve visualization of the main renal artery, in the evaluation of renal tumors to demonstrate altered flow architecture and to document global renal flow in cases of renal infection and ischemic disease.

Contrast is prepared immediately prior to the examination, mixing the powdered agent with a diluent to produce an emulsion or suspension. The contrast is injected into a peripheral vein and the scan plane aligned to the kidney or vessel to produce optimum sensitivity to flow. Observation over a period of several minutes will allow the demonstration of arterial filling, parenchymal perfusion and then contrast clearing. There are a number of approaches to optimum contrast demonstration. Early studies used color and power Doppler techniques to detect the microbubbles, and this remains appropriate for major vessels. However, it is now more common to use harmonic imaging for best visualization of parenchymal perfusion (Figure 1.37). The second harmonic coincides fortuitously with the oscillation of the microbubbles and therefore a strong signal is produced. In the kidney, stimulated acoustic emission is rarely used, although high mechanical index techniques are used to afford the demonstration of destruction and reperfusion techniques. These afford a dynamic assessment of renal perfusion, using processes of timed perfusion or destruction/reperfusion methods. It is possible with newer software programs to select regions of interest within the renal parenchyma and the hilum that afford the semiquantitative assessment of global and regional blood flow (Figure 1.38).

Spectral Doppler

Blood flow within the main renal arteries can be interrogated with spectral Doppler from a number of approaches. The axial position with the probe in the epigastrium angling to both right and to left may allow demonstration of blood flow at the origin of the renal arteries. Similarly, the coronal view will almost invariably demonstrate the origin of the right renal artery and frequently the origin of the left renal artery. Placing the sample volume within the renal artery at this level will allow the recording of sequential Doppler spectra (Figure 1.39). The sample volume may also be placed within the renal hilum, angling medially from the coronal view of the kidney on either the right or the left. Sampling here may therefore be within the main renal artery or within one or other of the segmental arteries. Similarly, sampling can occur then at any position within the renal parenchyma. Within the main renal artery, the Doppler spectrum has been likened to a ski slope. There is an initial rapid systolic rise and a gradual decay of flow throughout diastole, although flow persists to end diastole. A small spike may occur at the end of the systolic rise (early systolic peak). This early systolic peak is usually seen only in the main and segmental arteries.

A number of indices have been used to quantify Doppler parameters and these are outlined in Table 1.1. The pulsatility and resistance indices (RIs) reflect the ratio between a peak systolic velocity and diastolic velocities as does the diastolic systolic ratio, although the latter is now used infrequently. The renal/aortic ratio (RAR) compares

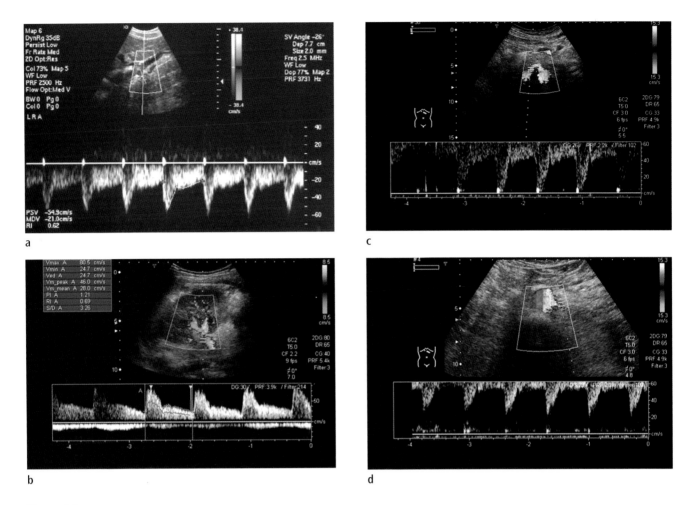

Figures 39
(a–d) Spectral recordings from the renal arteries at the origin, demonstrating the ski-slope pattern.

peak systolic velocity within the renal artery with that in the aorta. This value is usually less than 3.5 and increase in

excess of this implies high velocity flow within the renal artery, possibly reflecting renal artery stenosis.

Evaluation of the intrarenal vessels requires the assessment of different parameters that may reflect disease in the major vessels (Figure 1.40).

The TMS (time to maximum systole) and acceleration index are measures of the upstroke within the Doppler spectrum at systole. Delay in the systolic peak implies a proximal compromise of flow suggestive of renal artery stenosis.

In the solitary kidney the renal indices may not be directly comparable to those of paired kidneys. Studies of donors for renal transplantation have demonstrated normal RI values in the residual kidney of 0.73 ± 0.05 that persist at 12 weeks following surgery. It may be therefore inappropriate to use the same criteria for the evaluation of solitary kidneys. However, there are no data on long-term follow-up and no data on solitary kidneys consequent upon congenital absence.

Table 1.1 *Normal values for renal Doppler indices*

Pulsatility index	0.7–1.4
Resistance index	0.56–0.7
Peak systolic velocity	60–140 cm/s (>180*)
Diastolic/systolic ratio	0.26–0.4
RAR (renal/aortic ratio)	>3.5
TMS (time to maximum systole)	42–110 cm/s
Acceleration index	250–380 cm/s^2

*Cut-off peak velocity in screening for renal artery stenosis (RAS).

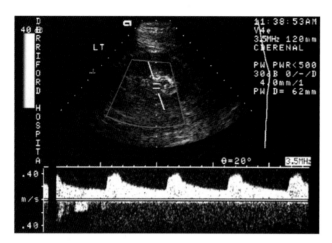

Figure 1.40
Spectral Doppler sampling at the renal hilum.

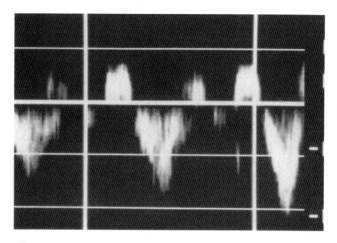

Figure 1.41
Pulsatile venous flow in the right renal vein produced by transmission from the heart.

There are rather fewer data with respect to analysis of the Doppler signal from renal vein flow. Although the Doppler signals from the renal vein are frequently assessed in a qualitative fashion to assess presence or absence of flow in certain pathologies, there has been little evidence to suggest that a quantitative assessment of blood flow within the renal vein will contribute to the diagnosis of more diffuse intrarenal pathology. However, alterations in flow patterns within the renal veins do occur. In the intrarenal vessels to the level of the hilar vein, venous flow is normally continuous with only very slight variation with respiration. This pattern is frequently altered in the main renal vein on the right by changes in flow characteristics within the inferior vena cava. The Doppler sonogram within the inferior vena cava is frequently pulsatile, reflecting the A, C and V waves of atrial and ventricular contraction and valve closure. Where these waves are prominent in the inferior vena cava (a fact related to body habitus as well as to cardiovascular and intra-abdominal pathology), then these will be transmitted into the proximal renal vein, sometimes as far as the hilum (Figure 1.41). On the left, however, the flow patterns in the renal vein are occasionally significantly damped, presumably by the effect of the course of the vein between the superior mesenteric artery and the aorta (Figure 1.42). There are no indices currently available for characterization and quantification of the Doppler signal of the renal veins, nor does an index appear appropriate with the current limitations of application.

It is possible to visualize and record a Doppler signal in as many as 95.5% of right renal arteries and 82% of left renal arteries.[1] Other authors have been less successful with yields of less than 60% technically adequate studies and infrequent visualization of accessory vessels.

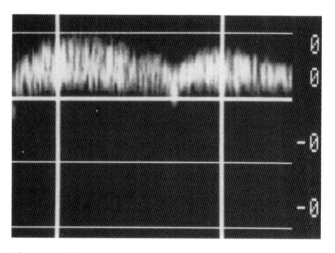

Figure 1.42
Damped flow in the left renal vein, presumably due to compression between the superior mesenteric artery and aorta.

Doppler indices

The initial promise of the use of Doppler indices to determine the nature and severity of disease has not been fulfilled. To a large degree, this has been due to a failure to acknowledge those physiologic parameters which contribute to resistance to blood flow, particularly in disease processes which exert multiple influences on renal physiology. The RI of the kidney depends upon certainly vascular resistance, but also vascular compliance; namely, that process which records the caliber change in the artery in systole and diastole. Vascular compliance will change with age and is also affected by hypertension. Similarly, the

Table 1.2 *Factors to take into account during assessment*
Cardiac output: low and high output states, valvular disease, etc.
Resistance and compliance of vessels proximal to the renal artery
Disease of the main renal artery
Disease of intrarenal arteries and arterioles
Renal obstruction: resultant changes in intrarenal pressure
Parenchymal disease of the kidney: interstitial infiltration and fibrosis or glomerular destruction
Conditions causing redistribution of blood flow within the kidney: tumors, arteriovenous fistulae, etc.
Peri- and pararenal pathology producing renal compression
Renal venous compromise: thrombosis, compression

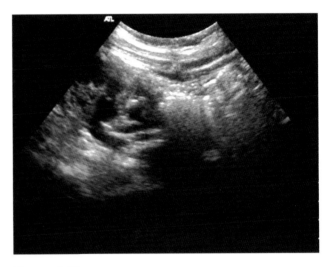

Figure 1.43
Proximal ureter. Oblique scan through the kidney demonstrating the origin of the ureter.

RI is dependent upon the cross-sectional area of the vessels within the kidney. High ureteral pressures will increase interstitial pressure within the kidney. This will affect a cross-sectional area of the vessel very markedly, particularly during diastole, but the distensability (or compliance) of the vessel is, if anything, more marked. Similarly, high intraureteric and intrapelvic pressures are not maintained at all stages of obstruction. Vascular resistance will be affected by interstitial fibrosis. Other factors which will affect Doppler indices within the kidney include direct pressure to the kidney, such as might be occasioned by perirenal fluid collection or adjacent masses and renal vein compromise.

Consequently, during the assessment of the Doppler indices within the renal vessels, account must be taken of a multiplicity of factors. These are summarized in Table 1.2.

Resistance and pulsatility indices are therefore a relatively crude tool for the assessment of global and regional renal perfusion and the identification of specific renal pathology.

The ureter

Only the proximal few centimeters of the ureter just beyond the pelviureteric junction can be visualized unless the ureter is significantly dilated (see Figure 1.11). The normal ureter measures between 1 and 3 mm in diameter. It appears as an echo-free tubular structure contiguous with the renal pelvis (Figure 1.43). The lower portion of the ureter can frequently be visualized posterior to the bladder in the pelvis. Oblique scans following the course of the ureter as it travels medially from the lateral pelvic wall to the trigone will frequently demonstrate an echo-free

tubular structure coursing towards the elevated projection of the vesicoureteric junction (see Figure 1.10). The separation of the vesicoureteric junction and the base of the trigone of the bladder can be demonstrated in the transverse plane (Figure 1.44).

When the patient is hydrated, both ureteric orifices sit proud and pout into the lumen of the bladder, and streams of echogenic fluid can be demonstrated pulsing into the bladder both in real time and, more particularly, on color flow Doppler (Figure 1.45). The jets are usually directed anteromedially and may exhibit discrete jet phenomena, ureteric streaming followed by rest periods. The phenomenon appears to be dependent upon the difference in the

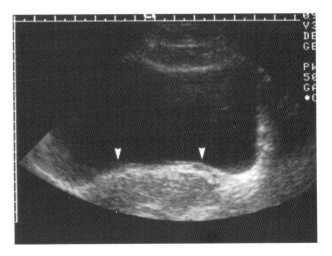

Figure 1.44
Transverse scan demonstrating the ureteric orifices (arrowheads) at the base of the trigone of the bladder.

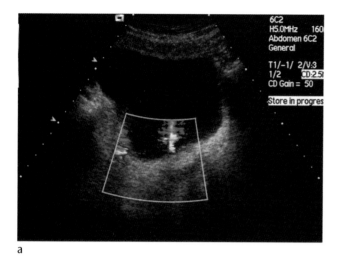

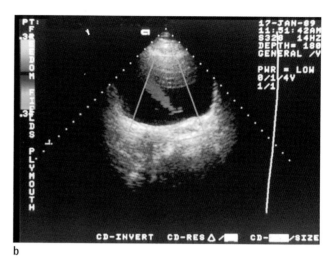

a

b

Figure 1.45
(a,b) Color flow Doppler demonstrating ureteric jets entering the bladder.

density or specific gravity between the urine entering the bladder and the urine already within the bladder. Flow velocity of the jets may reach between 1 and 1.74 m/s, with a mean of 57 cm/s. The interval between jets ranges between 2 and 150 s in the hydrated patient. The detection of jets and the characterization thereof may contribute to the diagnosis of poor renal function and particularly of renal obstruction. When the bladder is very poorly filled or overdistended, the jets may not demonstrate such marked streaming of flow (Figure 1.46).

CONGENITAL ABNORMALITIES OF THE KIDNEY

Embryology

It is not within the remit of this text to describe in detail the embryologic development of the kidneys. However, it is important to consider certain key aspects of the embryology of renal development in order to understand better some of the congenital abnormalities that occur.

Both the urinary and the genital tract have a common origin from the intermediate mesoderm. During embryonic folding in the horizontal plane, the dorsal body wall mesoderm is carried ventrally to lie on either side of the primitive aorta, where it becomes known as the urogenital ridge. It is at this stage that there is early division into the nephrogenic cord and the genital ridge. The former gives rise to the nephron, the excreting element of the urinary tract. Precursors of the final functioning metanephros are

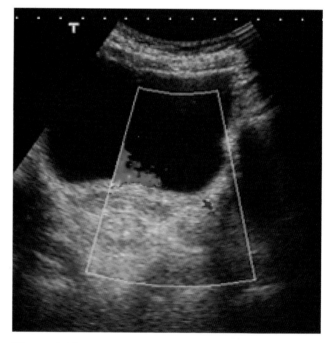

Figure 1.46
Poor ureteric jet demonstration in an inadequately filled urinary bladder.

the pronephrosis, which is transient, and the mesonephros. This latter only functions for a short time during embryonic life before the metanephros develops and assumes the excretory function; this forms the renal substance, the glomeruli, collecting tubules, etc. The urothelial tract, by contrast, from calyces to trigone, derives from the ureteric bud, which is part of the mesonephros. The ureteric bud penetrates the metanephric mesoderm, the resultant metanephric mass forming the renal pelvis and calyces.

Migration or ascent of the kidneys from the pelvis to the abdomen occurs as the body grows and is complete by the 9th week of gestation. During the ascent the kidneys rotate through 90° so that the hila become directed anteromedially. The vascular supply originally from the iliac arteries is finally from the upper part of the abdominal aorta.

Classification of congenital renal abnormalities

Classification of renal abnormalities is usually based on the following criteria:

1. Number
2. Position
3. Dysplasia or hypoplasia
4. Rotation and ascent
5. Fusion
6. Vessels
7. Duplication
8. Cystic disease
9. Ureteropelvic junction obstruction

Of these, cystic disease and ureteropelvic junction obstruction will be considered elsewhere under renal cystic disease and obstructive disease of the kidney.

Abnormalities of number

Supernumerary kidney

Only 60 cases are described in the literature of this rare abnormality which has its own ureter and is thought to result from the existence of two ureteric buds on the one side.

Renal agenesis

This occurs when the ureteric bud fails to penetrate the metanephros, with resultant failure of stimulation of development of the metanephric elements of the nephron. The ureter is frequently absent although there may be a short stump. Unilateral agenesis is relatively common, occurring in approximately 1 in 1000 newborns (Figure 1.47). Bilateral involvement is extremely rare and, with the widespread use of antenatal ultrasound for the diagnosis of structural fetal abnormalities, the incidence of this lethal condition, even in the newborn period, has become exceptional. Unilateral renal agenesis is not associated with

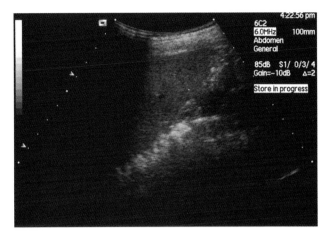

Figure 1.47
Absent right kidney. The right renal bed is empty.

symptoms unless the contralateral kidney is abnormal. Abnormalities of the contralateral kidney would include obstruction, abnormalities of ascent and rotation, etc. Features of unilateral agenesis are predominantly those of changes in the remaining organs. The contralateral kidney frequently exhibits compensatory hypertrophy (Figure 1.48), while in the renal bed other structures come to fill the renal fossa: this is usually bowel, but occasionally there is displacement of the pancreas, e.g. into the left renal bed. Renal agenesis may be associated with the VATER and VACTERL complex of congenital abnormalities. Clearly in this case there are symptoms predominantly relating to the other congenital abnormalities.

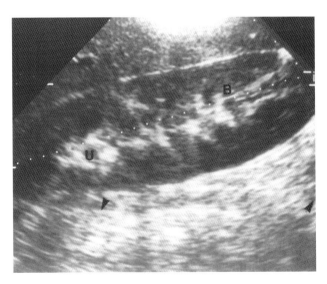

Figure 1.48
Compensatory hypertrophy of the right kidney in a patient with agenesis on the left.

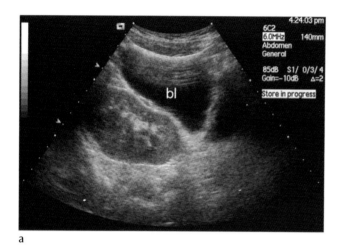

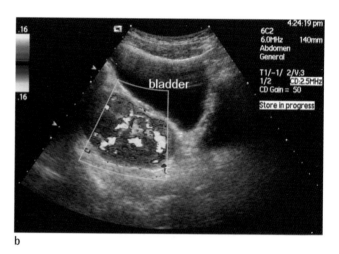

a   b

Figure 1.49
Sagittal section through the midline of the pelvis demonstrating a pelvic kidney (a). On (b) the malrotation and unusual shape are further evidenced by the direction of the renal hilum demonstrated by color flow Doppler.

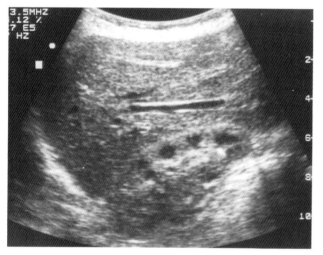

Figure 1.50
Upper pole of the right kidney abuts the diaphragm in this case of cranial ectopia.

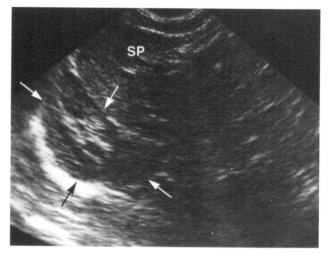

Figure 1.51
Cranial ascent of the left kidney. The left kidney (arrows) lies cephalad to the spleen (SP). In this case there probably was no true Bochdalek hernia but rather an eventration of the diaphragm, with the kidney remaining in intra-abdominal location.

Abnormalities of position

Renal ectopia results from an abnormality of ascent. This is most commonly incomplete ascent in which the kidney is located in the pelvis (Figure 1.49), but more rarely there is cranial ectopia where the kidney comes to lie adjacent to the hemidiaphragm (Figure 1.50), or even in an intra-

thoracic location when it is usually associated with a Bochdalek hernia (Figure 1.51). Occasionally, ascent causes the kidney to cross to the contralateral side. Crossed renal ectopia may be associated with renal fusion (Figure 1.52). The ultrasound features of abnormally located kidneys may reveal simply a structurally normal kidney in an abnormal location but more frequently there is an

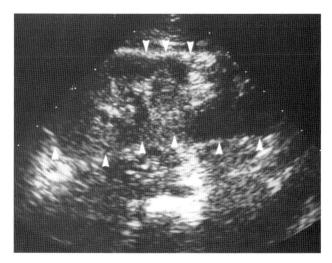

Figure 1.52
Crossed fused renal ectopia. The irregular fused renal mass is demonstrated on the right side of the abdomen, identified by the arrowheads.

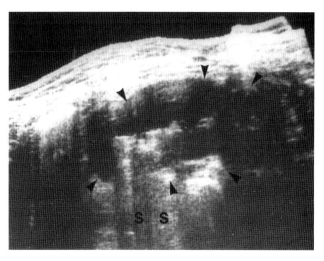

Figure 1.53
Crossed ectopia with calculi. In this case the ectopic kidney identified by the arrowheads lies just to the right of midline. Several calculi are noted in the right side of the ectopic kidney, producing distal acoustic shadowing (S).

associated malrotation: for example, a pelvic kidney lying in transverse oblique plane. There may be relative hypoplasia. Ectopic kidneys are more likely to be subject to certain pathologies such as renal calculi (Figure 1.53).

Abnormalities of fusion

During the course of the development of the metanephros, both kidneys lie in the pelvis and are closely related. At this stage, fusion of one part of the kidney with the other may occur, which will result in horseshoe kidney, cross-fused renal ectopia and the very rare 'lump' or 'cake' kidney. The horseshoe kidney occurs in 1 in 600 individuals, the lower poles being fused in the midline anterior to the aorta by an isthmus of varying composition. The presence of the isthmus tends to prevent the cranial migration of the horseshoe kidney and this therefore lies lower in the abdomen than normal kidneys. The axis of both kidneys is unusual, with the long axis lying parallel to the spine instead of diverted approximately 20° from the long axis, and the renal pelves being directed anteriorly. Apart from this change in rotation, the ultrasound appearances of a horseshoe kidney may be difficult to demonstrate, particularly if the isthmus is simply composed of fibrous tissue. However, a careful search for renal tissue along the lower poles of kidneys that demonstrate this unusual axis will usually reveal the lower pole fusion, particularly if high-frequency, high-resolution ultrasound probes are used (Figure 1.54).

The crossed, fused kidney is usually a polar fusion producing an S- or L-shaped structure within one or other flank. However, occasionally fusion may occur side by side.

The 'lump' or 'cake' kidney is a fused mass of renal tissue usually located in the pelvis and without obvious renal shape or form. It may be difficult to differentiate from other causes of pelvic or preaortic mass such as confluent lymphadenopathy, but the association between a mass and an 'empty' renal fossa will allow the diagnosis to be made.

Vessel abnormalities

Abnormalities of vascular supply to the kidneys are extremely common, occurring in more than 20% of adult kidneys. Usually there is only one additional vessel (Figure 1.55) but as many as four renal arteries can be present. Additional arteries are approximately twice as frequent as additional veins but neither are regularly demonstrated by ultrasound. Ultrasound demonstration of the renal vessels depends to some degree at least on the prior knowledge of the expected position of the artery relative to the origin of the celiac axis and the superior mesenteric artery, and its relationship with the inferior vena cava, e.g. on the right.

Accessory vessels may occur with an origin at any point along the ascent of the kidney, possibly arising from the distal aorta and even rarely from the iliac artery. Differentiation, therefore, of a small lower polar artery from a lumbar artery, for example, is extremely difficult. Color flow Doppler seems likely to improve this but it is unlikely that all supernumerary renal arteries will be demonstrated by ultrasound. The course of the left renal vein may be aberrant, crossing behind the aorta (Figure 1.56).

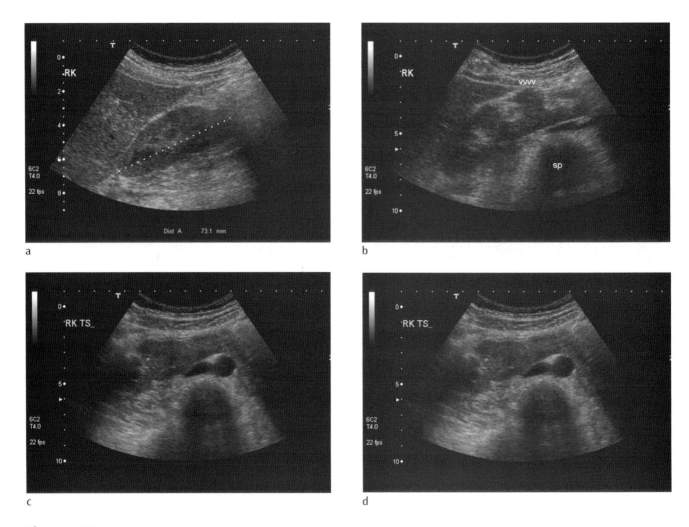

Figure 1.54

Horseshoe kidney. (a) The long axis scan through the right side demonstrates poor visualization of the lower pole of the kidney. (b and c) The renal tissue extends across the midline inferiorly over the spine, identified by arrowheads. (d) The relationship of the left-sided moiety partially obscured by bowel gas to the left of the aorta (arrowheads) is demonstrated.

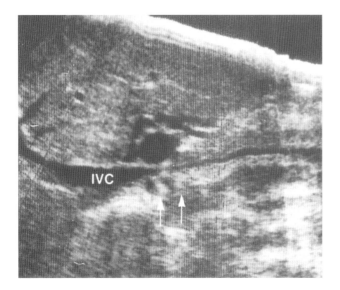

Figure 1.55

Multiple renal arteries. Two renal arteries are demonstrated (arrows) posterior to the inferior vena cava (IVC) as they course towards the right kidney.

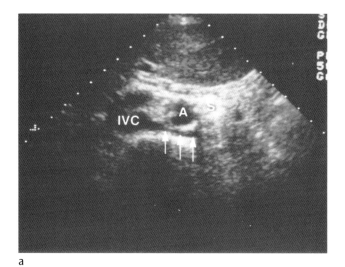

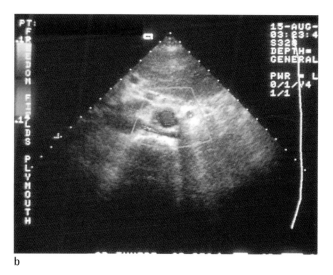

a

b

Figure 1.56
(a) **Retroaortic left renal vein.** There is a linear echo-free structure (arrows) posterior to the aorta (A) at the level of the superior mesenteric artery. IVC = inferior vena cava. (b) **Color flow Doppler shows flow in this structure towards the IVC, confirming the presence of a retroaortic left renal vein.**

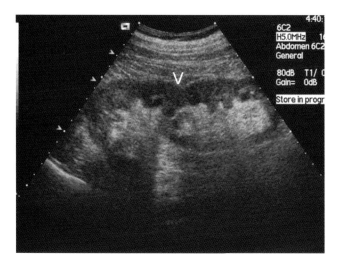

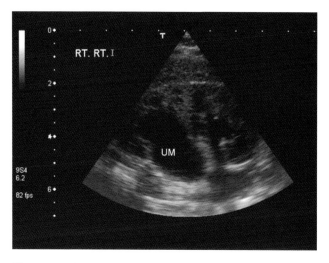

Figure 1.57
Renal duplication. The kidney is waisted, as identified by the arrowhead.

Figure 1.58
Dilated upper moiety (UM) in a duplex kidney.

Duplication of the ureter

Ureteric duplication is the result of duplication of the ureteric bud. Its extent depends upon the completeness of the bud division. However, ultrasound is an unreliable tool in the demonstration of ureteric duplication in the absence of dilatation. Ureteric duplication can usually only be inferred from separation of the renal sinus and 'waisting' of the kidney unless there is pathology affecting the collecting system of one or other moiety (Figures 1.57 and 1.58).

Renal dysplasia and hypoplasia

The diagnosis of renal dysplasia is rarely made in adult life. The unilateral small kidney with increased reflectivity, absence of corticomedullary differentiation and blending with the perirenal fat may be the result of renal dysplasia, including multicystic dysplastic kidneys, but equally could be the result of atrophy following infection, reflux, ischemia, etc. The specific diagnosis of renal dysplasia is therefore the province of the prenatal, perinatal and

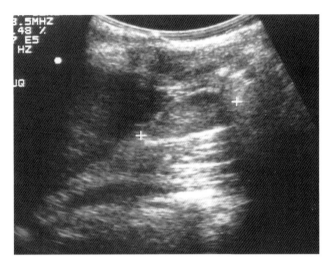

Figure 1.59
Hypoplasia of the right kidney. The kidney is structurally normal but small in size.

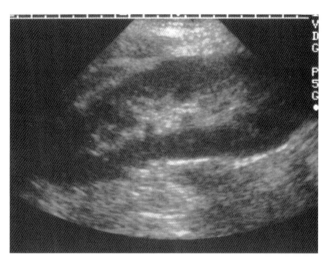

Figure 1.60
Congenital polar enlargement. The lower pole is significantly larger than the upper pole.

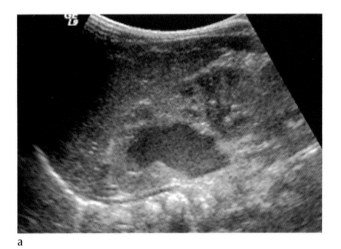

a

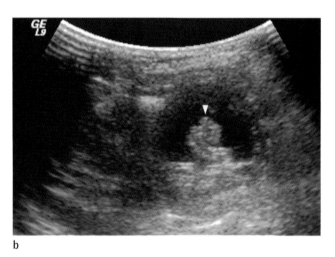

b

Figure 1.61
(a) Same case as Figure 1.58. There is a dilated upper moiety. **(b) Partially collapsed ureterocele within the bladder causing the upper tract obstruction.** The ureterocele is identified by the arrowhead.

pediatric sonographer and will be considered in the pediatric section of this book.

Hypoplasia of the kidney may also occur, one kidney being significantly smaller than its partner, but of otherwise normal sonographic appearance (Figure 1.59).

The existence of focal hypoplasia – the Ask Upmark kidney – may simply be the result of a segmental renal scar, perhaps secondary to vesicoureteric reflux, rather than a developmental congenital abnormality. The appearances are not dissimilar to those seen in other causes of renal scarring, although the cortical thinning usually involves a whole segment or a pole of the kidney.

Congenital polar enlargement, where either the upper pole or the lower pole is considerably larger than its mate, may be a variant of renal hypoplasia (Figure 1.60). Congenital abnormalities of the kidney may coexist with other abnormalities of the urogenital tract, including ureteric duplication. Similarly, ectopic insertion of the ureter into the urethra or vagina may occur particularly with renal duplication (Figure 1.61). Ureterocele may be an isolated abnormality or may coexist with renal ectopia or duplication. Abnormalities of the kidneys are also associated with genital abnormalities: in women with abnormalities of uterine development (e.g. bicornuate, absence) and in men with seminal vesicle abnormalities, abnormalities of testicular descent, etc.

ACQUIRED RENAL DISEASE

There are few characteristic ultrasound patterns that will allow the diagnosis of a specific disease process: benign and malignant tumors may have similar reflectivity and an abscess may be echo-free and thus mimic a simple cyst. Changes in parenchymal echogenicity occur as a function of age and this must be taken into account when evaluating diffuse parenchymal renal disease. Similarly, the echogenicity of mass lesions may approximate to normal renal parenchyma and occasionally to that of renal sinus fat, thus making the identification of small lesions difficult.

Consequently, evaluation of renal pathology must include an assessment of renal size, outline, the appearance of cortex, medulla and sinus, global and comparative echogenicity. The contribution of distribution of color flow may add to the diagnosis. The role of contrast enhancement has, for many pathologies, still to be established. The effect of pathology on adjacent structures within the kidney and outside the kidney, including perirenal fascia and adjacent organs, will be important in reaching a diagnosis.

In a text/atlas it is probably more appropriate to describe ultrasound appearances and relate these to possible differential diagnoses. Where there are specific features that may allow a particular diagnosis or may facilitate the differentiation of one pathology from another, these will be highlighted.

with obstruction of longer standing may present with a more diffuse loin pain, with a loin mass or, incidentally, without symptoms of obstruction (e.g. in prostatism). If infection supervenes, the patient may present with fever, malaise and rigors as well as the focal signs of obstruction.

Structural changes within the kidney

Renal pelvic and calyceal dilatation may occur in a number of conditions; conversely, in acute obstruction there may be no calyceal or pelvic dilatation, particularly in the early stages.

There are a number of features on ultrasound imaging which are characteristic of calyceal and pelvic dilatation. The cardinal feature is that of separation of the renal sinus. Although it has been stated that this can occur in up to 50% of patients during diuresis and secondary to back pressure with a full bladder (see Figure 1.26), it remains a highly sensitive technique in the detection, particularly, of long-standing renal obstruction. The dilated calyces and renal pelvis are usually best demonstrated in either the transverse or coronal plane, where the central echo-poor triangular pelvis may become dilated and rounded and may be seen to communicate with the peripherally placed fluid-containing calyces (Figure 1.62). Other features suggestive of renal obstruction may occur, including perirenal fluid, and increased echogenicity with heterogeneity of the perirenal fat similar to the stranding seen on CT (Figure 1.63). It is possible with ultrasound to grade the degree of obstruction (Figures 1.64).

Obstructive renal disease

The features of obstruction depend upon the use of all of the parameters available to the sonographer. These include the mode of clinical presentation, demonstration of the anatomy of the collecting system and the ureter, the effect of changing intrarenal pressure on Doppler indices within the renal vessels and the appearance and characteristics of ureteric jets.

The method of presentation

The symptoms with which a patient with obstructive renal disease presents depend upon the cause and duration of obstruction. Characteristically, acute calculus obstruction presents with symptoms of renal colic, whereas patients

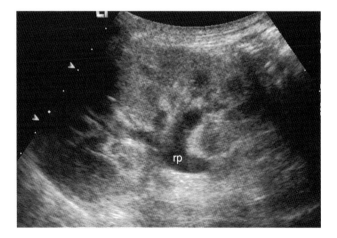

Figure 1.62
Early dilatation of the collecting system. The renal pelvis (RP) is distended.

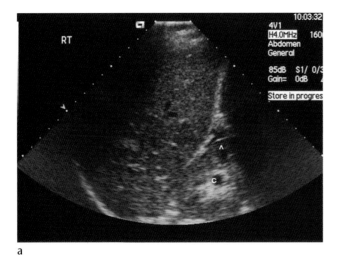
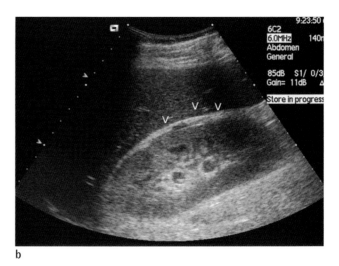

a

b

Figure 1.63

(a) Renal obstruction. A minimally dilated upper pole calyx is identified (c). There is free fluid in Morrison's pouch (arrowhead). **(b) Thickening and edema of the prerenal fascia (arrowheads) in acute obstruction.** This is similar to perirenal stranding on CT.

Grade 0	Normal
Grade 1	Minimal dilatation of the calyces
Grade 2	Visible papillae in a dilated system
Grade 3	Moderate dilatation of the calyces
Grade 4	Severe dilatation of the calyces

Occasionally, in Grade 2 hydronephrosis and in resolving obstruction, the papillae may be unusually prominent, mimicking papillary necrosis.

However, there is a wide possible differential diagnosis of these appearances. An extrarenal pelvis or a normal or capacious system can produce similar features. A recently relieved obstruction will still demonstrate a dilated collecting system, which will only return to normal after a period of hours or days, depending upon the severity and the duration of obstruction, or may remain dilated (Figure 1.65). Congenital megacalyx can mimic a focal obstruction to a segment of the kidney and compound calyces may produce similar diagnostic difficulties. Megacystis and megaureter represent dilatation of the collecting system without obstruction.

A parapelvic cyst may mimic pelvicalyceal dilatation (Figure 1.66). Although the cyst is commonly simply rounded and in the coronal and transverse plane can be distinguished from a dilated collecting system, frequently the cyst is lobulated, with the lobules extending into the region of the papillae and mimicking dilated calyces. Differentiation depends upon an evaluation of the shape of the cyst and the relative size of the locules extending into the renal sinus. A parapelvic cyst does not normally extend to the level of the renal cortex; there is usually a short 'infundibulum' of the locule and the locules appear more

bulbous than distended calyces. In some circumstances, however, it will be necessary to undertake additional imaging studies to resolve the diagnosis, particularly if the patient presents with loin pain.

The role of duplex sonography in renal tract obstruction

Currently ultrasound imaging has no functional correlate of intravenous urography (IVU) or of contrast-enhanced CT. It depends upon the effects of obstruction upon intrarenal anatomy: namely, calyceal dilatation and dilatation of the renal pelvis and ureter. There is, at present, no ultrasound contrast medium which is excreted in the urine.

However, the physiologic effects of obstruction on intrarenal pressure may also impact on Doppler ultrasound features and indices. During normal renal function, focal segments of high pressure are achieved within the ureter by muscular contraction. This propels urine along the ureter, while pressure within the renal pelvis remains low. In acute obstruction there is a rapid early change in intrarenal pressure, partly consequent upon back pressure, but partly consequent upon a diuretic response of the kidney. Intrarenal pressures of up to 70 mmHg are achieved within minutes of an acute complete obstruction. The intrarenal pressure, even in the presence of persistent obstruction, falls to normal, occasionally within hours, but more usually within days. The pressure rise is accompanied at first by an increase in peristaltic activity, which subsequently decreases. Renal blood flow increases for several

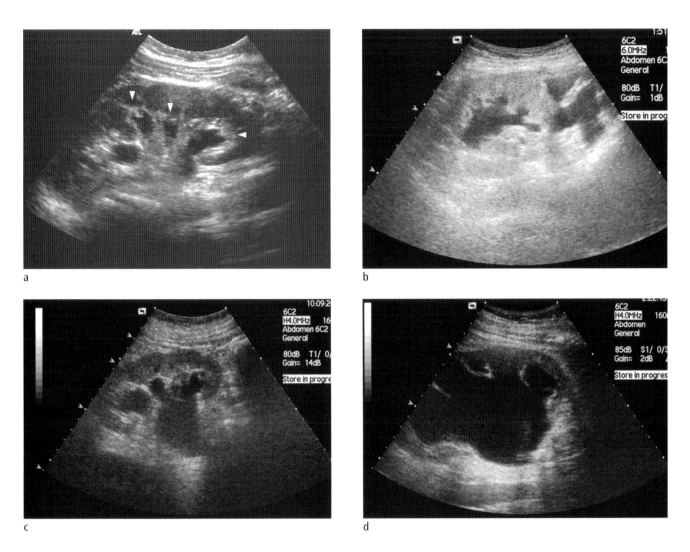

a   b

c   d

Figure 1.64

(a) **Early dilatation of the collecting system.** The renal papillae are prominent and outlined by fluid within the collecting system (arrowheads). (b) **Marked dilatation within the collecting system, but still demonstrating intercommunication of the fluid-filled spaces.** (c) **The calyceal dilatation is now moderate to severe with marked dilatation of the renal pelvis.** (d) **Gross dilatation of the calyces and of the renal pelvis.**

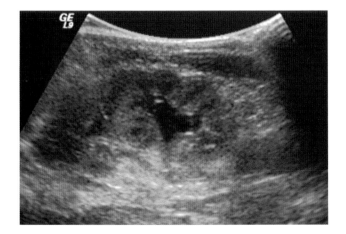

Figure 1.65

Persistent dilatation after relief of obstruction. Note the mucosal thickening of the papillae.

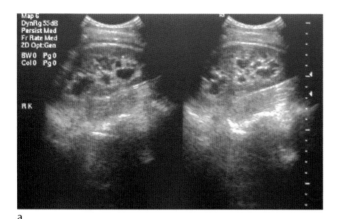

a

Figure 1.66
(a,b) Examples of parapelvic cysts mimicking hydronephrosis.

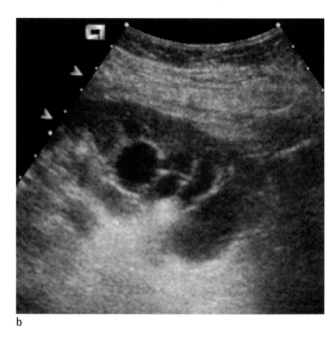

b

hours, probably reflecting the diuresis, and then subsequently decreases and may fall to normal or even less than normal in long-term obstruction. The effect of this on spectral Doppler does not exactly reflect experimental evidence of change in intrarenal pressure, but there are changes in pulsatility and resistance index which may contribute to the diagnosis of obstruction.

Dilatation of the collecting system ensues at a variable time after the initial onset of obstruction, and the degree of dilatation is normally dependent upon the nature and rapidity of onset of obstruction. Thus, the gradual increase in back pressure that occurs consequent upon benign prostate hypertrophy will produce marked pelvicalyceal dilatation as well as dilatation of the ureter, whereas a patient with a ureteric calculus exhibits calyces of normal or near-normal size.

The basis for the application of an assessment of Doppler spectra to the diagnosis of acute urinary obstruction has been based on animal research that demonstrated a biphasic hemodynamic response to complete ureteric obstruction. A short period (less than 2 hours) of prostaglandin-mediated vasodilatation occurs immediately after obstruction. After this period, renal blood flow decreases and renal vascular resistance increases. It is probable that the caliber changes within the renal vessels are consequent upon complex interactions between the mechanical effect of increase in collecting system pressure and the regulatory pathways of renin–angiotensin, kallikrein–kinin and prostaglandin–thromboxane.

The potential for Doppler ultrasound to detect these changes in intrarenal pressure has been widely investigated. Criteria for the diagnosis of obstruction have been developed using absolute values of resistance or pulsatility index, or differences between the resistance index between one kidney and another. Early work had suggested that the mean RI in kidneys with confirmed obstruction (0.77 ± 0.04) was significantly higher than the mean RI in kidneys with non-obstructive pelvicalyceal dilatation (0.64 ± 0.04). Moreover, these RI values return to normal after nephrostomy in the obstructed group. A discriminatory RI threshold of 0.7 has been proposed or an RI difference between the two kidneys of greater than 0.04. Initial work suggested sensitivities of approximately 90% (Figure 1.67). However, much of the early work has evaluated cases of complete ureteric obstruction. The demonstration of partial ureteric obstruction appears to be significantly limited.

Chen et al[2] suggests that the sensitivity of Doppler sonography for diagnosis of obstruction was only 52% when patients with a partial obstruction were included in the study group.

Other physiologic and pharmacologic factors may also compound the Doppler findings. There is, for example, a potential vasodilatory effect of nonsteroidal anti-inflammatory medication used for pain relief in early obstruction. Similarly, studies which have compared IVU with Doppler ultrasound have been challenged on the basis of a very significant vasoconstrictive effect of urographic contrast media. Furthermore, few of the studies have clarity of timing of the ultrasound evaluation. Opdenacker[3] in 1998 reported, in an experimental study, that changes in resistance index did not occur between 0 and 6 hours following acute obstruction and that increased RI was limited to a period of between 6 and 48 hours. After 48

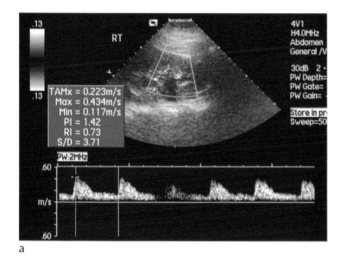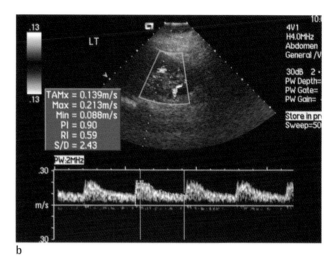

a b

Figure 1.67

(a) **Spectral Doppler in renal obstruction.** Note slightly raised pulsatility index and resistance index. (b) **Spectral Doppler in the contralateral kidney demonstrating normal resistance and pulsatility indices.** Although the indices are only slightly above normal limits in the affected kidney, the difference between the two sides is marked.

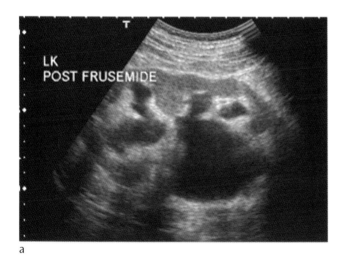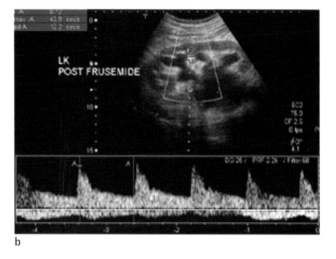

a b

Figure 1.68

(a) **Post-furosemide, there is marked dilatation of the collecting system with particular prominence of the renal pelvis.** (b) **Post-furosemide, the spectral pattern demonstrates an early diastolic notch in the intrarenal artery wave form consistent with obstruction.**

hours there was a gradual return to normal of RI. Other workers have suggested that the Doppler changes may persist for several months, even after release of obstruction.

A number of authors have advocated the combined use of Doppler ultrasound with a diuretic ± a water load, as a method of improving the sensitivity and specificity of Doppler assessment of obstruction, but there have been few confirmatory studies (Figure 1.68).

A pilot study, evaluating venous impedance indices by comparing obstructed and non-obstructed sides, suggested statistically significant differences. On average, the peak venous flow signal in the obstructed kidney was 69% higher than that of the non-obstructed kidney and 86% higher than that of the peak venous flow signal in controls. To date there has been no confirmatory evidence to support this finding.[4]

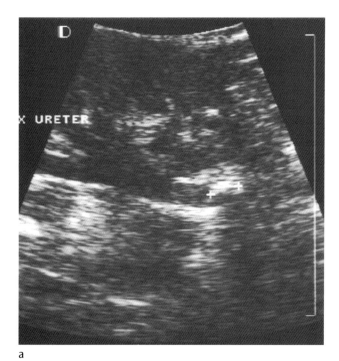

a

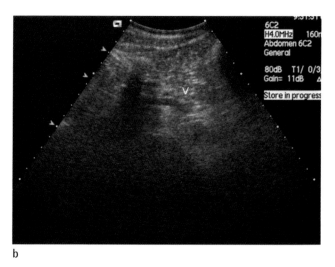

b

Figure 1.69

(a) **Proximal ureteric stone.** There is sludge proximal to this but little in the way of acoustic shadowing. (b) **Stone in the mid-ureter (arrowhead).** The stone distends the ureter but again produces little in the way of acoustic shadowing.

Direct visualization of the calculus

The ureter is notoriously difficult to demonstrate with ultrasound. Its course, lying anterior to the transverse processes of the lumbar vertebrae within the retroperitoneum, means that it is described as being largely inaccessible to ultrasound evaluation. Similarly, the reliability of ultrasound in the detection of calculi anywhere within the renal tract has been challenged. For example, Fowler et al[5] have indicated a sensitivity of only 24% and a specificity of 90% when using ultrasound to assess the presence or absence of multiple calculi within the kidney and indicate, consequently, that ultrasound is of limited value in the detection of renal calculi.

Ultrasound features of ureteric calculi are similar to calculi elsewhere, although the demonstration of acoustic shadowing is sometimes difficult, particularly in the mid ureter (Figure 1.69). Features include a highly echogenic focus within a mildly or moderately dilated ureter, demonstration of echogenic, presumed urinary sludge, proximal to the calculus and, occasionally, thickening of the ureteric wall (Figure 1.70).

Interpretation of ultrasound is now aided by a number of different processing technologies and these have not been fully evaluated in the detection of calculi. These include tissue harmonics, pulse inversion and phase inversion harmonics and the observation of comet tail twinkling artifacts on color flow and power Doppler. It is possible that these may contribute to improved visualization of renal calculi.

Visualization of the ureter is possible with ultrasound, particularly the first few centimeters distal to the renal pelvis and the distal ureter posterior to the bladder. Visualization of the ureter within the abdomen is acknowledged to be more difficult, but it is still possible in the presence of ureteric dilatation, even in patients less than ideal for sonographic evaluation (Figures 1.71 and 1.72).

The majority of ureteric calculi are located in the distal ureter close to the vesicoureteric junction and their demonstration by ultrasound is facilitated by a full urinary bladder. Indeed one study, using ultrasound in direct comparison with non-contrast-enhanced spiral CT, has suggested that ultrasound has a sensitivity and specificity similar to that of CT and of the order of 91–93% sensitivity and 95% specificity.

Ureteric jets

Flow of urine from the ureter into the bladder can be encountered during routine sonographic examination of the pelvis. Although demonstration may be compromised by an under- or overdistended urinary bladder, nonetheless, the characteristics of ureteric jets are modified by pathologies which produce complete or partial obstruction to the ureter. Similarly, ureteric jets may also be modified by other pathologies which affect renal function, and some have proposed that ureteric jets, when quantified, could be used to evaluate split renal function. This may have

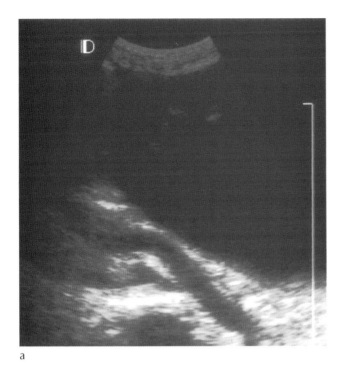

a

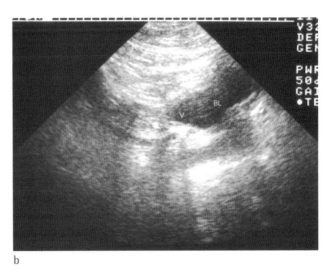

b

Figure 1.70

Stones in the distal ureter. (a) Stones in the distal ureter are more easy to demonstrate, particularly when the bladder is full. (b) However, even with a partially filled urinary bladder, a shadowing stone posterior to the trigone can be demonstrated.

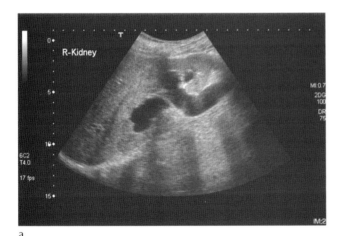

a

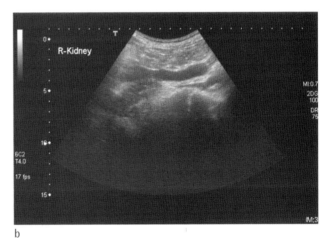

b

Figure 1.71

Figures (a–c) demonstrate the entire course of a dilated ureter due to outflow tract obstruction.

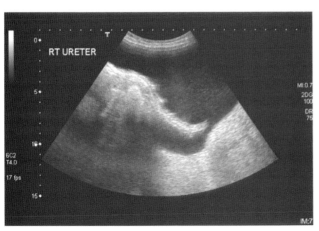

c

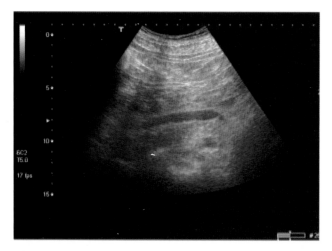

Figure 1.72
Visualization of the dilated mid-ureter by compression in the flank.

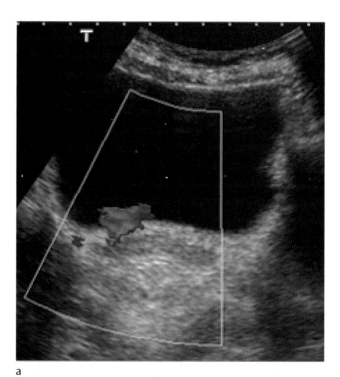

a

b

Figure 1.73
(a) Moderately filled urinary bladder. A ureteric jet is of low velocity and not typically directed. This feature followed recent passage of a stone. **(b) Local invasion of cervical carcinoma into the base of the bladder has caused distortion of the direction of the ureteric jet on the right.**

application in the assessment of vesicoureteric reflux but, more particularly, may also help to confirm partial or complete obstruction of the ureter by demonstrating the absence of jets or abnormality of periodicity, velocity or direction of flow in the ureter on the affected side (Figure 1.73).

Whereas ureteric obstruction may alter the presence or nature of ureteric jets, other conditions which affect the trigone may also alter the appearance of jets without necessarily producing obstruction. Local conditions such as cervical carcinoma may cause infiltration of the trigone of the bladder, producing distortion of flow direction within the ureteric jets (Figure 1.73b). Similar changes may occur postoperatively and following radiotherapy, although these potential changes have yet to be fully characterized.

As for all the criteria used to assess ureteric obstruction, evaluation of ureteric jets has produced variable results. However, the absence of jets correlates well with high-grade obstruction, and an assessment of jet frequency and flow velocity may also improve the applicability of this technique to the diagnosis of ureteric obstruction.

Application of sonographic criteria of obstruction

Unfortunately, the evaluation of all ultrasound parameters in the investigation of potential acute obstruction has received little attention.

Furthermore, the advent of non-contrast enhanced helical and now multislice CT has provided a rapid, reproducible and accurate alternative to the emergency IVU. The advantages of this approach are reported to be not only in high sensitivity and specificity for the detection of ureteric obstruction but also in the demonstration and characterization of other renal and non-renal pathologies. However, the widely increased use of spiral CT for a wide range of acute and non-acute conditions has the potential to increase significantly the radiation burden in our patient population. It is suggested that a combination of sonographic findings may achieve similar accuracies of diagnosis of ureteric obstruction to non-enhanced CT. Characteristics that should be considered are as follows:

- peri-renal stranding, fluid in or thickening of the renal capsule
- dilatation of the calyces and pelvis
- dilatation of the ureter
- demonstration of a ureteric calculus
- resistance indices within the affected kidney of greater than 0.7 or RI difference between the kidneys of greater than 0.4 (ΔRI)
- absent or abnormal ureteric jets.

Using this approach, a single group, Geavlete et al[6] have classified the ultrasound findings of renal colic into four groups:

1. The acute, completely obstructed kidney with a non-functional IVU. These present with pelvicalyceal dilatation, as compared with a normal contralateral kidney, and with demonstrable abnormalities of resistance index and absence of the ureteric jet in almost 90% of cases.
2. An acute, completely obstructed kidney with non-functional IVU but without evidence of pelvicalyceal dilatation. In this group, Doppler and ureteric jet findings were less reliable, but were still abnormal in over 80% of cases.
3. Incompletely obstructed kidney. The IVU demonstrate various degrees of pelvicalyceal and ureteric dilatation. (Doppler findings were least reliable, being abnormal in approximately 65% of patients, whereas the ureteric jets were asymmetrical in 74%.)
4. Normal findings on the IVU. In this group, the normal findings were replicated on Doppler and on evaluation of ureteric jets in over 90% of cases.

Evaluation of ureteric stents

It appears that ultrasound criteria for the evaluation of ureteric stents are unreliable. Documented changes in the degree of pelvicalyceal dilatation are dependent upon the degree of hydration and, unless a progressive change is observed, it is difficult to confirm obstruction. Similarly, the demonstration of ureteric jets depends upon the presence of peristaltic activity within the ureter. Since passive drainage (periprosthetic and luminal flow) is the principle mechanism of urine transport in the stented ureter, color Doppler ultrasound of ureteric jets is unreliable in the detection of stent obstruction.

Level of obstruction

While ultrasound combined with color flow and pulsed Doppler of the renal artery and the ureteric jet may combine to provide more accurate diagnosis of the presence of obstruction, the level of ureteric obstruction is less well demonstrated by ultrasound. The approach, then, to the demonstration of the level of obstruction using ultrasound should be first of all to assess the presence or absence of dilatation of the calyces and pelvis, and then to examine the urinary bladder and the pelvic course of the ureters to assess whether or not there is dilatation of the ureters at this level.

Causes of ureteric obstruction

The causes of obstruction are listed in Table 1.3. Most are considered elsewhere in the text.

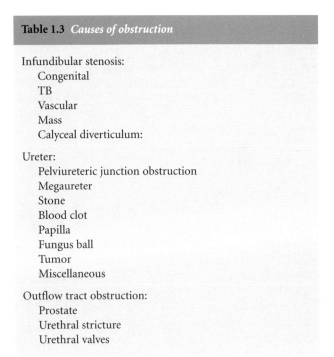

Table 1.3 Causes of obstruction

Infundibular stenosis:
 Congenital
 TB
 Vascular
 Mass
 Calyceal diverticulum:

Ureter:
 Pelviureteric junction obstruction
 Megaureter
 Stone
 Blood clot
 Papilla
 Fungus ball
 Tumor
 Miscellaneous

Outflow tract obstruction:
 Prostate
 Urethral stricture
 Urethral valves

The role of ultrasound in suspected obstruction

The limitations of ultrasound have been clearly set out, although the potential for the use of all ultrasound parameters has not been fully assessed. The judgment of the radiologist must be used to determine the most appropriate investigation in the individual case. This may be non-enhanced helical or multislice CT, intravenous urography or ultrasound, particularly in cases where there is a strong contraindication to the use of ionizing radiation or contrast media. Furthermore, ultrasound remains the investigation of first choice in patients with azotemia. In this situation, ultrasound affords the demonstration of renal obstruction and differentiation of other causes of renal failure and can be used to guide antegrade pyelography, percutaneous nephrostomy and, where necessary and appropriate, stent placement.

Dilatation of the renal tract in pregnancy

Dilatation of the pelvicalyceal system and of the ureters is well recognized in normal pregnancies. The etiology of this dilatation is not clear. Suggestions include that it may be physiologic, as a result of smooth muscle relaxation within the ureters, or anatomical, as a result of compression of the ureter by the fetus. Dilatation is usually more marked on the right than on the left and may reach massive dimensions; one case is reported where the renal pelvis measured 8.9 cm in diameter at 35 weeks without any evidence of functional renal compromise and with resolution of the dilatation following delivery of the infant. Indeed, comparison between pelvicalyceal dilatation in pregnancy where there is known renal infection and renal pelvic dilatation without intercurrent complication shows no difference in the degree of pelvicalyceal dilatation.

Duplex Doppler ultrasound has been proposed as a discriminating tool in the investigation of renal disease in pregnancy. Studies of time–velocity spectra in the renal arteries of normal pregnant women reveal a slight reduction of pulsatility and resistance indices, although most fall within the normal non-pregnant range. Furthermore, there is no difference between Doppler indices in dilated non-obstructed versus non-dilated systems.

Direct visualization, particularly of the distal ureter, is compromised by the position of the fetus, particularly in late pregnancy, but it remains possible to demonstrate jets in the majority of patients, particularly in the first and second trimester. Where a jet is absent, it is important to turn the patient on to the contralateral side. A previously absent or atypical jet will frequently return to normal. A combination of a ΔRI difference of greater than 0.04 (Figure 1.74) and/or abnormality of ureteric jets, allied to dilatation of the collecting system, will allow the selection of patients for further imaging. Features of complications of obstruction such as perirenal fluid are uncommon in the hydronephrosis of pregnancy. Similarly, demonstration of an unusual site of obstruction or the obstructing lesion will be useful in differentiation.

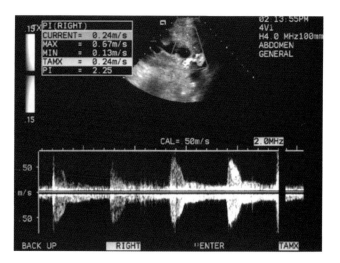

Figure 1.74
Raised pulsatility index (PI) in obstruction. The PI is noted to be 2.25.

Pelviureteric junction obstruction

Pelviureteric junction (PUJ) obstruction represents a particular form of obstruction to urine flow. The condition is exacerbated by a fluid load or other diuretic stimulants, the patient presenting with intermittent loin pain frequently occurring after a large fluid intake. The features on ultrasound are of dilated calyces, with a markedly rounded but occasionally patulous renal pelvis without evidence of demonstration of a dilated ureter. It is occasionally possible to demonstrate the irregularity of the PUJ, and in some cases where this is caused by a crossing vessel (Figure 1.75). PUJ obstruction may be associated with significant compromise of excretory function and with renal parenchymal loss. It is possible to calculate a ratio between the renal cortical area and the area of the renal pelvis, and a ratio of pelvic to parenchymal area of greater than 1.6 can be used to predict the need for surgery.

Doppler sonography may be of use in the diagnosis and follow-up of PUJ obstruction, and the sensitivity of the technique may be increased by use of intravenous furosemide to increase the intrarenal pressure in obstructed cases. In some cases, an early to mid-diastolic notch is demonstrated in the Doppler spectrum (Figure 1.76). The use of intravenous furosemide appears to be of particular importance following, for example, pyeloplasty, where assessment of changes in shape of the renal pelvis and dilatation of the collecting system is difficult. Furosemide will not normally alter the shape of the Doppler waveform in the normal kidney, although there may be a transient increase in 'renal perfusion' as demonstrated by color flow Doppler. In the patient with PUJ obstruction, administration of furosemide is accompanied by an increase in the RI.

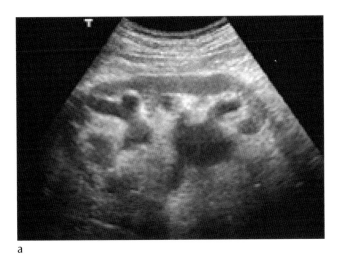

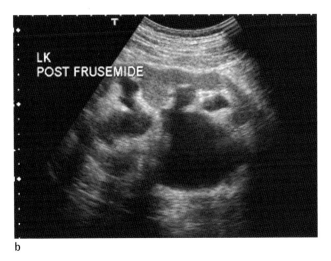

a   b

Figure 1.75
Pelviureteric junction obstruction. (a) The calyces and the pelves are dilated. (b) Following furosemide, there is marked dilatation of the renal pelvis. This coincided with reproduction of the patient's pain.

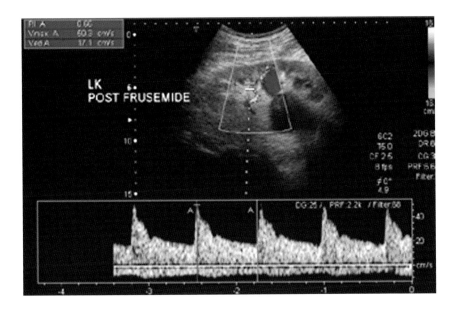

Figure 1.76
Spectral Doppler demonstrating an early diastolic notch in obstruction secondary to PUJ obstruction.

Prostatism

The investigation of patients with symptoms of benign prostatic hypertrophy has been the subject of significant controversy. The intravenous urogram, which has long been the mainstay of diagnosis, has been shown to have no significant advantage over ultrasound in the detection of hydronephrosis, post-obstructive atrophy, renal masses, renal calculi, bladder stones or bladder tumors. Since almost all patients with significant ureteric obstruction and hydronephrosis will have a biochemical abnormality, there is an argument that the only investi-

gation that is appropriate in a patient with prostatism is a plain abdominal X-ray, which will detect calculi and the occasional bone metastasis from an unsuspected prostatic carcinoma. The argument for performing other imaging investigations in simple, uncomplicated prostatism is not compelling. The serendipitous discovery of a renal tumor may be advanced as a reason for performing further investigation of the upper tracts, but there is scant evidence to support the postulate that renal carcinoma is more common in patients with prostatism than in age-matched controls without prostatic symptomatology (Figure 1.77).

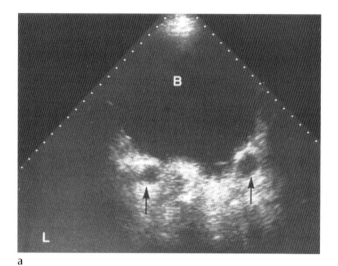
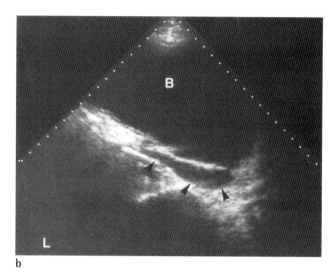

a

b

Figure 1.77
(a,b) Outflow tract obstruction. In (a), a transverse scan of the pelvis, the distended bladder (B) is demonstrated. The dilated distal ureters are identified by the arrows. In (b) an oblique scan through the pelvis demonstrates the distended bladder (B) and the dilated distal ureter identified by the arrowheads.

The rationale, therefore, for screening patients with prostatism for renal carcinoma is fairly tenuous. However, if any investigation other than a plain abdominal film is to be used in patients with prostatism, ultrasound should clearly be preferred because of the absence of ionizing radiation.

Renal and ureteric calculus disease

Vesical calculi, common for the last three centuries, are now rarely seen. Although the constituents of urine are commonly present in concentrations in excess of their solubility in water, it seems that certain predisposing conditions are necessary for stone formation. These include climate, urinary infection and stagnation as well as conditions producing hypercalciuria. In addition, certain congenital abnormalities such as cystinuria and hyperoxaluria, hyperuricaemia and the milk alkali syndrome may also predispose to renal calculus formation. Similarly, certain congenital, structural abnormalities of the kidney such as renal ectopia and horseshoe kidney are associated with an increased incidence of urinary tract calculi.

The calculi vary greatly in size from tiny sand-like grains to large staghorn calculi filling part or all of the renal pelvis and calyces. Staghorn calculi are usually associated with chronic infection and obstruction.

The clinical features vary, depending upon the presence or absence of obstruction or infection. Symptoms are therefore dependent upon the site of the calculus as well as its size. Renal parenchymal calculi are less commonly symptomatic than ureteric or renal pelvic calculi, although they may be associated with flank pain and hematuria. The classical symptoms of ureteric calculus are of renal colic associated with either frank or microscopic hematuria.

Diagnosis

The diagnosis of urinary tract calculi is dependent on clinical presentation and departmental protocol. The value of non-contrast helical CT in the detection of renal, ureteric and bladder calculi is well established in the literature. Certainly most authors would advocate this approach for the diagnosis of renal colic. Similarly, the detection of renal stones appears to be achieved with higher sensitivity with CT than with either ultrasound or plain abdominal film (KUB).

However, the sensitivity of ultrasound in the detection of renal and ureteric calculi remains uncertain, with reported sensitivities of 21–93%. Certainly, if the higher sensitivities are reproducible, ultrasound has a role when there is a contraindication to the use of the CT or intravenous urography.

Although ultrasound probably detects fewer renal calculi than CT, it is not clear whether the additional calculi so detected are clinically significant or amenable to therapy. Indeed, improved ultrasound equipment identifies smaller and smaller echogenic foci suggestive of calculi

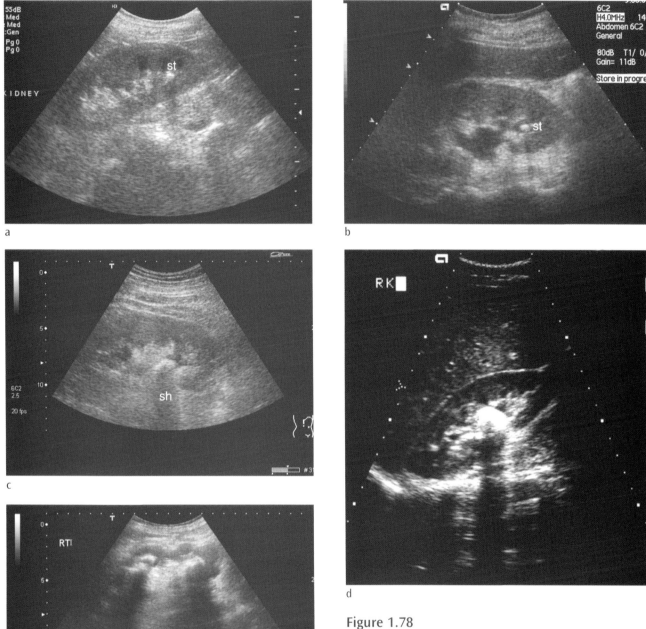

Figure 1.78

(a,b) **Calculus at the lower pole of the kidney within the collecting system (ST).** There is modest acoustic shadowing. (c) **Larger stone within the collecting system.** Again the shadowing (SH) is ill-defined and difficult to differentiate from shadowing deriving from the renal sinus itself. (d) **Sharp shadow from large stone within the central renal sinus.** (e) **Staghorn calculus.** The renal outline is difficult to identify and there are multiple shadowing foci from the renal bed.

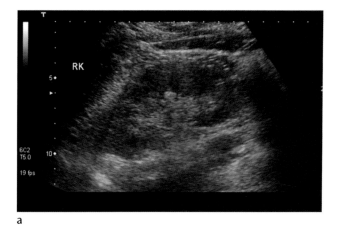

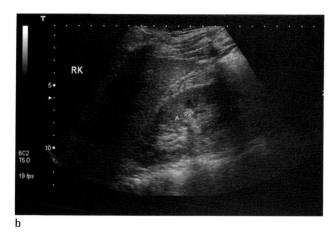

a

b

Figure 1.79
(a,b) Central renal calculus. (a) Little acoustic shadow. (b) Change of transducer position allows the demonstration of acoustic shadow.

which are below the size and/or in a location that would not afford intervention.

Extracorporeal shock wave lithotripsy (ESWL) requires accurate localization of renal calculi and regular assessment of the urinary tract at follow-up to ensure adequate fragmentation of the stones and their subsequent passage. Ultrasound is now the technique of choice for ESWL guidance and follow-up with reported sensitivity in the detection of renal parenchymal calculi of 95% compared with 92% for plain radiography.

Ultrasound appearances

Ultrasound features of renal calculi depend rather less on the composition than do those techniques using ionizing radiation. The characteristic features are those of a brightly reflective focus producing distal acoustic shadowing (Figure 1.78). The smaller the size of the calculus, the more difficult it is to recognize on ultrasound, and, indeed, for calculi less than 2.5 mm in diameter the sensitivity of detection decreases to approximately 85%. Although the brightness of the calculus and the degree of acoustic shadowing may differ between calcium phosphate, oxalate, magnesium ammonium phosphate and carbonate apatite stones when compared with cystine, urate, xanthine and matrix calculi which are non-opaque on plain radiography, this is not reported in the literature except for matrix calculi.

Since all calculi are highly reflective, ultrasound may be used in the differential diagnosis of non-opaque filling defects of the collecting system demonstrated at intravenous urography. Cystine and uric acid calculi can be differentiated from blood clot and urothelial tumor, for example. It is important to differentiate the discrete shadowing from a renal calculus from the rather diffuse shadowing that may occur from the normal rather echogenic renal sinus. This can be difficult since the reflectivity of stones located in the renal sinus may approximate to that of the renal sinus itself (Figure 1.79). It is vital in this situation to ensure that the highest frequency transducer possible is used, together with a focus located at the site of the suspected calculus. Other criteria of sonographic demonstration of calculi may be used. The shadowing artifact deriving from calculi is increased by non-linear ultrasound techniques such as tissue harmonic imaging, although there are other technical aspects of non-linear imaging which may compromise this theoretical advantage. Color and power Doppler may demonstrate unusual twinkling artifacts in renal calculi, which are manifest as a rapidly changing color complex behind stones with a pattern of a comet tail.

Urinary matrix calculi are rare. They have a 'putty-like' consistency, with a tendency to form a cast of the collecting system. There are few reports of matrix calculi in the literature, but the condition shows few of the classical features of a calculus (Figure 1.80). The mass is of relatively low echogenicity although there may be a brightly reflective layer at the margin and acoustic shadowing is said to be absent.

Calculi can occasionally be mimicked by milk of calcium present in small calyceal cysts or renal parenchymal cysts. As a general rule, the appearances of a cyst containing milk

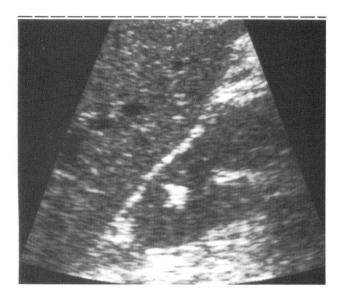

Figure 1.80
Matrix calculus at the upper pole of the right kidney. Ill-defined, somewhat irregular focus of increased reflectivity with no shadowing. This lesion is difficult to differentiate, for example, from a small angiomyolipoma.

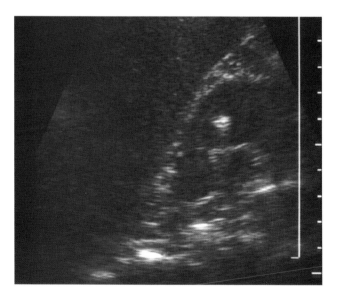

Figure 1.81
Milk of calcium cyst. Bright focus within the renal parenchyma, demonstrating reverberation and extending to a comet tail.

of calcium is of a cyst containing echogenic material which is frequently layered, although occasionally the cyst may be completely filled, and produce reverberation artifact. Clear-cut acoustic shadowing has been identified and in this situation differentiation from renal calculus is extremely difficult (Figure 1.81).

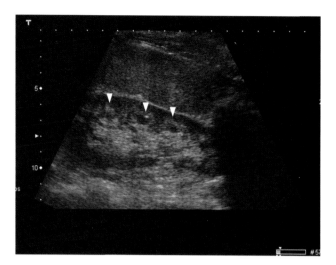

Figure 1.82
The Anderson–Carr kidney. Echogenic crescents surrounding the medullary pyramids (arrowheads).

The differential diagnosis of renal calculi would also include papillary necrosis. A sloughed papilla may produce a small echogenic mass within the collecting system. Occasionally, this may produce acoustic shadowing, particularly if there is calcification. The diagnosis is, however, usually obvious by the demonstration of other large abnormal papillae, occasionally calcified, projecting into the calyces from the apex of the renal pyramids.

The Anderson–Carr kidney represents the earliest appearances of renal calculus disease. This probably reflects the deposition of calcium within the tubule walls and is manifest on ultrasound by echogenic crescents marking the margin of the medulla with the cortex (Figure 1.82). There is usually no or little associated shadowing. Improvements in ultrasound technology allow the more frequent demonstration of this appearance, but equally in the younger patient margination of cortex and medulla is now frequently prominent and care must be exercised not to overdiagnose the condition.

Renal cystic disease

Cystic disease of the kidney represents not one entity but a wide variety of conditions with different etiologic, physiologic and genetic features. Certain cystic conditions of the kidney, such as multicystic dysplastic disease and obstructive dysplasia, occur only in the neonatal period and these are considered elsewhere in this book.

Renal cysts may arise from dilated glomeruli or tubules and their walls may consist of cuboid or columnar epithelium, which may or may not be hyperplastic. Therefore,

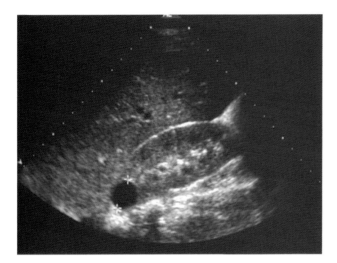

Figure 1.83
Simple cyst at the upper pole of the right kidney, demonstrating characteristic appearances. It is echo-free with clear anterior and posterior walls and acoustic enhancement.

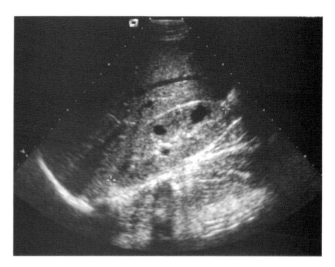

Figure 1.84
Multiple cysts within the kidney of a 75 year old. The cyst at the lower pole is somewhat irregular in outline and would therefore be classified as Bosniak 2.

classification based on histology is not entirely satisfactory; however, nor is it satisfactory to attempt a classification on radiologic characteristics. Cysts exhibiting entirely similar characteristics can occur in vastly different pathologies and one pathology can produce cysts of different appearances in different parts of the kidney. In this section, therefore, I shall not attempt to reproduce or create a classification of cysts. Instead, a description of commonly occurring cystic structures will be presented. Where appropriate, I will suggest how other conditions may mimic these appearances, and, where possible, differential diagnostic features will be presented. The complex or multilocular cystic mass in particular will be presented as a descriptive rather than a pathologic entity, since such masses normally present as a multilocular cyst rather than a cystic hypernephroma or 'localized cystic disease'.

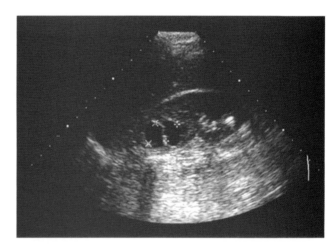

Figure 1.85
Septated cyst at the upper pole of the kidney. Incidental note is made of a calculus at the lower pole with acoustic shadowing.

Simple cysts

These are the most common of renal cysts. Their incidence increases with age; they are rare under the age of 40, whereas the incidence over the age of 70 reaches 60%. In 5% of cases there will be multiple bilateral cysts in this age group. The characteristic appearance of a cyst is of a unilocular echo-free structure of varying size, either within the substance or at the margin of the kidney (Figures 1.83–1.87). The cyst is normally spherical, with clear-cut anterior and posterior walls, acoustic enhancement and, frequently, lateral refraction artifact in common with any other cyst. Occasionally, the cyst may be somewhat angular if it is large and

compressed by adjacent structures; similarly, cysts may sometimes have an irregular, somewhat crenated margin, perhaps due to cyst rupture and reduction in size. Simple cysts may achieve a very large size (10 cm is not uncommon and some may reach 20 cm in diameter).

They have low intracystic pressures and are rarely symptomatic. Symptoms are usually caused either by space-occupation effects of larger cysts or as a result of complications such as intracystic hemorrhage.

Although reported to occur in as many as 6% of all renal cysts, intracystic hemorrhage is likely to be markedly less

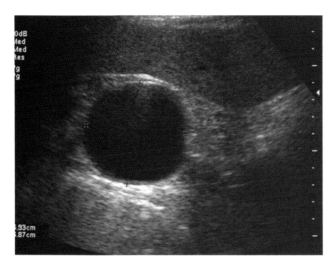

Figure 1.86
Large cyst at the upper pole of the kidney. Clear separation from the hepatic capsule is demonstrated, although on this image it would be difficult to differentiate from adrenal cyst.

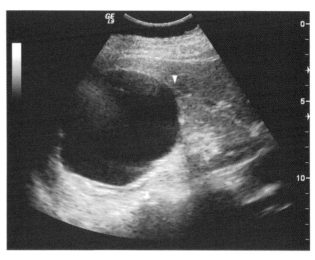

Figure 1.87
Large cyst at the upper pole of the right kidney. There is a 'claw sign' (arrowheads).

common than this considering the very high incidence of simple renal cysts that are now detected with cross-sectional imaging techniques. Where hemorrhage occurs, there may be a change in the reflectivity of the contents of the cyst, occasionally with layering debris (Figure 1.88): the cyst may become thick-walled and occasionally wall calcification ensues (Figure 1.89). Some renal cysts are remarkably exophytic in location. In this situation, there is little or no distortion of the renal outline and localization of the cyst to a renal origin depends upon careful evaluation of the kidney and cyst during quiet and occasionally deep respiration. Usually the cyst can be correctly located by the observation of movement of the cyst in concert with the rest of the kidney rather than with an adjacent structure such as the liver.

Infection of a simple renal cyst is uncommon. It may result from vesicoureteric reflux or hematogenous spread, or from iatrogenic infection either caused by cyst puncture or following surgery. An infected cyst is commonly indistinguishable from a simple cyst. There may be increased reflectivity of the cyst contents and loss of sharp margination of the cyst wall, and in this situation they are indistinguishable from abscesses from primary hematogenous renal infection.

Although many cysts are unilocular, cysts may be divided by septa, producing bilocular or occasionally multilocular septated cysts. These, when uncomplicated, demonstrate exactly the same features as unilocular cysts. The septa are fine, and highly reflective when imaged at right angles without alteration in the echo content of the cyst (Figures 1.90 and 1.91).

Simple cysts are not a premalignant condition, cystic tumors developing de novo rather than from pre-existing

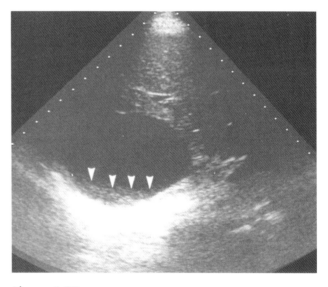

Figure 1.88
Complicated renal cyst. There is layering debris (arrowheads) in the most dependent portion of the cyst as a result of intracystic hemorrhage.

cysts. However, the differentiation of a simple cyst from a cystic malignancy is important. As a general rule, a cystic tumor will demonstrate a thicker wall, sometimes with a mural neoplastic nodule and irregularity of the wall margins (Figure 1.92). Occasionally, however, it is extremely difficult to differentiate the two conditions, particularly when the cyst is complicated either by partial cyst rupture, hemorrhage or infection. In these situations,

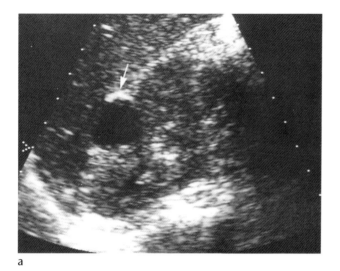

a

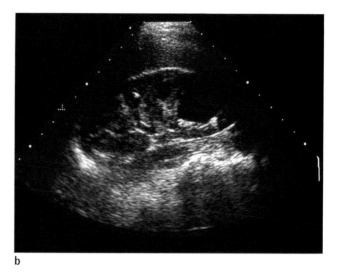

b

Figure 1.89
(a) Typical curvilinear calcification (arrow) in a cyst at the upper pole of the right kidney. (b) Irregular nodular margins of a cyst at the lower pole of the kidney suggestive of early calcification.

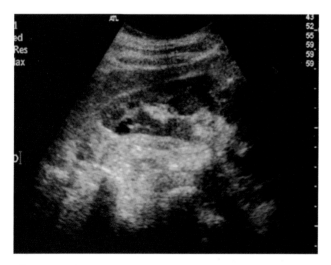

Figure 1.90
Small, but partly septated, cyst at the upper pole of the kidney.

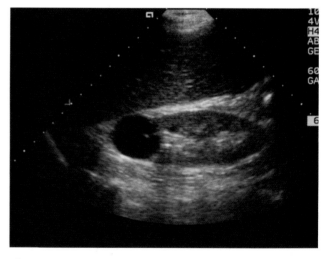

Figure 1.91
Ill-defined septum or mural irregularity of a cyst at the upper pole of the right kidney.

diagnostic cyst aspiration under ultrasound control usually allows an accurate cytologic diagnosis to be made.

Cysts of the renal sinus

These are otherwise known as parapelvic cysts (see Figure 1.66). Although as a general rule these are also echo-free, exhibiting distal acoustic enhancement, there are frequently unusual and atypical features. Parapelvic cysts are rarely purely spherical, their margins usually being shaped by the margins of the renal sinus. They can, therefore, closely mimic a hydronephrosis and particularly a PUJ obstruction. Similarly, because of their location in a highly reflective renal sinus, reverberation and beam width artifact are common, with the result that parapelvic cysts will often not appear purely echo-free, and acoustic enhancement is frequently difficult to demonstrate. It is possible to use a hydration test to attempt to resolve the differentiation between parapelvic cyst and hydronephrosis.

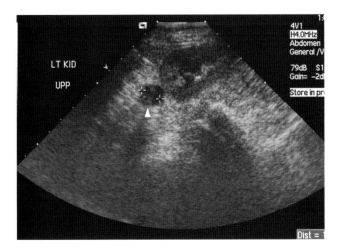

Figure 1.92
Cystic renal tumor. Exophytic mass immediately adjacent to the upper pole of the left kidney. There are echoes within the mass (arrowheads) and there is some sound attenuation.

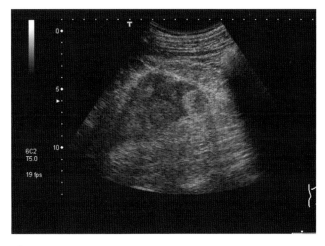

Figure 1.93
Tuberose sclerosis. The kidney contains multiple solid masses of varying echogenicity consistent with angiomyolipomata and adenomata.

Administering 1.5 liters of water orally will almost invariably yield a measurable alteration in the size of the dilated calyces but will not affect the appearance of parapelvic cysts. Sensitivity and specificity is reported to be in excess of 92% using this methodology. However, in situations where there remains doubt, it may be necessary to perform other investigations such as intravenous urography or CT.

Conditions predisposing to renal cyst and renal tumor formation

There are a number of conditions which predispose to renal cyst but also to renal tumor formation.

Von Hippel–Lindau disease

Von Hippel–Lindau disease is the association of retinal hemangiomas, cerebral hemangiomas and cysts of the kidney, pancreas, liver and epididymis. Renal cysts are usually multiple, varying between 5 and 30 mm in size, and rarely becoming large. There is a 35% incidence of renal carcinoma, which is bilateral in three-quarters of cases. The condition is also associated with pheochromocytomas.

Tuberose sclerosis

This is a neurocutaneous inherited condition in which sclerotic glial masses in the brain are associated with mental retardation, adenoma sebaceum and hamartomas

in various organs. In the kidneys, cysts or angiomyolipomata may occur either together or separately (Figure 1.93).

Ultrasound may be used as a procedure to screen first-order relatives of patients with either of these two conditions and also to monitor the kidneys for signs of development of solid lesions.

Acquired cystic disease of the kidney

The advent of cross-sectional imaging techniques has demonstrated that the end-stage kidney in patients who are being treated either by dialysis or with a renal transplant is the site of significant proliferative and occasionally endocrinologic activity. Acquired cystic disease of the kidney (ACDK) is extremely common, occurring in over 50% of long-term dialysis patients after 3–4 years of treatment. The etiology of the development of ACDK is unclear, but its importance relates to the occurrence of symptomatology and to the development of renal tumors in some cases.

The characteristic appearances of ACDK are usually of a few small cysts in a small echogenic kidney. The cysts range from 5 mm to 3 cm in size and in some cases there may be multiple cysts throughout the renal substance (Figures 1.94 and 1.95). In these cases, where the cysts enlarge the kidney, there may be difficulty in differentiating the condition from polycystic renal disease.

The demonstration of ACDK by ultrasound might prompt a program of regular imaging review. However, it is frequently difficult with ultrasound to differentiate between

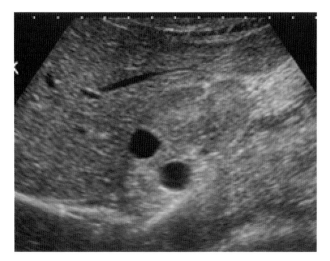

Figure 1.94
Early acquired cystic disease of the kidney. The kidney is small and echogenic and contains two cysts at the upper pole.

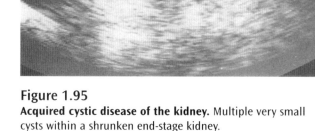

Figure 1.95
Acquired cystic disease of the kidney. Multiple very small cysts within a shrunken end-stage kidney.

hemorrhagic and infective complications of ACDK and the development of a malignant tumor of the kidney, which occurs in between 4 and 5% of cases. CT and MRI appear to be more reliable in the early detection of the development of solid tumors but it is difficult to justify regular screening CT in all patients on hemodialysis following renal transplantation and therefore CT is normally reserved for either those patients who present with symptoms or where the ultrasound findings are suspicious.

Complex cystic masses of the kidney

The presence of a cyst within the kidney containing two or more locules with irregular margins to the locules, although frequently with a well-defined capsule or pseudo-capsule, presents a wide differential diagnosis. Certain conditions such as cystic Wilms' tumor, mesoblastic nephroma, clear cell sarcoma of the kidney occur only in childhood and are therefore not considered here. For the most part, ultrasound alone is inadequate for the differen-tiation of pathologies presenting with a multilocular cystic mass and it must be used in conjunction with other imag-ing modalities, the history, cyst puncture cytology and, where necessary, needle biopsy. Occasionally, however, there are features which, while not necessarily allowing a specific diagnosis to be made, afford a more ordered differ-ential diagnostic list. Clearly, the presence of intravascular extension or distant metastasis will identify a malignant tumor, but equally the presence of areas of solid tissue within the mass are strongly in favor of a hypernephroma.

Increasingly, the role of contrast is becoming established in this situation. Late studies may demonstrate increased perfusion, or blush in hypervascular, malignant lesions or poor perfusion in hypovascular tumors, although, as yet, there are insufficient data to confirm the distinction from inflammatory processes.

The Bosniak classification of cystic renal masses

In 1986 Bosniak suggested that while radiologic features may not be specific for a particular diagnosis, management decisions could be made based on certain features. These categories are as follows:

- Category 1: the classic benign simple cyst.
- Category 2: minimally complicated cysts, including septated cysts, minimally calcified cysts and high-density cysts on CT. These require follow-up imaging at intervals rather than surgical intervention unless change is observed (Figures 1.96 and 1.97).
- Category 3: more complicated cystic lesions, including thick irregular calcification, a multiloculated mass with presence of nodularity and uniform thickening of the wall. These masses, while they have a potential for malignancy, can often be treated with conservative surgery sparing the adjacent normal renal tissue (Figures 1.98 and 1.99).
- Category 4: represents a cyst where there is prominent nodularity, large areas of solid tissue and an irregular thickened wall. Lesions of this nature have a high malignant potential and planned treatment should be for radical nephrectomy.

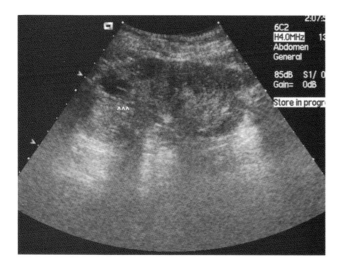

Figure 1.96
Complicated cyst with septa and margin irregularity (arrowheads).

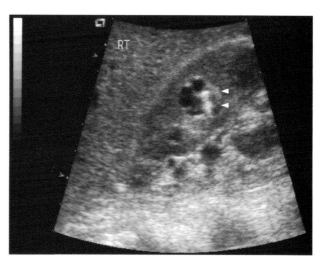

Figure 1.98
Mural nodularity and calcification together with septa (arrowheads) in a cyst at the upper pole of the kidney.

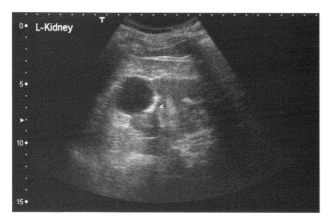

Figure 1.97
Cyst demonstrating mural calcification.

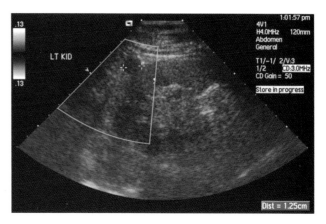

Figure 1.99
Exophytic mass with mural calcification and irregular echogenic content.

These two latter categories are best demonstrated by a combination of ultrasound and CT, since the absence of enhancement is a useful feature for differentiation of benign from malignant. There is some evidence that similar patterns of blood flow may be demonstrable using ultrasound contrast.

Benign multilocular cystic nephroma

This is a rare lesion with two peaks of incidence, one in childhood and one in middle age. It is a benign tumor without apparent malignant potential. Ultrasound features are those of multiple cystic masses separated by highly echogenic septa corresponding to masses of intervening fibrous tissue. The echogenic component may vary, but occasionally may produce a solid appearance to the mass that then makes it difficult to differentiate from Bosniak type 3. Cyst aspiration will yield clear fluid with negative cytology and instillation of contrast will show no communication with adjacent cysts (Figure 1.100).

Localized cystic disease of the kidney

This is a condition where multiple simple cysts involve only one portion of one kidney, producing an ill-defined

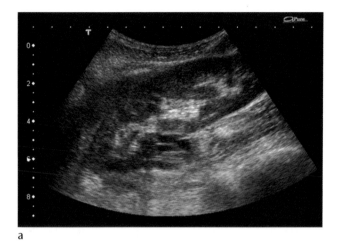

a

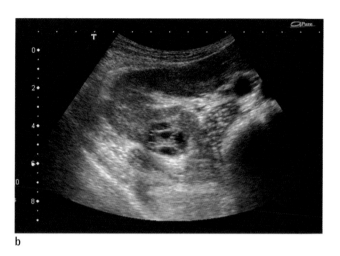

b

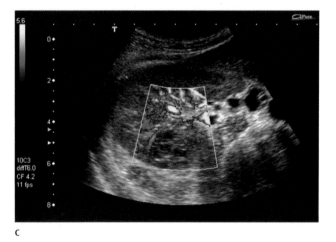

c

Figure 1.100
(a–c) Multilocular cystic nephroma. Several small cystic locules are separated by thick septa.

multiloculated mass without clear demarcation from the normal kidney and without a demonstrable capsule. There are no ultrasound features that will allow the differentiation of this lesion from more sinister pathology (Figure 1.101).

Hydatid disease

Hydatid disease of the kidney is uncommon in Western practice, being most prevalent in Africa, Mediterranean countries and the Middle East. The appearances are variable, including simple and complex cysts as well as solid masses. A detailed discussion is given elsewhere in this chapter.

Xanthogranulomatous pyelonephritis

This chronic infection is a granulomatous condition where the kidney becomes infiltrated with multiple lipid-containing macrophages. This condition is discussed elsewhere in the chapter.

Malakoplakia

One form of unusual infection may not produce all the features of a renal abscess. Malakoplakia is a granulomatous condition associated with *Escherichia coli* infection of the urinary tract. The condition most commonly affects the urothelial part of the urinary tract (renal pelvis and ureter), but may occasionally involve the renal parenchyma, when it commonly presents as a multilocular cystic mass. Malakoplakia usually occurs in immunocompromised patients, and where a multilocular cystic mass is associated with abnormality of the ureter or bladder the diagnosis should be suspected.

Other causes

Other causes of a multilocular mass include renal parenchymal abscess and an organizing hematoma. Usually in these cases the history, clinical signs and physical examination facilitate accurate diagnosis.

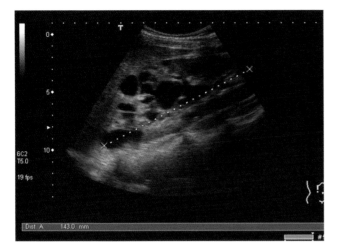

Figure 1.101
Localized cystic disease of the kidney. A pattern similar to polycystic renal disease is demonstrated within the upper pole, although the lower pole appears normal.

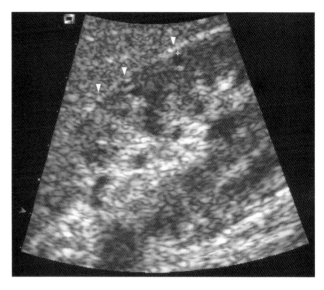

Figure 1.102
Early polycystic renal disease. Multiple tiny cysts are demonstrated just beneath the cortex (arrowheads).

Polycystic renal disease

Multiple renal cysts can be demonstrated in a variety of conditions. These include multiple renal cysts, cysts associated with inherited disorders such as tuberose sclerosis and multicystic dysplastic kidney (MCDK) disease. MCDK is diagnosed almost exclusively antenatally in the UK because of the use of routine prenatal ultrasound and will be considered elsewhere in this book. Other 'cystic pathologies' such as medullary sponge kidney are more appropriately considered in the section on diffuse parenchymal renal disease.

Adult or autosomal dominant polycystic kidney disease

ADPKD is thought to be carried in 1 in 1000 newborns. With 100% penetrance, it has been postulated that all carriers will develop the phenotype if they live long enough. Expression of the condition is, however, extremely variable. Some subjects maintain normal renal function into old age, although the majority develop varying degrees of renal insufficiency by the middle years. Clinical features include loin pain, hypertension, urinary tract infections, calculi and hematuria. Physical examination will frequently reveal bilaterally enlarged kidneys.

The characteristic appearance of ADPKD is of multiple cysts of varying size, in enlarged kidneys with or without cysts in other organs, including the liver, spleen, pancreas and seminal vesicles. The cysts are randomly distributed throughout the kidney and in advanced stages of the

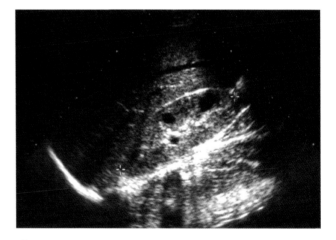

Figure 1.103
Multiple cysts within the kidney. Differentiation between multiple cysts and ADPKD depends upon age and clinical history.

disease no normal renal parenchyma can be identified (Figures 1.102–1.105).

Demonstration of the extent of involvement can be difficult. The effect of cysts of varying size with the attendant acoustic enhancement requires significant modification of machine settings in order to optimize the image. The sonographic characteristics of a cyst may be lost as enhancement from one cyst exaggerates the reverberation in the anterior wall of a posteriorly located cyst. Renal size may be

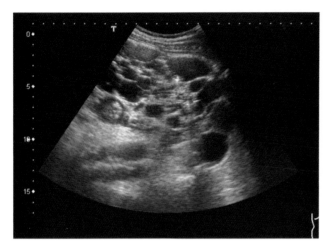

Figure 1.104
Multiple cysts of varying size, almost completely replacing renal parenchyma.

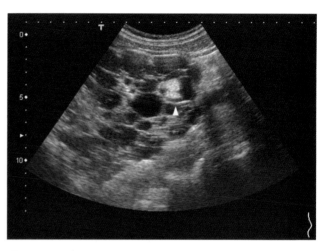

Figure 1.105
Haemorrhage into one of the cysts at the lower pole (arrowheads). It is difficult to differentiate this from the appearance of tumor within one of the cystic elements.

difficult to evaluate. Real-time probes will rarely afford the field of view adequate to demonstrate the entire kidney with a single scan plane. It is often therefore necessary to use the panoramic or extended field of view feature available on some machines to assess renal size.

Current high-resolution equipment will allow the demonstration of small cysts early in the evolution of the disease. Cysts have been reported in the neonate, although it is possible that cysts at this stage may regress. The earliest feature of ADPKD is the demonstration of tiny bright foci within the renal parenchyma (Figure 1.102). These probably correspond to the walls of a tiny cyst with associated acoustic enhancement. Subsequently, the cysts enlarge and exhibit more typical appearances. As the disease progresses, the kidney increases in size. Increase in size is more marked and more rapid in men, and the disease progression is more severe with greater incidence of renal dysfunction and severe hypertension. There is a direct correlation between renal volume and deteriorating renal function.

Screening for ADPKD in patients with a family history is a complex issue. Consideration should be given to the emotional, social, economic and family sequelae as well as the negative predictive value of ultrasound. Although features of ADPKD may be detected in childhood, some patients may not exhibit detectable cysts until the third decade. While this is probably useful from the perspective of prognosis (such individuals are more likely to experience a benign disease course), nonetheless, exclusion of the diagnosis cannot be reliably made until this age. We therefore counsel that patients should not be screened earlier than the third decade.

Severity of disease is correlated with the age of appearance of cysts and the size and growth of the kidneys. Appearance of cysts in adolescents may be associated with liver fibrosis, with an associated poor prognosis. The features will then include increased parenchymal echogenicity of the liver, loss of clarity of the portal tracts and coarsening of the echo pattern.

Diagnosis of ADPKD in the third decade depends upon the demonstration of two or more cysts in either kidney in the presence of a family history. Simple renal cysts, although rare in this age group, do occur. Consequently, the demonstration of a single cyst must be viewed with caution in a patient with a family history, and a follow-up examination performed. For patients in the 30–50 age group, the diagnosis is dependent upon the demonstration of two or more cysts in both kidneys. In the absence of a family history, the demonstration of two or more cysts is more difficult to manage. Gene mutations account for a significant minority of ADPKD and it is therefore difficult to discount the possibility of ADPKD arising de novo.

Doppler ultrasound has found little application in the evaluation of ADPKD. Although resistance and pulsatility indices are correlated with creatinine clearance, evaluation of the interlobar arteries is technically difficult and there has been no report of a predictive value of Doppler comparable to the morphologic features that have been described.

Similarly, however, the renal pelvis is frequently indistinguishable, and thus the diagnosis of coexisting obstruction requires the use of an intravenous urogram. Retrograde pyelography is necessary if the serum creatinine is high, since antegrade pyelography is rendered impossible by the presence of multiple cysts.

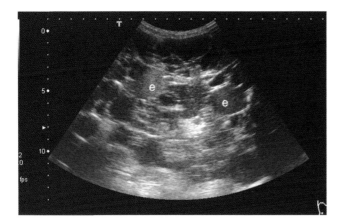

Figure 1.106
There are echoes within several of the cysts (e). It is likely that this is due to hemorrhage.

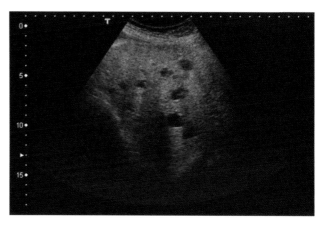

Figure 1.107
Multiple cysts are demonstrated in the liver in autosomal dominant polycystic disease of the liver.

Complications of polycystic renal disease

Symptoms from ADPKD are variable. Patients may experience discomfort consequent upon mass effect. This may be attributable to a large cyst and, in this case, percutaneous aspiration may be of value in symptom control although the cyst will often reaccumulate. The use of alcohol injection may afford the ablation of a particularly troublesome cyst, but this has received little attention in the management of cysts in the context of ADPKD. Acute pain may be the result of infection or hemorrhage within one of the cysts or consequent upon renal calculus disease. Pain is presumably caused by increased intracystic pressure, and percutaneous aspiration is reported to provide rapid symptomatic relief. However, signs suggestive of complication, such as echogenic content, fluid level, etc., are only infrequently reported (Figures 1.105 and 1.106). This is in part due to the subtle changes that the presence of blood or pus produce, but is also due to the difficulties in detecting these changes in the presence of the complex acoustic enhancement and bright reflections from the multiple intrarenal cysts. It is difficult to produce a 'good picture' of a polycystic kidney and yet more difficult to detect cyst complications. CT may allow the demonstration of increased attenuation of the cyst content and MRI will afford the identification of blood products. The demonstration of a complicating renal carcinoma requires the use of a multimodality approach. Although solid elements may be demonstrated by any of the imaging modalities, a combination of contrast-enhanced CT and gadolinium-enhanced MRI probably offers the greatest accuracy of detection.

Autosomal recessive polycystic kidney disease

This presents either antenatally or in childhood, with enlarged bright kidneys and usually, but not invariably, early significant renal impairment. This is considered elsewhere in this volume.

Polycystic disease of the liver

Polycystic disease of the liver (PCL) is a rare autosomal dominant condition. The multiple hepatic cysts derive from gradual dilatation of persisting intralobular bile ducts which fail to involute in the later embryologic development of the liver (Figure 1.107). Females are affected twice as commonly as males. Only 15% of cases are symptomatic, usually presenting as a result of mass effects, although hepatic dysfunction may occur. Fifty percent of cases occur in association with ADPKD, but the conditions are thought to be separate entities, the hepatic cysts occurring in classical ADPKD being of a different etiology and gene locus from those in PCL. Clearly, however, differentiation between the two conditions on the basis of imaging criteria is often difficult.

Renal tumor

Although renal tumors can be described as benign and malignant, truly benign tumors are rare and, whenever a

Table 1.4 *Classification of renal tumors*	
Simple cyst	*Complex cyst*
Single/multiple	Cystic nephroma:
Parapelvic	Carcinoma
Calyceal	Hemorrhagic
	Metastasis
Others – solid	Wilms' tumor
Renal cell carcinoma	Infected including TB:
Metastasis	Aneurysm
Lymphoma	AVM
Lobar nephronia	Abscess
Abscess	Xanthogranulomatous
TB	pyelonephritis
Xanthogranulomatous	Hematoma
pyelonephritis	TB
Pheochromocytoma	
Wilms' tumor	*Masses containing fat*
Oncocytoma	Angiomyolipoma
Fibroma	Lipoma and liposarcoma
Adenocarcinoma	Hibernoma
Granuloma	
Reninoma	
Leiomyoma and sarcoma	
Hematoma	
TCC	
Carcinoid	
Nephroblastomatosis	
Column of Bertin	

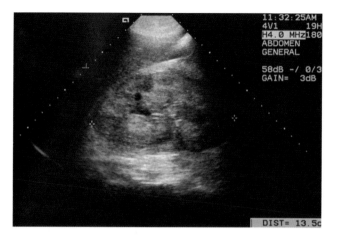

Figure 1.108
Multiple renal adenomata. Multiple masses are noted throughout the renal parenchyma.

renal mass is identified on ultrasound, caution needs to be exercised before identifying the lesion as potentially benign.

Classification may be based on tissue type, but for the purposes of imaging, a system which addresses imaging features is probably more appropriate (Table 1.4).

The kidney thus may be the seat of a number of different masses, including tumors, infection and pseudotumor. Different types of renal mass cannot be differentiated on ultrasound. The diagnosis will depend on clinical features and prevalence as well as on the demonstration of typical imaging signs.

Renal adenoma

Renal adenoma is described as a benign lesion, but more recent work has suggested that all renal adenomas have malignant potential. Adenomas are associated with the inherited abnormality Von Hippel–Lindau disease. The masses can be of varying size, but are usually solid and of similar echogenicity to normal renal parenchyma (Figure 1.108).

Metanephric adenoma

In this benign, but extremely rare, condition, tumors are said to be large and solid in appearance. There are no particular features that allow differentiation from renal cell carcinoma or other, more significant, pathologies.

Oncocytoma

Oncocytoma is a typically benign tumor of the kidney, which again is rare. Generally of small size and often echo poor, these tumors are reported to have a central scar with a spoke wheel pattern, although even this feature appears to be unreliable for differentiation from other more significant masses (Figures 1.109 and 1.110).

Angiomyolipoma

These benign renal harmartomata contain variable amounts of fat and muscle elements: 20% are discovered in patients with tuberose sclerosis. Although frequently asymptomatic and discovered incidentally or during screening of patients with tuberose sclerosis, they may present with spontaneous, massive, retroperitoneal hemorrhage known as Wunderlich's syndrome. The tumors may increase in size and occasionally extend into the perirenal tissues and into the renal vein.

The fat–muscle interface is recognized on ultrasound by a highly reflective mass with variable attenuation of the

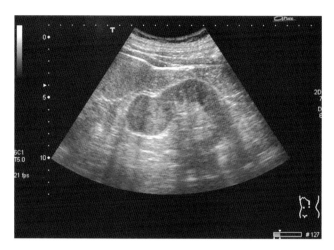

Figure 1.109
Solid oncocytoma arising eccentrically from the upper pole of the right kidney.

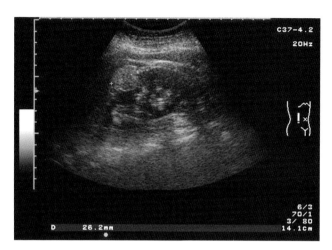

Figure 1.111
Echogenic mass situated peripherally in the kidney typical of an angiomyolipoma.

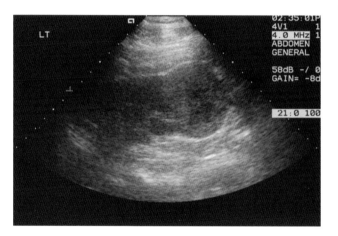

Figure 1.110
Oncocytoma demonstrating an ill-defined central scar.

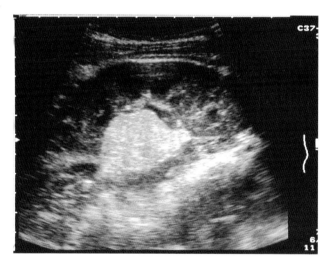

Figure 1.112
Centrally placed angiomyolipoma demonstrating typical increased reflectivity.

sound beam. This increase in reflectivity may make it difficult to differentiate the margins where the tumor abuts either the renal sinus or the perirenal fat (Figure 1.111).

Although the demonstration of a highly reflective and homogeneous mass may represent typical findings for an angiomyolipoma (Figure 1.112), occasionally there is significant heterogeneity. Similarly, a renal cell carcinoma can present with a highly reflective renal mass. Consequently, it is necessary to undertake renal CT in all patients presenting with masses of this nature. The demonstration of fat content is taken to represent evidence of a benign angiomyolipomatous lesion. The nature of local invasion by angiomyolipoma which occurs in large lesions is usually that of extension into the renal vein with associated venous thrombosis. However, extension into local lymph node with fatty content within the nodes can also be demonstrated. This represents a specific management problem, particularly given that these mimic the invasion pattern of renal cell carcinomata.

The demonstration of fat within the tumor, although identifying this as a hemangioma, will not predict the risk of complication such as retroperitoneal hemorrhage.

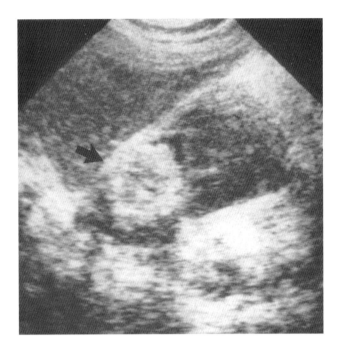

Figure 1.113
Focal postoperative fat replacement mimics a mass.
Reprinted by permission of Dr N Papanicalou, Massachusetts
General Hospital, Boston, MA, and of the American Roentgen
Ray Society.

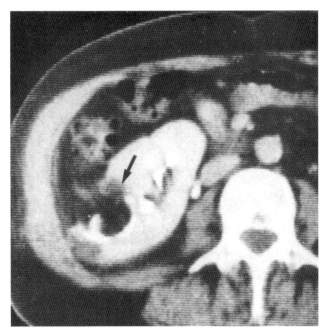

Figure 1.114
Focal postoperative fat replacement mimics a mass.
Reprinted by permission of Dr N Papanicalou, Massachusetts
General Hospital, Boston, MA, and of the American Roentgen
Ray Society.

Therefore, the use of surgical management must depend not
only on imaging criteria demonstrating apparently locally
aggressive angiomyolipoma but also on clinical features.

Differential diagnosis of subcentimeter, echogenic, renal cortical nodules

Frequently small, less than 1 cm, echogenic masses can be
demonstrated within the renal substance when an ultrasound examination is being performed for another indication. The differential diagnosis includes junctional
parenchymal defect, angiomyolipoma and postoperative
intraparenchymal fat after local cortical resection. The first
of these is associated with other features of persistent fetal
lobation (see above), whereas in intrarenal fat the history is
critical (Figures 1.113 and 1.114).

Where it is possible to exclude other diagnoses, these are
presumed to be angiomyolipomata. The management of
such lesions remains a dilemma (Figure 1.115). They are
usually too small for tissue resolution on CT. Annual
review with ultrasound appears to represent the most
appropriate policy. However, angiomyolipomata are
known to increase in size and, therefore, if such increase

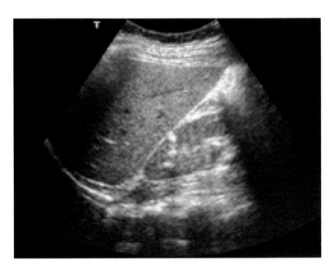

Figure 1.115
**Tiny peripheral echogenic lesion within the kidney
presumed to be an angiomyolipoma.** The lesion produces
some sound attenuation.

occurs, CT is used again to confirm the presence of fat
within the lesion.

There remains, however, considerable overlap for the
sonographic spectrum of renal cell carcinoma and angiomyolipoma. Renal cell carcinoma may be hyperechoic in up to

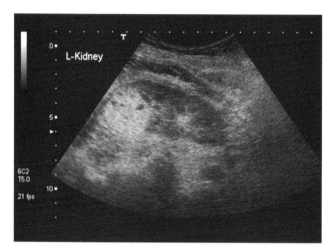

Figure 1.116
Echogenic lesion within the kidney, but which contains cystic elements suggestive of a renal cell carcinoma.

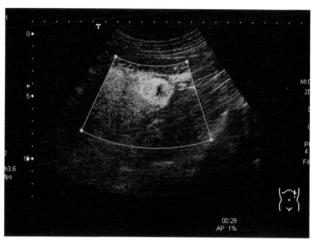

Figure 1.118
Contrast enhancement within an angiomyolipoma demonstrating late enhancement of the margin of the tumor consistent with hypervascularity.

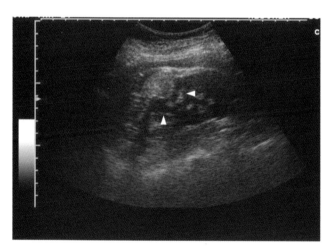

Figure 1.117
Echogenic lesion within the kidney demonstrating echo-poor rim (arrowheads).

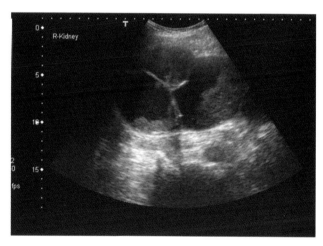

Figure 1.119
Multilocular cystic lesion of the kidney demonstrating septa and mural thickening. Differentiation of benign from malignant disease is difficult, but this must be considered a Bosniak category 3. This was an adult Wilms' tumor.

8% of cases, although they are usually larger and demonstrate some inhomogeneity or tiny cysts (Figure 1.116). Acoustic shadowing is seen in angiomyolipomata, but not renal cell carcinomas, although this is usually associated with lesions larger that 1.5 cm.[7,8] Finally, the demonstration of an anechoic rim to the tumor is strongly suggestive of an angiomyolipoma (Figure 1.117). Color flow Doppler is usually of little value in the assessment of angiomyolipoma but it may be that enhancement with microbubble contrast will allow increased confidence of diagnosis.

Angiomyolipoma is a hypervascular lesion and some studies suggest intense late enhancement (Figure 1.118).

Multilocular cystic lesions of the kidney

These lesions include benign, multilocular cystic nephroma, complicated renal cyst (hemorrhage, infection, etc.), atypical renal cell carcinoma and cystic Wilms' tumor. These lesions would be classified as category 3 in Bosniak's classification. Differentiation between benign and malignant tumors is difficult (Figure 1.119). Criteria that have been recommended include the demonstration of solid elements within the lesion, septal thickening and calcification. However, there appears to be no consistent relationship of any of these findings with benign or malignant lesions. Color flow Doppler has been used both to identify flow within solid elements and within the septa, and particularly when the spectral pattern exhibits intrarenal maximum velocities of 60 cm/s or greater, implies evidence of malignancy.[9]

Although the prevalence of cystic renal cell carcinoma is low, nonetheless, it is important to use an imaging algorithm that may help to determine management in these patients, particularly if there is a contraindication to surgery and if the features described above are present these should be used as an indication for further imaging.

Leiomyoma

This rare tumor of the kidney usually derives either from the capsule or from the renal sinus. The appearances are extremely variable, from cystic through solid.

Renal hemangioma

This uncommon benign tumor usually presents with gross hematuria. These tumors are mainly located at the pelvicalyceal junction or in the inner medulla, and are of varying echogenicity. There are, however, no specific signs that allow their differentiation, although on CT they demonstrate scant enhancement.

Renal cell carcinoma

Renal cell carcinoma is the third most common genitourinary neoplasm, representing approximately 3% of all adult malignancy. The incidence of renal cell carcinoma has been increasing at a rate of 3%/year since 1970. Although this is largely consequent upon the greater frequency of incidental discovery related to a greater use of cross-sectional imaging modalities, nonetheless there has probably also been a true increase in incidence of the tumor.

There are a number of different cell types which constitute renal cell carcinoma. The conventional cell type represents between 70 and 80% of all tumors, while tubulo-papillary 10–15%, chromophobic 4–5% represent the majority of the remainder. The very rare collecting duct and medullary carcinomas represent less than 1% of all renal carcinomas and have an extremely poor prognosis.

The classical triad of flank pain, hematuria and a palpable renal mass now represent the presenting signs in only a minority of patients. Indeed, they have been recently described as the 'too late' triad, in that they represent late findings of a renal cell carcinoma. The renal mass may not be initially recognized as such, the patient presenting with apparent hepato- or splenomegaly. Similarly, late findings are features suggestive of renal vein or inferior vena caval extension. Most tumors with direct symptoms exhibit tumor sizes of greater than 5 cm at the time of presentation.

The majority of patients, however, now present with paraneoplastic features. These include an elevated ESR (erythrocyte sedimentation rate), hypertension, anemia, weight loss and pyrexia. An unexplained elevation of the liver function test may be the presenting finding in up to 14% of cases in the absence of liver involvement either by direct extension or metastatic disease. The patients may also present with symptoms of hypercalcemia, polycythemia as well as a paraneoplastic neuromyopathy. Identification of such symptoms as potentially attributable to a renal cell carcinoma will allow the earlier diagnosis of the tumor; 75% of these patients will have tumors less than 5 cm in diameter and also a third less than 3 cm.

Renal carcinoma is staged either as a surgical staging or according to the TNM criteria. However, the most important two staging criteria are of a tumor size of less than 7 cm and a tumor contained within the renal capsule. For these tumors, a 70–90% 5-year survival would be expected.

Ultrasound features of renal tumors

The appearances of renal cell carcinomata are widely variable. The multilocular cystic renal cell carcinoma has already been described, although this is a rare manifestation of renal cell carcinoma, accounting for approximately 3% of all renal carcinomas. Echogenicity is predominantly related to the frequency of sonographic interfaces presented to the ultrasound beam. Thus, fat–muscle interfaces, vascularity and the presence or absence of necrosis will all contribute to the echogenicity of the tumor.

Tumors are variously described as hypoechoic, isoechoic or hyperechoic, compared with normal renal cortex, and this variable pattern is consistent across the major cell types (Figures 1.120–1.124).

Some degree of characterization of renal tumors, particularly when differentiating these from angiomyolipomas, is possible. This has already been alluded to above. The increased echogenicity and acoustic shadowing that occurs in large angiomyolipomas can be characterized using

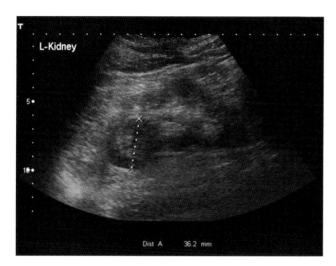

Figure 1.120
Solid lesion within the upper pole of the left kidney. The echo pattern is mixed, with a central area of increased reflectivity, perhaps reflecting necrosis.

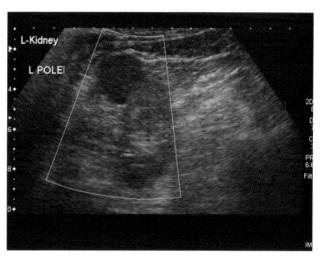

Figure 1.122
Echo-poor lesion distorting the margin of the kidney and extending into the medulla and renal sinus.

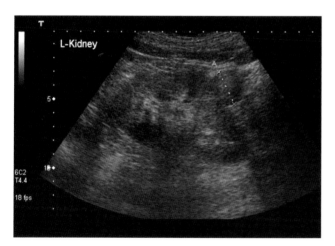

Figure 1.121
Small peripheral lesion with an echogenicity similar to that of the renal parenchyma.

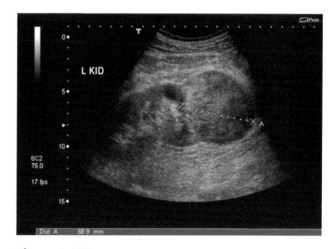

Figure 1.123
Large echogenic mass at the lower pole of the kidney with significant heterogeneity. There is an adjacent renal cyst.

frequency-dependent attenuation values. In most cases, frequency-dependent attenuation is significantly higher in angiomyolipomata. This affords the opportunity to differentiate even highly reflective renal cell carcinomas from angiomyolipomata.[10]

Angiomyolipomas tend to be more homogeneous. The presence of an anechoic rim or intratumoral cyst is strongly suggestive of a renal cell carcinoma, although oncocytomata may mimic these appearances (Figure 1.125).

On color flow Doppler, renal cell carcinomas typically have a peripheral vascular pattern or a mixed peripheral and penetrating pattern of blood flow. Angiomyolipomata and oncocytoma may demonstrate a similar pattern but a characteristic focal intratumoral 'spotty' flow or a single feeding vessel may be diagnostic in a small number of cases of angiomyolipoma.[11] Classic neovascular Doppler signals at the margins of renal tumors are of high velocity, measuring 3 kHz or more, and low impedance (low RI values of less than 0.6). Using these criteria, some workers indicated

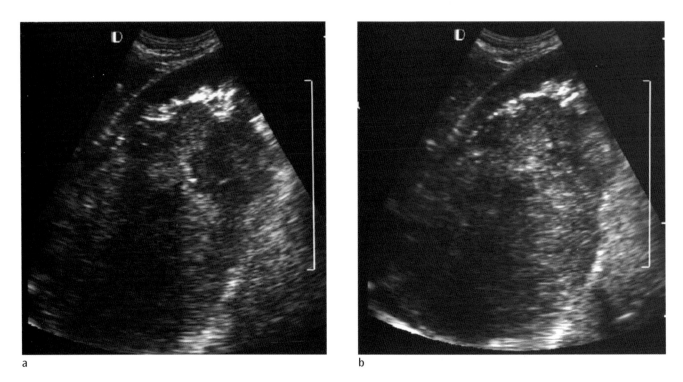

a   b

Figure 1.124
(a) Large heterogeneous mass destroying the upper pole of the kidney and invading adjacent structures. (b) Disruption of the renal sinus and the invasion of the posterior abdominal wall are noted.

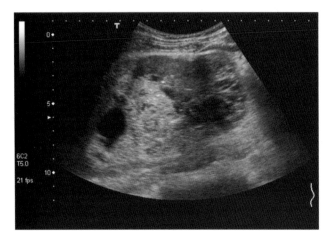

Figure 1.125
Heterogeneous mass within the kidney with both cystic and solid elements.

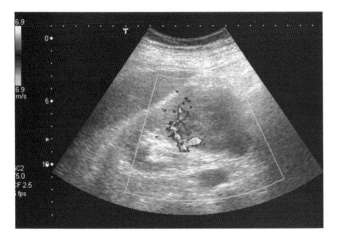

Figure 1.126
Renal cell carcinoma demonstrating irregular, large marginal vessels with a disordered blood flow pattern.

a sensitivity for the detection of neovascularity in malignant tumors of varying different organs as high as 94%, although in most studies suggesting such high accuracy patient mix did not include large numbers of patients with benign but neoplastic processes. Doppler ultrasound is therefore a useful tool in the evaluation of solid tumors of the kidney but the data derived from the Doppler signal must be interpreted with care (Figures 1.126–1.130).

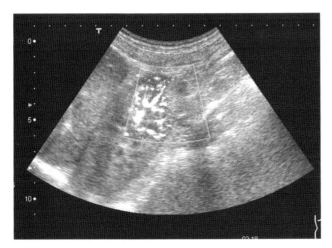

Figure 1.127
Irregular pattern of flow throughout a mass at the lower pole of the left kidney. There appears to be pooling of flow in a number of foci within the renal mass.

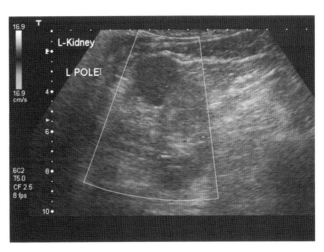

Figure 1.129
Mass, approximately 3 cm in diameter, but with no evidence of flow (black and white image). There is flow in the adjacent normal kidney.

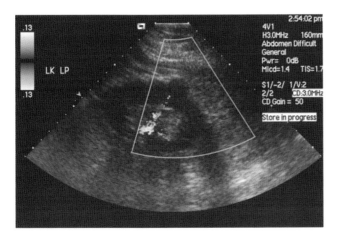

Figure 1.128
Small, marginal mass at the lower pole of the left kidney, but without evidence of flow on color power Doppler.

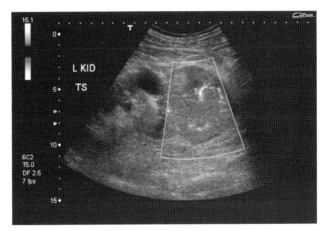

Figure 1.130
Irregular, almost serpiginous flow in a mass at the lower pole of the kidney.

The role of ultrasound contrast

There remains limited experience on the value of contrast enhancement of renal cell carcinoma. Although most solid renal cell carcinomata will demonstrate some enhancement, there is significant variability. It is important to observe the pattern of enhancement through arterial, parenchymal and late phases if the method is to contribute to diagnosis. Although it may have only a limited role in differentiation from angiomyolipoma, there is value in problem solving when differentiation of tumor from pseudotumor is difficult (Figures 1.131 and 1.132). Both cystic renal cell carcinoma and complex inflammatory cyst reveal intense contrast enhancement on a peripheral thick wall which decreases in the delayed phase,[12] whereas other authors have found no significant difference in diagnostic accuracy when compared to power Doppler.[13]

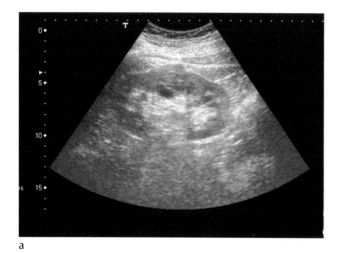

a

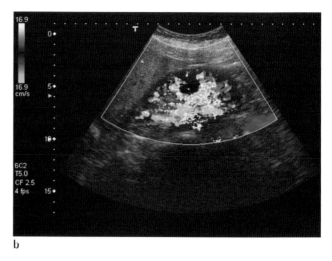

b

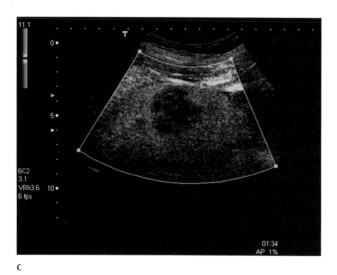

c

Figure 1.131
(a) An irregular, partially cystic lesion is demonstrated in the equatorial region of the kidney. (b) On color flow Doppler this is demonstrated to be poorly perfused. (c) This is confirmed on contrast-enhanced studies.

Staging of renal cell carcinoma

Staging of renal carcinoma can be broadly divided into four stages:

- stage 1 – within the capsule
- stage 2 – extension into the perinephric fat
- stage 3 – extension into lymph nodes and/or the renal vein
- stage 4 – extension into the adjacent organs with distant metastases.

Although a critical predictor of survival is tumor size at presentation, surgery represents the major therapeutic option capable of influencing survival following diagnosis. It is, therefore, important to assess local tumor extent, tumor size, lymph node metastases and caval invasion. The reported rates of invasion range from 8 to 15% and 1% will have tumor extending to the right atrium. Accurate assessment of the T stage with ultrasound is achieved in up to

85% of cases. Similarly, in the evaluation of a tumor thrombus, accuracy rates of 95% are recorded.

Demonstration of renal vein and inferior vena caval thrombus requires meticulous attention to technique. Whereas this is relatively easy for the right renal vein, the course of the left renal vein means that between the renal hilum and the superior mesenteric artery, the left renal vein may be difficult to image.

The features of renal vein and caval invasion include enlargement of the vessels, with absence of change during respiration, together with intraluminal echoes. These appearances may be significantly augmented by the use of color flow and color power Doppler. The intraluminal tumor or clot can be identified in silhouette against the color flow. It is important to attempt to identify the cephalad extent of the tumor; therefore, the evaluation of the inferior vena cava to the right atrium is necessary. While tumor thrombus may be of increased reflectivity, it is often of similar reflectivity to clotted blood and may be difficult

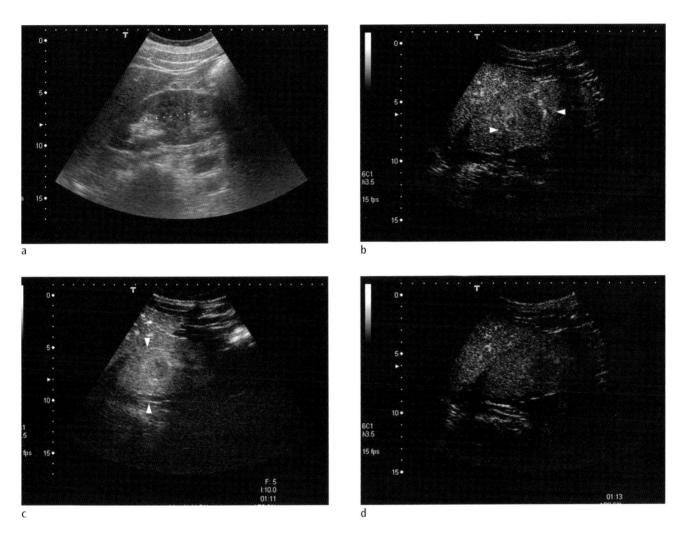

Figure 1.132

Renal tumor. A lesion is demonstrated in the equatorial region of the kidney. (a) It appears to distort the renal sinus, but does not produce distortion of the renal outline on contrast enhancement during the early parenchymal phase. (b) There is displacement of renal vessels, suggesting that this could represent a hypertrophied column of Bertin, although the vessels are somewhat irregular at the margin (arrowheads). (c) In the late phase the parenchymal blush is different from the adjacent renal cortex and there is a central area of heterogeneity (arrowheads). (d) In the late phase there is early wash out of the contrast compared with the adjacent normal renal parenchyma. Renal cell carcinoma.

to demonstrate in the absence of color or power techniques (Figures 1.133 and 1.134).

Occasionally the sudden onset of a varicocele will presage the development of a renal tumor and reflect the involvement of the renal and testicular veins, either by compression or invasion (Figure 1.135).

Screening for renal cell carcinoma

There is little doubt that the early diagnosis of renal cell carcinoma affords the identification of tumor contained within the renal parenchyma. More than 75% of patients with localized renal tumors achieve cure after surgical resection. Furthermore, in some centers, as many as two-thirds of patients with renal cell carcinoma have the diagnosis made incidentally as a consequence of investigation of other conditions. As a consequence, a number of authors have suggested the possibility of using cross-sectional imaging, and particularly ultrasound, as a method for screening for renal cell carcinoma. In one study of almost 10 000 patients, 0.1% were found to have a renal mass, of which 60% were shown to be renal carcinoma. The sensitivity for detection of renal cell carcinoma by this program was 82%.

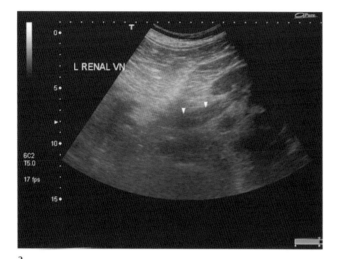

a

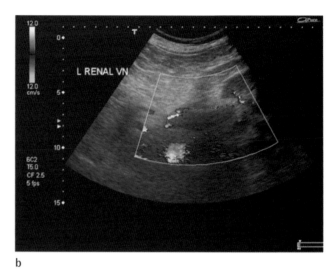

b

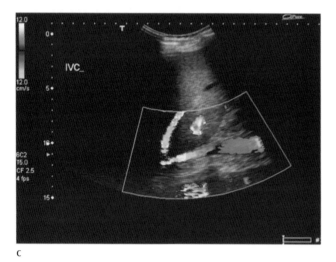

c

Figure 1.133
(a) **Axial scan through the left kidney at the left renal vein.** The left renal vein is distended and filled with echogenic material (arrowheads). (b) **Color flow Doppler demonstrates no flow within the left renal vein, although there is color at the margins of the vein.** (c) **There is no evidence of clot or thrombus within the inferior vena cava (IVC).**

It is, however, difficult to justify a screening program with such a low prevalence of disease, particularly as there are no reliable criteria for differentiation of benign from malignant lesions. Nonetheless, it must be recognized that most patients with renal carcinoma will present with non-specific symptomatology. It remains vital, therefore, that the kidneys are examined carefully in patients presenting with apparently unrelated symptoms. Prior to cross-sectional imaging, the frequency with which apparently occult renal carcinoma was discovered was reported to be as low as 4%. Most data would suggest that currently the numbers are between 50 and 70%.

Renal medullary carcinoma

Renal medullary carcinoma is a recently described, highly aggressive tumor occurring predominantly in young Afro-

Caribbeans with sickle cell trait. The tumor is centered on the renal sinus encasing the renal pelvis. There may be associated dilatation of the collecting systems. The outcome for this tumor is extremely poor. Most patients present late with hematuria, abdominal pain and weight loss and the tumor is frequently metastatic at the time of presentation.

Although the tumor may represent similar imaging findings to renal sarcoma, transitional cell carcinoma and collecting duct carcinoma of the kidney, the clinical background should allow the specific diagnosis.

Collecting duct carcinoma of the kidney

Collecting duct carcinoma derives from the renal medulla and has an infiltrative growth pattern. The tumor derives from the renal medulla and is usually hyperechoic to

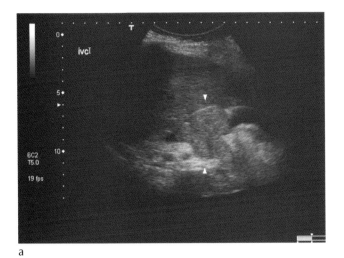

a

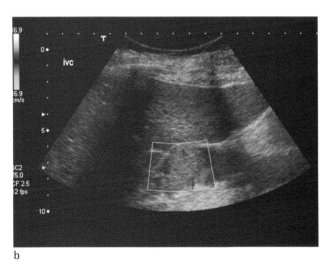

b

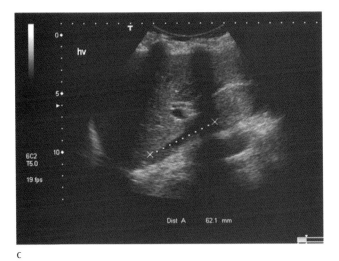

c

Figure 1.134

(a) Tumor thrombus is seen extending from the renal vein (lower arrowhead) into the inferior vena cava (upper arrowhead). (b) The IVC is filled with tumor. There is evidence of color flow at the margins of the tumor (black and white image). **(c) The distension of the IVC at the level of the renal veins is demonstrated.** However, 6 cm of IVC above the tumor mass has been measured, indicating a tumor-free area below the right atrium.

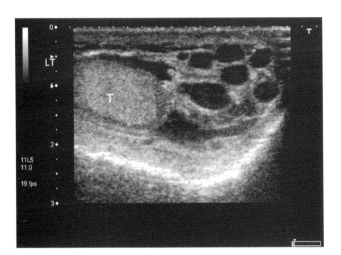

Figure 1.135

Ultrasound of the scrotum. Large varicocele, which was of sudden onset. There is a small hydrocele surrounding the testis (t).

normal renal parenchyma. When the tumor is of relatively large volume, it can usually be distinguished from other forms of renal cell carcinoma by its location and echogenicity. However, when the tumor enlarges, the outline may be distorted.

Over half of the patients will present with evidence of metastatic disease. It is possible to demonstrate lymph node involvement and local invasion with ultrasound. This is indistinguishable from metastasis and from other renal carcinoma cell types (Figure 1.136).

Adult Wilms' tumor

Adult Wilms' tumor is predominantly a tumor of infants and young children and will be considered elsewhere in this text. However, rarely, it may occur in young adults (Figure 1.137).

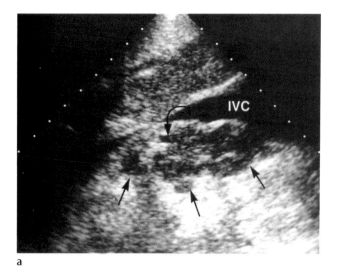

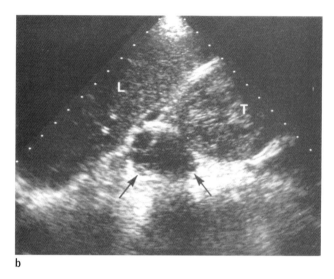

a

b

Figure 1.136

(a) **Lymph node involvement.** There is confluent lymphadenopathy (arrowheads) posterior to the inferior vena cava surrounding the right renal artery (curved arrow). (b) **Large adrenal metastasis (arrows) is demonstrated above the upper pole tumor (T).** The adjacent liver is demonstrated (L).

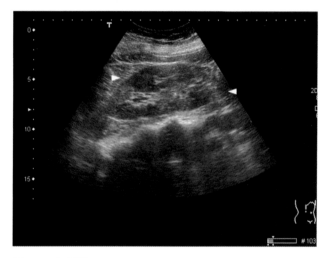

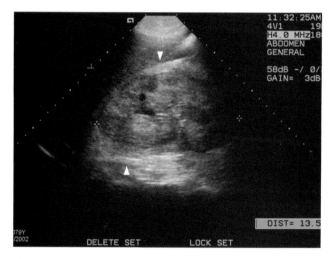

Figure 1.137

Adult Wilms' tumor. The lower pole of the kidney is replaced by an irregular heterogeneous mass (arrowheads). It is sonographically indistinguishable from other cell types.

Figure 1.138

Irregular heterogeneous replacement of renal parenchyma with focal nodules. There is thickening of the perirenal fascia, which may represent lymphomatous infiltration (arrowheads).

Renal lymphoma

Most cases of renal lymphoma reflect involvement of the kidney as part of a diffuse process of multi-organ disease. The majority of patients with renal lymphoma demonstrate a focal small nodular infiltrative pattern (Figure 1.138). Rather fewer patients demonstrate larger nodules of greater than 3 cm in diameter. Uncommonly, there is a perirenal infiltration, with the kidney encased by lymphomatous tissue. The kidney may also be diffusely enlarged without discrete nodules being demonstrable (Figure 1.139). Blood flow to the kidney is often compromised because of the compression by the infiltrated tissue (Figures 1.140 and 1.141).

Primary renal lymphoma is exceedingly rare because of the absence of lymphatic tissue within the normal kidney.

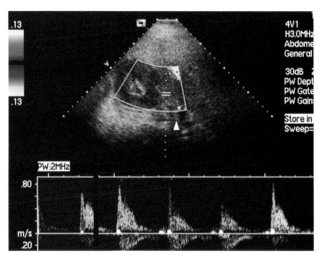

Figure 1.139
Renal lymphoma. The kidney is diffusely enlarged and echo-poor. There is a slightly lobulated outline.

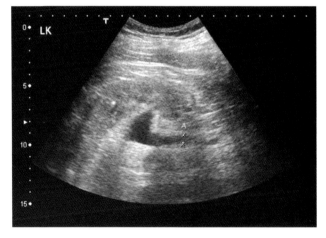

Figure 1.141
Spectral trace demonstrating almost no diastolic flow consequent upon increased intrarenal pressure. The flow in the right renal vein is demonstrated indicating that this is not occluded, although it was not possible to exclude compression of the renal vein (arrowhead).

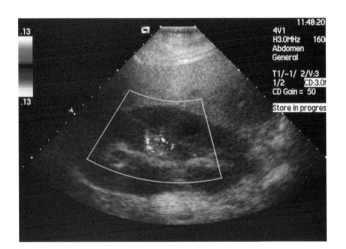

Figure 1.140
Color flow Doppler in the same case as Figure 1.139. Distortion of the interlobular vessels by the lymphomatous masses.

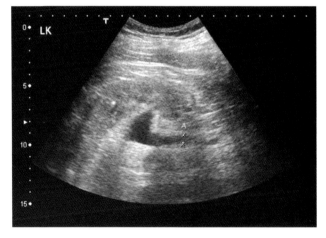

Figure 1.142
There is slight dilatation of the collecting system, but irregular thickening of the proximal ureter which is expanded. Transitional cell tumors are not usually of this infiltrative appearance and the differential diagnosis would include infection, infestation or malakoplakia.

The diagnosis of primary renal lymphoma requires the following criteria to be fulfilled:

1. Lymphomatous renal infiltration.
2. Non-obstructive, unilateral or bilateral renal enlargement.
3. No evidence of extrarenal lymphoma after complete diagnosis investigation, including renal biopsy, bone marrow biopsy and thoracoabdominal CT.

Tumors of the endothelium

Transitional renal cell carcinoma of the ureter

TCC of the ureter accounts for 2.5–5% of the transitional tumors involving the urinary tract (most arise in the bladder). Patients usually present with hematuria and/or flank pain. Appearances on ultrasound include an elongated soft

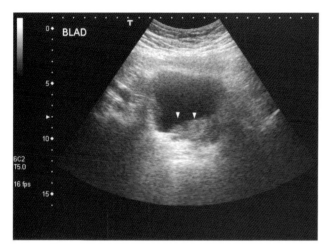

Figure 1.143
Same patient as Figure 1.142. Coexistent transitional cell carcinoma within the bladder invading through the bladder wall (arrowheads).

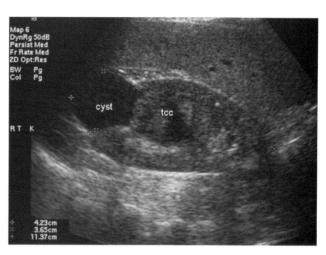

Figure 1.145
A large transitional cell carcinoma distorts the central renal sinus (tcc). Incidentally, there is a simple renal cyst at the upper pole of the kidney.

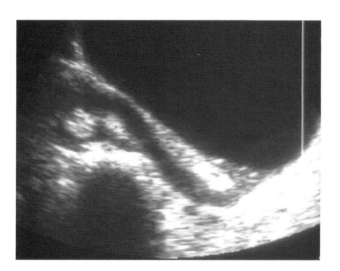

Figure 1.144
Transitional cell carcinoma involving the distal ureter and the ureteric orifice, causing obstruction.

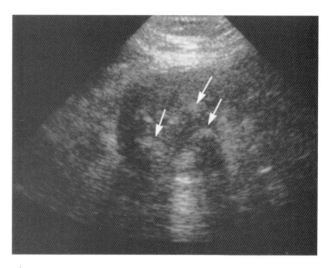

Figure 1.146
Keratin pearls are brightly reflective structures seen within the collecting system (arrows). These arise predominantly in squamous cell carcinoma of the urothelium.

tissue mass within the ureter measuring between 4 mm and 7 cm in length and outlined by fluid in the ureter. There is usually no associated acoustic shadowing and therefore the appearances can be differentiated from a renal calculus (Figure 1.142 and 1.143).

A sensitivity of 100% has been achieved for the detection of intraluminal tumor in association with hematuria and

flank pain in the presence of hydronephrosis and ureteric dilatation[14] (Figure 1.144). The ultrasound appearances are little different for tumors of any histologic nature. There is separation of the renal sinus by a solid mass whose echogenicity is usually equal to, or slightly greater than, that of the renal cortex, although occasionally the mass may be echo-poor (Figure 1.145). If the mass is obstructing the outflow of urine either by amputation of an infundibulum or by obstruction to the pelviureteric junction, then the margins of the mass can be demonstrated projecting into the dilated renal pelvis.

Occasionally, TCC and particularly squamous cell carcinoma of the renal pelvis and calyces can be difficult to differentiate from calculus disease. The formation of keratin pearls, particularly within squamous cell carcinomata, can produce focal bright reflectors within the collecting system together with acoustic shadowing. These can be indistinguishable from renal calculi (Figure 1.146).

The morphologic features of tumors affecting the renal sinus do not normally allow the distinction between tumors of different origin. Since the majority of tumors are likely to be of transitional or squamous origin, such differentiation is unlikely to be of management importance. Large transitional cell tumors can infiltrate large segments or the whole of the renal parenchyma, compromise the renal vein and produce lymph node metastases and thus be indistinguishable on ultrasound from renal cell carcinoma.

In most cases of lymphoma involving the renal sinus, there will be a history of, or evidence of, lymphoma elsewhere. An unusual form of renal sinus lymphoma has been described in which there is diffuse infiltration of the walls of the renal pelvis and proximal ureter, producing an echo-poor thickened wall with a central echogenic occluded calyceal or pelvic lumen. This appearance is rare but, when present, appears to be pathognomonic (Figure 1.147).

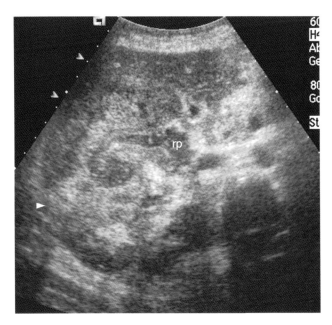

Figure 1.147
Renal sinus lymphoma. The kidney is enlarged, distorted and malrotated. The margins are identified by the arrowheads. The collecting system is filled with echogenic material (RP) and there is thickening of the urothelium.

Ultrasound in hematuria

The role of ultrasound in the investigation of hematuria is a complex one. Much of the evidence would suggest that ultrasound possesses inadequate sensitivity for the detection of tumors of the upper urothelial tract. However, since these constitute only 7% of all renal tumors, and since the accuracy of ultrasound in the detection of renal cell carcinoma and bladder tumors is either equivalent to or exceeds that of the intravenous urogram, most authors would now recommend ultrasound as the investigation of first choice in patients presenting with hematuria. If the ultrasound examination and cystoscopy are negative and the hematuria persists and/or there is abnormal urine cytology, then an intravenous urogram is indicated.

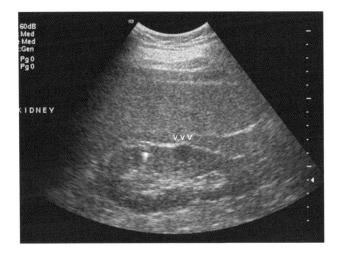

Figure 1.148
Isolated renal metastasis (arrowheads). The metastasis is echo-poor and causes mild distortion of the renal cortex. Reverberation from a presumed milk of calcium cyst is demonstrated in the upper pole.

Renal metastases

The incidence of renal metastases (Figure 1.148) is variously reported as between 2 and 20% at autopsy. The kidney can be the site of metastases from a number of different primary lesions, including colon, lung and breast, and from melanoma, of which lung is the most common primary. Few of these, however, are demonstrated by imaging modalities during life. Usually the metastases are small and multifocal but occasionally may be large and then may

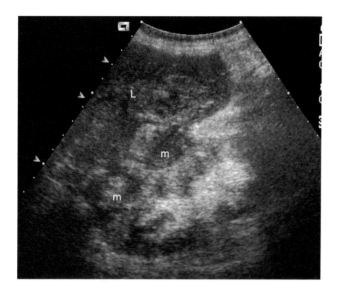

Figure 1.149
Multiple renal metastases (M) are associated with multiple hepatic metastases. L = liver.

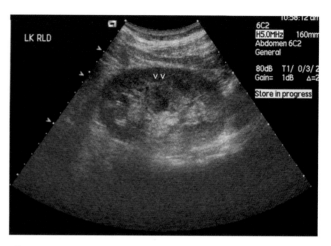

Figure 1.150
Hypertrophied column of Bertin. The invagination of the cortex and medulla into the renal sinus is identified by the arrowheads.

be indistinguishable from primary renal carcinomata. The echo pattern of secondary tumors is as variable as that of primary lesions, with solid, cystic and mixed appearances, although only rarely is there increased reflectivity (Figure 1.149). Metastases from melanoma may involve the perirenal space, even in the absence of demonstrable renal metastases.

Renal pseudotumors

Most anatomical variations of renal anatomy, such as congenital lobar enlargement and fetal lobulation, are unlikely to be confused with mass lesions of the kidney. Hypertrophied columns of Bertin, which in the past might have been mistaken for a renal mass, can almost invariably be distinguished from renal pathology by characteristic features. The lesion should be (a) located between two overlapping portions of the renal sinus, (b) co-located with a junctional line, (c) contain cortex and medulla and (d) the cortex should be continuous with the adjacent cortex of the kidney. This should allow the reliable identification of the column (Figure 1.150). Renal cell carcinoma may arise within or adjacent to a column, but this is exceptionally rare (Figure 1.151).[15]

Renal sinus lipomatosis will often produce distortion and stretching of the calyces on an intravenous urogram, but the appearances are normally sufficiently characteristic on ultrasound for a specific diagnosis to be made (Figure 1.152). Occasionally, however, the extent of the lipomatosis

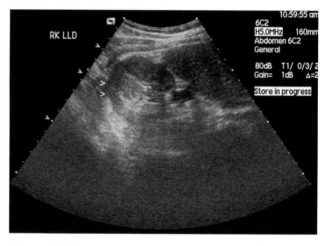

Figure 1.151
Renal cell carcinoma mimicking a hypertrophied column of Bertin. In this case (a transverse view of the right kidney), the neoplasm is identified by the differing echogenicity. The tumor is brighter than the adjacent cortex (arrowheads).

is so marked that it may produce an echogenic mass on ultrasound indistinguishable from other causes of echogenic tumor. Renal sinus lipomatosis may also produce appearances that suggest an alternative pathology. The echogenicity of the fat may be reduced when compared to normal sinus and to the renal parenchyma. In these cases the lipomatosis may be confused with renal sinus tumor or with hydronephrosis. However, the margins

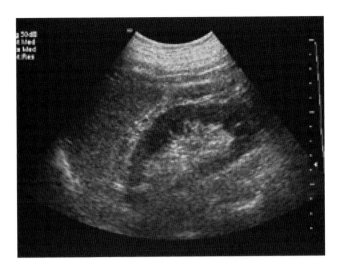

Figure 1.152
Normal appearance of the broadening of the renal sinus.
This occurs in obesity and in the elderly.

are usually ill-defined and there is evidence of posterior acoustic attenuation.[16]

Similar in content, but different in etiology, are fat-filled postoperative renal cortical defects which are the result of herniation of perirenal fat into surgical defects following a wedge resection, which can also mimic echogenic masses (see Figure 1.114). Although usually echogenic, rarely, these can be echo-poor, and therefore confused with renal cell carcinoma.[17]

Renal and perirenal infection

Infection of the renal parenchyma

In urinary tract infection, the role of ultrasound is predominantly the detection of obstruction, identification of complications, the diagnosis of abnormality predisposing to infection, such as horseshoe kidney, calculus disease, etc., characterization of infection in the presence of unusual organisms and the differentiation of urinary tract infection from other causes of urinary tract symptomatology.

Ultrasound is widely used in the investigation of children with suspected urinary tract infection, but this is considered elsewhere in this book.

The diagnosis of acute pyelonephritis is usually based on clinical grounds. Patients present with loin pain, dysuria, hematuria and fever, often with rigors. Ultrasound is indicated only if symptoms persist, or recur, in spite of antibiotic treatment, or the pattern of symptomatology is unusual.

Thus, although acute pyelonephritis is a relatively common clinical diagnosis, most of the cases are uncomplicated and ultrasound is only used infrequently to aid diagnosis.

Acute pyelonephritis is an infection involving both the collecting system and the parenchyma of the kidney. The organism most commonly isolated is *E. coli*, although *Proteus mirabilis* and *Klebsiella oxytoca* are found in a significant minority. The process of infection is thought to be predominantly ascending. Predisposing factors include diabetes, immunosuppression, vesicoureteric reflux and long-term catheterization.

Acute focal pyelonephritis, also known as acute bacterial nephritis or lobar nephronia, is described as a variant of pyelonephritis in which the acute infection causes an isolated area, or areas, of abnormality. However, focal and generalized parenchymal infection represent part of a continuum of renal involvement.

Ultrasound features of acute pyelonephritis

The sonographic features of acute pyelonephritis can be conveniently divided into anatomical distribution of abnormality, imaging features, features on color and power Doppler and features following contrast enhancement.

Renal infection usually produces enlargement, although this is difficult to document if both kidneys are affected (Figure 1.153).

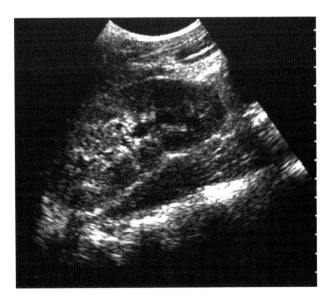

Figure 1.153
Focal pyelonephritis. The upper pole of the kidney is of increased reflectivity and is larger than the lower pole. The capsule has become ill-defined.

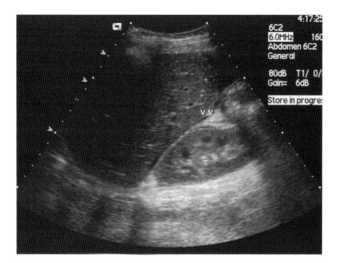

Figure 1.154
Thickening of the prerenal fascia in a patient with acute pyelonephritis (arrowheads). This pattern is non-specific and may relate to any inflammation in the right upper quadrant.

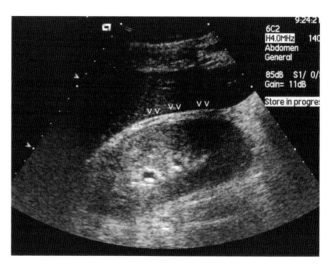

Figure 1.155
Acute pyelonephritis. Thickening of the prerenal fascia is demonstrated. There is associated enlargement of the right kidney and loss of definition of the corticomedullary junction. There is early pelvicalyceal dilatation.

In severe cases perirenal inflammation results in thickening and heterogeneity of Gerota's fascia and loss of definition of renal margins. This 'renal rind sign' is, however, non-specific and may also be seen in other inflammatory processes in the region of the kidney (Figure 1.154).

Mild dilatation of the calyces and ureter may occur as a result of atony and does not necessarily imply obstruction as a cause of the infection (Figure 1.155). Ultrasound demonstration of thickening of the renal sinus and increased echogenicity has been reported. This feature is more commonly seen in children, perhaps because of the relative paucity of sinus fat (Figure 1.156).

Occasionally, the increase in reflectivity of the renal sinus is sufficient to produce acoustic shadowing. This is not usually as sharp as shadowing from a renal calculus, and resolves with effective antibiotic therapy.

Parenchymal abnormalities

Multiple focal changes probably occur in all cases of severe acute pyelonephritis, although ultrasound abnormality reflects only part of the involved parenchyma.

Focal abnormalities may be echogenic, echo-poor or mixed. They may be wedge-shaped or mimic a renal mass, (solid or cystic) (Figure 1.157) or have a similar appearance to medullary pyramids. The presence of focal abnormality of the kidney on ultrasound examination does not appear to correlate with the subsequent development of renal scarring.

Lesions have been graded on a 5-point conspicuity scale: grade 0, not seen; grade 1, equivocal parenchymal defect;

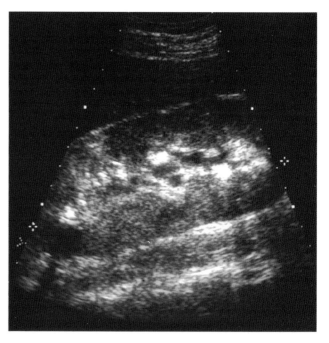

Figure 1.156
Increased reflectivity of the renal sinus in a patient with acute pyelonephritis.

grade 2, poorly demarcated defect; grade 3, moderately well-demarcated; grade 4, well-defined. Using these criteria, the detection of parenchymal lesions in patients with acute pyelonephritis is reported in 57% of patients using conventional ultrasound.

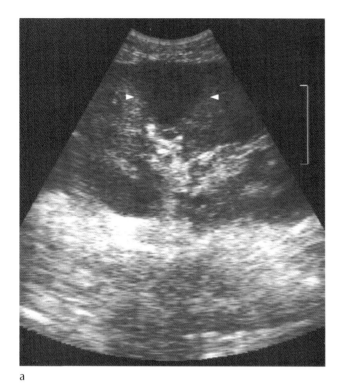

a

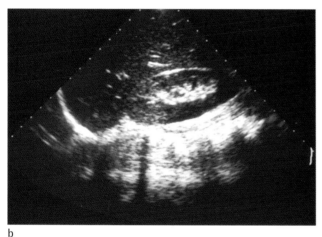

b

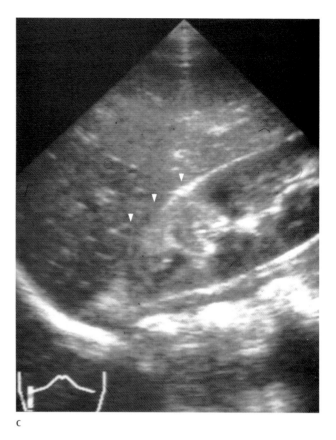

c

Figure 1.157

Focal pyelonephritis. (a) There is an almost wedge-shaped area of the kidney which is echo-poor and illustrates some swelling (arrowheads). (b) The upper pole of the kidney is of increased reflectivity and slightly enlarged. (c) Marked increase in reflectivity at the upper pole of the right kidney (arrowheads).

Note that tissue harmonic imaging may improve the demonstration of focal parenchymal abnormality.

The role of Doppler in acute pyelonephritis

Color and power Doppler may demonstrate an area of decreased blood flow within the parenchyma (Figures 1.158 and 1.159).

Although these techniques may have greater sensitivity than imaging alone (see Figure 1.159), there remain inher-ent difficulties, including attenuation of sound with depth and angle of incidence to the direction of flow (Figure 1.160). Thus, it is difficult to exclude perfusion defects at the renal poles. Blood flow within the interlobar vessels may be maintained or even increased in the early phase of infection as a consequence of hyperemia.

Demonstration of cortical perfusion by color or power Doppler requires optimum ultrasound imaging conditions and is compromised by adverse body habitus.

There are no reports of the use of spectral Doppler reflecting the hyperemic early phase of infection. Once

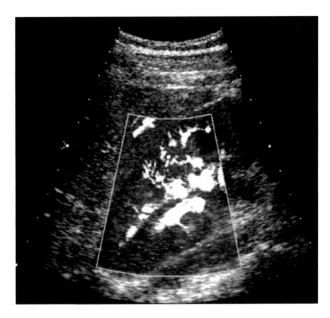

Figure 1.158
Focal pyelonephritis involving the upper pole of the kidney.
Power Doppler demonstrates diminished flow to the upper
pole.

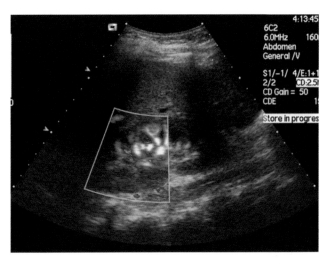

Figure 1.160
**Color power Doppler demonstrates poor perfusion to the
posterior aspect of the upper pole of the kidney.** This is due
to sound attenuation. The patient was asymptomatic.

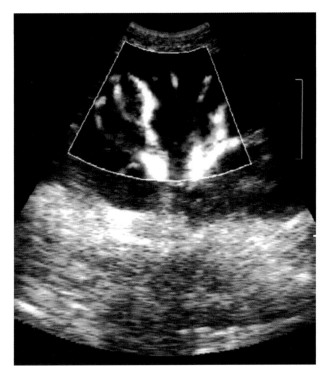

Figure 1.159
The same case as in Figure 1.157a. The focal abnormality
demonstrates poor perfusion on power Doppler.

renal enlargement is apparent, there is evidence of increase
in the resistance and pulsatility indices.

Early studies using microbubble contrast agents are
promising, but are based on small patient numbers.
Patients with acute pyelonephritis demonstrate perfusion
defects which are not apparent on precontrast examinations either on grayscale imaging or using color or power
Doppler. However, it is essential that specific contrast
imaging packages are available to achieve optimum sensitivity. Potential limitations of contrast-enhanced studies
are largely related to increased sound attenuation by the
microbubbles and the consequent false-positive detection
of areas of hypoperfusion in the more deeply situated renal
parenchyma (Figure 1.161).

Emphysematous pyelonephritis

Emphysematous pyelonephritis is an unusual infection
involving gas-forming organisms. The condition usually
occurs either in an obstructed system or in diabetics. The
symptoms of chills, fever, flank pain, lethargy and confusion are similar to those of acute pyelonephritis resulting
from infection with a more common organism, but the
ultrasound appearances are characteristic. The collecting
system and more deeply placed renal parenchyma are
obscured by the brightly reflective echoes from gas which
produce significant dirty distal acoustic shadowing (Figure
1.162). These appearances are demonstrated throughout
the renal sinus and pelvis but are also demonstrated usually

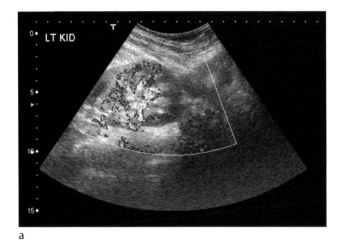
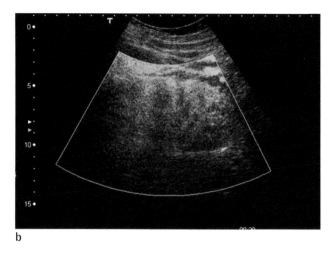

a   b

Figure 1.161

(a) **Lower pole of the left kidney is enlarged.** Color flow Doppler demonstrates normal flow within the segmental and interlobular vessels, but little perfusion of the cortex. (b) **The lower pole cortex appears to be normally perfused after contrast.** There are technical difficulties with demonstration of more deeply placed structures such as the posterior aspect of the kidney. Perfusion cannot be demonstrated to the posterior aspect of the lower pole.

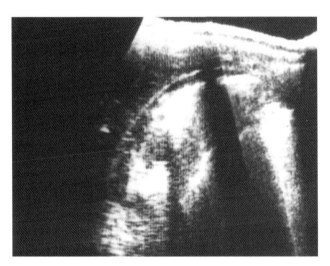

Figure 1.162

Emphysematous pyelonephritis. Much of the kidney is obscured by highly reflectvie gas within the collecting system producing distal dirty acoustic shadowing.

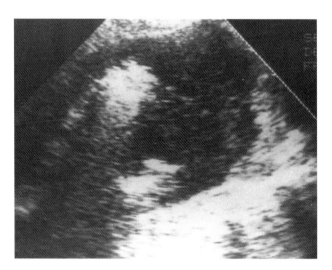

Figure 1.163

Renal carcinoma following embolization. Intrarenal gas is represented by highly reflectvie areas with distal dirty acoustic shadowing.

within the bladder lumen or within the wall. The combination of these two findings is pathognomonic of the condition. Occasionally, the condition of emphysematous pyelonephritis can be mimicked by other causes of gas within the collecting system. A vesicocolic fistula may produce gas shadowing within the bladder, but the gas rarely ascends the ureter into the collecting system of the

kidney. By contrast, however, we have demonstrated a large bowel tumor causing a fistulous connection between the renal pelvis and the lumen of the bowel, with the result that the renal sinus and calyces are filled with gas in the same way as in emphysematous pyelonephritis. Following embolization, the kidney may also contain gas and thus mimic gas-forming infection (Figure 1.163).

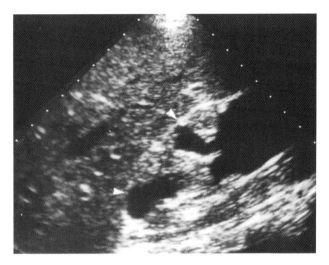

Figure 1.164
Chronic pyelonephritis. The kidney is small. There are clubbed calyces adjacent to significant cortical thinning (arrowheads).

Chronic pyelonephritis

Chronic pyelonephritis may be due to continued low-grade infection or recurrent attacks of acute pyelonephritis with scarring. Vesicoureteric reflux is also a major contributing factor in a large number of patients, and infection does not invariably have to be present to cause renal damage with scarring. The appearances of the kidney depend upon severity. There may be one or more focal scars of the kidney, producing significant loss of the cortex opposite a calyx (Figure 1.164). It is not always possible on ultrasound to demonstrate the dilated or clubbed calyx that is characteristic of a focal scar on an intravenous urogram, but there is an associated area of thickening and fibrosis characterized by an increased area of echogenicity (Figure 1.165). There is frequently an increase in the volume of renal sinus fat (Figure 1.166).

The role of ultrasound in the demonstration of renal scars is difficult to assess. Sensitivity is variously reported

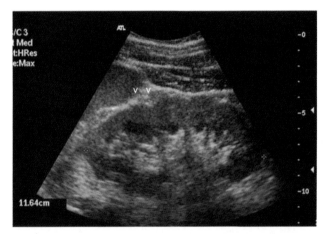

a

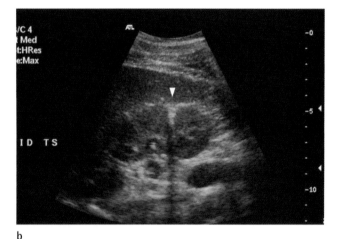

b

Figure 1.165
(a) **Focal cortical scar.** Triangular echogenic defect within the renal cortex (arrowheads). (b) Cortical scar at the lower pole of the right kidney (arrowheads). **Slight pelvicalyceal dilatation is evidenced by the prominent medullary papillae.** (c) Large cortical scar (arrowheads).

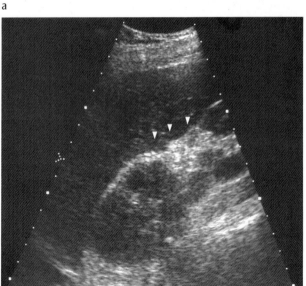

c

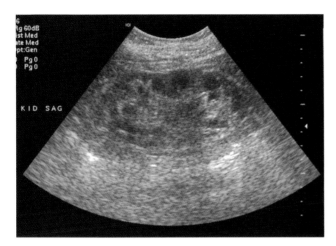

Figure 1.166
Chronic pyelonephritis. There is loss of renal cortex and broadening of the renal sinus.

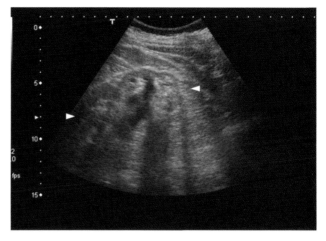

Figure 1.167
Chronic pyelonephritis. The kidney is small, difficult to demonstrate and irregular in outline (arrowheads). There is cortical loss and broadening of the renal sinus.

as between 37 and 100% and specificity as between 65 and 99%. However, comparison with DMSA suggests that for clinically significant scars ultrasound has acceptable sensitivity.

Doppler indices may further improve the value of ultrasound. There appears to be a relationship between renal scarring and increase in resistance indices. Those patients with reflux but no scarring yield normal RI values.

The patient with severe chronic pyelonephritis has a small irregular highly reflective kidney that may be indistinguishable from other causes of end-stage kidney (Figure 1.167).

Pyonephrosis

The infected obstructed kidney may result from any of the causes of renal obstruction. Loin pain may become more severe and more deep-seated and there is a fever and general debility. Ultrasound features may be variable and there are four distinct patterns described. The most characteristic pattern is that of multiple low-level echoes throughout the fluid contained within the dilated collecting system (Figure 1.168a,b). Occasionally, the echogenic debris within the collecting system may have a tendency to layer and, in the most extreme cases, there may be a fluid debris level (Figure 1.168c). If gas-forming organisms supersede, then the fluid within the dilating collecting systems may contain scattered, coarse, highly reflective foci with acoustic shadowing consistent with bubbles of gas within the infected fluid. Utilizing these signs, ultrasound

is up to 90% sensitive for the detection of pyonephrosis in an obstructed collecting system.

Renal abscess

Renal abscesses may occur as a result of focal or diffuse acute pyelonephritis, by direct extension of infection elsewhere in the retroperitoneal space or as a result of metastatic spread from a focus of infection elsewhere. Early in the development of an abscess the appearances are indistinguishable from those of focal pyelonephritis, with enlargement of the affected portion of the kidney, which is poorly marginated. Subsequently, the mass becomes more typically echo-free or echo-poor, sometimes with a content of fine diffuse echoes, posterior acoustic enhancement and a finely regular margin. There is frequently an associated peri- or pararenal abscess (Figure 1.169).

Atypical infections

Xanthogranulomatous pyelonephritis

XGP is an uncommon form of granulomatous inflammatory disease typified by the presence of lipid-laden macrophages, plasma cells, leukocytes and histiocytes. The condition exists in two forms: a diffuse form, which accounts for 85% of cases, and a focal form, which may be confused with renal tumor. The condition is associated

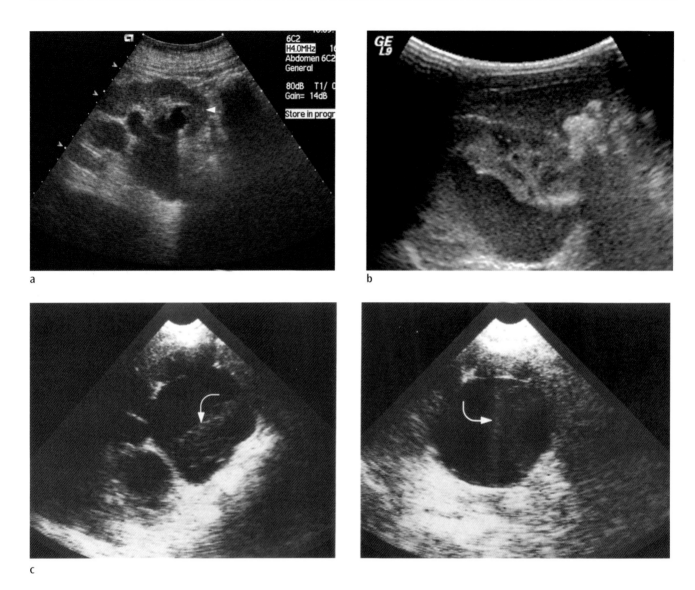

Figure 1.168
(a) **Dilated collecting system.** There are echoes within the calyces and within the pelvis, particularly within the lower pole calyx where there is some layering of material (arrowhead). (b) **Duplex collecting system.** Pyelonephrosis of the upper moiety. There is a fluid level within the kidney consistent with layering of pus. (c) **Pyonephrosis.** Left, layering debris is demonstrated within the renal pelvis (curved arrow). Right, when the patient is moved to a vertical position, the shift in the layering of debris is noted (curved arrow).

with chronic infection and focal deficiency of the immune system in an obstructed kidney or renal segment. Patients present with flank pain, fever, fatigue, weight loss and other non-specific urinary symptoms.

In the diffuse form, there is renal enlargement with pelvicalyceal dilatation and parenchymal destruction. The calyces may be filled with echogenic material returning low-level echoes. Calcification is evident, with bright echoes and distal acoustic shadowing, either from calculi or from peripheral calcification.

The focal form of the disease usually produces an echo-poor mass within the kidney, often distorting the renal outline. This may appear entirely solid, or may mimic an abscess with a thick wall and a complex fluid content. There is rarely a peritumoral halo and calcification appears to be less common in the focal form than in the diffuse form. There may be associated perirenal thickening and a perinephric fluid collection may be present in as many as 15% of cases.

In the diffuse form, the appearances are variously described as diffuse parenchymal, which is consequent

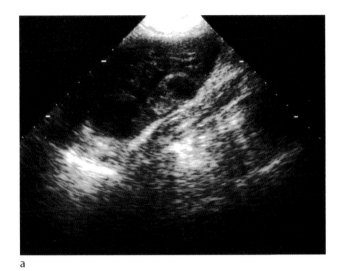

a

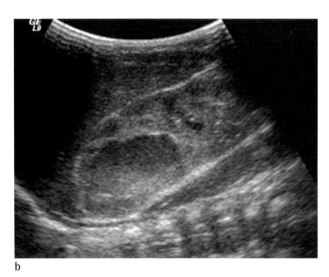

b

Figure 1.169
(a) Early renal abscess demonstrating focal increased reflectivity and an area of early necrosis. (b) Irregular abscess at the upper pole of the right kidney containing echogenic fluid.

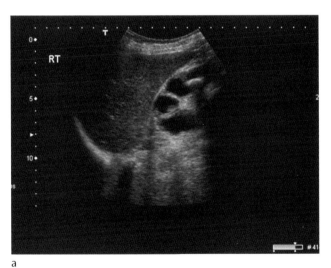

a

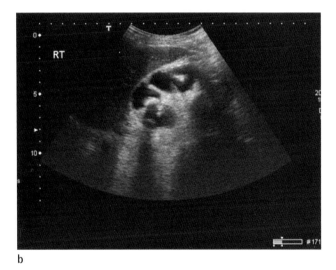

b

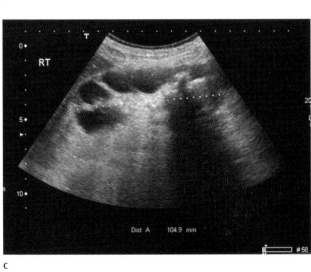

c

Figure 1.170
Xanthogranulomatous pyelonephritis. Figures a–c demonstrate the hydronephrotic form with distended calyces with cortical destruction and a central large, irregular calculus as well as further calculi within the renal parenchyma.

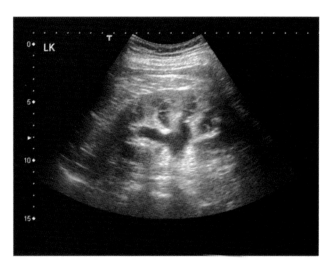

Figure 1.171
Malakoplakia. Diffuse thickening of the renal sinus with apparent elevation of the urothelium within the calyces and increased sinus reflectivity.

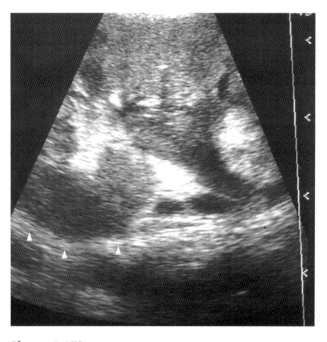

Figure 1.172
Malakoplakia. Urothelial thickening and debris. There is an ill-defined mass at the upper pole (arrowheads).

upon parenchymal loss and replacement of the corticomedullary junction with soft yellow nodules. These appear as echo-poor structures at the corticomedullary junction, similar to enlarged medullary pyramids. The diffuse hydronephrotic form more nearly mimics hydro- or pyonephrosis (Figure 1.170).

Malakoplakia

Malakoplakia is an uncommon inflammatory disorder with characteristic histopathologic findings of Michaelis–Gutmann bodies and von Hansemann cells. Patients present with fever, malaise, loin pain and, less commonly, a loin mass. Features consistent with renal parenchymal malakoplakia include diffuse enlargement of the kidney with diffuse increase in parenchymal echogenicity. This may be associated with the presence of one or more echo-poor lesions. Malakoplakia may also affect the ureter and the bladder with urothelial thickening, which is usually of polypoid nature when present in the bladder. The condition may produce papillary necrosis (Figures 1.171 and 1.172).

Renal tuberculosis

Tuberculosis (TB) is caused by *Mycobacterium tuberculosis*. Pulmonary infection is generally the primary focus. In most cases primary tuberculosis is a self-limited, mild pneumonic illness. Reactivation of infection occurs in those patients who are at risk, such as those who are immunosuppressed or those with diabetes or chronic renal failure. Genitourinary TB is the second most common form of extrapulmonary TB. Manifestations depend upon the site of urologic involvement. This may include the adrenal glands, producing adrenal insufficiency; the kidneys, leading to hematuria, pyuria, colic and renal failure; and the ureters and bladder, producing scarring and strictures. Renal tuberculosis develops following metastatic dissemination, producing microscopic foci of tuberculosis close to the glomeruli. A chronic inflammatory response ensues. This produces necrosis and sloughing of the renal papillae, as well as fibrosis of the collecting system and ureter (Figure 1.173). This latter produces focal or generalized hydronephrosis and, together with the renal necrosis, abscess formation may occur (Figure 1.174). Calcification occurs in as many as 25% of patients and, when extensive, is associated with 'autonephrectomy' (Figure 1.175).

Hydatid disease

Hydatid disease, which is caused by *Echinococcus granulosus*, is manifest by a slow-growing cystic mass. The infection is acquired by man by the ingestion of food or fluids contaminated by excreted eggs.

Renal hydatid is rare and, although it may be asymptomatic, most patients present with a flank mass, renal colic, fever and hematuria, which are all symptoms typical of renal disease but are not specific for renal hydatid. Findings usually are those of a unilocular or multilocular cyst or cysts, often with mural calcification and demonstrable daughter cysts. The cysts have been classified after Gharbi et al[18] as follows:

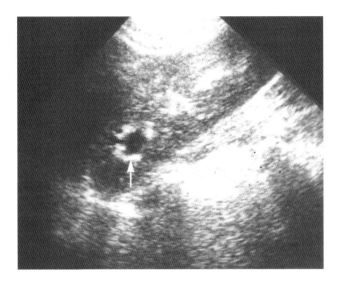

Figure 1.173
Early tuberculosis. Focal dilatation of an upper pole calyx (arrow) secondary to infundibular stricture.

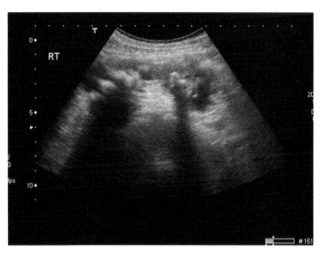

Figure 1.175
Extensive calcification in renal tuberculosis. There is marked cortical loss.

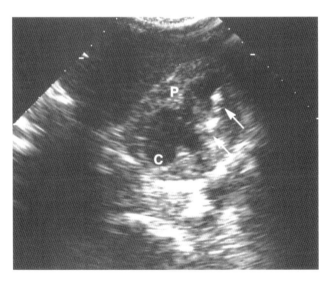

Figure 1.174
Tuberculous pyonephrosis. The kidney is small, with overall thinning of the parenchyma (P), which is of increased reflectivity. There is dilatation of the calyces (C), which contain ill-defined echogenic material. There are several foci of calcification (arrows).

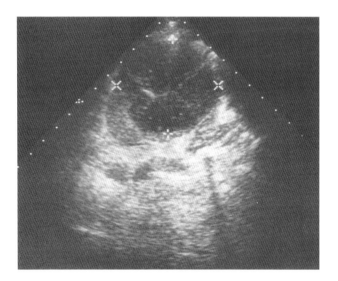

Figure 1.176
Characteristic spokewheel pattern of renal hydatid.

- Type 1 – well-defined, apparently simple cyst with distal enhancement.
- Type 2 – cyst with detachment of membrane (Figure 1.176).
- Type 3 – multilocular cyst or honeycomb pattern (Figure 1.177).
- Type 4 – heterogeneous cyst with solid elements.
- Type 5 – calcified cyst (Figure 1.178).

Differentiation of simple or multilocular cyst from other pathologies is difficult, although the type 2 is almost pathognomonic.

Schistosomiasis

This is a parasite infection consequent upon *Schistosoma haematobium*. Most of the manifestations are related to egg

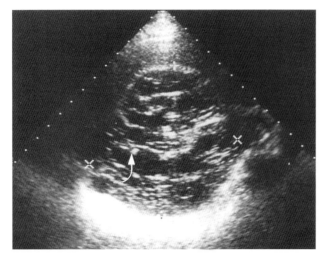

Figure 1.177
Renal hydatid. Complex cystic appearance within the kidney. There are cysts of multiple different sizes. At least one of the cysts, an inclusion body or scolex, can be identified (curved arrow).

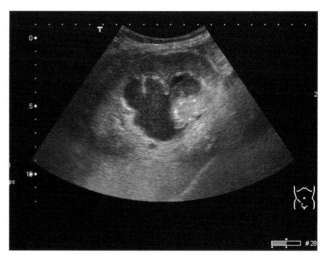

Figure 1.179
Renal candidiasis. Transplant kidney demonstrating thickening of the urothelium, irregular thickening of the proximal ureter and echoes within the dilated renal sinus.

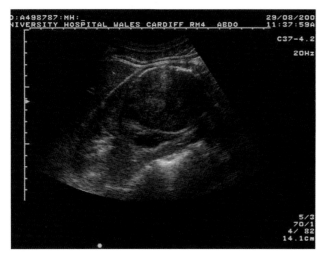

Figure 1.178
Renal hydatid. Large cyst at the lower pole of the kidney with marginal calcification. The apparent echoes within the hydatid cyst are caused by reverberation.

deposition and the formation of granulomas and fibrous tissue. The condition largely affects the lower urinary tract and the bladder, although it may produce upper tract dilatation, which is thought to be consequent upon polypoid lesions, either in the bladder or in the distal ureter.

Actinomycosis

This is a chronic infection which predominantly affects the cervicofacial and thoracic regions. Renal involvement is

extremely rare. Manifestations are those of either a solid or cystic mass, with thick irregular walls within the kidney, with extension to adjacent structures and particular involvement of perirenal fat. It is difficult, if not impossible, to differentiate on ultrasound imaging from renal tumor where there is evidence of local extension of the infection into the surrounding tissues with attending tissue destruction.

Fungi

Fungal infection of the kidney most commonly occurs in patients who are either suffering from a form of immune suppression, including AIDS or from diabetes. Ultrasound features are similar to pyogenic infections of the renal tract but there may be additional findings. Mucosal thickening of the renal pelvis and of the calyces has been reported to occur in candidiasis of the renal tract (Figure 1.179). Although similar appearances might be expected to be seen in early transitional cell carcinoma, malakoplakia, pyelitis cystica, epithelial hyperplasia, etc., the combination of a predisposing condition such as diabetes or AIDS might lead one to the presumptive diagnosis of a fungal infection of the kidney in the presence of these signs. Similar patterns may occur following the relief of obstruction, particularly in neonates and also in renal transplant rejection. The most characteristic abnormality seen in fungal infection of the kidney, however, is the presence of fungus balls within the collecting system (Figure 1.180). These are amorphous masses which exhibit varying degrees of echogenicity and attenuation of the sound beam,

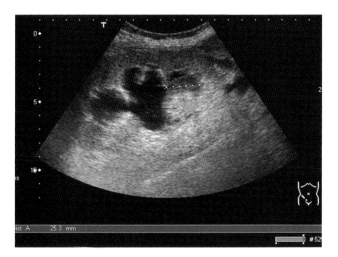

Figure 1.180
Renal transplant candidiasis. There is an amorphous mass identified in the lower pole calyx.

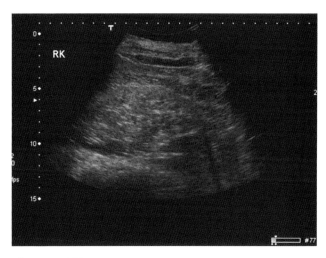

Figure 1.182
Renal amyloid. The kidney is not enlarged but there is irregular abnormality of the parenchymal texture.

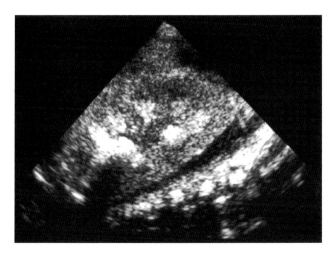

Figure 1.181
Candidiasis in a neonate kidney. There is an echogenic mass within the upper pole calyx which produces distal acoustic shadowing. This is presumed to be due to a mass of mycelia. *Candida* was identified within the urine.

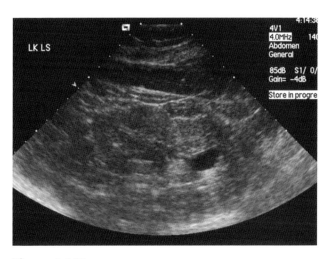

Figure 1.183
Renal amyloid. Left kidney enlarged, irregular in outline and ill-defined with diffuse parenchymal abnormality.

occasionally sufficient to produce slight acoustic shadowing (Figure 1.181). This will be seen not only in candidiasis but also in other fungal infections of the kidney.

Renal amyloid

Amyloidosis is characterized by deposition of fibrillar protein amyloid usually secondary to pre-existing pathology, particularly chronic infection. The condition is characterized by enlargement of the kidney and increased cortical reflectivity with enhanced corticomedullary differentiation, although if it is secondary to renal failure then the kidney may not be enlarged and there may be a diffuse abnormality of parenchymal texture (Figures 1.182 and 1.183). There is usually an associated abnormality of Doppler indices with increased resistance to flow.

Renal vascular disease

Anatomical variants

There are many variations in the vascular supply and drainage of the kidneys. Accessory renal arteries are present in over 20% of cases, although these are only infrequently demonstrated by current ultrasound techniques, including color flow Doppler. The position of the accessory artery may vary enormously, its origin from the aorta being related to the ascent of the kidney from the pelvis. Thus, accessory vessels may arise anywhere from the iliac arteries cephalad, although more commonly they arise within 2 cm of the main renal artery (see Figure 1.55). Certain congenital renal abnormalities, e.g. horseshoe kidney, are associated with arterial variants. Renal venous anomalies include double renal vein and retroaortic left renal vein (see Figure 1.56).

Renal arterial disease

Aneurysms of the renal artery occur but are uncommon. They may cause rupture, thrombosis embolization and dissection. They appear as a focal swelling of the vessel with a variable amount of intramural clot (Figure 1.184). Color flow Doppler will usually demonstrate flow within the aneurysm characterized by a swirling pattern of slow flow.

Renal artery aneurysms should not now be confused with the dilatation of the left renal vein that occurs as a result of the nutcracker effect of the superior mesenteric artery compressing the renal vein as it traverses between the superior mesenteric artery and the aorta.

Renal artery stenosis

Stenosis of the renal artery has achieved significant importance because of its association with the development of hypertension consequent upon increased renin production. Screening for arterial stenosis has therefore become an important aspect of the management of patients with systemic hypertension. This needs to be placed in perspective, however, since, although hypertension is common, its association with a renovascular problem is rare, being present in probably less than 1% of all cases of hypertension. Screening for renovascular hypertension, therefore, is predominantly reserved for patients who are young and/or have severe hypertension uncontrolled by normal therapeutic measures or have an accelerated form of hypertension. There exists significant dispute about the role of duplex Doppler in screening for renal artery stenosis.

Features of arterial stenosis

In its most severe form, arterial stenosis will significantly compromise perfusion of the kidney. In this situation, the kidney will decrease in size, usually in uniform fashion, with simultaneous loss of cortical and medullary thickness. Such reduction in size can clearly be demonstrated with ultrasound (Figure 1.185). Sequential measurements of the kidney may demonstrate a gradual reduction in renal size

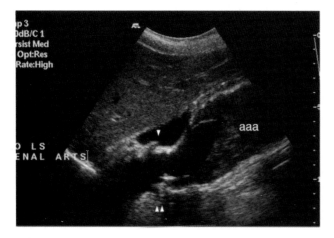

Figure 1.184
Oblique scans through the upper abdomen demonstrating an abdominal aortic aneurysm (AAA) arising distal to the renal arteries (arrowheads).

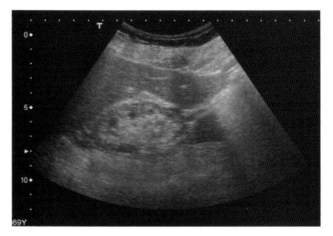

Figure 1.185
Small right kidney secondary to renal artery stenosis.

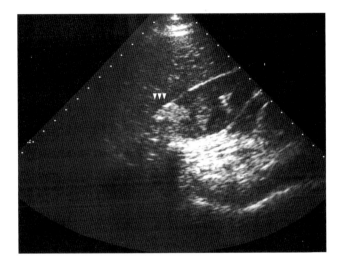

Figure 1.186
An upper pole cortical scar associated with parenchymal swelling (arrowheads).

over a period of time. Where the renal artery stenosis is accompanied by thromboembolic disease, as may occur in soft atheromatous plaque, the reduction in renal parenchyma may be focal with the production of a renal infarct. In this situation there is at first focal enlargement of the segment of the kidney, with initially a decrease in reflectivity, followed by a diffuse increase in reflectivity of the affected segment with loss of corticomedullary differentiation (Figure 1.186). Subsequently, the swelling diminishes, and the infarcted segment contracts and produces a focal cortical scar. This is usually a linear or wedge-shaped area of increased reflectivity with a cortical defect not dissimilar from that seen in chronic pyelonephritis. Although there is no relationship with a clubbed or dilated calyx, this feature is not always seen on ultrasound in any case, and the two conditions may be difficult to distinguish.

The demonstration of arterial stenosis before the development of such irreversible phenomena depends upon the use of Doppler spectral analysis. Sampling is usually performed in the main renal artery at the origin and at the hilum of the kidney (Figure 1.187). Features characteristic of a renal artery stenosis are: at the ostium, an increase in peak systolic velocities to greater than 1.8 m/s, spectral broadening and increase in maximum diastolic flow velocities (Figures 1.188–1.190). Whereas some authors have utilized the combination of increased velocity and spectral broadening to diagnose renal artery stenosis, others have used the renal to aortic ratio (RAR). This is the ratio of the systolic peak in the aorta to the systolic peak in the adjacent renal artery. An RAR of greater than 3.5 is reported as being sensitive in the detection of significant stenoses, i.e. those greater than 60%. Others have used flow sampling at the renal hilum, where similar features may be identified,

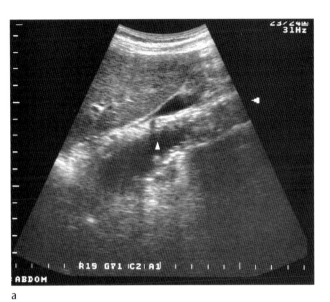

a

b

Figure 1.187
(a) Oblique scans through the aorta. There is significant atheroma. The right renal artery (arrowhead) is identified, but the left renal artery origin is compromised by atheromatous disease. **(b) Color Doppler (black and white image) identified flow within the main renal artery on the right.** No flow could be identified in the left renal artery.

although this depends on the distance from the stenosis. If sufficiently distant from the stenosis, the hilar signals may replicate those of the intrarenal vessels reflecting upstream stenosis (Figure 1.191).

Identifying the renal artery at its origin and reliably recording a Doppler signal from this site requires significant expertise and patience. In the best hands, satisfactory signals are achieved in up to 90% of cases. However,

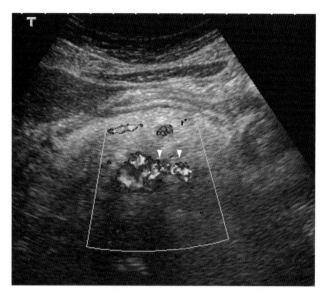

Figure 1.188
The origin of the left renal artery is characterized on this color flow image by extensive aliasing of the color signal within the renal artery in spite of an angle of incidence of close to 90° (arrowheads).

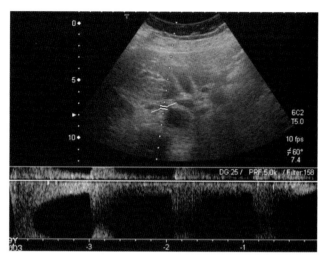

Figure 1.190
Renal artery stenosis. The right renal artery has been sampled. There is some 'cross-talk' between the channels because of difficult angle correction. However, flow velocities are greater than 2 m/s.

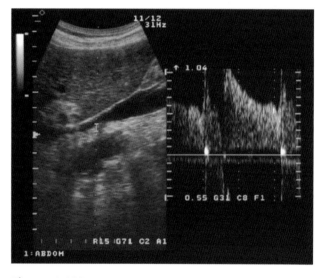

Figure 1.189
Spectral signal from the right renal artery in renal artery stenosis. There is marked aliasing of the signal with wrap around.

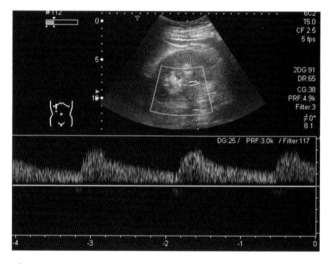

Figure 1.191
Renal artery stenosis: intrarenal findings. There is delay in the time to maximum systole. The interval between the onset of systole and peak systole is identified. This is the parvus tardus pattern.

particularly for the inexperienced, the technique can be time-consuming and frustrating. Sampling at the hilum, or in the interlobar vessels if effective, offers a rapid alternative technique requiring significantly less skill in its performance, particularly if color flow Doppler is available to facilitate the choice of optimum site for spectral analy-

sis. The characteristic features of renal artery stenosis when sampling distal to the site of the narrowing are shown in a delay in the rise to maximum systole. There is also a reduction in the pulsatility index with low flow velocities both in systole and diastole, the so-called parvus tardus pattern of proximal arterial stenosis (Figures 1.192 and 1.193).

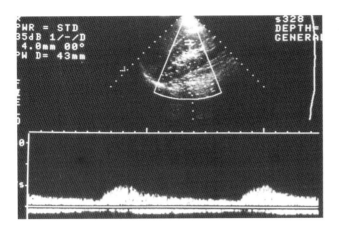

Figure 1.192
Sampling from the intrarenal vessels in renal artery stenosis.
There is marked delay in the systolic rise time and a decrease
in the pulsatility index, the so-called parvus tardus pattern.

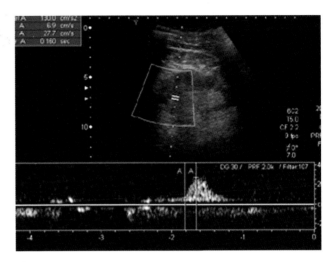

Figure 1.193
Renal artery stenosis. Difficult sampling because of patient
dyspnea (flash pulmonary edema). A prolonged TMS is,
however, demonstrated.

There is significant variation in the reported sensitivity
of duplex ultrasound and the renal hilum for the detection
of renal artery stenosis. Criteria of acceleration time and
resistance index are predominantly used. Utilizing an
acceleration time of greater than 80 ms, sensitivities as high
as 89% and specificities of 99% are reported for the diagnosis of renal artery stenosis of greater than 75% severity.
The results are reported to be better in patients over the age
of 50. Other workers, however, by contrast have suggested
that an acceleration time of greater than 100 ms demonstrates sensitivities of only 32% with a specificity of 100%.
In commenting on this, some authors suggest that the
isolated use of intrarenal Doppler sonographic criteria of
renal artery stenosis may lead to unacceptably high incidence of false-negative results.

Criteria of renal artery stenosis recorded from the main
renal artery are reported to be more accurate than
intrarenal indices. Thus, a peak systolic velocity of 2.2 m/s
or greater, together with evidence of post-stenotic turbulence, demonstrates sensitivities of 91%, specificity of 96%
and an overall accuracy of 92% for the detection of significant renal artery stenosis. However, neither intrarenal nor
main arterial studies will reliably detect polar vessels and
the stenosis associated with these, although occasionally
sampling adjacent to the renal hilum will allow the demonstration of stenosis of an accessory vessel (Figure 1.194).

Furthermore, there is an association between hypertension and raised peak velocity in all of the visceral arteries.
Similarly, there may be a relationship between hypertension and acceleration time even in the absence of renal
artery stenosis.

However, there does appear to be a role for renal
Doppler in the assessment of patients who are scheduled
for renal artery intervention. A renal artery RI of 0.8 or

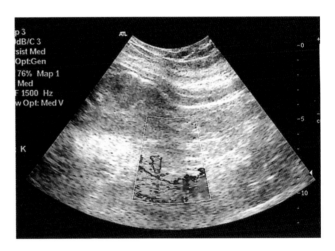

Figure 1.194
**Color flow Doppler of a lower polar renal artery on the left
demonstrates significant color aliasing consistent with
stenosis.**

greater reliably identifies patients with renal artery stenosis
in whom angioplasty or surgery will not improve renal
function, blood pressure or kidney survival. Where this is
combined with a renal length of less than 9 cm, the
outcome is universally poor.

Some workers have suggested that the use of captopril
may enhance the detection of renal artery stenosis by
duplex sonography, producing a reduction in the resistance
index in the affected artery only.

Contrast enhancement of the renal artery using
microbubble contrast agents has been reported to improve
the frequency with which the main renal artery can be

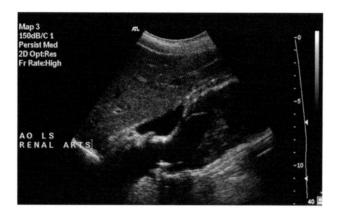

Figure 1.195
Abdominal aortic aneurysm arising below the level of the renal arteries.

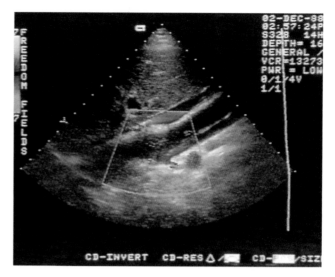

Figure 1.196
Aortic dissection. Flow down the true lumen is in the normal direction (in red). Underneath the intimal elevation there is reverse flow (in blue) and this supplies the left renal artery, producing significant compromise to the flow to the left kidney.

visualized with confidence, and therefore improve the sensitivity of evaluation of renal artery stenosis by direct interrogation of the main renal artery. However, it remains the case that other non-invasive techniques such as magnetic resonance angiography (MRA) and computed tomography angiography (CTA) may prove to have better sensitivities than duplex ultrasound and are certainly more reproducible.

Aortic aneurysm and dissecting aneurysm

Conditions affecting the aorta may also result in partial or complete compromise of the ostium of the renal arteries (Figure 1.195). Clearly, although the aortic aneurysm commonly arises below the level of the renal arteries, when these are involved in the aortic dilatation blood flow to the kidney may be compromised. Similarly, while aortic dissection extends into the abdomen in only a minority of cases, such intimal elevation may also compromise blood flow within the renal arteries (Figure 1.196).

Where an aortic dissection involves the ostium of the renal artery, flow characteristics can be variable from normal through marked diastolic spectral broadening, features characteristic of renal artery stenosis, abnormal eddy currents and complete occlusion. Duplex ultrasound may thus predict the potential for future renal function and for the development of severe hypertension.

Arteriovenous malformation and fistula

Arteriovenous malformations in the kidneys are uncommon, but usually present with severe intermittent hematuria with or without loin pain. The morphologic appear-

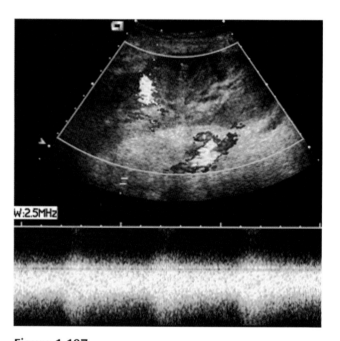

Figure 1.197
Renal transplant arteriovenous fistula. There is aliasing of color flow within the region of the fistula. Spectral Doppler shows pulsatile high-velocity flow. It is difficult to assess whether this is arterial or venous.

ances of the kidney are normal but there is a CFD (computational fluid dynamics) abnormality of the renal parenchyma manifest as a small color mosaic within the renal parenchyma. Arteriovenous fistula is most commonly the

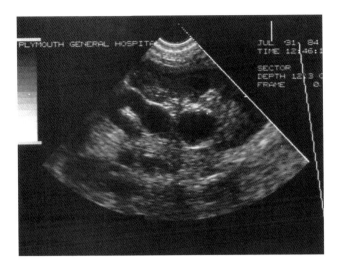

Figure 1.198
Traumatic arteriovenous fistula secondary to a stab wound.
There is massive enlargement of the left renal vein.

result of renal biopsy, although it may be due to another penetrating injury. A focal area of increased color flow at low color sensitivities in association with tissue vibration may be demonstrated. The ultrasound features are only infrequently demonstrated in the native kidney and are much more commonly seen in the renal transplant (Figure 1.197).

The appearances depend upon the degree of arteriovenous shunting. Rarely, where the shunt is large, there is an increase in the size of the supplying artery and the draining vein. Both vessels may become tortuous and are demonstrated as serpiginous echo-frec structures extending into the hilum of the kidney (Figure 1.198). Doppler-derived flow studies will demonstrate increased flow velocities in both the renal artery and the renal vein, frequently with arterialization of renal venous flow and absence of resistance to flow in diastole with low pulsatility indices.

Although intrarenal varices are uncommon, they may produce similar appearances. Similarly lienorenal varices will produce the appearance of distended vessels at the renal hilum, although it should be possible to trace the connection with the splenic vein.

Renal vein thrombosis

Renal vein thrombosis is unusual in the absence of associated focal disease of the kidney in adults, although it can, rarely, occur as a result of severe hypovolemic shock. More commonly, it occurs secondary to pathology which compromises the integrity of the renal vein, including compression, invasion by tumor, usually of renal origin,

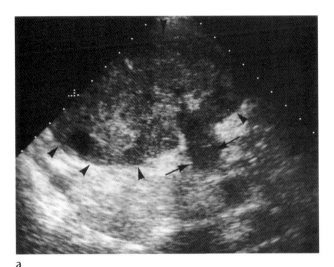

a

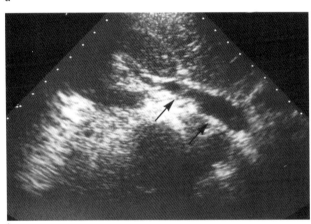

b

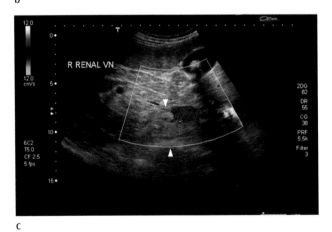

c

Figure 1.199
(a) **Renal vein thrombosis.** The kidney (arrowheads) is enlarged, globular and of inhomogeneous echo pattern. The renal vein (arrows) is distended and contains material of low echogenicity consistent with thrombus. (b) **Partial venous thrombosis.** The renal vein is distended. There is clot adherent to the wall of the renal vein but there remains a renal vein lumen. (c) **Partial occlusion of the right renal vein.** The vein is distended (arrowheads). There is some evidence of marginal flow demonstrated by the red and blue coloration.

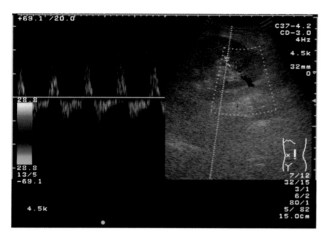

Figure 1.200
Renal vein thrombosis, native kidney. The spectral pattern demonstrates reverse flow in diastole. The W shape is not as characteristic as is usually demonstrated in the renal transplant.

and trauma. Features of renal vein thrombosis include diffuse enlargement of the kidney with decreased reflectivity and loss of corticomedullary differentiation (Figure 1.199a,b). The renal vein becomes distended with echogenic material and neither color flow nor spectral Doppler signal can be obtained. In partial renal venous thrombosis, color flow may be demonstrated around the margin of the thrombus (Figure 1.199c). In complete thrombosis of the renal vein, there is increased peripheral resistance to flow with reversal of flow in diastole, producing a W shape of the diastolic flow component similar to that seen in renal transplantation (Figure 1.200).

Renal trauma

Renal trauma may be the result of penetrating or blunt injury. Similarly, acceleration/deceleration injuries may result in trauma to the renal pedicle, with partial or complete avulsion. As a general rule, although the kidney is commonly involved in trauma, it usually heals spontaneously with few sequelae. The management depends therefore rather less upon features demonstrated by imaging techniques than upon patient well-being. Indications for surgical intervention depend more upon life-threatening hematuria than upon gross renal disruption demonstrated on ultrasound imaging, although surgical intervention in penetrating injury may be necessary to control hemorrhage. Furthermore, the management of patients with blunt renal injury depends more upon associated injuries to other organs than on renal trauma itself.

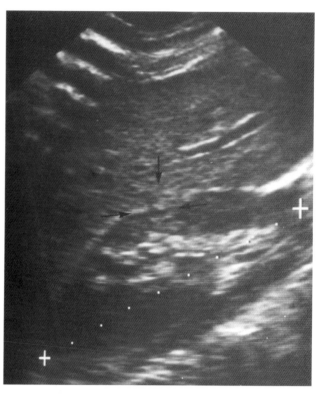

Figure 1.201
Minor renal trauma. There is a shallow cortical laceration identified by the arrows. The renal capsule is disrupted and there is echogenic hematoma extending as far as the medullary pyramids.

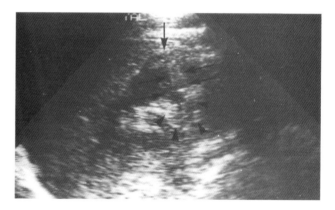

Figure 1.202
Renal trauma. In this case the laceration extends through the renal parenchyma (arrows) to produce a forniceal rupture (arrowheads). There is a small subcapsular hematoma.

The degree of renal trauma may be described as minor or major. In minor trauma, the kidney may simply be contused, in which case ultrasound examination is frequently normal. There may be shallow cortical laceration or a forniceal disruption (Figures 1.201 and 1.202). It

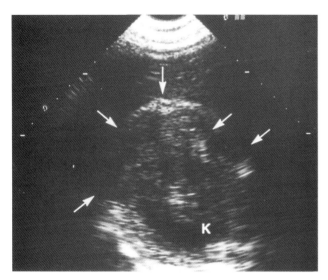

Figure 1.203
Same patient as Figure 1.202 36 hours later. Transverse scan demonstrating the kidney (K). The anterior hematoma (arrows) has increased markedly in size.

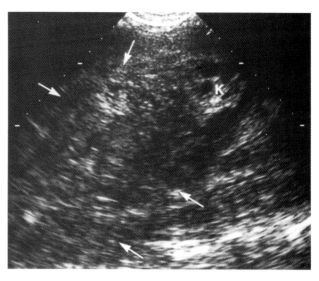

Figure 1.205
Shattered kidney. The upper pole of the kidney (K) is completely unrecognizable. There is extensive hematoma, which involves the retroperitoneum as well as the renal substance (arrows).

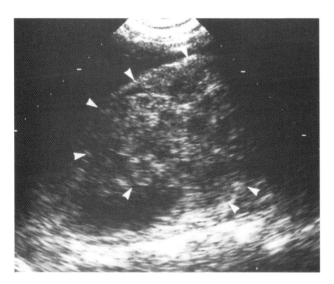

Figure 1.204
Major renal trauma. Deep laceration into the mid-pole of the kidney with disrupted fragments. The upper pole retains its normal morphologic features. There is extensive hemorrhage into the lower pole (arrowheads).

may be difficult to differentiate shallow from deep cortical laceration, except where there is disruption of the renal fragments (Figures 1.203 and 1.204). Such multiple deep lacerations will produce a shattered kidney. In any of these conditions, there may be not only an adjacent hematoma but also a urine leak (Figure 1.205). Damage to the renal pedicle is difficult to demonstrate on ultrasound imaging (Figure 1.206). However, vascular compromise of the traumatized kidney may be detectable using color flow and spectral Doppler examination.

Rupture of the parenchyma produces a focal linear or wedge-shaped area within the kidney of increased or decreased reflectivity. When there is disruption of the fragments of the kidney, a hematoma between the fragments can be demonstrated, either as an echo-free collection of fluid or, depending upon the degree of development of clot, by a variable degree of inhomogeneity of the echo pattern. In minor cases of renal laceration the hematoma is frequently contained within the renal capsule. Where the laceration is more severe, the hematoma will extend into Gerota's fascia as a pararenal hematoma (Figure 1.207).

Although ultrasound may lack the sensitivity of CT in the demonstration of the extent of trauma, there remain major advantages. Ultrasound can be performed in the emergency room during resuscitation. It can be used rapidly to assess major degrees of intra-abdominal trauma in the severely injured patient, to assess the contribution of renal and other intra-abdominal injury to the patient's condition and thus focus clinical attention. CT will invariably be required in the severely injured patient, but the initial assessment of the severity and site of abdominal injury allows time for resuscitation and planning of initial management (Figure 1.208). If there is no intraperitoneal fluid, no sign of renal abnormality or perirenal fluid collection, nor any features to suggest injury to another organ,

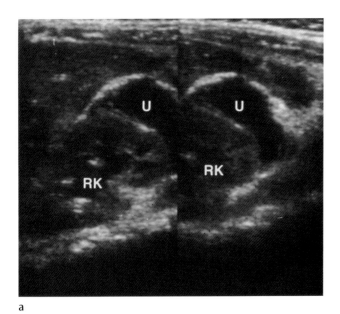

a

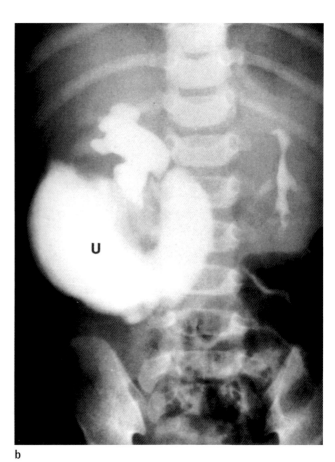

b

Figure 1.206
(a) Longitudinal ultrasound scan through the right kidney (RK) which demonstrates dilatation of the collecting system and a urinoma (U) at the lower pole. The linear array partially overlapping composite scan demonstrates the extent of the urinoma. **(b) Intravenous urogram 48 hours later.** The urinoma has increased in size (U).

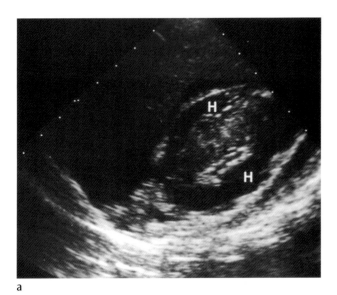

a

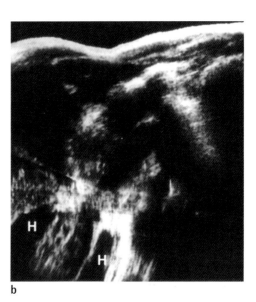

b

Figure 1.207
Longitudinal (a) and transverse (b) scans of different patients with renal pedicle compromise. There are large perirenal hematomata (H) but the kidney is small. We have seen this appearance in two cases of trauma to the renal pedicle.

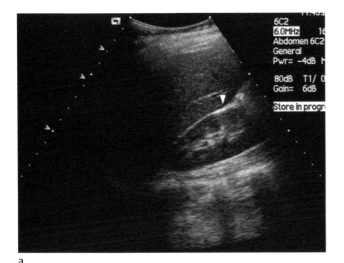

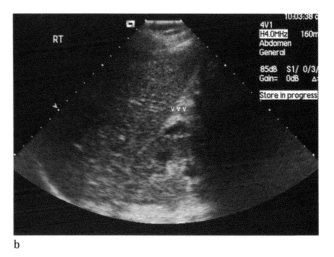

a

b

Figure 1.208
Abdominal trauma. (a) There is a small amount of anterior pararenal fluid (arrowhead). (b) There is complex fluid anterior to the kidney (arrowheads), with mild irregularity of the anterior renal parenchyma.

and the patient is clinically stable, then no further examination needs to be performed, although follow-up with ultrasound may be indicated, depending upon the clinical condition.

Page kidney

Page kidney is the association between hypertension and either acute or chronic unilateral, subcapsular or perinephric hematoma. It is usually associated with a history of blunt trauma to the kidney, although it may be consequent upon penetrating trauma.

In generalized severe injury, particularly where there is crush injury involving muscles, acute renal failure will ensue. There is an association between the renal failure associated with crush injury and abnormality of RI. Patients with severe crush injury present with RIs of the order of 0.8 or greater. The rate of change of the RI correlates well with the speed of recovery of the acute renal failure.

Medical renal disease

Ultrasound examination of the kidney is the examination of first choice in patients presenting with acute and chronic renal failure. Acute renal failure is defined as a rapid decline in glomerular filtration rate with accompanying accumulation of nitrogen waste products. The etiology may be prerenal, consequent upon renal hypoperfusion; renal, usually associated with renal parenchymal disease; or postrenal,

consequent upon obstruction. In prerenal failure, morphologic features of the kidney will usually be normal. There is no change in size or echogenicity. Doppler characteristics may reflect the hypovolemia and poor cardiac output with diminished velocities of arterial flow.

Diffuse parenchymal renal disease

In the diffuse parenchymal diseases, findings are inconstant. The acute nephritides, such as acute glomerulonephritis, may produce an increase in renal size as is the

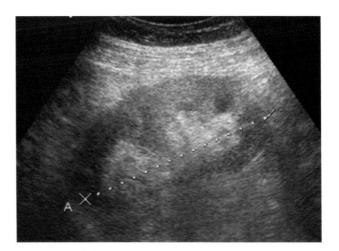

Figure 1.209
Diabetic nephropathy. The kidney is enlarged and of increased reflectivity.

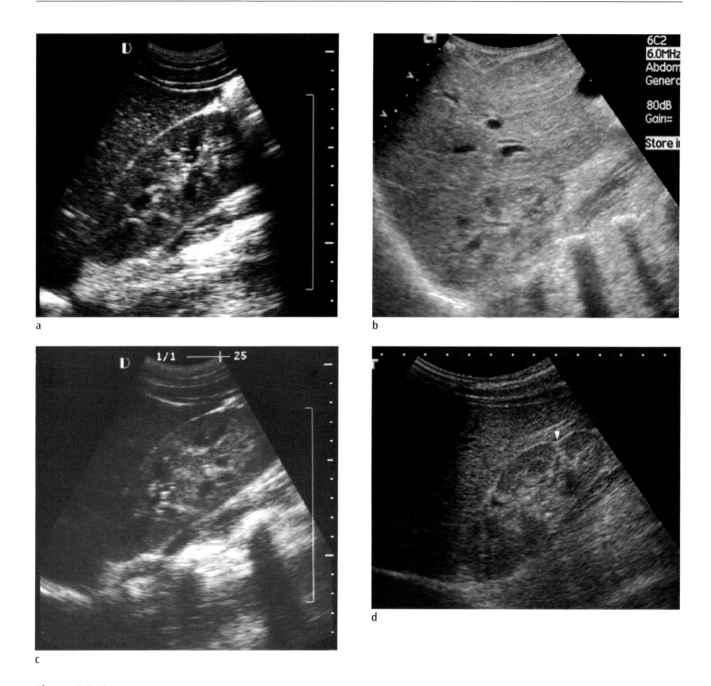

Figure 1.210
Medical renal disease. (a) The echogenicity of the cortex is equivalent to that of the adjacent liver. (b) The echogenicity of the kidney is equivalent to that of the adjacent liver. It becomes difficult to identify the kidney separate from the liver, particularly when the echogenicity is close to that of the renal capsule. (c) The echogenicity of the renal parenchyma is greater than that of the adjacent liver. There is prominence of the medullary pyramids. (d) Diabetic kidney. The echogenicity of the renal cortex is increased, but this is difficult to assess because of increased reflectivity of the adjacent liver, presumably due to fatty change. Incidental note is made of a cortical scar at the lower pole (arrowhead).

case in the diuretic phase of diabetic nephropathy (Figure 1.209). Changes in cortical reflectivity are also variable. Classically, there is an increase in cortical reflectivity with some loss of clarity of the margins between the cortex and the medullary pyramids, although the pyramids themselves may be enlarged and echo-poor. Cortical echogenicity is usually assessed by comparison with the adjacent liver or spleen and therefore requires prior knowledge of the status of these organs. Where there is increased reflectivity of the liver consequent upon fatty replacement or chronic

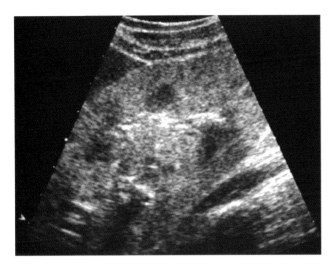

Figure 1.211
Medical renal disease. Increased reflectivity of the cortex with echo-poor medullary pyramids but with poor definition of the margins.

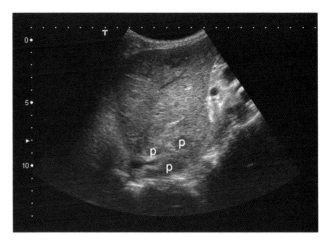

Figure 1.212
Medical renal disease. The kidney is apparent only because of the presence of prominent medullary pyramids (P).

liver disease, for example, this may influence the ability to assess renal cortical and medullary echogenicity. The echogenicity of the renal cortex is described as either equal to or less than the echogenicity of the liver parenchyma (Figure 1.210). It is important to assess these at exactly the same depth in the patient given the sound attenuation that occurs with depth. It is possible to quantify renal cortical echogenicity by an assessment of the mean pixel density. Utilizing this method, the echogenicity of normal kidneys is demonstrated to be significantly less than that of the liver, with a range of 0.810–0.987. Clearly, with a ratio close to 1 at the upper end of the range, these kidneys would have cortices indistinguishable in echogenicity from the adjacent liver. Thus, while there is clearly a role for ultrasound when cortical echogenicity is increased when compared to the liver, in identifying diffuse parenchymal renal disease there is a significant area of overlap between normal and abnormal when cortical echogenicity approximates to that of the liver.

Since glomeruli in the adult kidney only occupy approximately 8% of the cortex, it is possible that early changes of renal disease which are confined to the glomerulus will not produce changes in echogenicity of the cortex. Thus, vascular and tubulo interstitial abnormalities of the kidney would be more likely to produce changes in echogenicity.

Prominence of the medullary pyramids is a non-specific finding, but is less commonly seen than cortical changes. It is presumed to result from congestion and edema of the medulla, although with increasing number of hyaline casts the pyramids become less distinct and the corticomedullary differentiation is lost (Figures 1.211 and 1.212).

Conditions causing increased cortical echogenicity and prominent corticomedullary differentiation

The classical picture of the kidney in diffuse parenchymal renal disease is that of an enlarged or normal-sized kidney whose cortical echogenicity is greater than that of the adjacent liver (Table 1.5), approaching that of the renal sinus but with prominent echo-poor medullary pyramids.

Table 1.5 *Causes of diffuse renal disease detected by ultrasound*

Membranous and chronic glomerulonephritis

Nephrosclerosis

Amyloidosis

Leukemic infiltration

Acute tubular necrosis

Alport's syndrome

Lupus nephritis

Polycythemia

Glomerulosclerosis

Diabetic renal disease

Preeclampsia

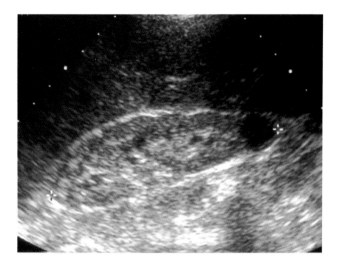

Figure 1.213
AIDS-related renal disease. There is cortical hyperechogenicity with echogenic bands.

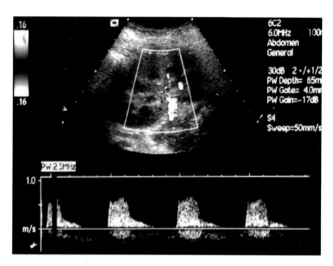

Figure 1.214
Medical renal disease. Absent diastolic flow in severe acute glomerulonephritis.

AIDS

Patients with AIDS are more susceptible to a wide variety of renal disease. These include pyelonephritis, abscess formation, tuberculosis and fungal infection. In addition, patients with AIDS have a predisposition for the development of non-Hodgkin's lymphoma and Kaposi's sarcoma. While nodal involvement may occur, parenchymal involvement is also apparent.

Renal obstruction can occur as a consequence of infection and obstruction consequent upon tumor.

In addition, patients with AIDS may develop an AIDS nephropathy. In approximately half of these patients with deteriorating renal function, ultrasound appearances of the kidney are normal. However, in the remainder there is increased cortical echogenicity, which is related to glomerulosclerosis, interstitial infiltration and/or proliferative glomerulonephritis. There is associated tubular dilatation. The changes of increased reflectivity are, however, indistinguishable from parenchymal renal disease in non-AIDS sufferers. However, in some patients with AIDS-related nephropathy, the pattern of cortical hyperechogenicity exhibits a particular finding of heterogeneity, with a feature of echogenic bands that extend from the central kidney to the cortex (Figure 1.213). The renal sinus becomes less apparent.

Opportunistic infection typically will produce focal echogenic densities scattered throughout the cortex and to the medulla. Some of these are sharp, while others are less well-defined. They may vary in size and, in some cases, develop rapidly. They have been reported in diseases caused by *Pneumocystis carinii* and *Mycobacterium avium-intracellulare* and in histoplasmosis.

Doppler studies in parenchymal renal disease

Doppler signal recording from the main and branch renal arteries in parenchymal renal disease may yield specific spectral changes. There is loss of diastolic flow and a gradually increasing resistance or pulsatility index correlating with the rising serum creatinine. In one series, RIs in parenchymal renal disease were reported as high as 0.82, whereas in controls the normal value was 0.63 (Figure 1.214). In contrast, however, Mostbeck et al found little correlation between renal parenchymal disease and Doppler indices and only weak correlation with the serum creatinine.

The only form of renal disease shown to have any significant correlation with altered RI in this study was in those patients with arteriosclerosis. There is little doubt that blood flow characteristics will alter in certain parenchymal renal diseases and that the severity of renal disease is often reflected in the degree of abnormality of the Doppler spectrum. However, these are neither sufficiently sensitive to detect renal disease nor sufficiently specific to exclude other pathologies. There may be a role in the evaluation of disease progress but, largely, this is more effectively and simply performed using biochemical parameters.

Acute cortical necrosis

Acute cortical necrosis is a rare cause of acute renal failure secondary to shock as a result of sepsis, myocardial

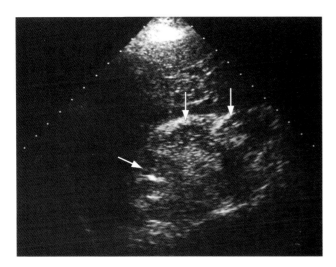

Figure 1.215
Cortical calcification (arrows) is seen in this case of acute cortical necrosis.

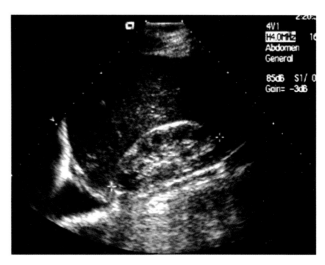

Figure 1.216
Lupus nephritis. There is increased echogenicity of the cortex with a somewhat lobular pattern.

infarction, hypovolemia, etc. The appearances on ultrasound are said to be characteristic, with loss of the corticomedullary junction and marked increase in echogenicity of the outer rim of the cortex even in the absence of calcification. The appearances are said to correlate with the area of cortical necrosis seen at histology (Figure 1.215).

Lupus nephritis

In some cases of systemic lupus erythematosus, a characteristic appearance is said to occur. In addition to the hyperechoic renal cortex, several areas of focal abnormality within the cortical substance produce localized hypoechoic areas with consequent distortion of renal anatomy (Figure 1.216). This appears to be associated with a particularly aggressive form of systemic lupus erythematosus.

Increased medullary echogenicity

The normal renal medulla has lower echogenicity than the cortex. In a number of conditions there is significant increase in medullary echogenicity. Commonly, this is due to calcification within the renal medulla and is therefore associated with any of the causes of medullary nephrocalcinosis (Table 1.6).

The earliest signs of nephrocalcinosis and other pathologies causing increased medullary echogenicity are reported to be the appearance of echogenic rings in the periphery of the medullary pyramids. These rings appear to outline the margin of the medullary pyramids, are not

Table 1.6 *Hyperechoic renal medulla*	
Nephrocalcinosis	Medullary sponge kidney, hyperparathyroidism, sarcoidosis, tubular acidosis, milk alkali syndrome, Sjögren's syndrome
Gout	Secondary to urate deposition and including Lesch–Nyhan syndrome
Primary aldosteronism	Secondary to hypokalemia
Pseudo-Bartter syndrome	Secondary to hypokalemia

accompanied by acoustic shadowing and appear to be the precursor of full-blown medullary hyperechogenicity (Figures 1.217–1.219).

Cortical calcification

This is a rarely reported phenomenon but occurs in oxalosis, metastatic tumors, islet cell neoplasms, chronic glomerulonephritis, renal cortical necrosis and Alport's syndrome.

Papillary necrosis

In this condition the papillae of the pyramids undergo ischemic necrosis, become enlarged, may slough and

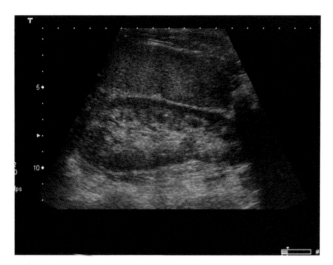

Figure 1.217
Early medullary calcinosis. There is marginal increased echogenicity around the medullary pyramids.

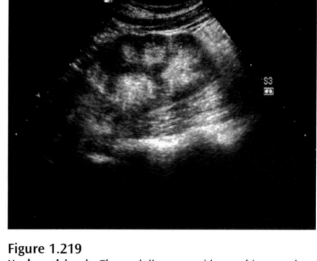

Figure 1.219
Nephrocalcinosis. The medullary pyramids are of increased reflectivity and exhibit ill-defined acoustic shadowing.

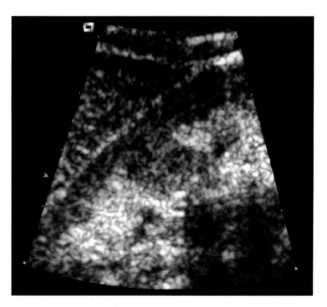

Figure 1.218
Magnified view of medullary pyramids in medullary sponge kidney.

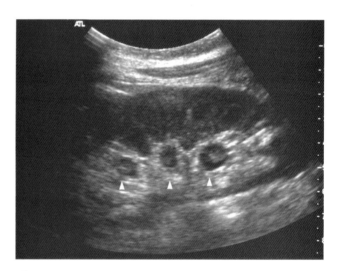

Figure 1.220
Papillary necrosis. Large edematous papillae are identified within the center of the renal calyces (arrowheads).

cause obstructive symptoms (Figure 1.220). They may become calcified (Figure 1.221). The condition is secondary to a variety of pathologic causes, including phenacetin abuse, diabetes mellitus, sickle cell disease, pyelonephritis, acute tubular necrosis and long-term renal obstruction. The features of the condition are variable but include prominent papillae projecting into the calyces. These may or may not be calcified and thus

produce an acoustic shadow. When no acoustic shadow is present, it is difficult to differentiate the prominent abnormal papilla from a normal papilla projecting into the calyx in obstruction. When the papilla has sloughed, round or triangular fluid-filled spaces are demonstrated at the apices of the pyramids, communicating with the calyces. Sloughing of the papillae may result in obstructive appearances, which are then difficult to distinguish

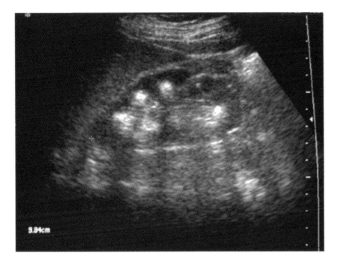

Figure 1.221
Papillary necrosis. The renal papillae are now of increased reflectivity and exhibit acoustic shadowing consistent with calcification.

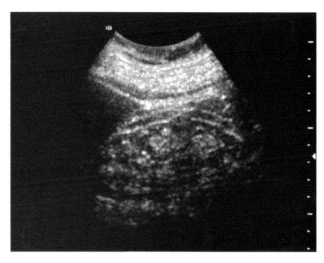

Figure 1.223
Papillary necrosis. The kidney is small and difficult to identify. The medullary pyramids appear bright, although acoustic shadowing is difficult to identify.

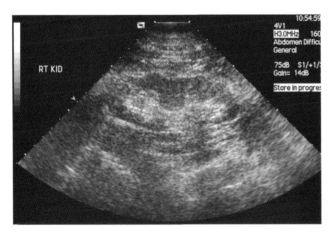

Figure 1.222
Chronic renal disease. The kidney is small and of slightly increased echogenicity. There is irregularity of the margin. There is broadening of the renal sinus. These appearances are of postobstructive atrophy.

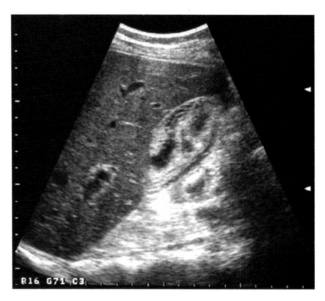

Figure 1.224
End-stage kidney. The kidney is small and of increased reflectivity. There is dilatation of the calyces and focal cortical loss at the upper pole. The patient had chronic pyelonephritis.

from other causes of obstruction unless other calcified papilli are demonstrated within the kidney.

Chronic renal disease

In chronic renal failure, differentiation between different causes becomes increasingly difficult. The patient with increased cortical echogenicity due to, for example, glomerulonephritis, will gradually develop a loss of the corticomedullary differentiation. Subsequently, further increased echogenicity of the cortex will occur until the echogenicity of the cortex, medulla and renal sinus blend. The kidney reduces in size and the end-stage kidney – small, shrunken and of an echogenicity equivalent to that of perirenal fat – is frequently almost unidentifiable within

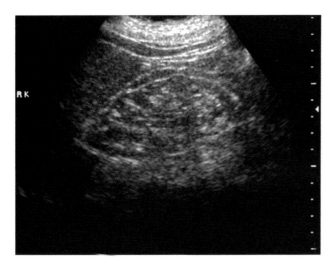

Figure 1.225
End-stage kidney. The kidney, while not of marked increased reflectivity, is extremely similar to the surrounding perirenal fat. Differentiation of internal structure is difficult.

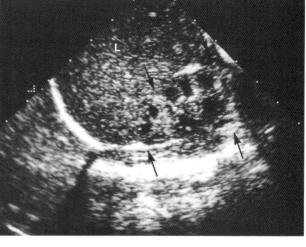

Figure 1.227
The kidney (arrows) almost blends with the adjacent liver (L) in this case of lupus nephritis.

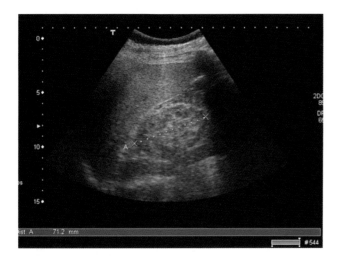

Figure 1.226
Chronic glomerulonephritis. The kidney is small and echogenic.

the renal fossa. The end-stage kidney is the final feature of renal disease from a variety of causes (Figures 1.222–1.227).

As chronic renal failure ensues, the Doppler findings become increasingly abnormal. Blood flow characteristics in the main and branch renal arteries show progressive loss of diastolic flow with its eventual absence. In the end-stage kidney, systolic velocities are also low and may be undetectable even with the use of color flow capability.

In one case under our care, this pattern in a patient with chronic renal failure reverted to near normal with higher systolic velocities and reinstatement of diastolic flow with the development of a renal carcinoma.

References

1. Robertson R, Murphy A, Dubbins PA. Renal artery stenosis: the use of duplex ultrasound as a screening technique. Br J Radiol 1988; 61(723): 196–201.
2. Chen JH, Pu YS, Liu SP, Chiu TY. Renal hemodynamics in patients with obstructive uropathy evaluated by duplex Doppler sonography. J Urol 1993; 150(1): 18–21.
3. Opdenakker L, Oyen R, Vervloessem I, et al. Acute obstruction of the renal collecting system: the intrarenal resistive index is a useful yet time-dependent parameter for diagnosis. Eur Radiol 1998; 8(8): 1429–32.
4. Bateman GA, Cuganesan R. Renal vein Doppler sonography of obstructive uropathy. AJR Am J Roentgenol 2002; 178(4): 921–5.
5. Fowler KA, Locken JA, Duchesne JH, Williamson MR. US for detecting renal calculi with nonenhanced CT as a reference standard. Radiology 2002; 222(1): 109–13.
6. Geavlete P, Georgescu D, Cauni V, Nita G. Value of duplex Doppler ultrasonography in renal colic. Eur Urol 2002; 41(1): 71–8.
7. Mindell HJ. Do all homogeneously echogenic renal lesions that are smaller than 1.5 cm and are seen incidentally on sonograms (lesions presumed to be angiomyolipomas) require CT to confirm fat content of such lesions? AJR Am J Roentgenol 1996; 167(6): 1590.
8. Siegel CL, Middleton WD, Teefey SA, McClennan BL. Angiomyolipoma and renal cell carcinoma: US differentiation. Radiology 1996; 198(3): 789–93.
9. Hirai T, Ohishi H, Yamada R, et al. Usefulness of color Doppler flow imaging in differential diagnosis of multilocular cystic lesions of the kidney. J Ultrasound Med 1995; 14(10): 771–6.

10. Taniguchi N, Itoh K, Nakamura S, et al. Differentiation of renal cell carcinomas from angiomyolipomas by ultrasonic frequency dependent attenuation. J Urol 1997; 157(4): 1242–5.

11. Jinzaki M, Ohkuma K, Tanimoto A, et al. Small solid renal lesions: usefulness of power Doppler US. Radiology 1998; 209(2): 543–50.

12. Quaia E, Siracusano S, Bertolotto M, Monduzzi M, Mucelli RP. Characterization of renal tumours with pulse inversion harmonic imaging by intermittent high mechanical index technique: initial results. Eur Radiol 2003; 13(6): 1402–12.

13. Ascenti G, Zimbaro G, Mazziotti S, et al. Usefulness of power Doppler and contrast-enhanced sonography in the differentiation of hyperechoic renal masses. Abdom Imaging 2001; 26(6): 654–60.

14. Hadas-Halpern I, Farkas A, Patlas M, et al. Sonographic diagnosis of ureteral tumors. J Ultrasound Med 1999; 18(9): 639–45.

15. Yeh HC, Halton KP, Shapiro RS, Rabinowitz JG, Mitty HA. Junctional parenchyma: revised definition of hypertrophic column of Bertin. Radiology 1992; 185(3): 725–32.

16. Yeh HC, Halton KP, Shapiro RS, Rabinowitz JG, Mitty HA. Junctional parenchyma: revised definition of hypertrophic column of Bertin. Radiology 1992; 185(3): 725–32.

17. Millward SF, Lanctin HP, Lewandowski BJ, Lum PA. Fat-filled post-operative renal pseudotumour: variable appearance in ultrasonography images. Can Assoc Radiol J 1992; 43(2): 116–9.

18. WHO Informal Working Group. International classification of ultrasound images in cystic echinococcosis for application in clinical and field epidemiological settings. Acta Trop 2003; 85(2): 253–61.

19. Mostbeck GH, Kain R, Mallek R, et al. Duplex Doppler sonography in renal parenchymal disease. Histopathologic correlation. J Ultrasound Med 1991; 10(4): 189–94.

Further reading

General and anatomy

Akpinar IN, Altun E, Avcu S, et al. Sonographic measurement of kidney size in geriatric patients. J Clin Ultrasound 2003; 31(6): 315–18.

Dalla Palma L, Bazzocchi M, Cressa C, Thommasini G. Radiological anatomy revisited. Br J Radiol 1990; 63: 680–90.

Emamin SA, Nielsen MB, Pedersen JF, Ytte L. Sonographic evaluation of renal appearance in 665 adult volunteers. Correlation with age and obesity. Acta Radiol 1993; 34(5): 482–5.

Gillard JM, Talner LB, Pinckney L. Normal renal papillae simulating calyceal filling defects on sonography. AJR Am J Roentgenol 1987; 148: 895–6.

Harrison RG. The urogenital system. In: Romanes GJ, ed. Cunningham's textbook of anatomy. London: Oxford University Press, 1964: 475–86.

Millward S, Lanctin H, Lewandowski B, Lum P. Fat filled post-operative renal pseudo-tumor, variable appearance in ultrasonography images. Journal de l'association Canadien des Radiologiste 1992; 43(2): 116–19.

Ninan VT, Koshi T, Niyamthulla MM, et al. A comparative study of methods of estimating renal size in normal adults. Nephrol Dial Transplant 1990; 5: 851–4.

Patriquin H, Lefaivre JF, Lafortune M. Fetal lobation, an anatomo-ultrasonographic correlation. J Ultrasound Med 1999; 191–7.

Shokeir AA, Abubieh EA, Dawaba M, El-Azab M. Resistive index of the solitary kidney, a clinical study of normal values. J Urol 2003; 170(2 Pt 1): 377–9.

Yeh HC, Halton KP, Shapiro RS, Rabinowitz JG, Miti HA. Junctional

parenchyma, revised definition of hypertrophied column of Bertin. Radiology 1992; 185(3): 325–32.

Zubarev A. Ultrasound of renal vessels. Eur Radiol 2001; 11: 1902–15.

Ultrasound contrast

Ascenti G, Zimbaro G, Mazziotti S, et al. Contrast enhanced power doppler ultrasound in the diagnosis of renal pseudo-tumors. Eur Radiol 2001; 11: 2496–9.

Kim JH, Eun HW, Lee HK, et al. Renal perfusion abnormality. Coded harmonic angio-ultrasound with contrast agent. Acta Radiol 2003; 44(2): 166–71.

Puls R, Hosten N, Lemke M, et al. Perfusion abnormalities of kidney parenchyma: microvascular imaging with contrast-enhanced colour and power Doppler ultrasonography – preliminary results. J Ultrasound Med 2000; 19(12): 817–21.

Robbin M, Lockhart M, Barr R. Renal imaging with ultrasound contrast: current status. Radiol Clin North Am 2003; 41: 963–78.

Congenital

Banerjee B, Brett I. Ultrasound diagnosis of horseshoe kidney. Br J Radiol 1991; 64: 898–900.

Gritzmann N, Czembirek H, Karnel F. Pulsed duplex sonography in the detection of lower pole arteries in hydronephrosis. Radiologe 1986; 26: 503–5.

Lubat E, Hernanz-Schulman M, Genieser NB. Sonography of the simple and complicated ipsilateral fused kidney. J Ultrasound Med 1989; 8: 109–14.

MacPherson RI. Supernumerary kidney typical and atypical features. Can Assoc Radiol J 1987; 38: 116–19.

Saxey R. Sonographic findings in crossed renal ectobia without fusion. AJR Am J Roentgenol 1990; 154: 657.

Obstruction

Asrat T, Roossin MC, Miller EI. Ultrasonographic detection of ureteral jets in normal pregnancy. Am J Obstet Gynaecol 1998; 178(6): 1194–8.

Bateman GA, Cuganesan R. Renal vein Doppler sonography of obstructive uroprothy. AJR Am J Roentgenol 2002; 178(4): 921–5.

Cronan JJ, Tublin ME. Role of the resistive index in the evaluation of acute renal obstruction. AJR Am J Roentgenol 1995; 164(2): 377–8.

Cvitkovic, Kuzmic A, Brkljacic B, Rados M, Galesic K. Doppler visualisation of ureteric jets in unilateral hydronephrosis in children and adolescents. Eur J Radiol 2001; 39(3): 209–14.

Dubbins, PA, Kurtz AB, Darby J, Goldberg BB. Ureteric jet effect, the echographic appearance of urine entering the bladder. A means of identifying the bladder trigone and assessment of ureteral function. Radiology 1981; 140(2): 513–5.

Geavlet E, Georgescu D, Cauni V, Nita G. Value of duplex Doppler ultrasonography in renal colic. Eur Urol 2002; 41(1): 71–8.

Juul N, Torp-Pedersen S, Nielsen H. Abdominal ultrasound versus intravenous urography in the evaluation of intravesically obstructed males. Scand J Urol Nephrol 1989; 23: 89–92.

Mirk P, Maresca G, Fileni A, et al. Sonography of normal lower ureters. J Clin Ultrasound 1988; 16: 635–42.

Nicolau C, Vilana R, Del Amo M, et al. Accuracy of sonography with a hydration test in differentiation between excretory renal obstruction and renal sinus cysts. J Clin Ultrasound 2002; 30(9): 532–6.

Opdenakker L, Oyen R, Vervloessem I, et al. Acute obstruction of the renal collecting system: the intrarenal resistive index is a useful yet time dependent parameter for diagnosis. Eur Radiol 1998; 8(8): 1429–32.

Patel U, Kellet MJ. Ureteric drainage and peristalsis after stenting studied using color Doppler ultrasound. Br J Urol 1996; 77(4): 530–5.

Platt JF. Urinary obstruction. Radiol Clin North Am 1996; 34(6): 1113–29.

Renowden SA, Cochlin DL. The potential use of diuresis Doppler sonography in PUJ obstruction. Clin Radiol 1992; 46: 94–6.

Shokeir AA, Abdulmaaboud M. Prospective comparison of nonenhanced helical computerized tomography and Doppler ultrasonography for the diagnosis of renal colic. J Urol 2001; 165(4): 1082–4.

Shokeir AA, Mahran MR, Abdulmaaboud M. Renal colic in pregnant women: role of renal resistive index. Urology 2000; 55(3): 344–7.

Vigayaraghavan SB, Kandasamy SV, Mylsamy A, Prabhakar M. Sonographic features of necrosed renal papillae causing hydronephrosis. J Ultrasound Med 2003; 22(9): 951–6.

Wachsberg RH. Unilateral absence of ureteral jets in the third trimester of pregnancy. Pitfall in colour Doppler ultrasound diagnosis of urinary obstruction. Radiology 1998; 209(1): 279–81.

Renal and ureteric calculus disease

Howler KA, Locken JA, Duchesne JH, Williamson MR. Ultrasound for detecting renal calculi with non-enhanced CT as a reference standard. Radiology 2002; 222(1): 109–13.

Marumo MK, Horiguchi Y, Nakagawa K, et al. Significance in diagnostic accuracy of renal calculi found by ultrasonography in patients with asymptomatic microscopic hematuria. Int J Urol 2002; 9(7): 363–7.

Patlas M, Farkas A, Fisher D, et al. Ultrasound versus CT for the detection of ureteric stones in patients with renal colic. Br J Radiol 2001; 74(886): 901–4.

Renal cystic disease

Aronson S, Frasier HA, Baluch JD, et al. Cystic renal masses usefulness of the Bosniak classification. Urol Radiol 1991; 13: 83–90.

Fick-Brosnahan GM, Belz MM, McFann KK, et al. Relationship between renal volume growth and renal function in autosomal dominant polycystic kidney disease: a longitudinal study. Am J Kidney Dis 2002; 39(6): 1127–34.

Gasparini D, Sponza M, Valotto C, et al. Renal cysts: can percutaneous ethanol injections be considered an alternative to surgery? Urol Int 2003; 71(2): 197–200.

Kier R, Taylor KJW, Feyock AL, Ramos IM. Renal masses: characterisation with Doppler US. Radiology 1990; 176: 703–7.

Kondo A, Akakura K, Ito H. Assessment of renal function with colour Doppler ultrasound in autosomal dominant polycystic kidney disease. Int J Urol 2001; 8(3): 95–8.

Melekos MD, Kosti P, Zarakovitis IE, Dimopoulos PA. Milk of calcium cysts masquerading as renal calculi. Eur J Radiol 1998; 28: 62–6.

Narla LD, Slovis TL, Watts FB, Nigro M. The renal lesions of tuberose sclerosis (cysts and angiomyolipoma) – screening with sonography and computerized tomography. Pediatr Radiol 1988; 18: 205–9.

Ravine D, Gibson R, Walker R, et al. Evaluation of ultrasonographic diagnostic criteria for autosomal dominant polycystic kidney disease. Lancet 1994; 343: 824–7.

Terada N, Ishioka K, Matsuta Y, et al. The natural history of simple renal cysts. J Urol 2002; 167(1): 21–3.

Renal tumor

Ascenti G, Zimbaro G, Mazziotti S. Usefulness of power Doppler and contrast-enhanced sonography in the differentiation of hyperechoic renal masses. Abdom Imaging 2001; 26(6): 654–60.

Bos S, Mensink H. Can duplex Doppler ultrasound replace computerised tomography in staging patients with renal cell carcinoma. Scand J Urol Nephrol 1998; 32: 87–91.

Casper KA, Donnelly LF, Chen B, Bissler JJ. Tuberose sclerosis complex: renal imaging findings. Radiology 2002; 225(2): 451–6.

Choyke PL, White EM, Zeman RK, et al. Renal metastases, clinico-pathologic and radiologic correlation. Radiology 1987; 162: 359–63.

Cittadini G, Mucelli F, Danza F, et al, Aggressive renal angiomyolipoma. Acta Radiol 1996; 37: 927–32.

Filipas D, Spix C, Schulz-Lampel D, et al. Screening for renal cell carcinoma using ultrasonography: a feasibility study. BJU Int 2003; 7: 595–9.

Gorg C, Weide R, Schwerk WB. Sonographic patterns in extra-nodal and abdominal lymphomas. Eur Radiol 1996; 6: 855–64.

Gossios K, Argyropoulou M, Vazakas P. Bilateral papillary renal carcinoma. Eur Radiol 2001; 11: 242–5.

Hadas-Halpern I, Farkas A, Patlas M, et al. Sonographic diagnosis of ureteral tumors. J Ultrasound Med 1999; 18: 639–45.

Hartman DS, Davis CJ, Sanders RC, et al. The multiloculated renal mass: considerations and differential features. Radiographics 1987; 7: 29–52.

Hartman DS, Davidson AJ, Davis CJ Jr, Goldman SM. Infiltrative renal lesions: CT–sonographic–pathologic correlation. AJR Am J Roentgenol 1988; 150: 1061–4.

Jantschek G, Putz A, Feichtinger H. Renal transitional cell carcinoma mimicking stone echoes. J Ultrasound Med 1988; 7: 83–6.

Jinzaki M, Ohkuma K, Tanimoto A, et al. Small solid renal lesions: usefulness of power Doppler US. Radiology 1998; 209: 543–50.

Khan A, Thomas N, Costello B, et al. Renal medullary carcinoma, sonographic computed tomography, magnetic resonance and angiographic findings. Eur J Radiol 2000; 35: 1–7.

Lee HS, Koh B, Kim J, et al. Radiologic findings of renal hemangioma. Report of 3 cases. Korean J Radiol 2000; 1(1): 160–3.

McGahan JP, Blake LC, Devere-White R, et al. Colour flow sonographic mapping of intravascular extension of malignant renal tumors. J Ultrasound Med 1993; 12: 403–9.

Nassir A, Jollimore J, Gupta R, et al. Multilocular cystic renal cell carcinoma. A series of 12 cases and review of the literature. Urology 2002; 60(3): 421–7.

Pickhardt PJ, Siegel CL, McLarney JK. Collecting duct carcinoma of the kidney. AJR Am J Roentgenol 2001; 176: 627–33.

Quaia E, Siracusano S, Bertolotto M, et al. Characterisation of renal tumors with pulse inversion harmonic imaging by intermittent high mechanical index technique – initial results. Eur Radiol 2003; 13(6): 402–12.

Russo P. Localised renal cell carcinoma. Curr Treatment Options Oncol 2001; 2(5): 447–55.

Seong CK, Seung HK, Jong SL, et al. Hypoechoic normal renal sinus and renal pelvis tumors. Sonographic differentiation. J Ultrasound Med 2002; 21: 993–9.

Siegel CL, Middleton WD, Teffey SA, McClennan BL. Angiomyolipoma and renal cell carcinoma: US differentiation. Radiology 1996; 198(3): 789–93.

Stallone G, Infante B, Manno C, et al. Primary lymphoma does exist: case report and review of the literature. J Nephrol 2000; 13: 367–72.

Taniguchi N, Itoh K, Nakmura S, et al. Differentiation of renal cell carcinomas from angiomyolipomas by ultrasonic frequency dependent attenuation. J Urol 1997; 157: 1242–5.

Tikkakoski T, Paivansalo M, Alanen A. Radiologic findings in renal oncocytoma. Acta Radiol 1991; 32: 363–7.

Yamashita Y, Ueno S, Makita O, et al. Hyperechoic renal tumors: anechoic rim and intratumoral cysts in US differentiation of renal cell carcinoma from angiomyolipoma. Radiology 1993; 188(1): 179–82.

Renal infection

Alan HA, Walsh JW, Brewer JW, et al. Sonography of emphysematous pyelonephritis. J Ultrasound Med 1984; 3: 533.

Chen JJ, Changchien CS, Kuo CH. Causes of increasing width of right anterior extra space seen in ultrasonographic examinations. J Clin Ultrasound 1995; 23(5): 287–92.

Cheng CH, Tsau YK, Hsu SY, Lee TL. Effective ultrasonographic predictor for the diagnosis of acute lobar nephronia. Pediat Infect Dis J 2004; 23(1): 11–14.

Coleman BG, Arger PH, Mulherne CB, et al. Pyonephrosis sonography in the diagnosis and management. AJR Am J Roentgenol 1981; 137: 939.

Dubbins P. Ultrasound in renal infection. BMUS Bull November 2003; Vol 11, No. 4.

Farmer KD, Gellett LR, Dubbins PA. Sonographic appearance of acute focal pyelonephritis. Eight years experience. Clin Radiol 2002; 57: 483–7.

Horchani A, Nouira Y, Kbaier I, Attyaoui F, Zribi AS. Hydatid cyst of the kidney. A report of 147 controlled cases. Eur Urol 2001; 38(4): 461–7.

Horvath K, Porkolab Z, Palko A. Primary renal and retroperitoneal actinomycosis. Eur Radiol 2000; 10: 287–9.

Kiersi DA, Karabacakoglu A, Odev K, Karakose S. Uncommon locations of hydatid cysts. Acta Radiol 2003; 44: 622–36.

Kim J. Ultrasonic graphic features of focal xanthogranulomatous pyelonephritis. J Ultrasound Med 2004; 23: 409–16.

Odev K, Kilinc M, Arslan A. Renal hydatid cysts and the evaluation of their radiologic images. Eur Urol 1996; 30: 40–9.

Roebuck DJ, Howard RG, Metreweli C. How sensitive is ultrasound in the detection of renal scars? Br J Radiol 1999; 72(856): 345–8.

Salah MA, Boszormenyi-Nagy G, Alabsi M, et al. Ultrasonographic urinary tract abnormalities in *Schistosoma hematobium* infection. Int Urol Nephrol 1999; 31(2): 163–72.

Tain YL. Renal pelvic wall thickening in childhood urinary tract infections. Evidence of acute pyelitis or vesico-ureteral reflux. Scand J Urol Nephrol 2003; 37(1): 28–30.

Tiu CM, Chou WH, Chiou HJ, et al. Sonographic features of xanthogranulomatous pyelonephritis. J Clin Ultrasound 2001; 29(5): 279–85.

Venkatesh SK, Mehrotra N, Gujral RB. Sonographic findings in renal parenchymal malakoplakia. J Clin Ultrasound 2000; 28: 353–7.

Wise G, Marella V. Genito-urinary manifestations of tuberculosis. Urol Clin North Am 2003; 30: 111–21.

Vascular disease

Demirpolat G, Ozbek SS, Parildar M. Reliability of intrarenal Doppler sonographic parameters of renal artery stenosis. J Clin Ultrasound 2003; 31: 346–51.

Dubbins PA, Wells IP. Renal artery stenosis, duplex Doppler evaluation. Br J Radiol 1986; 59: 225–9.

Johansson M, Jensen G, Aurell M, et al. Evaluation of duplex ultrasound and captopril renography for detection of reno-vascular hypertension. Kidney Int 2000; 58(2): 774–82.

Martin KW, MacAlistair WH, Shackleford GD. Acute renal infarction: diagnosis by Doppler ultrasound. Pediatr Radiol 1988; 18: 373–6.

Metser U, Friedman Z, Even-Sapier E, et al. Renal multigated spectral Doppler imaging before and after captopril challenge. Invest Radiol 2001; 36(4): 234–9.

Motew SJ, Cherr GS, Craven TE, et al. Renal duplex sonography. Main renal artery versus hilar analysis. J Vasc Surg 2000; 32(3): 462–9, 469–7.

Naganuma H, Ashida H, Konno K, et al. Renal arterial venous malformation: sonographic findings. Abdom Imaging 2001; 26: 661–3.

Radermacher J, Chavan A, Bleck J, et al. Use of Doppler ultrasonography to predict the outcome of therapy for renal artery stenosis. N Engl J Med 2001; 344(6): 410–17.

Ripolles T, Aliaga R, Morote V. Utility of intrarenal Doppler ultrasound in the diagnosis of renal artery stenosis. Eur Radiol 2001; 40(1): 54–63.

Robertson R, Murphy A, Dubbins PA. Renal artery stenosis. Use of duplex ultrasound as a screening technique. Br J Radiol 1988; 61: 723.

Soulez G, Therasse E, Qanadli SD, et al. Prediction of clinical response after renal angioplasty. Respective value of renal Doppler sonography and scintigraphy. AJR Am J Roentgenol 2003; 184(4): 1029–35.

Van weel V, van Bockle JH, van Wissen R, van Baalen JM. Intraoperative renal duplex sonography: a valuable method for evaluating renal artery reconstructions. Eur J Vasc Endovasc Surg 2000; 20(3): 268–72.

Yucel C, Ozdemir H, Akpek S, et al. Renal infarct: contrast-enhanced power Doppler sonographic findings. J Clin Ultrasound 2001; 29(4): 237–42.

Trauma

Furtschegger A, Egender G, Jakse G. The value of sonography in the diagnosis and follow up of patients with blunt renal trauma. Br J Urol 1988; 62: 110–16.

Guerriero WG. Aetiology, classification and management of renal trauma. Surg Clin North Am 1988; 68: 1071–84.

Ivory CM, Dubbins PA, Wells IP, Hammonds JC. Ultrasound assessment of local complications of percutaneous stone removal. J Clin Ultrasound 1989; 17(5): 345–51.

Sato M, Yoshii H. Reevaluation of ultrasonography for solid-organ injury in blunt abdominal trauma. J Ultrasound Med 2004; 23(12): 1583–96.

Diffuse medical renal disease

al-Murrani B, Cosgrove DO, Svensson WE, Blaszczwk M. Echogenic rings – an ultrasound sign of early nephrocalcinosis. Clin Radiol 1991; 44: 49–51.

Braden GL, Kozinn DR, Hampf FE Jr, et al. Ultrasound diagnosis of early renal papillary necrosis. J Ultrasound Med 1991; 10(7): 401–3.

Buturovic-Ponikvar J, Visnar-Perovic A. Ultrasonography in chronic renal failure. Eur J Radiol 2003; 46(2): 115–22.

Di Fiori JL, Rodrigeu ED, Kaptein EM, Ralls PW. Diagnostic sonography of HIV-associated nephropathy: new observations and clinical correlation. AJR Am J Roentgenol 1998; 171(3): 713–16.

Dubbins P. Colour flow doppler of the renal tract. BMUS Bull 1994; 2(3): 10–14.

Huntington DK, Hill SC, Hill MC. Sonographic manifestations of medical renal disease. Semin Ultrasound CT MR 1991; 12(4): 290–307.

Kay CJ. Renal diseases in patients with AIDS: sonographic findings. AJR Am J Roentgenol 1992; 159(3): 551–4.

McCune T, Stone W, Breyer J. Page kidney: case report and review of the literature. Am J Kidney Dis 1991; 18(5): 593–9.

Page JE, Morgan SH, Eastwood JB, et al. Ultrasound findings in renal parenchymal disease: comparison with histological appearances. Clin Radiol 1994; 49(12): 867–70.

Platt JF, Rubin JM, Ellis JH. Lupus nephritis: predictive value of conventional and Doppler US and comparison with serologic and biopsy parameters. Radiology 1997; 203(1): 82–6.

Roebuck DJ. The significance of hypoechoic renal rims. Australas Radiol 1994; 38(4): 345.

Sasagaw I, Terasawa Y, Imai K, et al. Acquired cystic disease of the kidney and renal carcinoma in hemodialysis patients: ultrasonographic evaluation. Br J Urol 1992; 70(3): 236–9.

Toyoda K, Miyamoto Y, Ida M. Hyperechoic medulla of the kidneys. Radiology 1989; 173(2): 431–4.

Tublin ME, Bude RO, Platt JF. Review of the resistive index in renal Doppler sonography. Where do we stand? AJR Am J Roentgenol 2003; 180(4): 885–92.

Van den Noortgate N, Velghe A, Petrovic M, et al. The role of ultrasonography in the assessment of renal function in the elderly. J Nephrol 2003; 16: 658–62.

Yassa NA, Ping M, Ralls PW. Perirenal lucency ('kidney sweat'): a new sign of renal failure. AJR Am J Roentgenol 1999; 173(4): 1075–7.

2

The ureters

Dennis Ll Cochlin

Relevant anatomy

The anatomy presented here is intentionally brief and incomplete. The purpose is to present only the anatomy that is relevant to the text. If the reader wants more detail, many excellent anatomy texts are available.

We will start with the renal pelvis. This is not part of the ureter, but is relevant. The renal pelvis is the sac formed by the confluence of the renal infundibula. Its position and shape are variable. It may lie completely within the renal tissue or partially or completely outside the kidney (extrarenal pelvis). Congenital anomalies include partially or completely double or duplex pelves, anterior pointing pelves and pelviureteric junction obstruction.

The ureter starts at the pelviureteric junction (PUJ). Variations in the renal pelvis are relevant because they affect the positions of the junction. With an intrarenal pelvis, the ureter starts close in at the renal hilum. With an extrarenal pelvis, the PUJ lies a variable distance medial and caudal to the renal hilum. In the case of a large extrarenal pelvis, the PUJ may even lie below the lower pole of the kidney. A bifid or duplex renal pelvis raises the possibility of double (duplex) ureters. An anterior-pointing renal pelvis found in malrotated or horseshoe kidneys leads to an anterior position of the upper ureter.

The ureter is divided, for descriptive purposes, into three sections: the abdominal or lumbar, iliac and pelvic ureter. The pelvic ureter is further divided into the intramural vesical ureter, and the extravesical portion that lies outside the bladder wall.

The ureter is an endothelial-lined muscular tube, which undergoes regular peristaltic contractions. It has an outer diameter of 4–6 mm and a luminal diameter of between 0 and 2–4 mm, depending on peristalsis.

The abdominal ureter

The abdominal ureter starts at the pelviureteric junction and runs in the retroperitoneal space anterior to the psoas muscles. Most ureters lie at the level of the tips of the trans-verse process of the lumbar vertebrae, but many are more lateral or medial. The descending part of the duodenum lies anterior to the right ureter, the sigmoid colon anterior to the left, together with mesentery and omentum. It is these anterior relations that make it difficult, particularly in large patients, to visualize the ureters by ultrasound.

The iliac ureter

The ureter crosses anterior to the iliac blood vessels, lateral to the bifurcation into internal and external on the right, anterior to the bifurcation on the left. This short portion is termed the iliac ureter.

The pelvic ureter

The pelvic ureter runs along the posterior pelvic wall, running downwards but also backwards and lateral to follow the contour of the posterior pelvis. At the level of the ischial spine, it changes direction and runs forward and medially to enter the bladder wall.

The ureter then becomes the intramural vesicle ureter. This portion crosses obliquely through the bladder wall. It then runs beneath the bladder mucosa for about 1 cm, and enters the bladder at a small protrusion, the ureteric eminence, at the corner of the trigone.

Ultrasonic imaging of the ureters

The normal ureters lie in the retroperitoneal space. They lie posterior to the bowel and peritoneum, and anterior to the retroperitoneal muscles. The bowel tends to obscure the ureters when scanning from an anterior approach, whereas the muscles of the back degrade the ultrasound beam to the extent that the ureters are not visible when scanning from the posterior. This makes the ureters inaccessible to ultrasound for most of their length. In general, therefore, ureteric imaging is best achieved by computed tomography (CT: contrasted, when looking primarily at the ureters; uncontrasted, when looking for calculi) or intravenous urography (IVU). In practice, however, evaluation of the ureters is often an essential part of the urinary tract ultrasound study, even if some patients subsequently proceed to CT or IVU.

More detailed examination of ureteric anatomy reveals that three sections of the ureter are amenable to ultrasound study: the proximal ureter, at and immediately below the pelviureteric junction; the distal ureter, at and immediately proximal to the vesicoureteric junction (VUJ); and, less reliably, the sections of the ureter that cross anterior to the iliac vessels. In addition, it is sometimes possible, in a slim patient, to visualize the mid ureter as it lies anterior to the psoas muscle, but this is the exception rather than the rule.

In addition to anatomical ultrasound study of the ureters, significant physiologic information may be gained from the study of the jets of urine that enter the bladder from the ureters (ureteric jets).

Imaging technique[1–4]

The pelviureteric junction and proximal ureter may be visualized by scanning from a lateral oblique approach through the lower pole of the kidney, using the kidney as a window (Figure 2.1a). The longitudinal plane is usually used, although in some patients, the axial plane may be effective, following the ureter down in real time (Figure 2.1b). Using this technique, a variable length of proximal ureter, typically only about 1 cm, may be studied before it is 'lost' behind the bowel. However, a sufficient length is seen to assess whether or not there is ureteric dilatation (Figure 2.1c).

The distal ureter is best visualized by scanning through the semi full bladder, angling towards the bladder base in the transverse plane. Good landmarks for the position of the ureters are the small bulges into the bladder where the intramural ureters enter the bladder, and the ureteric jets. The distal ureters are seen posterior to these landmarks (Figure 2.2). Blood vessels may be distinguished from the ureters by utilizing color Doppler. Peristalsis may sometimes be observed in the ureter, but is not seen often enough to be a reliable marker. If the distal ureters are dilated, then the lower centimeter or so may be imaged by rotating the transducer into the longitudinal plane of the ureter (Figure 2.2). If the ureter is not dilated, however, longitudinal imaging is rarely possible.

The portions of the ureters that cross the iliac vessels may be studied in slim patients, by identifying the iliac vessels and then scanning in either a transverse plane or in the line of the ureter. The ureter is seen crossing anterior to

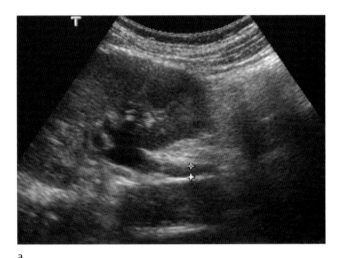

a

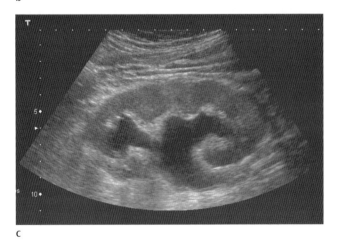

b

c

Figure 2.1
Upper ureter. The upper ureter is seen using the lower pole of the kidney as a sonic window: (a) longitudinal; (b) transverse (ureter arrowed); and (c) reasonable length of upper ureter seen in a case of ureteric obstruction.

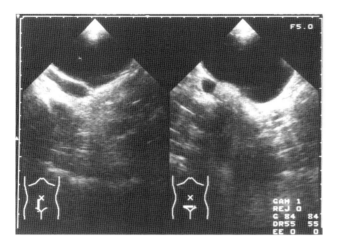

Figure 2.2
Lower ureter. The lower end of the ureter is dilated as far as the vesicoureteric junction, indicating that the obstruction must be vesicoureteric or outlet obstruction.

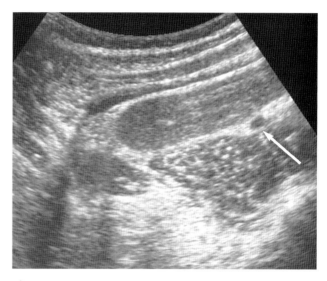

Figure 2.4
Ureter anterior to the psoas muscle. Transverse section. The ureter is arrowed.

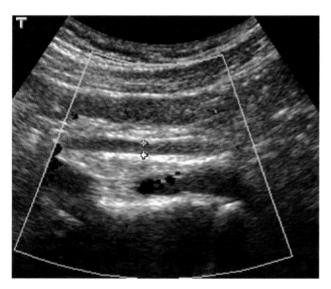

Figure 2.3
Ureter crossing the iliac vessels. The ureter (calipers) is seen crossing the iliac vessels.

the vessels (Figure 2.3). These portions of the ureter are important in the study of hydronephrosis of pregnancy. In pregnant women, they are most often well visualized by turning the patient into a 45° oblique position and using the posterior uterine wall as a sonic window.

The other portions of the ureter may not be reliably imaged, although, in slim patients, the ureter may sometimes be seen anterior to the psoas muscle (Figure 2.4). The technique of scanning the ureteric jets is discussed later.

The ureters may also be studied by ultrasound using intraluminal transducers. These produce highly detailed cross-sectional views of the ureters. Three-dimensional views are also possible. Possible applications include the study of ureteric tumors and mapping of the blood vessels around a pelviureteric obstruction. These studies are still at the trial stage, although clinical use may follow.

Hydroureter (obstruction dilatation)

Terminology

The terms hydroureter and dilated ureter mean widening of the ureteric lumen, from any cause. The term obstruction means an increase in the resistance to urinary flow and, consequently, an increase in pressure proximal to the obstruction. Dilatation may be due to obstruction or other causes, such as reflux or dilatation of pregnancy. Obstruction, while usually causing dilatation, does not necessarily do so, particularly in acute cases.

Obstruction may be acute, chronic or intermittent. Acute obstruction may be complete or incomplete.

Physiologic changes

The physiologic changes that occur in acute obstruction are important to the understanding of the imaging appearances and also the damage that occurs to the kidney. Acute obstruction causes an increase in pressure. An increase of about 5-fold – from 10 to 50 mmHg – is needed to initiate the other changes. Incomplete obstruction causing a lower pressure increase does not do so. The increased pressure is accompanied by a brief period of hyperperistalsis, followed by hypoperistalsis or aperistalsis. There is an immediate, short-lived increase in the renal blood flow. Three to five hours later, there is vasoconstriction of the glomerular capillaries, causing a reduced glomerular filtration rate. This accounts for the fact that some cases of acute obstruction do not have pelvicalyceal or ureteric obstruction in the early phase. The vasoconstriction persists for 24 hours after the obstruction is relieved. If obstruction with increased pressure persists for a significant period, progression of renal damage occurs with loss of nephrons. Complete obstruction, however, does not necessarily cause continuously high pressure, as rupture of the calyceal fornices causes temporary reduction in pressure and return of glomerular function. Frequently, such ruptures may occur during an obstructive episode. The time scale for renal damage is not precisely known for humans, but Kerr[5] showed that, in dogs, renal damage starts after 7 days and, after 6 weeks, the kidney is effectively non-functioning.

Hydronephrosis and hydroureter[6–11]

Hydronephrosis is readily identified on an ultrasound scan, and is discussed in Chapter 1. When a hydronephrosis is identified, the cause needs to be established. An important part of this is to establish whether, and to what level, the ureter is dilated. While this may ultimately need a CT or IVU study, much may be determined on the initial ultrasound study.

Basically, ultrasound can usually determine whether the proximal and distal ureter is dilated, and whether the bladder empties completely. Based on this, and the clinical history, it is possible to make a presumptive distinction between dilatation from obstruction or non-obstructive causes, and, in the case of obstruction, to determine the level of obstruction as being at the pelviureteric junction, ureteric level, the vesicoureteric junction or the bladder outlet. The degree of certainty varies. It depends on how well the ureters are seen. This, in turn, depends on the patient habitus, the amount of bowel gas present and the degree of ureteric dilatation. In many cases, it is necessary to confirm the level by CT or IVU.

The cause of obstruction is also sometimes, although not invariably, demonstrated by the ultrasound study. Ureteric calculi may be seen when they lie at the pelviureteric junction or at the vesicoureteric junction, but are only rarely seen in the rest of the ureter. PUJ obstruction is assumed when there is a dilated renal pelvis and non-dilated upper ureter. Bladder tumors, enlarged prostate, retroperitoneal or pelvic pathology may be seen. In many cases, however, further investigation is necessary to demonstrate the cause of obstruction or to confirm a diagnosis suggested but not proven on the ultrasound study. The following sections discuss causes of hydronephrosis and hydroureter in turn.

Pelviureteric junction obstruction

Clinical considerations

PUJ obstruction is a condition in which there is a functional obstruction to the passage of urine at the PUJ. This leads to an increase in pressure and dilatation of the pelvicalyceal system down to the PUJ. In many (probably most) cases, following dilatation, the pressure reduces. This probably occurs for two reasons. The first reason is a reduction in function, and hence urine output, of the kidney. This may, in some cases, be very small, but enough to reduce the pressure. The second reason is the dilatation of the system, particularly if there is an extrarenal pelvis, which can dilate to a considerable size. This dilatation has the effect of evening out peaks of high pressure. The majority of patients reach a state where they have a dilated system but normal pressure and no symptoms. Such cases are detected only when they undergo imaging procedures for other reasons. A smaller group present with loin pain after a fluid load, typically beer drinking. These patients have a normal intrarenal pressure for most of the time. The fluid load causes increased renal output, increased pressure and dilatation and pain. Another group that usually, but not invariably, have episodes of loin pain; have increased intrarenal pressure, which may lead to deterioration in renal function. These patients may present at any age. As the condition is congenital, these patients probably have another, at present unrecognized, factor that changes them from a stable condition to one of high pressure.

Cause

PUJ obstruction is not a mechanical obstruction. It is due to lack of peristaltic movement at the PUJ.

Ultrasound appearances

The typical ultrasound appearances are of calyceal and infundibular dilatation, with a large renal pelvis and normal-sized ureter (Figure 2.5). In most cases the renal pelvis is very large, although intrarenal pelves cannot distend to the degree of extrarenal pelves.

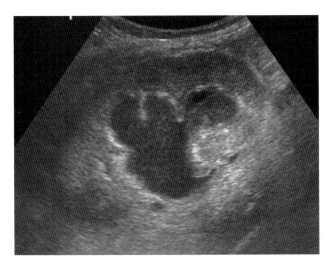

Figure 2.5
Pelviureteric (PUJ) obstruction. There is a hydronephrosis. The upper ureter is narrow, indicating that this is a PUJ obstruction.

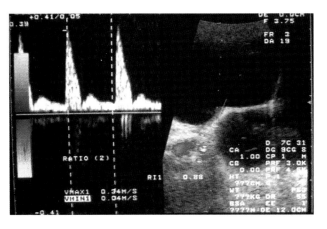

Figure 2.6
PUJ obstruction – response to furosemide.

Although the ultrasound appearance may be highly suggestive of the diagnosis, many centers will confirm the diagnosis with a CT study or an IVU. It is also necessary to distinguish those cases that have normal pressure, that do not require any treatment, from those with high pressure that require some form of pyeloplasty to prevent continuing deterioration of renal function. The distinction is normally made by isotope renography. The Whitaker test is theoretically superior but is invasive and is, therefore, not routinely used in most centers. Platt has shown that increased intrarenal pressure is associated with decreased diastolic velocities (increased resistance index) in the intrarenal arteries. This may be utilized to study PUJ obstruction, particularly if furosemide is used to exaggerate the effect by increasing renal output (Figure 2.6). Although well documented, however, this test has not gained widespread acceptance. It is isotope renography with furosemide that is almost universally used.

The treatment of PUJ obstruction is by pyeloplasty, in which the width of the pelviureteric junction is increased surgically. This may be done by open surgery or laparoscopically, or using a minimally invasive procedure that cuts or splits the pelviureteric junction via a catheter approach. In the case of a cutting procedure (such as 'acucide') it is important to document the relationships of the renal blood vessels to the PUJ, so as not to cut into the vessels. Ultrasound is not sufficiently accurate to achieve this, at least in most hands, and contrasted CT angiography is utilized.

Ultrasound studies following treatment often show little or no change in the degree of calyceal or pelvic dilatation, even though the treatment is effective in lowering the pressure.

Calculus obstruction[12,13]

Calculi may be detected by ultrasound study if they are intrarenal (Figure 2.7a), within the renal pelvis (Figure 2.7b), at the pelviureteric junction or at the vesicoureteric junction (Figure 2.7c–e). Calculi lying within the rest of the ureter, although occasionally seen, are not reliably detected by ultrasound (Figure 2.8). Calculi are characterized on ultrasound as highly echogenic structures with posterior shadowing.

This chapter is concerned with the ureter. Let us start, however, with the kidney itself. The reason for including intrarenal calculi is that, in cases of ureteric obstruction, the demonstration of intrarenal calculi suggests that a calculus is the probable cause of the ureteric obstruction, even if a ureteric calculus is not seen. There is a problem within the kidney because the parenchymal or renal sinus fat may be of high echo density, often with very high echo density 'flecks', presumably due to fat–fibrous tissue interfaces. These may approach or even equal the echo density of a calculus (Figure 2.9). This is the main factor that limits the sensitivity and specificity of ultrasound in the detection of intrarenal calculi. Most calculi produce a dense acoustic shadow. Very small calculi, of less than about 1 mm, however, do not cast a shadow but rather produce a comet tail artifact. Shadowing is best shown by using tissue harmonic imaging. Care must be taken in some machines that utilize spatial compounding, as this decreases the size of the acoustic shadow and should, therefore, not be used when assessing calculi. Renal sinus fat flecks produce only very weak shadows.

Ureteric calculi may be relatively easily shown at the PUJ, where the dilated pelvis acts as a landmark, and at the VUJ, where they may be seen through the full bladder.

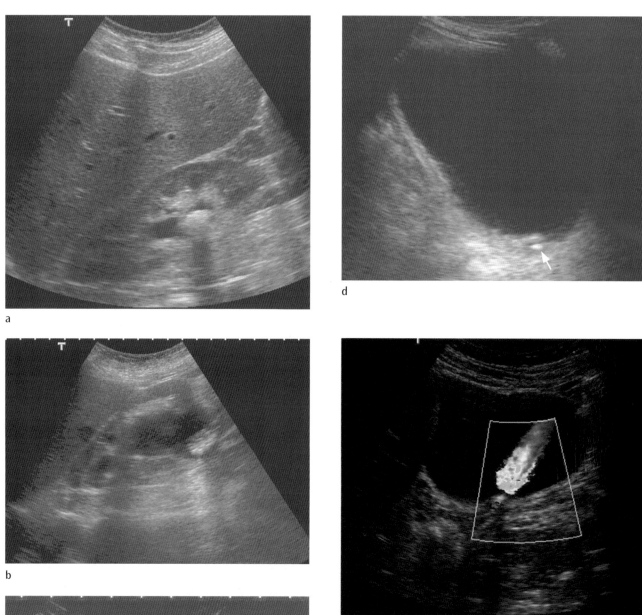

Figure 2.7
Renal calculus. (a) Renal calculus lying in the upper pole calyx.
(b) Calculus in the renal pelvis. (c–e) Longitudinal and
transverse views of a calculus (arrowed) at the vesicoureteric
junction.

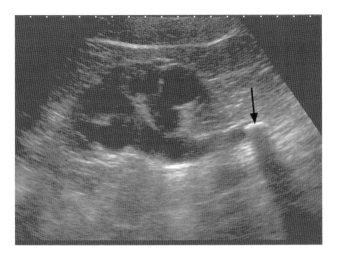

Figure 2.8
Midureteric calculus. A calculus is seen in the mid-portion of a dilated ureter (arrows). Ultrasonic visualization of calculi in such a position is, however, exceptional.

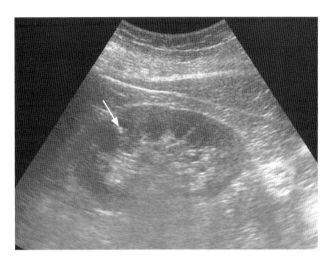

Figure 2.9
Echogenic renal sinus fat.

Elsewhere in the ureter calculi are generally only seen if the ureter is dilated down to the calculus, and even then are not reliably shown. Thus, in the majority of patients with ureteric obstruction due to calculi, a hydronephrosis and hydroureter are shown on the ultrasound study (although a normal system does not exclude obstruction), but the calculus is not demonstrated. The addition of a plain abdominal film (KUB) may show a radio-opaque calculus, but most often the definitive diagnosis is made by an uncontrasted CT scan or an IVU.

Bladder pathology causing ureteric obstruction

Bladder tumors that involve the trigone may cause ureteric obstruction (Figure 2.10), as may ureteroceles (Figure 2.11). Bladder outlet obstruction may cause hydroureter and obstructive uropathy. Ureteroceles are discussed later in this chapter. Bladder tumors and outlet obstruction are dealt with in Chapter 3.

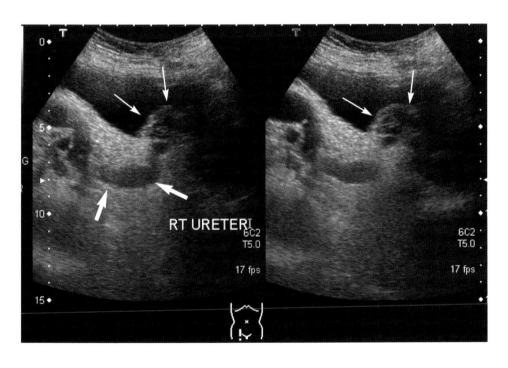

Figure 2.10
Bladder tumor obstructing the ureter. There is a transitional cell cancer (narrow arrows) obstructing the ureter (wide arrows).

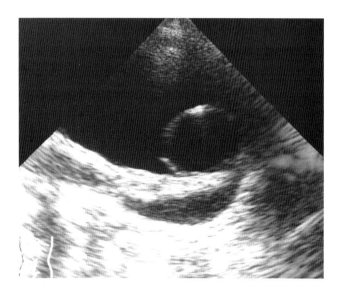

Figure 2.11
Ureterocele obstructing the ureter. There is a ureterocele with a dilated obstructed ureter.

Table 2.1 *Retroperitoneal fibrosis: causes*

Findings	Percent
Idiopathic	67.8
Methysergide	12.4
All malignancies	7.9
Mediastinal fibrosis	3.3
Periaortic inflammation/arteritis	2.4
Mesenteric fibrosis	2.0
Sclerosing cholangitis	1.6
Abdominal aortic aneurysm	1.6
Crohn's disease	1.2
Thrombophlebitis	1.0
Reidel's thyroiditis	0.8
Others	5.3

From: Koepl L, Zuidena GD, The clinical significance of retroperitoneal fibrosis. Surgery 1977; 81: 250.

Other causes of ureteric obstruction

There are many possible causes of ureteric obstruction. It is not very productive to discuss all of them here. The point to be made, however, is that these causes should be actively sought. As well as studying the kidneys, ureters and bladder, the ultrasound scan should include a study of the retroperitoneal space that is as thorough as possible, dependent on the amount of bowel gas present, and also a study of the pelvic contents.

Retroperitoneal tumors are diverse in ultrasound appearance and there is little point in listing all possible appearances. Any retroperitoneal tumor or mass may obstruct the ureters. Retroperitoneal fibrosis, however, deserves a special mention.

Retroperitoneal fibrosis[14–17]

Retroperitoneal fibrosis is a condition in which fibrous tissue is laid down mainly in the retroperitoneal space. Its relevance to urology is that it causes functional obstruction of the ureters, resulting in hydronephrosis, renal failure and sometimes renovascular hypertension.

Most cases are of unknown etiology and are classified as idiopathic, whereas others may be related to the collagen diseases, use of certain drugs and other retroperitoneal pathologies (Table 2.1).

Retroperitoneal fibrosis occurs most commonly between 40 and 60 years of age, but may occur at any age from infancy to old age. Early symptoms are those of pain, gastrointestinal disturbance, diarrhea, weight loss, anorexia and fever. It is in advanced disease that ureteral obstruction or hypertension occurs, these conditions affecting nearly half of such cases.

Malignancy and retroperitoneal fibrosis

Primary malignant processes of the retroperitoneum, notably fibrosarcoma and nodular sclerosing Hodgkin's disease, may mimic retroperitoneal fibrosis, whereas metastatic disease, often from breast or lung, may provoke a form of retroperitoneal fibrosis by a desmoplastic response. These processes may be indistinguishable from retroperitoneal fibrosis on imaging of the retroperitoneum, although the clinical picture usually indicates the nature of the disease.

Inflammatory disease and retroperitoneal fibrosis

Inflammatory bowel disease, such as Crohn's disease, appendix abscess or paracolic abscess, may provoke a fibrotic reaction around the ureters. Thickened bowel may

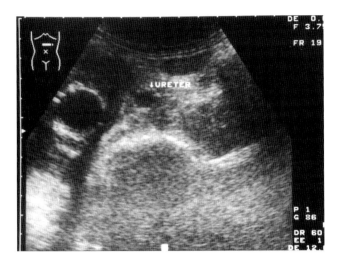

Figure 2.12
Retroperitoneal fibrosis following aortic graft insertion. The low echodensity fibrosis surrounds the graft. The dilated left ureter is seen down to the level where it is obstructed by the fibrosis.

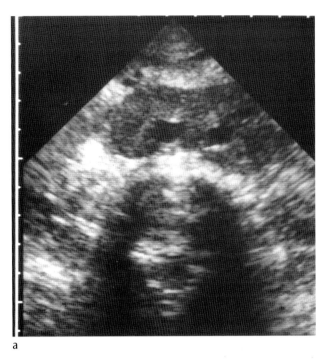

a

be seen in Crohn's disease; in appendix or paracolic abscess, the abscess itself may be imaged ultrasonically. The fibrotic process that causes ureteric obstruction is more chronic and is not usually visible ultrasonically. Abscesses may also produce functional ureteric obstruction, the inflammation causing paralysis of the ureter. This reverses when the inflammation subsides. Appendicitis, without abscess, may also provoke this change, and must always be borne in mind as a differential diagnosis in suspected right ureteric colic.

Postoperative retroperitoneal fibrosis

Any retroperitoneal operation may lead to ureteric obstruction from scarring. The most common is aortic graft insertion. In these cases, ultrasound or CT rarely demonstrate fibrosis (Figure 2.12). Ultrasound is often used, however, as a screening test 3 and 6 months post aortic graft insertion to detect or exclude the development of calyceal dilatation.

Imaging of retroperitoneal fibrosis (Figures 2.12–2.16)

Retroperitoneal fibrosis may appear ultrasonically as a band of fairly homogeneous medium-echodensity tissue

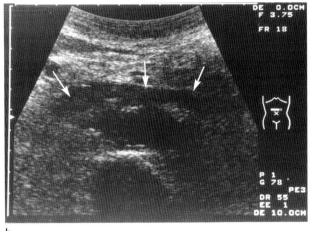

b

Figure 2.13
Retroperitoneal fibrosis. (a) A medium-echodensity band surrounds the two iliac arteries. In this case the fibrosis is easily distinguished from the more echogenic fat. (b) A band of medium-echodensity tissue (arrows) lies anterior to the aorta and vena cava. In this case distinction from the surrounding fat is less clear.

anterior to and enveloping the aorta and vena cava. Often the vena cava is compressed and difficult to see.

Fibrotic tissue is difficult to distinguish from fat on ultrasound, however, and retroperitoneal fat in obese subjects, particularly males, may be misdiagnosed as retroperitoneal fibrosis. The presence of bilateral

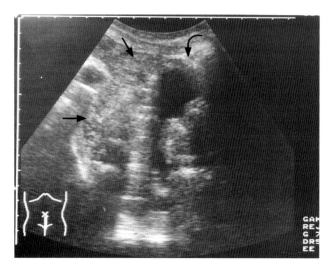

Figure 2.14
Retroperitoneal fibrosis presenting as a circumscribed mass.
This patient presented with renal failure and was found to have
bilateral hydronephroses. There is a poorly circumscribed mass
(straight arrows) above the bladder (curved arrow). This was
thought to be a pelvic malignancy but surgery revealed
retroperitoneal fibrosis.

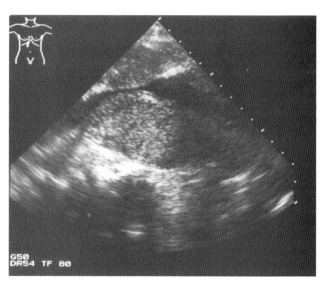

Figure 2.15
**Severe retroperitoneal fibrosis causing a high
retroperitoneal mass.** A rather atypical mass is seen high in
the retroperitoneal space. There was also fibrosis lower in the
retroperitoneum causing a hydronephrosis. Although the
previous cases are more typical, retroperitoneal fibrosis may
sometimes cause a rounded mass as in this case rather than
the more typical sheets of tissue.

hydronephrosis, of course, suggests retroperitoneal fibrosis, but may be due to a coincidental cause. Retroperitoneal
fat tends to be more extensive than fibrosis.
Retroperitoneal fibrosis is typically confined to the lumbar
regions, although it may rarely extend to the thorax and to
the pelvis and even into the scrotum.

Despite these differences, ultrasound may not clearly
distinguish fibrosis from fat, especially in obese subjects, in
whom the retroperitoneum may be difficult to visualize.
Because of these problems, CT or MRI (magnetic resonance imaging) are far better than ultrasound at diagnosing or excluding retroperitoneal fibrosis. The diagnosis
may be suggested on ultrasound by a combination of
hydronephrosis and a retroperitoneal tissue band, but
confirmation by CT or MRI is advisable.

Appendicitis[18]

Inflammatory conditions close to a ureter can cause functional obstruction. The most common of these is acute
appendicitis. Pain of acute appendicitis may also mimic the
loin to groin pain that typifies ureteric colic caused by a
calculus. This should always be considered. A full description of the ultrasound appearances of appendicitis is
outside the scope of this book but illustrative examples are

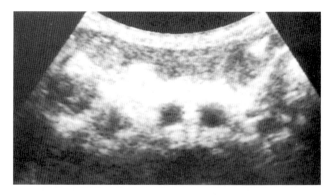

Figure 2.16
Retroperitoneal fibrosis secondary to pancreatic carcinoma.
Very echodense tissue surrounds the iliac arteries in the
transverse plane. Surgery revealed dense desmoplastic
retroperitoneal fibrosis secondary to carcinoma of the
pancreas. The extreme echodensity in this case is unusual
although not excessively rare.

included of the more severe cases with significant periap-
pendiceal inflammation that cause functional ureteric
obstruction and right-sided hydronephrosis (Figure 2.17).

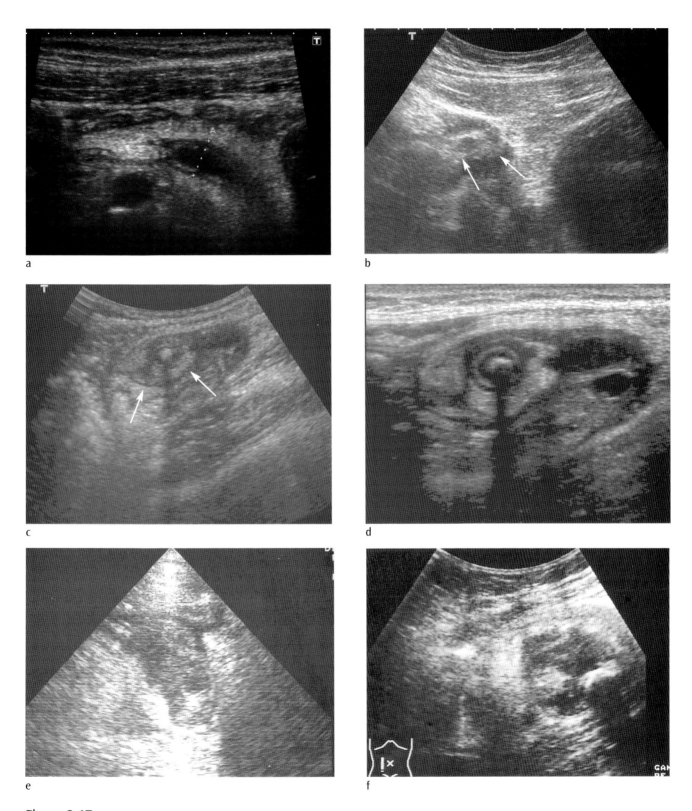

Figure 2.17

Appendicitis. (a) The appendix is moderately swollen (10 mm) with free fluid around it. (b) The appendix is seen in transverse section and is swollen at 21 mm. (c) The appendix is markedly swollen and the fat posterior to it is edematous and echogenic. (d) An echodense mass of edematous fat and omentum surrounds the appendix. (e) As the phlegmon progresses to an abscess, the image of the appendix becomes lost within a complex mass. (f) There is a typical thick-walled cavity with inhomogeneous contents. The echogenic area with shadowing could be gas or a faecolith.

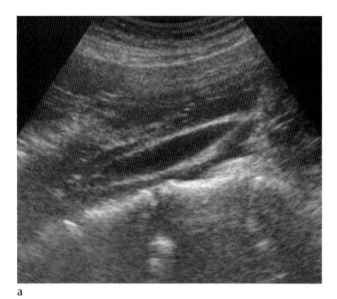

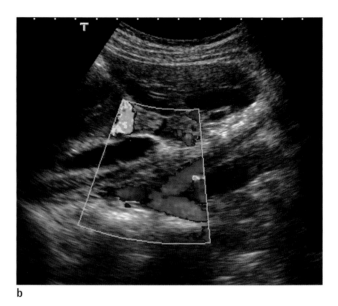

a

b

Figure 2.18
Hydronephrosis of pregnancy. (a) The right ureter is dilated down to the iliac vessels and not beyond. (b) Color Doppler helps to distinguish the ureter from blood vessels.

Hydronephrosis of pregnancy[19–23]

Dilatation of the calyceal system and ureters is very common during pregnancy. It may start as early as the 10th week. The incidence increases throughout pregnancy, affecting about 90% of women by the third trimester. The cause has been stated to be hormonal (progesterone and gonadotropin both cause smooth muscle relaxation) and compression by the gravid uterus. The fact that pelvic kidneys and kidneys with reimplanted ureters do not dilate has been taken as support for the compressive theory, although hormone-mediated smooth muscle relaxation may also play a part. The majority of cases are asymptomatic. A minority, however, may have mild, or less commonly, severe loin pain. These cases are problematic for two reasons. First, the choice of treatment is a problem. Secondly, although straightforward 'physiologic' dilatation of pregnancy may well be the cause of the pain, other causes, principally ureteric calculus but also non-urologic causes such as appendicitis, need to be excluded. Furthermore, diagnostic tests are limited by the reluctance to use ionizing radiation during pregnancy. Thus, ultrasound is the primary imaging modality of choice in these cases, the secondary modality being MR urography. The limited IVU still has a place, but CT urography may not be used because of the unacceptably high radiation dose.

Imaging appearances

Physiologic dilatation of pregnancy produces a varying degree of calyceal and ureteric dilatation. The degree of dilatation tends to be higher in multipara. The right side is affected more frequently, and with a greater degree of dilatation than the left. The reason is unknown. The characteristic of ureteric dilatation is that the ureters are dilated down to the level that the lumbar ureter crosses the iliac vessels. At this point, the ureters taper, and the ureter below this is of a normal caliber. Narrowing above this level or dilatation below is highly suspicious of a pathologic cause, usually calculus. It is thus essential to attempt to visualize the whole of the ureters by the ultrasound study. Fortunately, the gravid uterus may be used as a sonic window for visualizing the lumbar ureters. The patient is placed in an oblique position, and the ureters are scanned by placing the transducer in the iliac fossa and scanning across the back of the fetus, using the uterine wall, placenta and amniotic fluid as a sonic window. Using this technique, MacNeily et al[23] have shown that the right lumbar ureter is seen in 52% and the left in 88% of pregnant women with hydronephrosis (Figure 2.18).

Calculus obstruction in pregnancy

Urolithiasis is more common during pregnancy, though the incidence is still low at 0.03–0.6%, the incidence increasing with multiparity. Unlike physiologic dilatation, the incidence of calculus obstruction is equal on both sides. Symptoms are the same as those in non-pregnant patients. Macroscopic hematuria may be an important sign, occurring in 75–100% of cases. This apart, the other symptoms and signs may mimic pain from physiologic dilatation.

A careful ultrasound study may show an obstructing calculus, the appearances being the same as those described from the non-pregnant patient. In many cases, however, the calculus is not seen. In these cases, a calculus is suspected if the narrowing of the ureters is at any point other than where it crosses the iliac vessels. Another pointer is if the pain is left sided, or if the left system is dilated more that the right. In such cases a judgment has to be made whether to obtain a plain abdominal radiograph (KUB). Only 80% of renal or ureteric calculi are radio-opaque. Also, in later pregnancy the fetal skeleton may obscure a calculus. Thus, while a positive KUB is useful, a negative one is not.

As stated, while careful ultrasound technique may often show the whole ureters, there is a significant technical failure rate. In such cases, an MR urogram – a heavily T2-weighted study that visualizes the hydrogen-rich urine in the system – is the appropriate next modality. The same consideration as to the level of narrowing, and the more dilated side, apply. While calculi may sometimes be seen as a signal void, they are not reliably shown by MRI. The limited IVU has little to offer over ultrasound and MR urography, and is now more often used.

Platt et al[6] have shown that acute ureteric dilatation decreases the diastolic velocities in the intrarenal arteries, measured as an increase in the resistance index to above 0.7. Physiologic dilatation of pregnancy does not affect the resistance index. This may, therefore, also be used as an indicative test, although its sensitivity and specificity are uncertain.

Table 2.2 *Ureteral malformations*
Renal and ureteral agenesis
Ectopic ureter
Ureterocele
Vesicoureteric reflux
Megaureter
Reduplicated ureter

Treatment

The treatment of symptomatic hydronephrosis and hydroureter in pregnancy is problematic, whatever the etiology. In patients with mild to moderate pain, the treatment is symptomatic, in the hope that this will tide the patient through the pregnancy. If pain is severe, however, then reduction of the intrarenal pressure is necessary. This may be achieved by placement of a percutaneous nephrostomy drain, which may be performed under ultrasound control without any use of ionizing radiation. Alternatively, retrograde stenting may be performed, which has the advantage of being internal with no external tubing or bags. In the case of calculus obstruction, removal of the calculus by ureteroscopy may be performed with careful monitoring of fetal well-being during the procedure.

Ureteric malformations[24–27]

A number of congenital malformations of the ureters occur (Table 2.2). The more common and important ones are discussed.

Renal and ureteric agenesis

Most cases of renal agenesis are associated with total absence of the ureters and hemitrigone. In others, some may be a blind-ending lower ureter. The blind-ending ureter is often dilated and may sometimes be seen on a

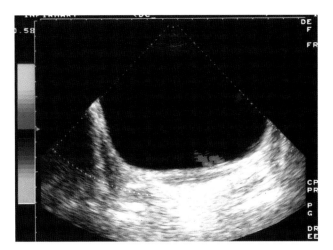

Figure 2.19
Duplex ureter – double uerteric jets. The color Doppler image shows two jets from duplex ureters opening separately into the bladder. Although this is an interesting image, ultrasound plays little part in the investigation of duplex ureters.

bladder scan. Renal agenesis may be associated with absent vas deferens and epididymis, absence or undescended ipsilateral testes or, in females, uterine agenesis, hypoplasia, unicornuate or bicornuate uterus, and vaginal aplasia.

the ejaculatory duct, seminal vesicles or vas deferens; and in females, the vestibulum or distal vagina, the cervix or the broad ligament. Ultrasound studies have little to offer in the study of ectopic ureters (Figure 2.19). Contrast CT, IVU or MRI may all be used in their investigation.

Ectopic ureter

Ectopic ureters may open into any part of the system that develops from the Wolffian duct. This includes an abnormal position in the bladder, such as the bladder neck; in males,

Ureterocele

A ureterocele is a thin-walled dilatation of the lower end of the ureter that bulges into the bladder. The orifice may lie

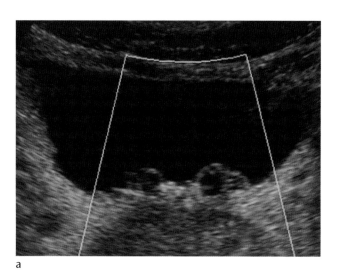

a

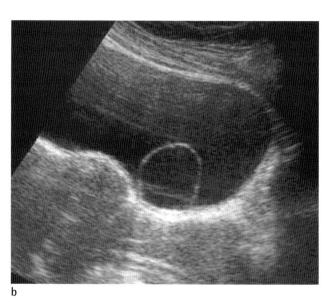

b

Figure 2.20
Ureterocele. (a) Small bilateral ureteroceles. (b) Larger unilateral ureterocele.

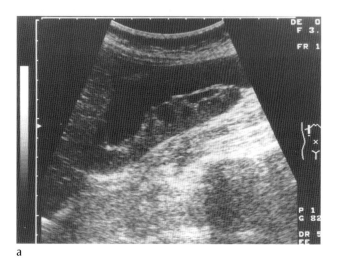

a

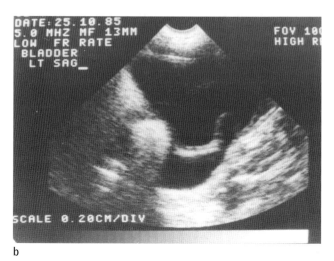

b

Figure 2.21
Duplex kidney with a megaureter draining the upper moiety and ureterocele. This is a common association. (a) Kidney with anterior proximal megaureter, (b) distal megaureter with an ureterocele.

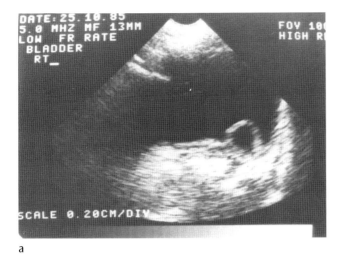

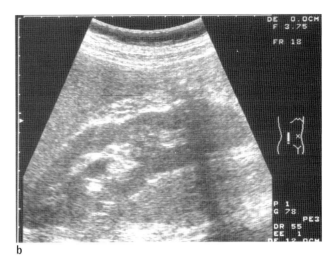

a   b

Figure 2.22
Ureterocele with crossed renal ectopia. The ureterocele (a) is on the ureter draining the normally placed upper kidney, which is mildly hydronephrotic. The ectopic lower kidney is drained via a ureter which crossed to the other side of the bladder and did not have a ureterocele. Ureteroceles are often associated with renal ectopia and may occur on the normal or ectopic side. (b) Shows the fused moieties of the crossed renal ectopia.

at its tip, superior or inferior surface, and open into the bladder (intravesical ureterocele), or the dilated part of the ureterocele may lie in the submucosa of the bladder, with a narrow part extending into the bladder neck or urethra where the orifice lies (ectopic ureterocele).

The site of the orifice is, however, rarely demonstrated on ultrasound, although the ureteric jet seen in real time on color Doppler imaging may sometimes reveal its site.

Ureteroceles may occur in a single (non-duplex) ureter, in which case they are usually intravesical, asymptomatic and present as incidental findings in adult life. A minority are ectopic, may cause obstruction because of a stenotic orifice, or may become sufficiently large to cause bladder neck obstruction.

Ureteroceles in duplex ureters are most frequent on the upper pole ureter; next in frequency is a ureterocele in the common stem of a duplex ureter, and least common is a ureterocele on a lower pole ureter. Ureteroceles in upper pole ureters are often ectopic, and may be blind ending. They are often associated with a very hydronephrotic upper pole moiety, which may by dysplastic and produce little urine. Any type of ureterocele may, however, occur at any site, and the moiety drained by the affected ureter may be normal or dysplastic, hydronephrotic or non-dilated.

Ultrasound appearances (Figures 2.20–2.25)

The intravesical portion of the ureterocele is seen as a thin-walled structure extending into the bladder. The shape is usually rounded but may vary with the state of filling of the bladder. The ureterocele is often compressed in an overfull

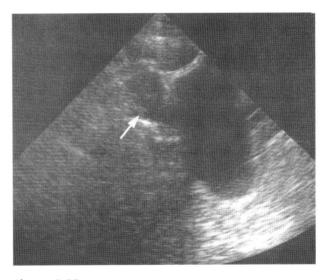

Figure 2.23
Inverted ureterocele. The lesion (arrow) was initially thought to be a bladder diverticulum. Cystoscopy later revealed a ureterocele which was inverted at the time of the scan.

bladder and may invert on micturition, giving an ultrasonic appearance similar to a diverticulum. This inverted appearance is more often seen in IVU, although it may be seen on ultrasound scanning in young children.

The ureter draining via the ureterocele may be dilated to a varying degree, depending on the severity of stenosis, and in a duplex system the upper pole moiety may be dysplastic, in which case a sac is seen with little surrounding renal

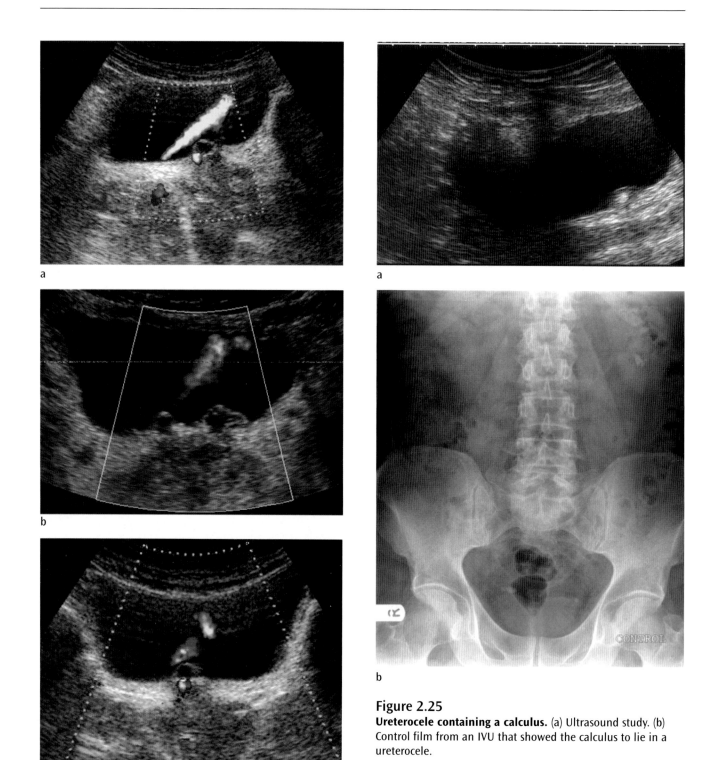

a

b

c

Figure 2.24
Ureterocele emptying from its base. (a) The color Doppler image shows the left-sided ureterocele emptying into the bladder from its base. There is a poor jet. Compare the normal jet on the right. Such ureteroceles often cause partial obstruction, (b,c) shows ureteroceles emptying from their tips but with abnormal jet angles.

a

b

Figure 2.25
Ureterocele containing a calculus. (a) Ultrasound study. (b) Control film from an IVU that showed the calculus to lie in a ureterocele.

tissue. In other cases, the moiety may be hydronephrotic with normal tissue or may be normal with no hydronephrosis. The appearance of a fluid-filled sac representing the upper pole strongly suggests a ureterocele. The finding of a ureterocele also raises the possibility of renal ectopia, as there is a strong association.

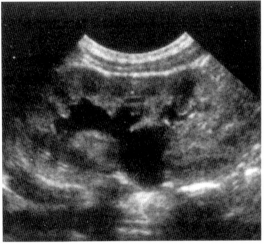 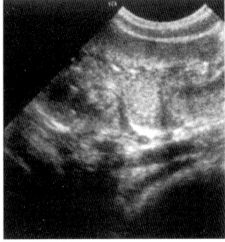

a   b

Figure 2.26
Vesicoureteric reflux.
Contrast studies (a) show a dilated calyceal system. (b) The renal pelvis has filled with ultrasound contrast, indicating reflux. (Reproduced with permission from Piaggio G, Degl'Innocenti ML, Toma P, Perfumo F. Cystosonography and voiding cystourethrography in the diagnosis of vesicoureteral reflux. Pediatr Nephrol 2003; 18(1): 18–22.

Vesicoureteric reflux[28–30]

The normal ureters enter the bladder obliquely through the muscular bladder wall, then run a short submucosal course before opening into the bladder lumen. This arrangement acts as a valve that allows urine to enter the bladder but not to reflux from the bladder back into the ureters. In some patients this arrangement is imperfect, with the ureters running a less oblique course through the bladder wall. Most such ureters enter the bladder lateral and cephalad to their normal position but ectopic ureters that enter the bladder below the normal position also usually reflux. Part of the valvular mechanism is the submucosal part of the ureters. This elongates with growth. This elongation may correct childhood reflux in most cases. This explains why reflux is, in most cases, a condition of children, with only the most severe cases persisting into adulthood.

In some cases, reflux occurs in normal ureters, due to voiding dysfunction or bladder outlet obstruction. In these cases the valvular mechanism at the vesicoureteric junction is normal but the bladder pressure exceeds its capacity.

Reflux may start in utero, possibly due to transient anatomical obstruction, or it may start in older children, particularly girls, because of voiding dysfunction. Thus, reflux is usually found in the investigation of uropathy detected on antenatal scans, or in the investigation of childhood urinary tract infections.

Congenital abnormalities of the vesicoureteric junction, although usually isolated, are sometimes associated with renal dysplasia, agenesis, PUJ obstruction, multicystic dysplastic kidney or fused kidneys. If any of these conditions are detected, investigations for reflux are indicated.

Reflux has a familial tendency, and siblings of children with reflux should be investigated.

Although the treatment of reflux is still very controversial, it is generally accepted that children with suspected reflux should be investigated.

Table 2.3 *Grading of vesicoureteric reflux*	
I	Ureter only
II	Intrarenal pelvis and calyces – no dilatation
III	Intrarenal pelvis and calyces – mild dilatation
IV	Intrarenal pelvis and calyces – moderate dilatation
V	Intrarenal pelvis and calyces – marked dilatation, tortuous ureter

Imaging of reflux

The gold standard remains micturating cystourethrography, despite the need for urethral catheterization and ionizing radiation. Ultrasound studies are often the modality that detects the signs that initially suggest reflux. Calyceal dilatation occurring either prenatally or in children, renal dysplasia, renal scarring or poor bladder emptying suggest the possibility of reflux. Ultrasound may also monitor the affects of reflux such as calyceal dilatation and increasing scarring. Attempts to use ultrasound for the investigation of reflux itself have, however, been disappointing. Dilatation of the calyceal system occurs, and increases during micturation in grade IV and V reflux (Table 2.3). However, the study of the phenomenon by ultrasound is insensitive. It is possible to study reflux by introducing ultrasound contrast agents (stabilized gas microbubbles) into the bladder and scanning the kidney during micturition to detect reflux of the contrast (Figure 2.26). This does not detect the grade I reflux, which is into the ureter only. Although this investigation has its proponents, it still requires urethral catheterization and can be difficult in a moving child. Also, only one side can usually be studied at a time. Refilling the bladder is necessary to study the other side. Thus, conventional voiding

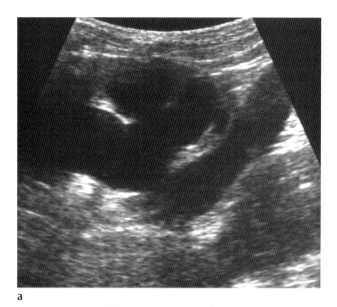

a

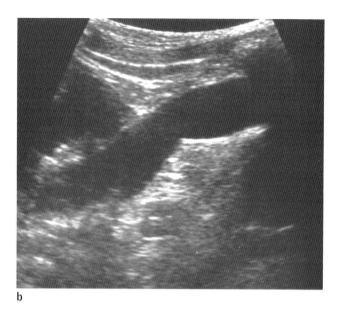

b

Figure 2.27
Megaureter. (a–c) Hydronephrosis and hydroureter sufficiently large to call it a megaureter.

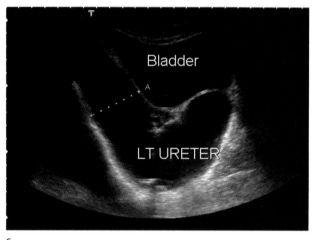

c

cystourethrography remains the usual method in most centers. Ultrasound is, however, widely used in the follow-up of reflux nephropathy.

Megaureter[31]

The general term megaureter means a dilated ureter due to any cause (Figure 2.27). Primary megaureter is a specific pathologic entity. There is an aperistaltic segment of lower ureter which results in dilatation of the ureter proximal to it, usually only the distal ureter but sometimes the whole ureter. Secondary megaureter is dilatation of the ureter due to reflux or obstruction. The term tends to be used for marked dilatation as opposed to mild dilatation, which is termed hydroureter, although there is no logical distinction between the two. Megaureters, because of their size, are usually visible on an ultrasound study. One thing to appreciate is that megaureters are often tortuous, so that they may appear as multiple ovoid fluid-filled lesions, as opposed to a single tube. Primary megaureters have increased peristalsis of the lower ureteric segment, with to and fro motion, which may be seen on real-time ultrasound. Below the dilatation is a segment of ureter with a narrow thread-like lumen. This is seen on IVU, but is not usually visible on an ultrasound study.

Reduplication of the ureter

Duplex kidneys may be obviously duplex on an ultrasound study. More often, they are suspected although not proven when a kidney appears long with or without a dividing septum. It is not usually possible on an ultrasound study,

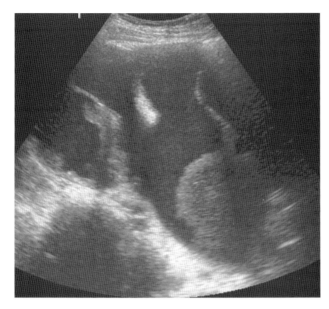

Figure 2.28
Uroepithelial tumor. There is a transitional cell cancer in the upper pole calyx and another at the pelviureteric junction that is causing obstruction.

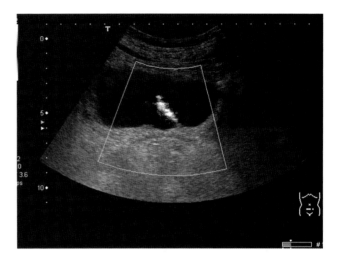

Figure 2.29
Normal ureteric jet. There is a strong jet, indicated by a long jet length. The angle is normal. See also Figure 2.24.

however, to determine whether the ureters are reduplicated. When a ureter from an upper pole moiety is dilated it may be seen crossing the lower moiety (see Figure 2.21a), but this is an exception. Twin ureteric jets may also be seen in the bladder (see Figure 2.19). This, however, is so inconstantly seen as to be a curiosity rather than a diagnostically useful sign.

Intraluminal pathologies[32]

Ureteric calculus is the most common intraluminal pathology to cause ureteric obstruction, and has already been discussed. Uroepithelial tumors are only usually seen ultrasonically when in the renal pelvis or bladder. Such tumors may themselves cause obstruction. The presence of uroepithelial tumors in parts of the renal pelvis or bladder that do not cause obstruction is sometimes accompanied by hydronephrosis. In these cases, a second ureteric tumor should be suspected, although such tumors are extremely rarely seen on an ultrasound study (Figure 2.28).

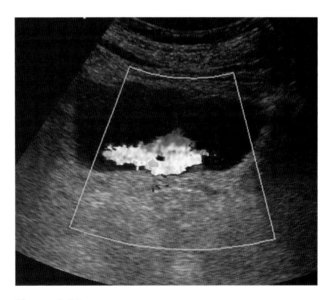

Figure 2.30
Jet from a ureter with vesicoureteric reflux. There is a narrow angle between the jet and the bladder base.

The ureteric jets

The jets of urine that project from the ureteric orifices into the bladder may be clearly seen on a real-time ultrasound study. While color Doppler is the easiest way to demonstrate

them, they are seen on the gray-scale image, presumably due to the difference in density between the urine in the jets and the residual urine within the bladder. The presence, positions and angle of the jets may be observed in this way. Additionally, spectral Doppler studies of the jets, obtained in the same way as is used to study blood flow, reveal the

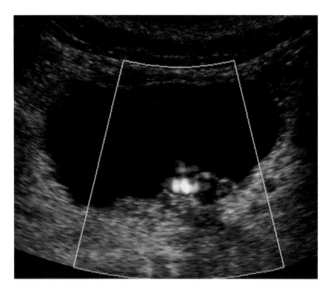

Figure 2.31
Jet from partially obstructed ureter. There is a ureterocele draining from its base and causing partial obstruction. The jet is weak, indicated by a short length. See also Figure 2.24.

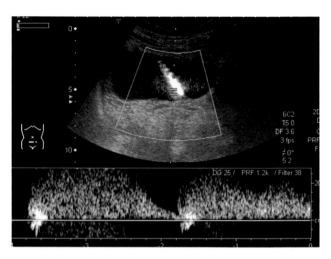

Figure 2.32
Ureteric jet – normal spectral pattern. There is a normal biphasic flow pattern.

temporal flow pattern of the jets. The position of the jets depends on the position of the ureteric orifices, and this may be potentially useful in the study of ectopic ureters. The angle of the jets depends on the angle of the intramural ureter, which may be shallower in cases of reflux. The jets may be absent in complete ureteric obstruction, or weak in partial obstruction. The jet may be modified, in angle or form, by tumor or ureterocele. The temporal pattern of the jet depends on the combined effects of ureteric peristalsis and the sphincteric action of the intramural portion of the ureter (VUJ). The normal jet waveform in adults is intermittent, the frequency depending on urine output, which, in normally functioning kidneys, mainly depends on the degree of hydration. Each individual jet consists of several peaks, normally between 2 and 4. This is presumed to be due to the effect of the sphincteric (antireflux) action of the intramural ureter (VUJ). The jet becomes continuous and prolonged in a forced diuresis. A monophasic jet is, however, abnormal in adults. The monophasic jet is a normal waveform in infants, and may be regarded as an immature waveform. The monophasic pattern is almost universal up to the age of 6 months. It persists in some children to a varying age, up to 14 years. Beyond this age, it is abnormal. Although the monophasic waveform may be regarded as normal in children from 6 months to 14 years, a greater proportion of children with a monophasic waveform have vesicoureteric reflux than those with polyphasic waveforms.[33–35]

Valuable information may, therefore, be gained from observing the ureteric jets. Caution must, however, be exer-

cised. In cases of suspected ureteric obstruction, the presence of a strong ureteric jet obviously excludes complete obstruction. Incomplete obstruction is not, however, excluded. Conversely, an apparently absent jet may be due to poor hydration, poor renal function or technical failure – looking in the wrong place. A poor, i.e. low-velocity jet, is suggestive of incomplete obstruction.

In the study of vesicoureteric reflux much has been written about the angle of the jet, a less-horizontal jet indicating a shorter intramural ureter that is more likely to reflux. More recently, the monophasic jet has been shown to be associated with reflux. These observations undoubtedly give valuable scientific information about the mechanism of vesicoureteric reflux. They have not, however, proved to be very valuable in the routine clinical investigation of reflux and are not in widespread clinical use (Figures 2.29–2.32).

References

1. Mirk P, Maresca G, Fileni A, Vincenzoni M. Sonography of normal lower ureters. J Clin Ultrasound 1988; 16(9): 635–42.
2. Pfister RC, Newhouse JH. Radiology of ureter. Urology 1978; 12(1): 15–39.
3. Holm HH, Torp-Pedersen S, Larsen T, Dorph S. Transabdominal and endoluminal ultrasonic scanning of the lower ureter. Scand J Urol Nephrol Suppl 1994; 157: 19–25.
4. Roshani H, Dabhoiwala NF, Verbeek FJ, et al. Anatomy of ureterovesical junction and distal ureter studied by endoluminal ultrasonography in vitro. J Urol 1999; 161(5): 1614–19.

5. Kerr WS Jr. Effects of complete ureteral obstruction in dogs on kidney function. Am J Physiol 1956; 184: 521–6.

6. Platt JF, Rubin JM, Ellis JH, DiPietro MA. Duplex Doppler US of the kidney: differentiation of obstructive from nonobstructive dilatation. Radiology 1989; 171: 515–17.

7. Platt JF. Advances in ultrasonography of urinary tract obstruction. Abdom Imaging 1998; 23(1): 3–9.

8. Webb JA. Ultrasonography and Doppler studies in the diagnosis of renal obstruction. BJU Int 2000; 86(Suppl 1): 25–32.

9. Tublin ME, Bude RO, Platt JF. Review. The resistive index in renal Doppler sonography: where do we stand? AJR Am J Roentgenol 2003; 180(4): 885–92.

10. Akcar N, Ozkan IR, Adapinar B, Kaya T. Doppler sonography in the diagnosis of urinary tract obstruction by stone. J Clin Ultrasound 2004; 32(6): 286–93.

11. Renowden SA, Cochlin DL. The potential use of diuresis Doppler sonography in PUJ obstruction. Clin Radiol 1992; 46(2): 94–6.

12. Yilmaz S, Sindel T, Arslan G, et al. Renal colic: comparison of spiral CT, US and IVU in the detection of ureteral calculi. Eur Radiol 1998; 8: 212–17.

13. Onishi K, Watanabe H, Ohe H, et al. Ultrasound finding in urolithiasis in the lower ureter. Ultrasound Med Biol 1986; 122: 15.

14. Erden A, Aytac S, Cumhur T, et al. Retroperitoneal fibrosis: evaluation by ultrasonography and color Doppler imaging. Urol Int 1995; 55(2): 111–14.

15. Amis ES Jr. Retroperitoneal fibrosis. Urol Radiol 1990; 12(3): 135–7.

16. Sanders RC, Duffy T, McLoughlin MG, et al. Sonography in the detection of retroperitoneal fibrosis. J Urol 1977; 118: 944–6.

17. Amis ES. Retroperitoneal fibrosis. AJR Am J Roentgenol 1991; 157: 321–9.

18. Jones W, Barie P. Urological manifestations of acute appendicitis. J Urol 1988; 139: 1325–8.

19. Irving SO, Burgess NA. Managing severe loin pain in pregnancy. BJOG 2002; 109(9): 1025–9.

20. Grenier N, Pariente JL, Trillaud H, et al. Dilatation or the collecting system during pregnancy: physiological vs obstructive dilatation. Eur Radiol 2000; 10: 271–9.

21. Murthy LN. Urinary tract obstruction during pregnancy: recent developments in imaging. Br J Urol 1997; 80(Suppl 1): 1–3.

22. Haddad MC, Abomelha MS, Riley PJ. Diagnosis of acute ureteral calculus obstruction in pregnant women using color and pulsed Doppler sonography. Clin Radiol 1995; 50(12): 864–6.

23. MacNeily AE, Goldenberg SL, Allen GJ, et al. Sonographic visualization of the ureter in pregnancy. J Urol 1991; 146: 298–301.

24. Hernanz-Schulman M, Genieser N, Ambrosino M, Hanna M. Bilateral duplex ectopic ureters terminating in the seminal vesicles: sonographic and CT diagnosis. Urol Radiol 1989; 11(1): 49–52.

25. Schaffer RM, Shih YH, Becker JA. Sonographic identification of collecting system duplications. J Clin Ultrasound 1983; 11(6): 309–12.

26. Griffin J, Jennings C, MacErlean D. Ultrasonic evaluation of simple and ectopic ureteroceles. Clin Radiol 1983; 34(1): 55–7.

27. Madeb R, Shapiro I, Rothschild E, et al. Evaluation of ureterocele with Doppler sonography. J Clin Ultrasound 2000; 28: 425–9.

28. Marshall JL, Johnson ND, De Campo MP. Vesicoureteric reflux in children: prediction with color Doppler imaging. Work in progress. Radiology 1990; 175(2): 355–8.

29. Kuzmic AC, Brkljacic B. Color Doppler ultrasonography in the assessment of vesicoureteric reflux in children with bladder dysfunction. Pediatr Surg Int 2002; 18(2–3): 135–9.

30. Radmayr C, Oswald J, Klauser A, et al. [Contrast-medium enhanced reflux ultrasound in children. A comparison with radiologic imaging up to now]. [German] Urologe (Ausg. A) 2002; 41(6): 548–51.

31. Vereecken RL. Proesmans W. A review of ninety-two obstructive megaureters in children. Eur Urol 1999; 36(4): 342–7.

32. Hadas-Halpern I, Farcas A, Patlas M, et al. Sonographic diagnosis of ureteral tumors. J Ultrasound Med 1999; 18: 639–45.

33. Jequier S, Paltiel H, Lafortune M. Ureterovesical jets in infants and children: duplex and color Doppler US studies. Radiology 1990; 175(2): 349–53.

34. Burge HJ, Middleton WD, McClennan BL, Hildebolt CF. Ureteral jets in healthy subjects with unilateral calculi: comparison with color Doppler US. Radiology 1991; 180: 437–42.

35. Leung VY, Metreweli C, Yeung CK. Immature ureteric jet doppler patterns and urinary tract infection and vesicoureteric reflux in children. Ultrasound Med Biol 2002; 28: 873–8.

3

The bladder

Dennis Ll Cochlin

Embryology

As this chapter deals with the adult bladder, a brief discussion of embryology will be given as it applies to those congenital abnormalities that escape detection and remain undiscovered until adulthood.

Bladder development is a two-stage process beginning with the terminal end of the primitive gut, the embryonic cloaca. The cloaca is divided into an anterior and posterior portion by the urorectal septum. The anterior portion will form the primitive bladder and the posterior portion forms the anal rectal canal. The mesonephric ducts insert into the anterior portion of the cloaca, dividing it into a superior portion, the primitive bladder, and an inferior portion, the urogenital sinus. As the mesonephric ducts are incorporated into the bladder, they maintain separate openings near the lower portion, giving rise to the ureters. The upper portion of the cloaca or primitive bladder is continuous with the allantois. The urachus is the superior connection with the allantois which will degenerate into a cord-like structure called the median umbilical ligament in the adult.

At birth, the neonatal bladder occupies a much more superior location in the pelvis than the adult bladder. With maturation, the bladder assumes a lower position within the true pelvis. The surrounding anatomical structures seen on ultrasound will vary with the sex of the patient.

Sonographic technique and anatomy[1,2]

Successful ultrasound imaging of the bladder requires adequate distension by urine. The average adult bladder will hold approximately 500 ml of urine, and to achieve good distension the patients are instructed to drink 1 liter (8–16 ounces) of fluid 1 hour before their arrival in the ultrasound department. The patient is examined in the supine position.

Scanning is initiated by placing the transducer approximately 1 cm above the symphysis pubis, either in the sagittal or transverse orientation. Once the bladder is identified, real-time scanning is done in a systematic fashion in both the transverse and sagittal planes as well as oblique sagittal planes. The transducer must be angled behind the symphysis pubis to image the anterior basal portions of the bladder. Sometimes body habitus will preclude visualization of this region of the bladder and it is especially problematic for measurements of bladder volume. In addition, transabdominal scanning may be limited in the postsurgical patient by sutures, bandages and open wounds. A patient with an indwelling catheter may have iatrogenic air in the dome of the bladder, which will limit through transmission of the ultrasound beam. In these cases, a transrectal or a transperineal approach may yield useful information with respect to the base of the bladder. Unfortunately, the apex and dome of the bladder may be suboptimally imaged.

The sex of the patient determines the anatomical structures adjacent to the bladder. Ultrasonographically, the bladder in either sex appears as an anechoic structure with a variable shape governed to a large degree by the amount of distension. When the well-distended bladder is imaged in the transverse plane, it usually takes the shape of a tetrahedron. In the sagittal or oblique sagittal plane, it may have an oval to pyramidal shape.

The adult bladder lies in the bony true pelvis. Dome, apex, superior lateral and posterior one-third of the bladder are covered by peritoneum. In the male, the peritoneal reflection posteriorly forms the deepest recess within the pelvis, the rectovesical pouch. Anteriorly, the bladder is separated from the symphysis pubis by the prevesical fascia or cavum retzii. The base of the bladder lies on the prostate and the prostatic urethra courses through the prostate, exiting at the prostatic apex to form the membranous portion of the male urethra. Posterior to the bladder, the fluid-filled seminal vesicles and the medially positioned, tubular-shaped vas deferens may be imaged (Figure 3.1).

In the female, the bladder lies anterior to the uterus. The pouch of Douglas will represent the deepest posterior recess between the rectum and uterus. The short female urethra exits from the bladder base. The muscles and adjacent structures in the female are similar to those in the male. These important muscular and bony lateral boundaries surround the bladder and are common to both sexes. At the level of the acetabular roofs, the hypoechoic paired

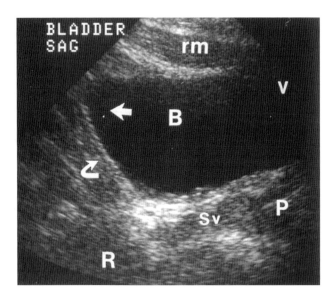

Figure 3.1
Sagittal transabdominal image of the male bladder. In this image the male bladder (B) is located superior to the prostate (P) and anterosuperior to the seminal vesicle (Sv). The peritoneum (curved arrow) reflects over the dome (arrow) and it will descend to its deepest point in the pelvis to form the retrovesical pouch between bladder and rectum (R). The vertex (V) of the bladder is posterior to the symphysis and is often hidden by acoustic shadowing. Anteriorly, a portion of the hypoechoic rectus abdominis muscle (rm) is imaged with hyperechoic adipose tissue posteriorly.

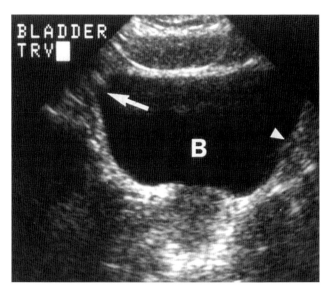

Figure 3.2
Transverse transabdominal image of the bladder. The bladder (B) is imaged in the transverse plane, with the right iliopsoas (arrow) and the left obturator internus (arrowhead) forming the hypoechoic muscular borders of the bladder.

obturator internus muscles are seen adjacent to the bladder wall. Anteriolaterally, the iliopsoas muscles can be seen as they exit the pelvis. The paired external iliac artery and vein are seen adjacent to these muscles. The oval-shaped, hypoechoic rectus abdominis muscles are easily identified landmarks of the anterior abdominal wall. The bony portions of the pelvis will be seen as echogenic reflectors which block thorough transmission of sound (Figure 3.2).

Bladder wall thickness[3–5]

The sonographic appearance of the bladder wall varies with the degree of bladder distension and the ultrasound system used. Sonographically, the mucous, submucous, muscular and serous coats of the bladder wall are usually not recognized as distinct entities, but the echogenic mucosa and more sonolucent muscular coat may be identified. Measurement of bladder wall thickness has been problematic and may vary depending on bladder distension. The maximum thickness of the bladder wall has been said to be no more than 7–8 mm, but this figure is probably an overestimation since it includes perivesical fat. More recently, the upper limits of the bladder wall have been redefined as 3 mm for a full bladder and 5 mm for an empty bladder. It has been noted that measurement location is also critical (Figure 3.3).

Bladder volume estimation[6–10]

Quantification of the overall bladder volume is important in patients who have urinary retention. Attempts to measure the various dimensions of the bladder and then derive accurate volume measurements have met with limited success. So far, none of these methods produces an exact volume. The lack of accuracy has been attributed to the variations in bladder shape secondary to filling and inability to image the anterior aspect of the bladder base. In practice, however, ultrasonic estimation of bladder volume is perfectly satisfactory for clinical use.

Numerous formulae for the measurement of volume have been derived based on mathematical models for ellipses and from linear regression analysis of laboratory data. Common to all of them is the requirement for measuring the various distances from the sagittal and transverse planes. The sagittal plane provides the cranio-caudad (height) and the anteroposterior distances. The transverse image of the bladder at its widest dimensions yields the width. In practice the formula

$$\left(0.54 = \frac{\pi}{6}\right) a \times b \times c \times 0.54$$

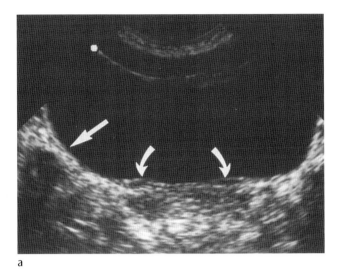

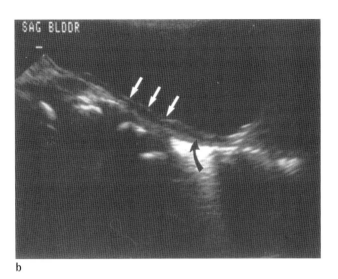

a

b

Figure 3.3

Normal bladder wall. The sonographic appearance of the wall (arrow) of the adult bladder in (a) is described as echogenic with no clear separation made between the normal anatomical layers. The ureters enter the wall of the bladder at the ureterovesical junction (curved arrows). On the other hand, the echogenic mucosa (arrows) and the hypoechoic to sonolucent muscular layer (curved arrow) may be imaged as two distinct layers (b).

where *a*, *b* and *c* are the three orthogonal bladder measurements, is almost universally used and is adequate for clinical purposes (Figure 3.4).

Congenital anomalies

The majority of congenital anomalies of the bladder are encountered during the neonatal period. These rare anomalies include congenital diverticula, complete duplication

of the bladder and complete absence of the bladder. Another rare anomaly, extrophy of the bladder, presents with other renal abnormalities and it is often associated with absence of the abdominal musculature.

Urachal cyst[11–14]

It is the urachal malformations, in particular the urachal cyst, which escape detection until adult life. As previously

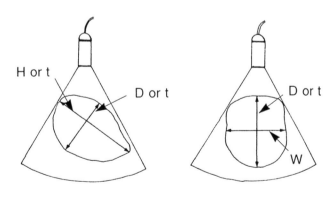

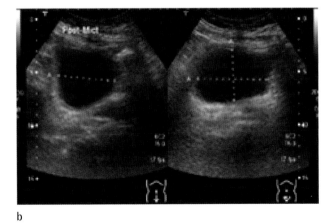

a

b

Figure 3.4

Bladder volume estimation. (a) Line drawing of the various dimensions that are measured for height (H), depth (D or t) and width (W or q), and then substituted into the formulae for calculating bladder volumes. (b) Images of measurements as outlined in (a).

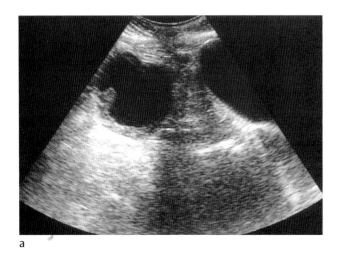

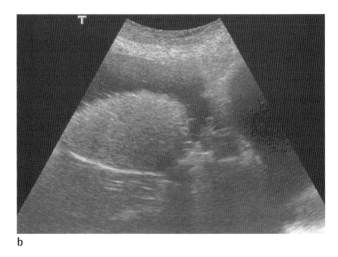

a

b

Figure 3.5
Urachal cyst. (a) There is an anechoic cyst cephalad to the bladder. The thick posterior wall caused concern that there may be malignant change. Histology after excision, however, showed non-specific inflammatory change only. (b) A large urachal cyst containing mucus.

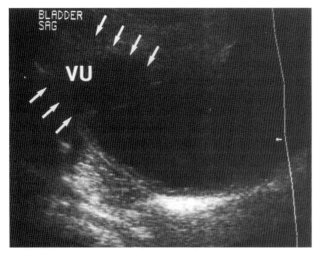

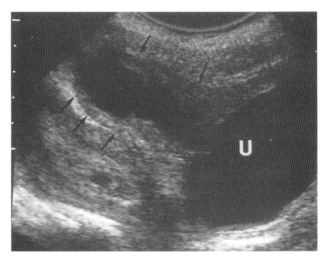

Figure 3.6
Vesicourachal diverticulum. A vesicourachal diverticulum (VU) is imaged in the sagittal plane. There is a sonolucent cystic structure with echogenic walls (arrows) just posterior to the anterior abdominal wall. The communication with the bladder lumen is seen.

Figure 3.7
Infected vesicourachal diverticulum. The patient presented as a case of cystitis, and the cystosonogram reveals a thick-walled, infected vesicourachal diverticulum (arrows) superior to the urinary bladder (U).

mentioned, the urachus is the primitive connection between the true bladder and the allantois. Much of it lies extraperitoneally and only its pelvic portion lies intraperitoneally.

The basic problem with urachal development is either complete or incomplete failure of regression of this structure. Non-regression of the urachus produces a patent urachus, resulting in a fistulous connection between the

bladder and umbilicus. Segmental failures or incomplete regression produce the vesicourachal diverticulum (patency of the caudal segment of the urachus), urachal sinus (patency of the cephalic portion of the urachus with the umbilicus) or urachal cyst (patency of only the mid-portion of the urachus). This midline cyst lies silently beneath the anterior abdominal wall, often escaping detection until

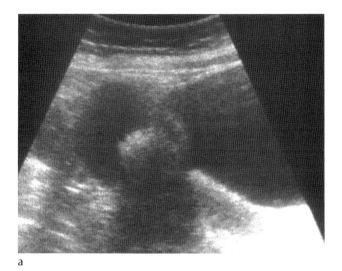

a

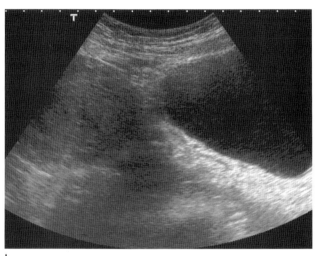

b

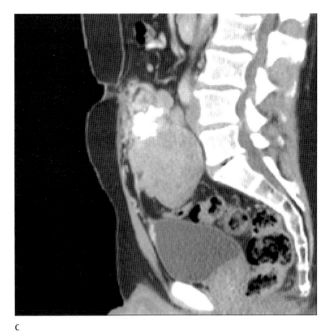

c

Figure 3.8
Urachal cyst with malignant change. (a) A urachal
diverticulum with a solid element posteriorly indicating
malignant change. (b) A tumor above the bladder.
Communication with the umbilicus could be demonstrated. (c)
A sagittal MRI study of the same tumor.

adulthood. Occasionally a urachal cyst may present early
after it spontaneously drains into either the umbilicus or
bladder as a complication of a secondary infection.
Sometimes a patient with one of these conditions will present with vague abdominal or urinary symptoms and in such
cases the anomaly may be identified with ultrasound.

Ultrasonographically, the urachal cyst occupies an
extraperitoneal location and is in the expected line of the
median umbilical ligament. It is an oval-shaped, sonolucent and echo-free cyst when it is not complicated by infection (Figure 3.5). The vesicourachal diverticulum presents
as a sac-like midline projection from the superior aspect of
the bladder (Figure 3.6). Infection causes a thick wall, similar to the bladder wall in cystitis (Figure 3.7). In 2% of
cases, this epithelial-lined structure undergoes neoplastic
transformation into adenocarcinoma. These are medium-
echodensity masses; 70% contain mucin and dystrophic
calcification, resulting in areas of low echodensity, and
areas of shadowing (Figure 3.8).

Acquired abnormalities

Micturition disorders[8–12]

The most common micturition disorder is bladder outlet
obstruction. In men this is most often attributed to
prostate enlargement, although even in the presence of an
enlarged prostate, the mechanism of outlet obstruction is
often complex and also involves bladder dysfunction. In
women, outlet obstruction is less common, and usually
due to bladder dysfunction.

There is also the large group of patients with neurogenic
bladders, due to spinal injury, multiple sclerosis, spina
bifida or a long list of other neurologic conditions.

The most common reason for requesting ultrasound is
to assess bladder emptying. Often all that is needed to
plan management, and for follow-up, is assessment of the
upper tracts for hydronephrosis, and measurement of

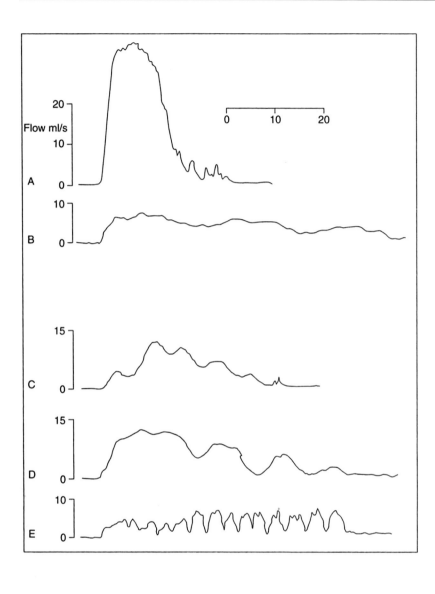

Figure 3.9
Typical urinary flow rate studies. (A) Normal, (B) obstruction, (C) underactive detrussor muscle, (D) anxious bladder syndrome, and (E) atonic bladder. (Reproduced from Halpern EJ, Cochlin DL, Goldberg BB, eds. Imaging of the prostate. London: Martin Dunitz, 2002.)

postmicturition bladder volume. It should be realized that an overfull bladder may sometimes cause distension of normal pelvicalyceal systems. If mild distension is seen with a very full bladder, the kidneys should be rechecked after micturition. Return to normal probably indicates normality. Assessment of residual bladder volume is often preceeded with a urine flow-rate measurement. The patient micturates into a device that produces a graph of the urine output, from which flow rates may be measured (Figure 3.9). In many cases, this provides sufficient information to plan management. In complex cases, however, more information about bladder function may be needed. In these cases urodynamic studies are performed. Fine catheters are placed in the bladder and rectum, and pressures measured during micturition. Subtraction of the rectal pressure (abdominal pressure) from the bladder pressure gives the true bladder pressure. Micturition is normally monitored by filling the bladder with contrast and radiographic screening. Ultrasound has, however, been

used for this purpose. A discussion of urodynamic interpretation is outside the scope of this book, but an idea of what is involved may be obtained from Figure 3.10.[15,16]

Postmicturition bladder volumes are measured as outlined earlier in the chapter. It is important to have a reasonably full bladder premicturition, as some claim that a false residue may result if the premicturition volume is too small. The patient should empty the bladder in whatever way is normal for him; single or double micturition, activation of incontinence device, self-catheterization or other. In cases of condom drainage or nappies, the bladder volume at the time of the scan is recorded. What constitutes a normal postmicturition residue is debatable. Theoretically, the normal bladder should empty completely. In practice, however, a small residue of less than about 20 ml in an adult and less than 10 ml in a child is accepted as insignificant. It is also important to remember that, with a fluid load, the bladder fills at about 4 ml/min, so even a fairly short delay in obtaining the measurement may result in a spuriously large volume.

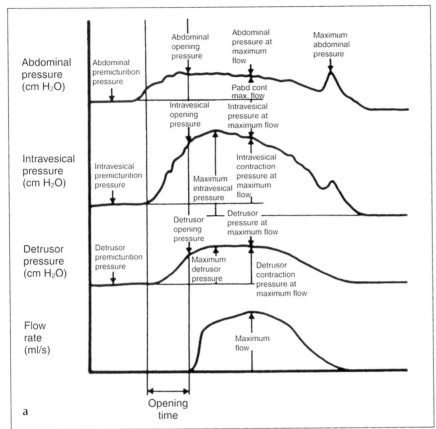

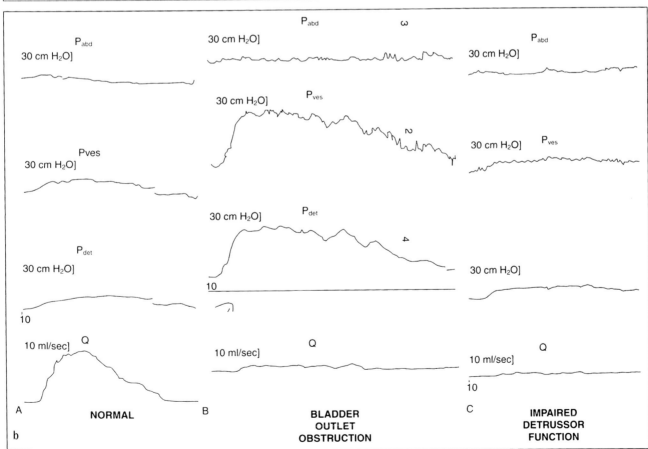

Figure 3.10
Typical urodynamic studies. (a) The parameters that should be measured according to the International Continence Society. (b) Patterns found in normal and abnormal states. (Reproduced from Halpern EJ, Cochlin DL, Goldberg BB, eds. Imaging of the prostate. London: Martin Dunitz, 2002.)

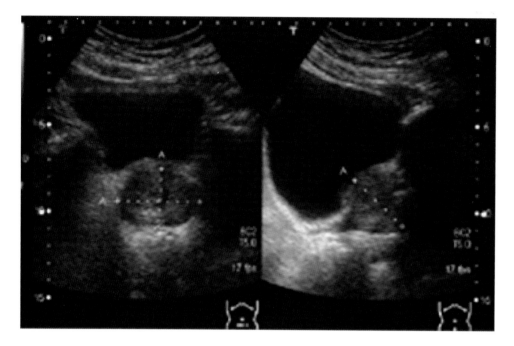

Figure 3.11
Transabdominal measurement of prostate volume. The prostate was measured as shown. Although not as accurate as transrectal measurements, transabdominal measurements give a good approximation of prostate size.

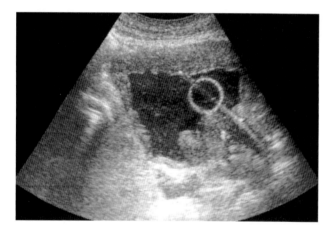

Figure 3.12
Outlet obstruction: thick-walled bladder. There is bladder outlet obstruction caused by prostatic enlargement. The bladder wall is significantly thickened.

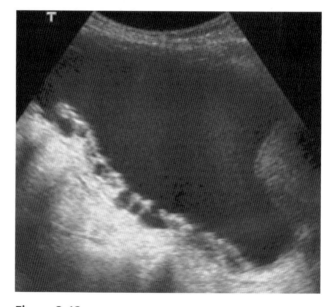

Figure 3.13
Trabeculation. There is marked trabeculation. This is more clearly shown on the posterior wall, partly as this is in the best focal zone of the transducer.

In patients with prostate enlargement, a good estimate of prostate volume may be obtained from the bladder scan by angling downwards to visualize the prostate (Figure 3.11). The volume is calculated by the same formula as is used for bladder volume. It is customary in many centers to report the prostate size in grams. As prostatic tissue has a specific gravity of nearly 1, the weight in grams is approximately the same as the volume in ccs. Transabdominal ultrasound usually reveals little about the nature of prostate enlargement, although locally invasive cancer may be diagnosed if extensive. Nor does transabdominal scanning measure volume as accurately as transrectal ultra-

sound. However, the approximation obtained is sufficiently accurate to be useful in clinical management.

The type of dysfunction present will depend on the level of the lesion. This will affect appearances. In bladder outlet obstruction, ultrasound demonstrates a dilated, thick-walled bladder (Figure 3.12). In some cases the hypertrophied muscle bundles form a pattern resembling a thick net or web,

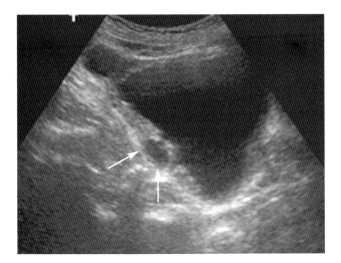

Figure 3.14
Pseudodiverticulum. The trabeculation has caused an appearance superficially resembling a diverticulum (arrows). Unlike a true diverticulum, it does not extend through the muscularis layer.

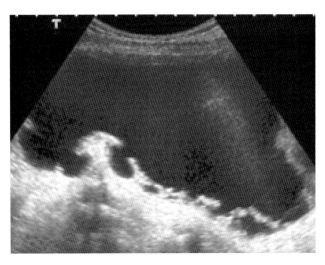

Figure 3.15
Neurogenic bladder. The muscular hypertrophy has caused a coarse trabeculation. On a single slice this appears as shown on the posterior bladder wall. (See also Figure 3.22.)

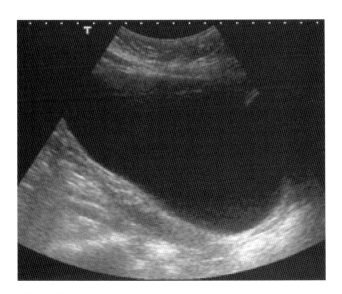

Figure 3.16
Distended neurogenic bladder. A large thin-walled bladder.

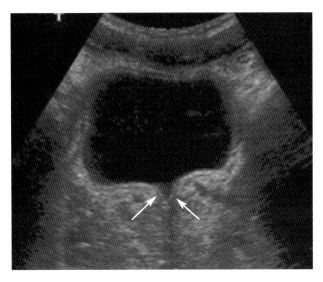

Figure 3.17
Open bladder neck. The bladder neck (arrows) is open.

called trabeculation (Figure 3.13). The redundant mucosa may falsely appear to project beyond the wall, forming pseudodiverticula, which are not true diverticula (Figure 3.14).[5,17,18]

If bladder dysfunction is secondary to an underlying neurologic problem, then the sonographic appearance of the bladder may vary depending on the level of the lesion and the duration of the effect. For low lesions involving the cauda equina or conus of the spinal cord, the bladder may initially dilate and then become hypertrophied and trabeculated when detrusor activity is regained (Figure 3.15). In

spinal lesions above the sacral level, bladder distension may be dominant, with trabeculation and hypertrophy occurring as a result of superimposed infection. Cerebral lesions may result in a thin-walled atrophic bladder that is often overdistended (Figure 3.16).[19–22]

Patients who have incurred a spinal injury are prone to bladder dysfunction. The resulting bladder dysfunction and urinary tract complications are a frequent cause of death. Neuromuscular dysfunction may produce detrusor–sphincter dyssynergia, detrusor–bladder neck

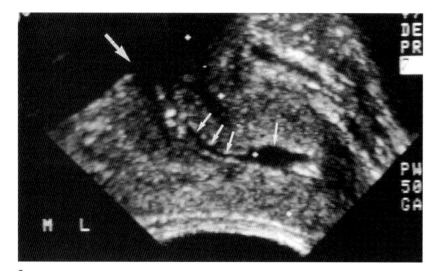

a

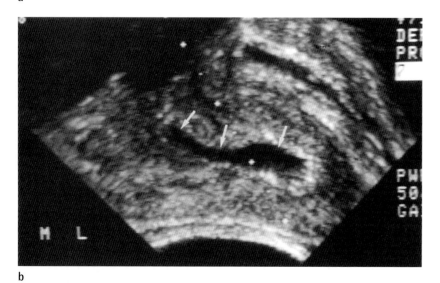

b

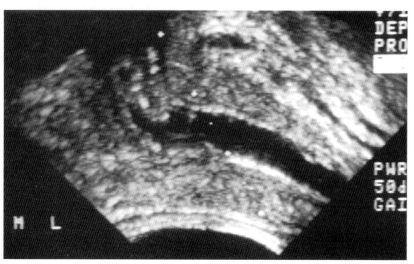

c

Figure 3.18
Transrectal voiding urethrosonography. (a) Voiding is begun. There is flattening of the base plate of the bladder (large arrow) and the C-shaped prostatic urethra begins to dilate (arrows). (b) As voiding proceeds, the prostatic urethra becomes straighter and more dilated (arrows). (c) Finally, the urethra becomes fully dilated during full stream.

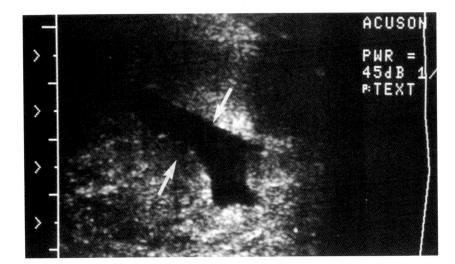

Figure 3.19
Spinal cord injury. As this spinal cord injury patient attempts to void, the bladder neck becomes straightened and dilated (arrows) but no urine passes beyond the region of the detrusor.

dyssynergia, central cord syndrome, or anterior cord syndromes. Detrusor–sphincter dyssynergia arises from failure of the periurethral striated sphincter to relax as the detrusor muscle contracts. If the bladder neck does not relax during detrusor contraction, then detrusor–bladder neck dyssynergia occurs. If a cauda equina lesion leads to disruption of the pelvic parasympathetic nerves and the higher sympathetic root nerves remain intact, a lower motor neuron lesion yields detrusor–bladder neck dyssynergia. In the anterior cord syndrome, the sympathetic fibers within the lateral horns are affected, leading to a widely patent bladder neck (Figure 3.17).

Patients with lesions above the T5 level and, in some cases, abnormalities between the T5 and T8 levels, may have autonomic dysreflexia. If the bladder is irritable and contracts vigorously, patients may develop hypertension, bradycardia, sweating and headaches. If the rapidly rising blood pressure is not controlled, then acute cerebral hemorrhage may be a catastrophic complication for the patient. This response can be precipitated by small volumes of urine or by catheterization.

Transrectal cystosonography can be helpful in delineating voiding abnormalities, especially in individuals suffering from spinal cord injury (Figures 3.18 and 3.19).[23] Furthermore, cystosonography has been utilized in the evaluation of alpha-adrenergic blocking agents such as phentolamine and phenoxybenzamine. These agents block the overactivity of alpha-adrenergic receptors of the sympathetic nervous system which play a role in detrusor–bladder neck dyssynergia. Moreover, many of these patients require chronic intermittent catheterization to relieve bladder distension. Some of these patients will develop catheterization difficulties secondary to mechanical obstruction created by short and long soft tissue shelves at the bladder neck. Transrectal ultrasound has been able to demonstrate them in real time as the patient is catheterized (Figure 3.20).

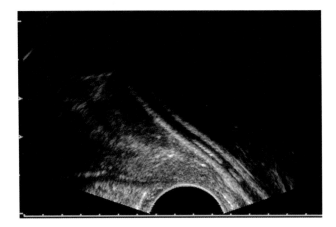

Figure 3.20
Transrectal guidance of bladder catheterization. The catheter is clearly seen.

Pelvic floor weakness in women[13–18]

Stress urinary incontinence is a common symptom in women. These women are subject to involuntary passage of urine, the result of rising bladder pressure which overcomes urethral resistance. Lack of anatomical support for the bladder base is primarily responsible. It usually follows parturition with injury to the pudendal and perineal nerves. It has also been associated with vaginal and bladder neck surgery, but may occur in older women with none of these causes. Evaluation has included plain cystography and cystometric studies. Ultrasound may also be used to investigate the problem by observing movement of the bladder floor and urethra on straining. This may be combined with full urodynamic studies or just with residual bladder volume estimation. The advantages of using ultrasound are that there is no need for bladder catheterization if urodynamics are not performed, and the lack of

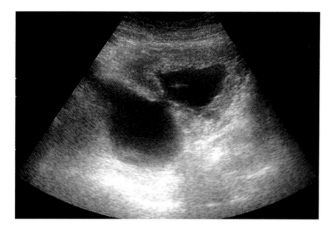

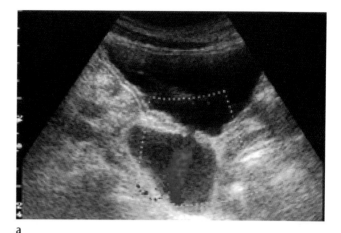

a

Figure 3.21
Bladder diverticulum. There is a diverticulum in a typical paraureteral position in a thick-walled neurogenic bladder.

ionizing radiation. The usual scanning method is by the perineal or introital route. Transvaginal or transrectal scanning give better views of the bladder base and urethra, but are less physiologic, as the presence of the transducer may modify the bladder floor movement.

The technique requires a full bladder. Midline sagittal views of the bladder base and urethra are obtained at rest and during pelvic floor contraction and maximal straining. The views are obtained in the lateral decubitus position and standing.

The bladder neck should remain closed during these maneuvers. A line is drawn perpendicular to the symphysis pubis. The bladder base should lie above this line at rest, and should not descend more than 1 cm during pelvic floor contraction or straining. A linear displacement of the urethral vesical junction on straining greater than 1 cm has been associated with poor pelvic support. On surgical correction, a less than 1 cm linear displacement showed good correlation with urodynamic and clinical cure of stress urinary incontinence.[24–30]

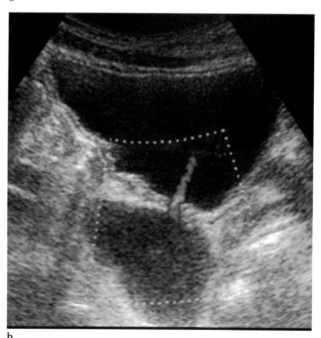

b

Figure 3.22
Diverticulum jet. (a,b) Jets through the diverticulum neck when pressure is increased then released.

Bladder diverticula

Most bladder diverticula are acquired secondary to chronic bladder outlet obstruction, although rarely they can be a congenital anomaly. Generally, acquired diverticula are found in males of more than 50 years of age with bladder outlet obstruction secondary to benign prostatic hyperplasia. These diverticula frequently reside in a paraureteral location (Figure 3.21), although they may occur anywhere posteriorly or laterally, rarely anteriorly.

Sonographically, these anechoic sacs vary in size and will lie adjacent to the bladder wall. The wall of the bladder may be thickened and trabeculated. The opening onto the

diverticulum may be identified and they may increase in size during voiding. The opening is sometimes difficult to see. In these cases, color Doppler may show a urine jet through the opening. With laterally placed diverticula, the jets may be spontaneous and pulsatile, caused by transmitted iliac arterial pulsation. In other cases, the jet may be produced by pressing on the bladder with the transducer (Figure 3.22).* Within the diverticulum, calculi, blood

*I am indebted to Mr Michael Pritchard, senior radiographer and sonographer at the University Hospital of Wales, who first observed this phenomenon.

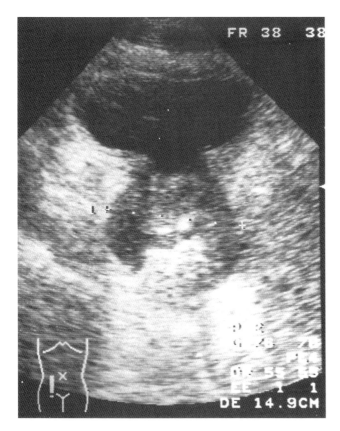

Figure 3.23
Diverticulum with malignant change. A mixed echodensity tumor in the diverticulum. (Courtesy of Dr David Lloyd, University Hospital of Wales.)

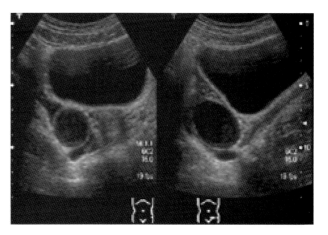

Figure 3.24
Incontinence device balloon reservoir. This was initially thought to be either a bladder diverticulum or an ovarian cyst. A brief question to the patient about previous surgery solved the problem – there was no mention of an incontinence device on the request form.

clots and neoplasms have been encountered (Figure 3.23). If the opening of the diverticulum is not identified, then different possibilities include extrinsic cystic masses such as an ovarian cyst, hematoma or lymphocele.[31] Ureteroceles and portions of a megaureter may also be confused with a diverticulum (Figure 3.24).

Calculi, clots, pus and other debris

Most bladder calculi are acquired secondary to passage of upper tract stones into the bladder. Stones may also form within the bladder from retained blood clots or necrotic debris. Formation can be aided by the presence of infection with urea-splitting organisms or underlying urinary stasis. Metabolic stones are also found in the bladder and are similar to those that form in the upper tracts.

On ultrasound images, a bladder stone or calculus possesses an increased echogenicity with a discrete posterior acoustic shadow. A stone is usually mobile, changing location as the patient is turned into an alternative posi-

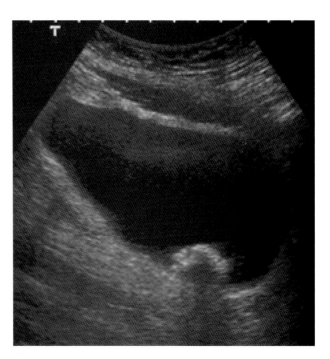

Figure 3.25
Bladder calculus. There is a typical strong crescentic echo and shadowing. It moved on turning the patient.

tion, but occasionally it may adhere to the bladder wall. It may serve as a focus for infection and it rarely produces bladder outlet obstruction (Figure 3.25).[32]

A blood clot may result from hemorrhage within the upper tract passing down the ureter into the bladder, or it may arise within the bladder from an intrinsic process

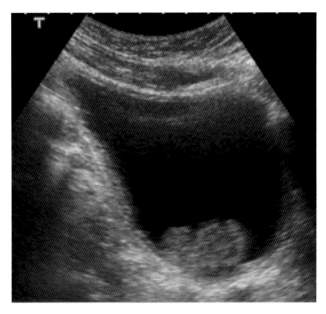

Figure 3.26
Blood clot. There is a medium-echodensity lobulated mass in the bladder lumen which had no demonstrable Doppler flow. Cystoscopy confirmed a blood clot.

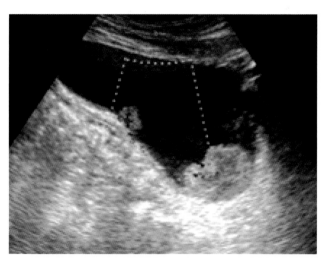

Figure 3.28
Blood clot: Doppler image. The mass at the bladder base shows no demonstrable vasculature on color Doppler. It was a blood clot. The smaller mass higher in the bladder is vascular, indicating that it is a tumor.

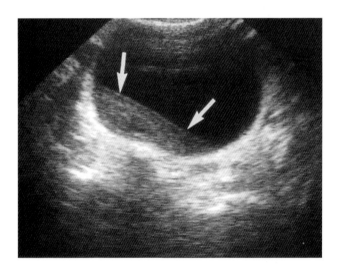

Figure 3.27
Blood in the bladder. A transverse image of the bladder with the low-level echoes of layered hemorrhage (arrows).

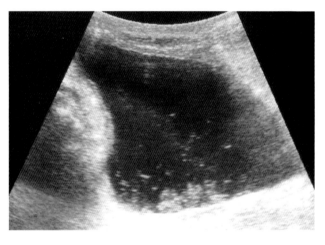

Figure 3.29
Debris in a poorly emptying bladder. There is echogenic debris in the bladder.

such as a neoplasm (Figure 3.26). Depending on the quantity of blood present, a clot may be focal and mobile or adherent. When hemorrhage is profuse, a blood layer may be imaged as a medium echogenic layer on the dependent portion of the bladder wall. This fluid–blood product level will also change its location with alterations in the patient's position (Figure 3.27). If the hemorrhage is primarily from the bladder, then a neoplasm should be

sought intensively. A common problem is differentiating bladder clot from tumor, and both often coexist. One useful differentiator is the demonstration of blood vessels within the lesion by color Doppler (Figure 3.28). The demonstration of vessels indicates tumor. Non-demonstration of vessels, however, does not exclude tumor, as tumor vessels may be very small and below the resolution of the ultrasound system.

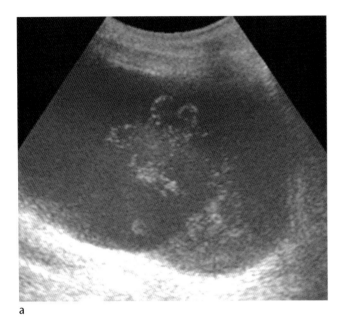

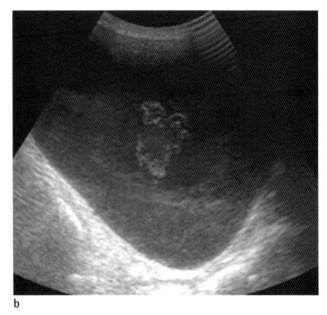

a

b

Figure 3.30
Pyocystis. The patient was in renal failure. (a) There is urine in the bladder, making the echogenic mass of pus easier to see. (b) In this plane, an echogenic layer of debris is seen.

In patients with incomplete bladder emptying, small echogenic particles of debris may be seen in the bladder (Figure 3.29). These are seen in infected and non-infected cases.

Pus within the bladder (pyocystis) does not occur in a normally functioning system, presumably because any pus formed is voided before it accumulates to form a visible mass. In patients with renal failure who are anuric or oliguric, and patients with urinary diversion with retained bladder, pus may accumulate within the bladder to form medium-echogenic masses or fluid–fluid levels, the layer or mass of pus being more echogenic than any urine present. There is often accompanying echogenic cellular debris (Figure 3.30). It is important to recognize pyocystis, as failure to treat the condition may lead to septicemia and death. Treatment is by bladder irrigation and intravesical antibiotics.

Cystitis

Cystitis usually results from a descending upper tract infection or an ascending urethral infection. Primary infection of the bladder is unusual, since the bladder is a fairly resistant organ. However, other types of cystitis also occur, as listed in Table 3.1. The diagnosis is usually based on clinical and laboratory findings without the need for ultrasound. In some cases, however, an ultrasound study first reveals the condition.

Table 3.1 *Causes of cystitis*
Infections Bacterial: *Escherichia coli, Staphylococcus aureus, Streptococcus faecalis.* Less common: *Proteus* spp., *Pseudomonas aeruginosa*, malakoplakia Protozoal: schistosomiasis Fungal: *Candida*, actinomycetes Viral: herpes, adenovirus
Non-infectious Foreign body: catheter, stent, self-inserted object. Calculus Pelvic infection, adjacent inflammatory bowel
Toxic Cyclophosphamide
Radiotherapy
Allergic Interstitial Eosinophilic

Cystitis – ultrasound appearances[33–35]

If cystosonography is performed, in many cases the bladder appears normal. In some, the bladder wall is generally diffusely thickened (Figure 3.31), although focal thickening also occurs. Occasionally, the diffusely thickened bladder wall may exhibit lesions which are thicker than the surrounding regions of abnormality (Figure 3.32). Cystitis

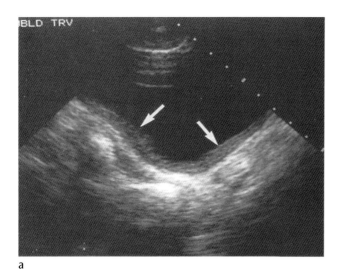

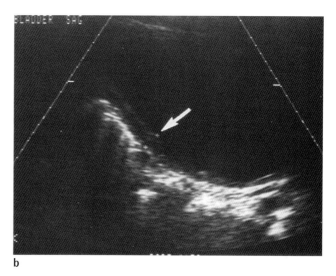

a

b

Figure 3.31
Cystitis. (a) From an individual with cystitis, exhibiting diffuse thickening of the bladder wall (arrows). (b) A patient with pyouria with a focally thickened bladder wall (arrow). This is a less common presentation for cystitis.

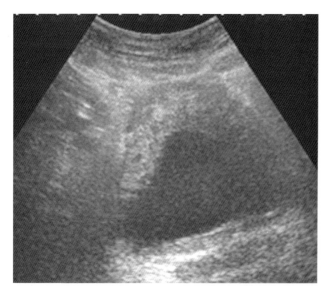

Figure 3.32
Focal cystitis. There is an area of focal thickening in the anterior bladder wall.

Table 3.2 *Types of cystitis*
Whole bladder involvement
Focal
Polypoid
Bullous
Emphysematous
Hemorrhagic
Cystica
Glandularis
Squamous metaplasia
Alkaline encrustation

may occur in a number of forms, listed in Table 3.2. The ultrasonic appearances of each type will not be described here and, indeed, there is large overlap in appearances. The way in which the ultrasound appearances may vary in the different types may be inferred from their descriptive names (see Figures 3.33 and 3.34). Pyocystis may be regarded as an extreme form of cystitis and is found in anuric or oliguric patients, and patients with urinary diversion. It is discussed in the previous section.

Emphysematous cystitis[36,37]

Emphysematous cystitis results when gas permeates the bladder wall and is secondary to gas (carbon dioxide and hydrogen) produced by bacterial fermentation. It is frequently found with *Escherichia coli*, although any of the aforementioned pathogens may serve as a causative agent. It usually afflicts females with diabetes, and chronic urinary retention is an associated condition. Sonographically, the bladder wall will be increased in thickness, with foci of increased echogenicity that cast distal acoustic shadows. The acoustic shadow from gas is usually not as well defined as the one accompanying a

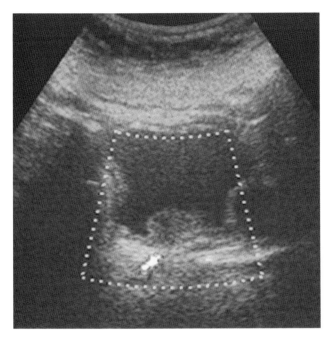

Figure 3.33
Polypoidal cystitis. There is a polypoidal lesion with vessels, thought to be a carcinoma. Excision biopsy showed it to be polypoidal cystitis.

stone (Figure 3.35). This abnormality must be distinguished from primary pneumaturia, where the gas lies intraluminally and is usually iatrogenic in origin.

Fungal infections

Fungal infections may cause fungal balls in the bladder or the renal collecting system (Figure 3.36). These are medium-echodensity masses casting weak shadows. They are usually rounded, occasionally irregular.[38] The diagnosis is made by examining the urine for fungal fragments.

Schistosomiasis[39–41]

Parasites may infect the bladder, one of the most common being *Schistosoma haematobium*. Although schistosomiasis is uncommonly seen in Western countries, it may be the most common cause of renal failure worldwide. Schistosomiasis of the urinary tract typically affects the lower ureters, causing strictures and hydronephrosis. The bladder may also be affected. Granuloma formation within the wall may lead to sonographic findings of polypoid-like thickening of the wall (Figure 3.37). Calculi may be encountered and, with chronic infestation, the resulting fibrosis can lead to a small thick-walled non-calcified blad-

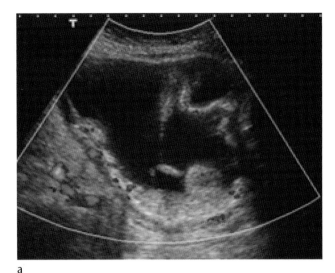

a

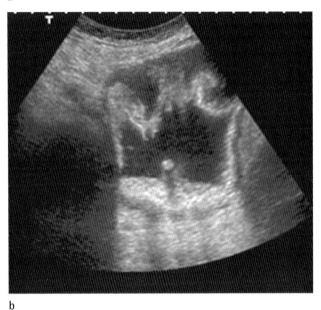

b

Figure 3.34
Hemorrhagic cystitis. A bizarre appearance of mucosal thickening and lifting of the mucosa due to hemorrhage. Cystoscopy made the diagnosis of hemorrhagic cystitis. (a) Sagittal view, (b) axial view.

der. A large number of chronic cases develop squamous cell carcinoma. These tumors may be difficult to distinguish sonographically from the granulomatous changes. Any suspicion should be checked by cystoscopy.

Tuberculosis[42,43]

Tuberculosis of the bladder occurs by direct spread from the kidneys. It is therefore accompanied by changes in the kidneys that are described in Chapter 1. In the bladder,

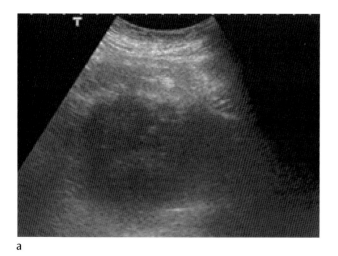
a

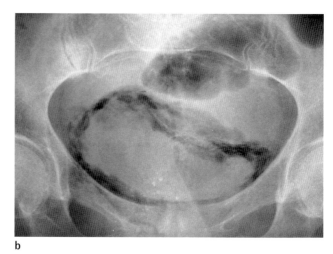
b

Figure 3.35
Emphysematous cystitis. (a) There is 'dirty' shadowing partly obscuring the bladder. The cause was uncertain. (b) A few days later, the cause is revealed as gas in the bladder wall. This had increased, as on a repeat ultrasound at this time the bladder was totally obscured.

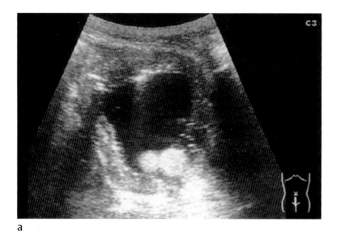
a

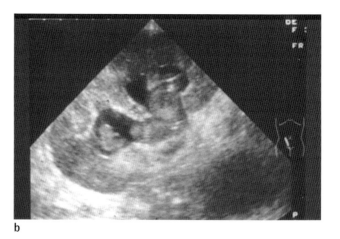
b

Figure 3.36
Fungal cystitis. (a) There are fungal balls in the bladder in a patient with a renal transplant on immunosuppressive therapy. (b) There are also fungal balls in the renal collecting system.

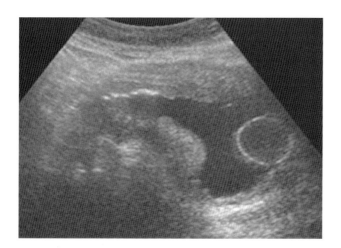

Figure 3.37
Schistosomiasis. There is marked thickening of the bladder wall.

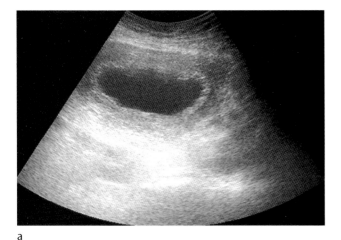

a

Figure 3.38
Tuberculosis. (a) Sagittal and (b) axial views of a thick-walled bladder due to late-stage tuberculous cystitis. Some early calcification in the posterior wall with shadowing is shown in (b).

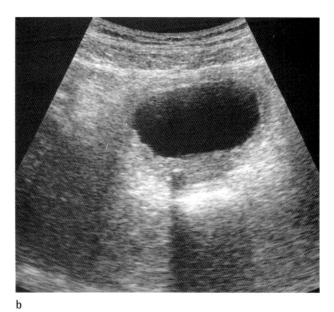

b

bullous edema and granulation occur, usually starting at the ureteral orifice and spreading in severe cases to involve the whole bladder. Healing is by fibrosis and calcification. At the ureteral orifices, in most cases, there is ureteral narrowing and sometimes fibrosis. In some cases, the fibrosis holds the orifice open, causing reflux. The cystoscopic appearances of this are described as 'golf-hole ureter'. The early ultrasound appearances are similar to those of any cystitis, with focal or global mucosal thickening. In healed cases or whole bladder involvement, the bladder muscle is replaced by fibrous tissue, often with calcification. Ultrasonically, this appears as a small thick-walled bladder, with a low-echodensity wall with areas of shadowing from calcification (Figure 3.38). When calcification is extensive, the whole bladder casts a shadow.

Malacoplakia[44]

Malakoplakia is an uncommon condition occurring in the genitourinary tract, and rarely the skin, of immunocompromised patients. It is thought to be caused by incomplete phagocytosis of bacteria, because of compromised phagocyte or monocyte activity. This results in development of the characteristic yellow plaques. Bladder ultrasound reveals non-specific mucosal plaques that are usually misdiagnosed as transitional cell carcinoma (Figure 3.39). Diagnosis is suspected when cystoscopy reveals the yellow-colored plaques, and is confirmed by biopsy.

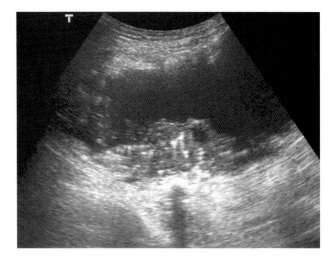

Figure 3.39
Malakoplakia. There is a mass lesion indistinguishable from a tumor. The patient was immunocompromised with a poorly emptying augmented bladder.

Catheter cystitis[45]

Patients who have a chronic indwelling catheter may develop a catheter-induced cystitis. Ultrasonographically, focal thickening of the bladder wall is seen adjacent to the balloon of the indwelling catheter. The thickened mucosa

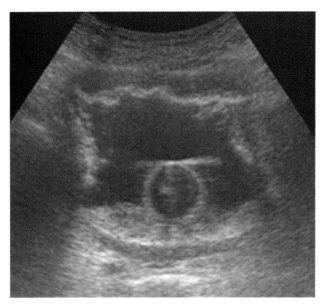

Figure 3.40
Catheter cystitis. There is focal thickening of the bladder wall adjacent to the catheter, which is consistent with catheter-induced cystitis.

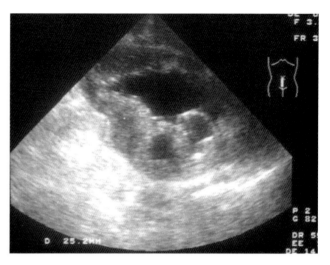

Figure 3.41
Cyclophosphamide-induced cystitis. There is marked bladder wall thickening with some calcification.

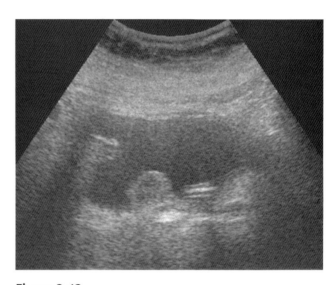

Figure 3.42
Eosinophilic cystitis. There are polypoidal masses simulating carcinoma. The diagnosis was made by cystoscopy and biopsy.

may have a hypoechoic appearance secondary to increased fluid content. Depending on the direction of catheterization, thickening may be diffusely present (Figure 3.40). These changes must be distinguished from other focal processes such as carcinoma. The presence of catheterization suggests the diagnosis, but definitive differentiation from carcinoma often requires cystoscopy and biopsy.

Cyclophosphamide cystitis[46]

Chemotherapeutic agents may result in cystitis and the most notable hemorrhagic cystitis results from treatment with cyclophosphamide. The degradation products of cyclophosphamide are responsible rather than the drug itself. On ultrasound, the bladder may be thick-walled and contracted. Debris may be identified within the bladder lumen secondary to blood clots. Focal areas of calcification may also be seen within the bladder wall (Figure 3.41).

Eosinophilic cystitis[47]

Eosinophilic cystitis is an allergic cystitis usually occurring in severely atopic adults and children; it is also reported following intravesical mitomycin C therapy and in elderly men with prostatism. It is self-limiting, but resolution is helped by steroids. It causes a grossly thickened edematous bladder wall and sometimes polypoidal masses that resem-

ble tumors (Figure 3.42). On CT scan, inflammatory stranding of the perivesical fat is characteristically seen, but this is not apparent on ultrasound.

Bladder tumors

Tumor types

Both benign and malignant tumors occur in the bladder (Table 3.3). Primary malignant tumors are mostly

Table 3.3 *Tumor types*		
Status	*Common*	*Uncommon*
Benign	Leiomyoma Fibroepithelial polyp	Hemangioma Adenoma Pheochromocytoma
Malignant	Transitional cell carcinoma Squamous cell carcinoma	Adenocarcinoma, small cell cancer (carcinosarcoma) Sarcoma, lymphoma (pediatric)

transitional cell cancers; most benign tumors are papillomas. Less common tumors include squamous cell cancers, neurofibromas and, in the pediatric age group, sarcomas and lymphomas. Patients usually present with painless hematuria, sometimes with voiding symptoms. Direct invasion of the bladder may occur in prostate cancer, or any pelvic malignancy. Endometriosis may also occur in the bladder wall, although the mechanism of implantation is not fully understood.

The most common primary bladder malignancy in Western countries is transitional cell carcinoma, which accounts for about 96% of bladder tumors. Arising from the transitional epithelium, it accounts for approximately 4% of all male cancers and approximately 2% of female cancers. Cigarette smoking is a predisposing factor in 50% of cases. It is sometimes associated with occupations involving aniline dyes and toxic substances with the metabolic byproducts of *a*- and *p*-naphthylamine, benzidine and 4-aminobiphenyl. There is often a lag period between the time of exposure and presentation of the transitional cell carcinoma. Two percent of bladder tumors are squamous cell cancers, 1–2% are adenocarcinomas and other tumors are rare. In countries where schistosomiasis is endemic, 75% of tumors are squamous cell cancers.

Detection by ultrasound[48–53]

Ultrasound has shown a high degree of accuracy for the detection of transitional cell carcinomas, although cystoscopy remains the gold standard. Detection accuracies have ranged from 80 to 95%. The ultrasound technique does, however, have its limitations. Tumors within the dome of the bladder may be missed secondary to gas shadowing from interposed loops of bowel or reverberation artifacts in the lumen of the bladder. Tumors located along the posterior wall, lateral wall and trigone region are less easily missed. Detection frequently depends on degree of bladder filling, patient body habitus and the presence of associated mimics of transitional cell carcinoma.

Sonographically, transitional cell carcinomas have been described as flat, polypoidal, ellipsoid, massive, obliterating

Table 3.4 *Bladder cancer: descriptive types*	
Small, flat	Not usually seen on ultrasound
Polypoidal	Broad-based, stalk-, or frond-like
Ellipsoid	Smooth or irregular surface
Massive	Usually lobulated surface
Obliterating	Obscure bladder
Infiltrating	Spread into or through bladder wall

and infiltrating (Table 3.4). If the lesion is superficial, it may present as a flat shallow projection from the bladder wall. Flat tumors are, however, often missed on ultrasound and, when seen, the appearances are often equivocal. Polypoidal tumors appear as frond-like echogenic or hyperechoic projections from the bladder wall. The base may be narrow or broad (Figure 3.43). Tumor size may influence detection, with tumors greater than 1 cm being more easily detected than those less than 5 mm (Figure 3.44). Ellipsoid, massive and obliterating tumors appear as their descriptions suggest (Figures 3.45–3.47). Tumors may be encrusted, causing shadowing (Figure 3.48). This may cause confusion with calculi. The shape is often more irregular than calculi. Calculi may be shown to be mobile by turning the patient, but not all calculi move. More deeply infiltrating tumors will obliterate the normal bladder wall, and the transition between normal and abnormal wall may be abrupt (Figure 3.49).

A sonographic differential diagnosis must be considered whenever the diagnosis of transitional cell carcinoma is entertained. Focal cystitis, especially in individuals with chronic indwelling catheters, needs to be differentiated from focal transitional cell carcinoma. Mobility of blood clots often distinguishes them from the non-mobile neoplasms, but clots can be adherent. Absence of demonstrable blood vessels on color Doppler makes clot more likely, although it does not totally exclude tumor. Ventrally located nodules of benign prostatic hyperplasia or invasive

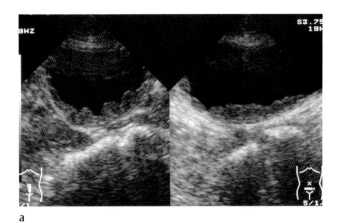

a

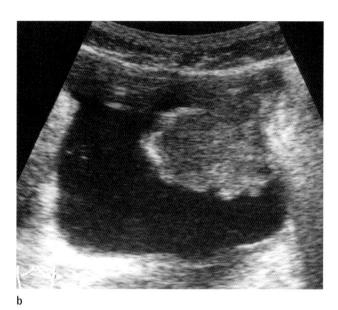

b

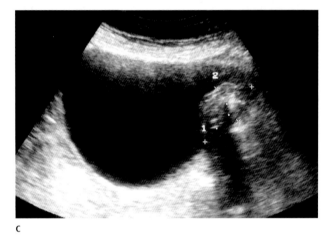

c

Figure 3.43
Varieties of bladder tumor. (a) A flat broad-based transitional cell carcinoma. (b) A polypoidal transitional cell carcinoma. There is early surface encrustation causing an echogenic line around the surface. (c) Pedunculated tumor with a broad stalk. There is calcification within the tumor.

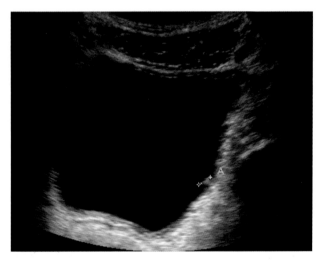

Figure 3.44
Small tumor. The tumors shown in Figure 3.43 are relatively large and not easily missed. Tumors the size shown in this figure are, however, easy to miss. Histology showed it to be a benign fibroepithelial polyp.

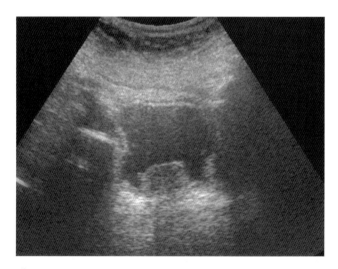

Figure 3.45
Ellipsoid tumor. A tumor with an ellipsoid shape; this was an adenocarcinoma.

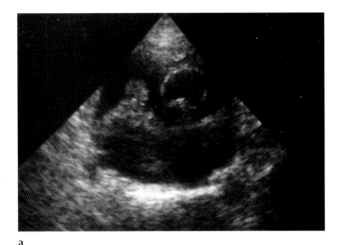

a

Figure 3.46
Massive tumor. (a) This was a transitional cell cancer of the
bladder. A study of the upper tracts (b) showed a further
transitional cell cancer in the kidney (arrowed).

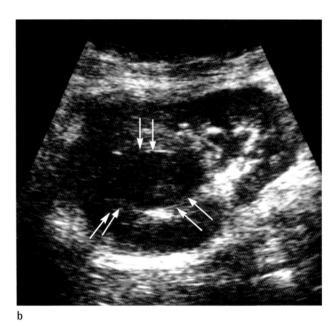

b

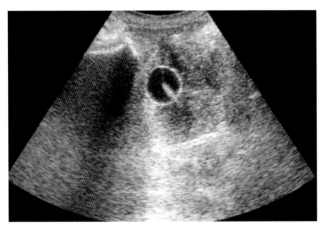

Figure 3.47
Tumor obliterans. The tumor fills the bladder. Its relation to
the bladder is only seen by the position of the urinary catheter.

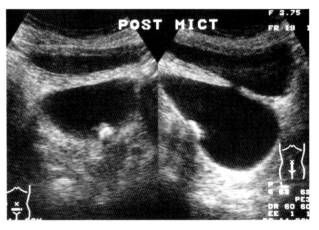

Figure 3.48
Encrusted tumor. The encrustation on the surface of the small
tumor causes shadowing. It resembles a calculus. It did not
move and has an irregular surface, making tumor more likely.
Tumor was confirmed by cystoscopy. (See also Figure 3.43.)

prostatic carcinoma may mimic transitional cell carcinoma
(Figure 3.50). The central location of these prostatic lesions
usually helps distinguish them from the invasive bladder
cancer but it is often difficult to exclude a coexisting bladder cancer close to the prostate. In cases of doubt,
cystoscopy is indicated. Benign bladder wall trabeculation
may be confused with small neoplasms. Trabeculations
usually measure 1–3 mm in size and it is rare for small
polypoid transitional cell carcinoma of this size to be identified. Ultimately, cystoscopy with biopsy is necessary for
definitive diagnosis.

Squamous cell cancer

Squamous cell carcinoma of the bladder is unusual,
accounting for only 2% of all primary neoplasms of the
bladder in Western countries. It has been associated with
chronic inflammation of the bladder due to infection,
calculi or strictures, and it may arise in bladder diverticula
as a result of chronic inflammation. Neither racial nor
occupational associations are known. However, a 3:2 male
to female sex ratio has been described. Sonographically,
these neoplasms may have a similar appearance to

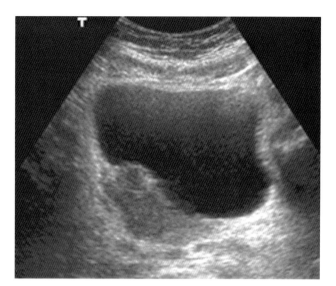

Figure 3.49
Infiltrating transitional cell cancer. The tumor has invaded through the muscularis layer. The transition between tumor and normal bladder wall is clearcut. Although the tumor is clearly shown to be T3A in this case, in general ultrasound is inaccurate at tumor staging and MRI or CT should be used.

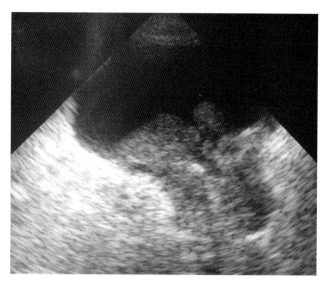

Figure 3.50
Prostate cancer. This tumor invading the bladder base has been clearly shown in this plane to be arising from the prostate. The situation is not always as clear, and both prostate cancer and benign prostatic enlargement can simulate bladder cancer.

transitional cell carcinoma. In schistosomiasis endemic areas, 75% of malignant bladder tumors are squamous cell cancers. In these cases, other signs of schistosomiasis, small thick-walled bladder and hydronephrosis from lower ureteric strictures, may also be seen.

Adenocarcinoma

Adenocarcinomas account for only 1–2% of malignant bladder tumors. They are nearly always invasive. Their appearances are otherwise similar to squamous cell cancers.

Staging

Treatment and outcome is related to depth of infiltration, histopathologic type, grade of malignancy and lymphatic invasion. Tumors may be staged based on the TNM system. Tumors involving the mucosa and submucosa are classified as stage Tl. Stage T2 tumors invade the superficial muscle layer. If the tumor invades the deep muscular layer, then it is a stage T3a lesion, and it is a T3b lesion if it extends beyond muscle into the perivesical fat but not beyond. Stage T4 lesions have extension into the adjacent perivesical tissues. If lymph nodes are involved, then it is stage N, and in cases of distant metastasis, it is stage M (Table 3.5).

Staging by transabdominal sonography has been problematic. Various investigators have met with different

Table 3.5	*Bladder cancer: TNM classification*
T1S	Carcinoma in situ Papillary non-invasive tumor
T1	Papillary tumor with lamina propria invasion
T2	Superficial muscle invasion
T3A	Deep muscle invasion
T3B	Perivesical fat invasion
T4A	Invasion of contiguous viscera
T4B	Invasion of pelvic or abdominal wall
N4	Regional lymphadenopathy
M1	Distal metastases

degrees of success. Accuracies have ranged as high as 100% for deeply invasive tumors and 55% for more superficial tumors.[54] Ultrasound has not proved to be sufficiently accurate for clinical staging. MRI is the best staging test, although CT may also be used.

Hematuria

Ultrasound is widely used in the investigation of hematuria, often combined with IVU (or CT). It is the

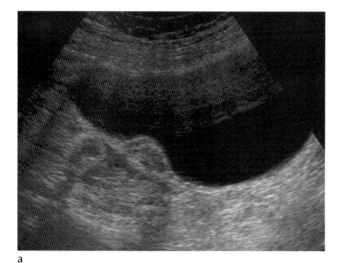

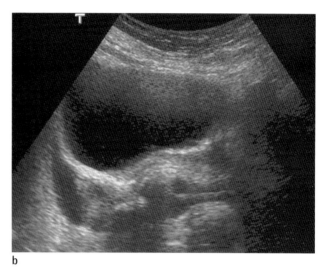

a

b

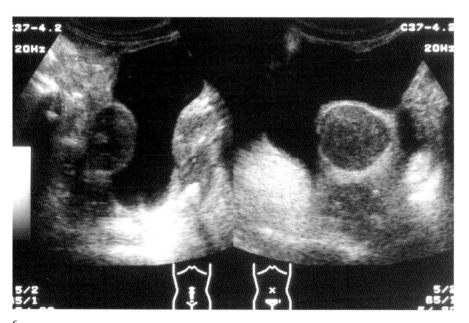

c

Figure 3.51
Endometriosis. (a,b) Sagittal and coronal planes. The patient had the typical symptoms of hematuria and bladder irritation at the time of her periods. There is a medium-echodensity mass, with even texture lying within the bladder wall, which was an endometrioma. There is a pelvic endometrioma outside the bladder immediately adjacent to it. (c) A different patient. Two bladder endometriomas. The position within the bladder wall is clearly seen.

ultrasound study, therefore, that often provides the initial diagnosis of bladder tumor. Confirmation and histologic staging is then obtained by cystoscopy and biopsy. Further TNM staging is then obtained by MRI (or CT). Follow-up is, at present, by cystoscopy. The possibility of follow-up by ultrasound is attractive, being less invasive and cheaper. So far, ultrasound has not been shown to be sufficiently sensitive. However, the constant improvement in ultrasound imaging may ultimately change this.

Endometriosis[55–58]

Endometriosis in the bladder classically, although not always, presents with hematuria at the time of the periods. Ultrasound shows a non-specific mass within the bladder wall, often extending outside the bladder (Figure 3.51). There may also be other evidence of pelvic endometriosis. Endometriosis of the bladder is usually caused by implantation following surgery, typically cesarean section. It also occurs without a history of surgery. In such cases, the mechanism of implantation is not known.

The augmented bladder

Some patients have voiding symptoms due to poor bladder volume and/or poor detrusor compliance. Some bladder tumors are amenable to partial bladder resection. In both these cases, bladder reconstruction or augmentation may be performed. There are several ways of achieving this. Most

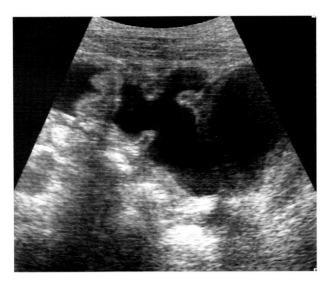

Figure 3.52
Augmented bladder. Enterocystoplasty–Clam procedure. The dome of the bladder has been opened out and a loop or cecum and colon incorporated.

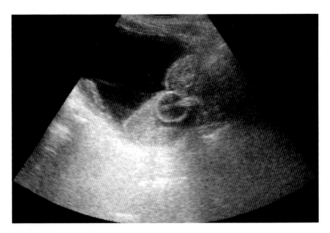

Figure 3.53
Poorly positioned catheter. The catheter was draining poorly. It lies in the prostatic urethra. It was easily repositioned during the ultrasound scan.

involve isolating a loop of bowel, with intact blood supply, and incorporating this into the bladder (enterocystoplasty, cecocystoplasty, ileocystoplasty). A variant of cecocystoplasty is the Mitrofanoff procedure in which the appendix is opened onto the skin surface as a stoma for self-catheterization. Less commonly, part of the stomach may be used (gastrocystoplasty). Although there are differences, which may be deduced from the nature of the reconstruction, the ultrasound appearances of the different types of augmented bladder are remarkably similar. The component that is the original bladder may be seen, while the bowel component contains haustra, valvulae conniventes or rugae (Figure 3.52). Large bowel components sometimes contain mucous strands. The normally functioning reconstructed bladder empties nearly completely at micturition. Bladder volume is difficult to measure in these cases because of the bladder's irregular shape. In practice, an adequate approximation may be obtained from measuring an ellipsoid that approximately fits the shape. In patients with very dilated ureters, part of the ureter may be used to augment the bladder (ureterocystoplasty). These bladders look more like normal bladders on ultrasound studies.

Ileal conduit

In some cases of renal tract pathology, the ureters cannot drain into the bladder, and need to be diverted to another site. A common method is to isolate a loop of ileum, close one end, and open the other onto the skin surface as a stoma. The ureters are implanted into this bowel loop. This is termed an ileal conduit. Ultrasound may be requested when there is suspected abscess or hernia at the stomal site. Such studies are difficult, as the stoma impedes access. Scanning close to the stoma and angling the transducer appropriately is, however, usually successful. The conduit itself looks like any loop of ileum, with a variable volume of fluid in the lumen.

Artificial sphincters and penile erection devices

Ultrasound has little part to play in the investigation of these devices. The urethral cuff of an artificial sphincter may be seen on a transrectal scan, and the erectile tubes of a penile erection device may be seen on a penile scan. Functional failure of either device is investigated by plain X-ray to check continuity of the connecting tubes and fullness of the reservoir, which is filled with contrast. The reason for including this section is that the reservoir, which is a spherical balloon, is usually placed in the pelvis, lateral to the bladder. It appears on ultrasound scan as an approximately 2 cm round cyst-like object. It may be slightly irregular if there is a leak in the system. It is often mistaken for an ovarian cyst or a bladder diverticulum. The true nature of the object is deduced from the clinical knowledge that a device is present, and from the absolutely spherical shape of the normal (non-leaking) reservoir (see Figure 3.24). The activating bulbs of these devices are usually placed in the scrotum in the male, and the labia in the female. These also often cause diagnostic confusion.

Urinary catheters

Ultrasound may occasionally be used to check the position of urinary catheters in problematic cases. In other cases, misplacement of catheters is found when scanning for other purposes.[59] Misplacement of catheters is readily recognized (Figure 3.53). Ultrasound may be used to assist catheterization in difficult cases. This is discussed earlier in this chapter. Suprapubic catheters are usually inserted 'blind', using palpation and percussion to locate the distended bladder. Ultrasound guidance may, however, be used. The balloons of long-standing catheters sometimes fail to deflate, thus preventing removal. The balloon may be burst with a fine needle advanced suprapubically through the bladder under ultrasound guidance.

Acknowledgments

I would like to thank Archie A Alexander, author of the chapter entitled 'Bladder and Urethra', which appeared in the first edition of *Urogenital Ultrasound: a text atlas*. His work has formed the basis of this chapter.

References

1. Djavan B, Roehrborn CG. Bladder ultrasonography. Semin Urol 1994; 12(4): 306–19.
2. Cochlin DL. Urinary system. Ultrasound Med Biol 2000; 26(Suppl 1): S76–8.
3. Yang JM, Huang WC. Bladder wall thickness on ultrasonographic cystourethrography: affecting factors and their implications. J Ultrasound Med 2003; 22(8): 777–82.
4. Jequier S, Rousseau O. Sonographic measurements of the normal bladder wall in children. AJR Am J Roentgenol 1987; 145: 563–5.
5. Hakenberg OW, Linne C, Manseck A, Wirth MP. Bladder wall thickness in normal adults and men with mild lower urinary tract symptoms and benign prostatic enlargement. Neurourol Urodyn 2000; 19(5): 585–93.
6. Griffiths CJ, Murray A, Ramsden PD. Accuracy and repeatability of bladder volume measurement using ultrasonic imaging. J Urol 1986; 136: 12–16.
7. Hakenberg OW, Ryall RL, Langlois SL, et al. A determination of bladder volume by sonocystography. J Urol 1983; 130: 249–53.
8. Kiely EA, Hartnell GG, Gibson RN, et al. Measurement of bladder volume by real-time ultrasound. Br J Urol 1987; 60: 33–6.
9. McLean GK, Edell SL. Determination of bladder volumes by gray scale ultrasonography. Radiology 1978; 128: 181–4.
10. Naya Y, Kojima M, Honjyo H, et al. Intraobserver and iterobserver variance in the measurement of ultrasound-estimated bladder weight. Ultrasound Med Biol 1998; 24(5): 771–3.
11. Ueno T, Hashimoto H, Yokoyama H, et al. Urachal anomalies: ultrasonography and management. J Pediatr Surg 2003; 38(8): 1203–7.
12. Mengiardi B, Wiesner W, Stoffel F, et al. Case 44: adenocarcinoma of the urachus. Radiology 2002; 222(3): 744–7.
13. Robert Y, Hennequin-Delerue C, Chaillet D, et al. Urachal remnants: sonographic assessment. J Clin Ultrasound 1996; 24(7): 339–44.
14. Holten I, Lomas F, Mouratidis B, et al. The ultrasonic diagnosis of urachal anomalies. Australas Radiol 1996; 40(1): 2–5.
15. Heesakkers JP, Vriesema JL. The role of urodynamics in the treatment of lower urinary tract symptoms in women. Curr Opin Urol 2005; 15(4): 215–21.
16. Artibani W, Cerruto MA. The role of imaging in urinary incontinence. BJU Int 2005; 95(5): 699–703.
17. Hendrikx AJ, Doesburg WH, Reintjes AG, et al. Effectiveness of ultrasound in the preoperative evaluation of patients with prostatin. Prostate 1988; 13(3): 199–208.
18. Ukimura O, Iwata T, Ushijima S, et al. Possible contribution of prostatic anterior fibromuscular stroma to age-related urinary disturbance in reference to pressure–flow study. Ultrasound Med Biol 2004; 30(5): 575–81.
19. Brandt TD, Neiman HL, Calenoff L, et al. Ultrasound evaluation of the urinary system in spinal-cord-injury patients. Radiology 1981; 141: 473–7.
20. Perkash I, Friedland GW. Catheter-induced hyperreflexia in spinal cord injury patients: diagnosis by sonographic voiding cystourethrography. Radiology 1986; 159: 453–5.
21. Perkash I, Friedland GW. Transrectal ultrasonography of the lower urinary tract: evaluation of bladder neck problems. Neurourol Urodyn 1986; 5: 299–306.
22. Petritsch PH, Colombh TH, Rauchenwald M, et al. Ultrasonography of urinary tract and micturition as an alternative to radiologic investigations in the spinal-cord-injured patient. Eur Urol 1991; 20: 97–102.
23. Shapeero LG, Friedland GW, Perkash I. Transrectal sonographic voiding cystourethrography: studies in neuromuscular bladder dysfunction. AJR Am J Roentgenol 1983; 141: 83–90.
24. Bergman A, Vermesh M, Ballard CA, Platt LD. Role of ultrasound in urinary incontinence evaluation. Urology 1989; 33(5): 443–4.
25. Yang JM, Huang WC. Discrimination of bladder disorders in female lower urinary tract symptoms on ultrasonographic cystourethrography. J Ultrasound Med 2002; 21(11): 1249–55.
26. Kuo HC, Chang SC, Hsu T. Application of transrectal sonography in the diagnosis and treatment of female stress urinary incontinence. Eur Urol 1994; 26(1): 77–84.
27. Dietz HP. Ultrasound imaging of the pelvic floor. Part I: two-dimensional aspects. Ultrasound Obstet Gynecol 2004; 23(1): 80–92.
28. Dietz HP. Ultrasound imaging of the pelvic floor. Part II: three-dimensional or volume imaging. Ultrasound Obstet Gynecol 2004; 23(6): 615–25.
29. Tunn R, Petri E. Introital and transvaginal ultrasound as the main tool in the assessment of urogenital and pelvic floor dysfunction: an imaging panel and practical approach. Ultrasound Obstet Gynecol 2003; 22(2): 205–13.
30. Bergman A, McKenzie CJ, Richmond J, et al. Transrectal ultrasound versus cystography in the evaluation of anatomical stress urinary incontinence. Br J Urol 1988; 62: 228–34.
31. Wang CW, Chang YL, Horng SG, et al. Pitfalls in the differential diagnosis of a pelvic cyst: lessons from a post-menopausal woman with bladder diverticulum. Int J Clin Pract 2004; 58(9): 894–6.
32. Rosenfield AT, Taylor KJW, Weiss RM. Ultrasound evaluation of bladder calculi. J Urol 1979; 121: 119.
33. Benson M, Li Puma JP, Resnick MI. The role of imaging studies in urinary tract infections. Urol Clin North Am 1986; 13(4): 605–25.
34. Gooding GA. Varied sonographic manifestations of cystitis. J Ultrasound Med 1986; 5(2): 61–3.
35. Friedman EP, de Bruyn R, Mather S. Pseudotumoral cystitis in children: a review of the ultrasound features in four cases. Br J Radiol 1993; 66(787): 605–8.
36. Choong KK. Sonographic detection of emphysematous cystitis. J Ultrasound Med 2003; 22(8): 847–9.
37. Kauzlaric D, Barmeir E. Sonography of emphysematous cystitis. J Ultrasound Med 1985; 4: 319–20.

38. McDonald DF, Fagan CJ. Fungal balls in the urinary bladder. AJR Am J Roentgenol 1972; 114: 753–7.

39. Abdel-Wahab MF, Strickland GT. Abdominal ultrasonography for assessing morbidity from schistosomiasis. 2. Hospital studies. Trans R Soc Trop Med Hyg 1993; 87(2): 135–7.

40. Al-Shorab MM. Radiological manifestations of genitourinary bilharziasis. Clin Radiol 1968; 19: 100–4.

41. Jorulf H, Linfstedt E. Urogenital schistosomiasis: CT evaluation. Radiology 1985; 157: 745–9.

42. Vijayaraghavan SB, Kandasamy SV, Arul M, et al. Spectrum of high-resolution sonographic features of urinary tuberculosis. J Ultrasound Med 2004; 23(5): 585–94.

43. Premkumar A, Latimer J, Newhouse JH. CT and sonography of advanced urinary tract tuberculosis. Am J Roentgenol 1987; 148: 65–9.

44. Baumgartner BR, Alagappian R. Malakoplakia of the ureter and bladder. Urol Radiol 1990; 12(3): 157–9.

45. Abu-Yousef MM, Narayana AS, Brown RC. Catheter-induced cystitis: evaluation by cystosonography. J Radiol 1984; 151(2): 471–3.

46. Kumar A, Aggarwal S. The sonographic appearance of cyclophosphamide-induced acute haemorrhagic cystitis. Clin Radiol 1990; 41(4): 289–90.

47. Verhagen PC, Nickels PG, de Jong TP. Eosinophilic cystitis. Arch Dis Child 2001; 84(4): 344–6.

48. Abu-Yousef MM, Narayana AS, Franken EA Jr, et al. Urinary bladder tumors studied by cystosonography. I. Detection. Radiology 1984; 149: 563–70.

49. Itzcha KY, Singer D, Fischelovitch Y. Ultrasonographic detection of bladder tumors. I. Tumor detection. J Urol 1981; 126: 31–7.

50. Cronan JJ, Simeone JF, Pfister RC, et al. Cystosonography in the detection of bladder tumors: a prospective and retrospective study. J Ultrasound Med 1982; 1(6): 237–41.

51. Denkhaus H, Crone-Munzebrock W, Muland H. Noninvasive ultrasound in the detection and staging of bladder carcinoma. Urol Radiol 1982; 7: 121–8.

52. Bahnson RR, Zaontz MR, Maizels M, et al. Ultrasonography and diagnosis of pediatric genitourinary rhabdomyosarcoma. Urology 1989; 33: 64–8.

53. Malone PR. Transabdominal ultrasound for surveillance of bladder cancer. Urol Clin North Am 1989; 16: 823–8.

54. Abu-Yousef MM, Narayana AS, Brown RC, et al. Urinary bladder tumours studied by cystosonography. Part II: Staging. Radiology 1984; 153: 227–31.

55. Thijs I, Bhal PS, Shaw R, Kynaston H. Isolated vesical endometriosis in the absence of previous surgery. J Obstet Gynaecol 2002; 22(4): 448–9.

56. Savoca G, Trombetta C, Troiano L, et al. [Echographic, MRI and CT features in a case of bladder endometriosis]. [Italian] Archivo Italiano di Urologia, Andrologia 1996; 68(5 Suppl): 193–6.

57. Kumar R, Haque AK, Cohen MS. Endometriosis of the urinary bladder: demonstration by sonography. J Clin Ultrasound 1984; 12: 363–5.

58. Goodman JD, Macchia RJ, Macasaet MA, et al. Endometriosis of the urinary bladder: sonographic findings. AJR Am J Roentgenol 1980; 135: 625–6.

59. Janus C. Sonographic appearance of the abnormally positioned Foley catheter. J Ultrasound Med 1982; 4: 439–42.

4

The prostate and seminal vesicles

Ethan Halpern

Anatomy

The normal adult prostate is a walnut-sized organ situated between the bladder and the muscles of the pelvic floor. As the urethra exits from the bladder, it courses caudally and anteriorly through the long axis of the prostate. The cranial aspect of the prostate just under the bladder is denoted as the base of the prostate. The base of the prostate is clearly defined against the bladder by sonography. The apex of the prostate, adjacent to the muscles of the pelvic floor, is situated just posterior to the pubic symphysis. The apex of the prostate merges into the corpora spongiosum without a well-defined sonographic landmark to define the inferior margin of the prostate.

Measurements of the prostate are obtained in the midline sagittal plane as well as in the axial plane. The urethra should be visible on the sagittal midline imaging plane used for the anterior–posterior and craniocaudal measurements (Figure 4.1). The transverse diameter is measured in an axial plane between the base and mid-gland, at a level that demonstrates the maximum transverse diameter of the prostate. Mean dimensions of the young adult prostate are 3.3 cm in height, 2.4 cm in thickness and 4.1 cm in width,[1] with a sonographic volume of 12.9–37.1 ml.[2]

The urethra provides the most important sonographic landmark within the prostate. The crista urethralis is a posterior midline crest that extends along the urethra. At approximately the mid-portion of the crista urethralis, the verumontanum (also known as the colliculus seminalis) is a local protuberance of the urethral crest that contains the openings of the prostatic utricle and the two ejaculatory ducts. The young adult urethra measures approximately 15 mm proximal to the verumontanum and 15 mm distal to the verumontanum. In the setting of benign prostatic

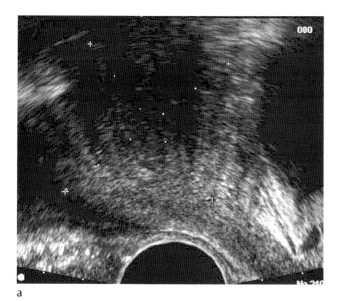

a

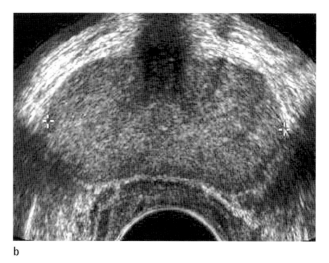

b

Figure 4.1
Prostate measurements. (a) Craniocaudal and anterior–posterior measurements of the prostate are obtained on the midline sagittal image. The normal urethra is often difficult to visualize. (b) Transverse measurements are obtained on an axial image of the prostate.

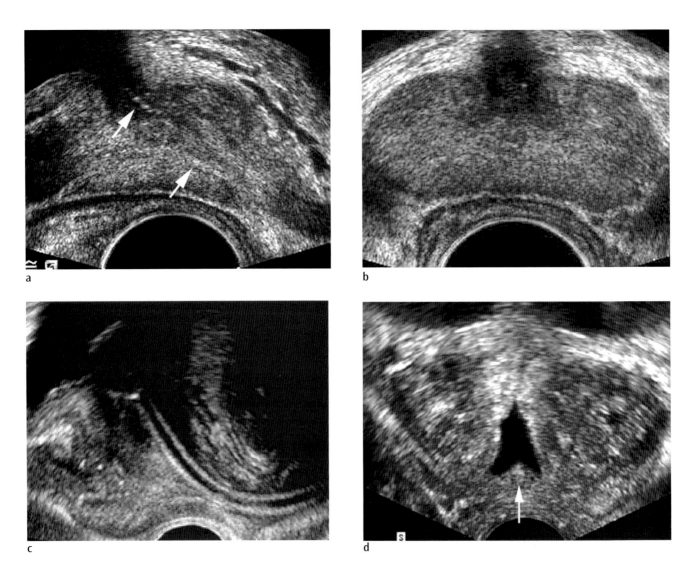

Figure 4.2
Normal appearance and course of the urethra. (a) The urethra is followed down from the bladder neck through the midline sagittal plane of the prostate (arrows). (b) The normal urethra is not easily visualized on a transverse image of the prostate. (c) Midline sagittal image with a Foley catheter in place to demonstrate the course of the urethra. Note the concave course of the urethra in the normal prostate. (d) Transverse image of the prostate in a patient with a dilated urethra. The crista urethralis presents as a posterior bulge within the urethra (arrow).

hyperplasia, the proximal portion of the urethra is stretched and the verumontanum is displaced caudally. The normal young adult prostatic urethra demonstrates an anterior concavity because it is angulated about 35° at the level of the verumontanum (Figure 4.2). The internal sphincter of the bladder extends from the bladder neck into the base of the prostate, and surrounds the prostatic urethra above the verumontanum. Sonographically, the smooth muscle of the internal sphincter may present as a hypoechoic ring around the upper prostatic urethra (Figure 4.3).

The seminal vesicles and vasa deferentia are paired structures on either side of midline just above the prostate (Figure 4.4). These structures extend cranial to the prostate and posterior to the bladder. Often, both seminal vesicles may be imaged together on a single axial image. However, in some cases the orientation of the seminal vesicle requires independent imaging of each side. The two seminal vesicles should be relatively similar in size, and each seminal vesicle should taper in caliber as it approaches the midline, producing a 'beak sign'.[3] The typical size of a seminal vesicle is 27–50 mm in length and 12–15 mm in thickness.[4,5] The vas deferens is generally visible just superior to the body of the ipsilateral seminal vesicle. The ampullary portion of the vas, adjacent to the midline, is the largest and most easily visualized portion of the vas deferens. The

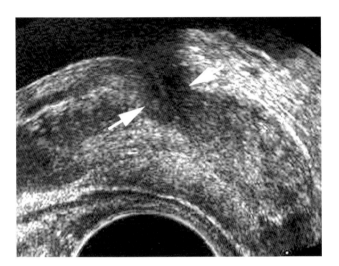

Figure 4.3
Hypoechoic ring around the proximal prostatic urethra on this midline sagittal image corresponds to the smooth muscle of the internal sphincter.

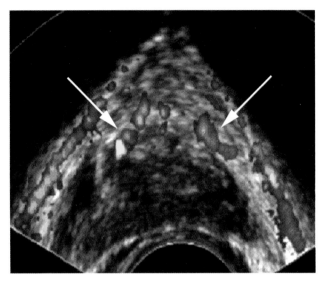

Figure 4.5
Transverse power Doppler image near the apex of the prostate. The vessels anterior to the prostate represent the venous plexus of Santorini (arrows).

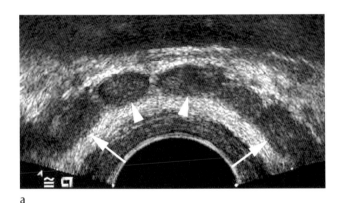

a

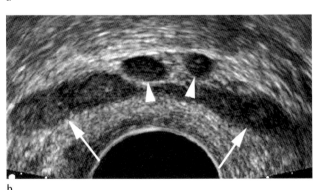

b

Figure 4.4
(a,b) Transverse images above the base of the prostate. The seminal vesicles (arrows) and vasa deferentia (arrowheads) are paired structures on either side of midline.

distal vas deferens courses medial to the seminal vesicle, and joins with the ipsilateral seminal vesicle to form an ejaculatory duct as it enters the base of the prostate. The two ejaculatory ducts course through the base of the prostate to enter the urethra at the verumontanum.

Although there is no true epithelial capsule around the prostate, a thin layer of fibromuscular stroma (no more than half a millimeter in thickness) surrounds the prostate, resulting in a smooth glandular contour. The fascial planes surrounding the prostate are a caudal continuation of the hypogastric sheath and contain many neurovascular structures. Sonographically, these fascial planes appear as well-defined echogenic tissue around the prostate. Vascular structures are often visible within these planes with color Doppler imaging. The venous plexus of Santorini is contained within the fascia of Zuckerkandl anterior to the prostate (Figure 4.5). The prostatic arteries are within the lateral pelvic fascia on either side of the prostate. The neurovascular bundles responsible for male potency usually lie between the prostate and the rectum, along Denonvilliers' fascia (Figure 4.6). Small perforating vessels and neural structures enter the prostate from the neurovascular structures in the adjacent fascial planes, and represent a potential pathway for spread of prostate cancer through the prostatic capsule.[6]

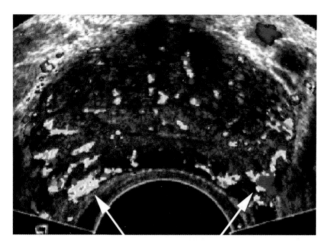

Figure 4.6
Transverse image of the prostate with color Doppler. The neurovascular bundles are demonstrated along the posterolateral aspect of the prostate (arrows).

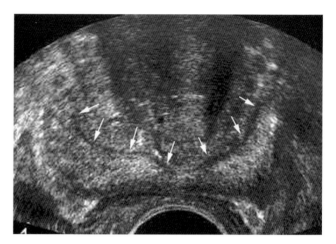

Figure 4.7
Transverse image of the prostate in a patient with benign prostatic hyperplasia. The outer gland is homogeneously echogenic. The inner gland is more heterogeneous, and is separated from the outer gland by a hypoechoic surgical capsule (arrows).

Zonal anatomy

For the purposes of zonal anatomy, we consider the young adult prostate prior to the onset of benign prostatic hyperplasia. The anterior one-third of this ideal prostate is composed of non-glandular tissue – the anterior fibromuscular stroma. This fibromuscular stroma is stretched around the lateral and posterior margins of the gland as a thin capsule. Few pathologic processes involve this fibromuscular stroma. The remaining two-thirds of the prostatic parenchyma is glandular tissue. The zonal anatomy of this tissue has been described in detail by McNeal.[7,8]

The zonal anatomy defined by McNeal divides the glandular tissue of the prostate into four zones:

1. Periurethral glands with limited glandular development empty into the urethra through lateral line ducts along the course of the prostatic urethra. The glands of this periurethral zone are confined within the muscular tissue that surrounds the urethra. This muscular tissue may limit glandular development in this zone. The periurethral zone accounts for 1% of the glandular tissue in the prostate.
2. Transition zone tissue is composed of two lobes of glandular tissue on either side of the urethra. The transition zone glands drain into the urethra at the verumontanum, just above the ejaculatory duct openings. In the absence of benign prostatic hyperplasia, transition zone glands are found only above the level of the verumontanum, and the transition zone accounts for no more than 5% of the glandular tissue in the prostate.
3. Central zone glands surround the ejaculatory ducts as they course toward the verumontanum. The central zone exists only above the verumontanum, and ducts from this zone empty into the urethra at the verumontanum. The central zone accounts for 25% of the glandular tissue in the prostate.
4. Peripheral zone glands surround the central zone at the base of the gland, and also form the bulk of the glandular parenchyma below the level of the verumontanum. These glands drain into the urethra on either side of the verumontanum as well as below the verumontanum along the crista urethralis – a posterior midline crest that extends along the urethra. The peripheral zone accounts for 70% of the glandular tissue in the prostate.

A short-axis section of the prostate below the level of the verumontanum will demonstrate anterior fibromuscular stroma anteriorly and peripheral zone glandular tissue posteriorly. A short-axis section of the prostate above the level of the verumontanum should demonstrate periurethral tissue, transition zone tissue, central zone tissue and peripheral zone tissue.

The distinction between central and peripheral zones is based upon microscopic glandular appearance as well as the different locations where their ducts enter along the urethra. The central and peripheral zones cannot be distinguished by sonography. For sonographic purposes, the periurethral and transition zones comprise the inner gland, whereas the central and peripheral zones comprise the outer gland (Figure 4.7). The inner gland and outer gland can be distinguished from each other by differences

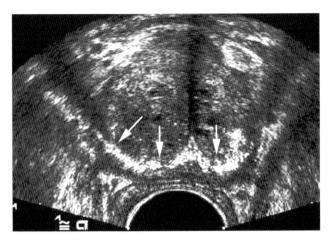

Figure 4.8
Transverse gray-scale image of the prostate in a patient with benign prostatic hyperplasia. The surgical capsule appears echogenic due to deposition of corpora amylacea (arrows).

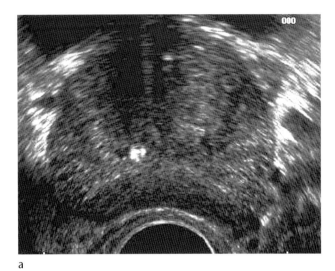

a

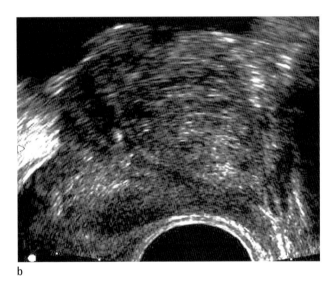

b

Figure 4.9
Benign prostatic hyperplasia (BPH) is manifest by enlargement of the inner gland, visible on (a) transverse and (b) sagittal images.

in their echotexture. The normal outer gland is homogeneously echogenic, and is usually more echogenic than the inner gland. The inner gland is often heterogeneous in its appearance due to the presence of benign prostatic hyperplasia. The inner gland and the outer gland are separated by the surgical capsule, which defines the plane of enucleation for suprapubic prostatectomy. The surgical capsule is not a true anatomical structure, but is often defined by linear deposition of corpora amylacea or calcification that is sonographically visible (Figure 4.8).

Benign diseases

Benign prostatic hyperplasia

The zonal anatomy as defined by McNeal is observed in the young adult prostate after puberty. As a male ages, the glandular distribution changes due to benign prostatic hyperplasia.[9] Benign prostatic hyperplasia results in enlargement of the inner gland due to an increase in the number of glandular elements as well as hypertrophy of the tissues.[10] Benign prostatic hyperplasia is most marked in the transition zone, but is also noted in the periurethral zone. Since prostate cancer is a disease of older men, most men with prostate cancer demonstrate some degree of benign prostatic hyperplasia.

Benign prostatic hyperplasia results in a nodular enlargement of the inner gland (Figure 4.9). Often the two lobes of the transition zone are seen to enlarge on the two sides of the midline. Enlargement of the transition zone stretches and thins the outer gland tissue, and may stretch the urethra and deviate it posteriorly. The enlarged transition zone displaces the verumontanum inferiorly, but may also extend below the level of the verumontanum. When the periurethral glands are involved, the resulting hyperplasia may result in an enlarged 'median lobe'. Although there is no true median lobe, this term is used to refer to midline enlargement of the prostate that bulges into the base of the bladder (Figure 4.10).

Enlargement of the prostate with benign prostatic hyperplasia may result in a marked change in the overall shape and position of the prostate. The enlarged transition zone may become the dominant glandular component of

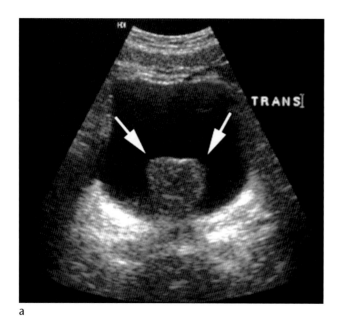

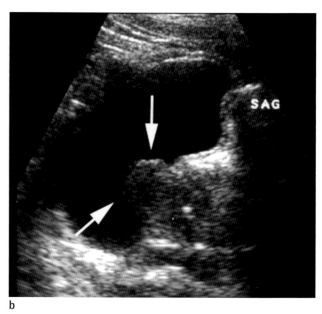

a   b

Figure 4.10
Median lobe hypertrophy is the term applied to BPH that extends into the bladder, resulting from hyperplasia of periurethral tissue. (a) Transverse and (b) sagittal images of median lobe hypertrophy.

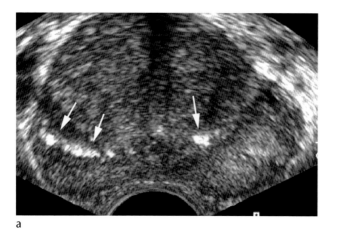

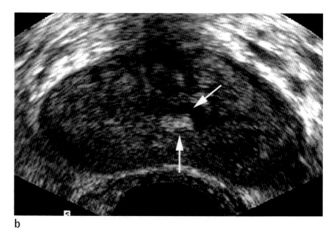

a   b

Figure 4.11
Calcifications in BPH are often present (a) along the surgical capsule or in (b) periurethral tissues (arrows).

the prostate. As the gland becomes more globular in shape, it may extend anteriorly over the symphysis pubis. Among patients referred for brachytherapy, benign prostatic hyperplasia is an important cause of pubic arch interference to the introduction of seeds through a perineal approach.

In addition to the glandular enlargement associated with benign prostatic hyperplasia, this process also results in a more heterogeneous appearance of the gland. Hypoechoic hyperplastic nodules visible within the inner gland may be indistinguishable from hypoechoic masses of cancer. Due to the high prevalence of benign prostatic hyperplasia in middle-aged to elderly males, it is impossible to use gray-scale sonographic criteria to detect cancer within the inner gland.

Prostatic calcifications are often related to the presence of benign prostatic hyperplasia. Calcification is commonly seen along the surgical capsule as well as in the periurethral tissues (Figure 4.11), but dystrophic calcification may be present throughout the hyperplastic inner gland.

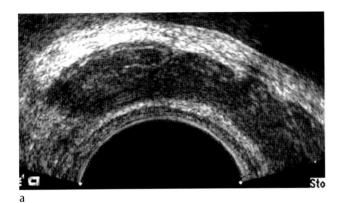

a

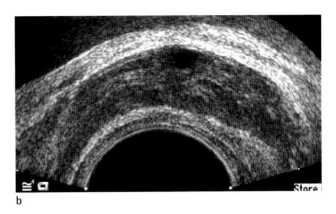

b

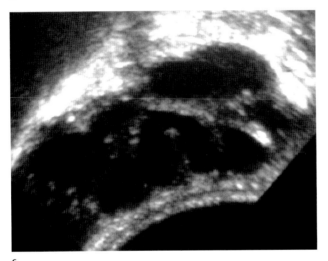

c

Figure 4.12
Seminal vesicles with ductal ectasia. (a) Right seminal vesicle and (b) left seminal vesicle with mild ductal ectasia. (c) Left seminal vesicle with severe ductal ectasia.

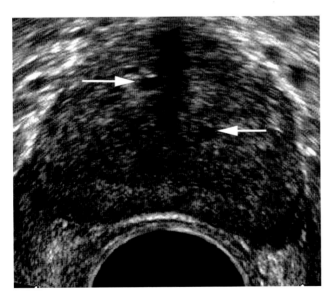

a

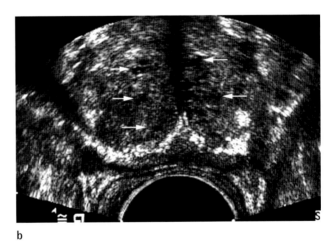

b

Figure 4.13
(a,b) Benign prostatic hyperplasia with scattered cystic changes (arrows). Also see similar cystic changes in Figure 4.8.

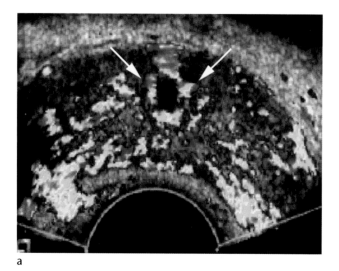

a

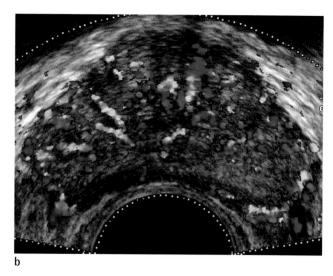

b

Figure 4.14
Normal Doppler flow patterns. (a) Transverse color Doppler image of the young adult prostate demonstrates extensive capsular flow, with a radial pattern of vessels extending toward the dilated urethra, as well as a ring of periurethral flow (arrows). (b) Transverse color Doppler image in a patient with mild BPH demonstrates the normal radial pattern of vessels extending from the capsule toward the urethra.

Acoustical shadowing from these calcifications may complicate visualization of the more anterior aspect of the prostate.

Ductal ectasia of the seminal vesicles is commonly associated with benign prostatic hyperplasia (Figure 4.12). The enlarged inner gland compresses the ejaculatory ducts as they course to the verumontanum, resulting in relative obstruction. The tubules within the seminal vesicles as well as the vasa deferentia may dilate secondary to this obstruction. In a patient with cancer of the prostate, it is often impossible to determine whether obstruction of the seminal vesicles is related to benign prostatic hyperplasia or to the cancer.

Cystic changes are often found in areas of benign hyperplasia (Figure 4.13). Although this finding is most commonly found in the inner gland, cystic areas of hyperplasia may be seen within the outer gland as well. Both cystic change and calcification of the glandular parenchyma may also be related to prostatitis. In my experience, cystic changes in the prostate are overwhelmingly associated with benign disease.

Finally, benign prostatic hyperplasia is associated with a distortion of the normal pattern of blood flow within the prostate. The young adult prostate demonstrates capsular flow, with perforating branches that radiate toward the urethra at the center of the gland, as well as a small amount of periurethral flow (Figure 4.14). Enlargement of the inner gland associated with benign prostatic hyperplasia distorts this radial pattern of flow, and results in increased flow to the hyperplastic inner gland (Figure 4.15). Areas of

increased Doppler flow in the inner gland may mimic the increased flow associated with prostate cancer.

Congential anomalies and cysts

Cysts of the prostate and seminal vesicles should be recognized by their characteristic appearance and location. Certain types of cysts may be significant because of their association with infertility or with other genitourinary anomalies. Most cysts are asymptomatic and should be recognized as benign entities that require no further intervention.

Müllerian duct cysts are the most common congenital cyst of the prostate. The Müllerian duct cyst is a remnant of the Müllerian tubercle, and is commonly seen in the midline, near the base of the prostate. Müllerian duct cysts may extend or arise above the prostate (Figure 4.16). Müllerian duct cysts are benign and generally asymptomatic unless they become superinfected. In rare cases, Müllerian cysts may be associated with infertility related to pressure effect and obstruction of the adjacent ejaculatory duct.[11]

The seminal vesicles, vas deferens and ejaculatory duct arise from the mesonephric (Wolffian) duct. Congenital anomalies of the seminal vesicle, including cysts and agenesis, may be associated with other Wolffian anomalies. Cysts of the seminal vesicles are associated with ipsilateral renal agenesis in two-thirds of cases.[12] Cysts of the seminal

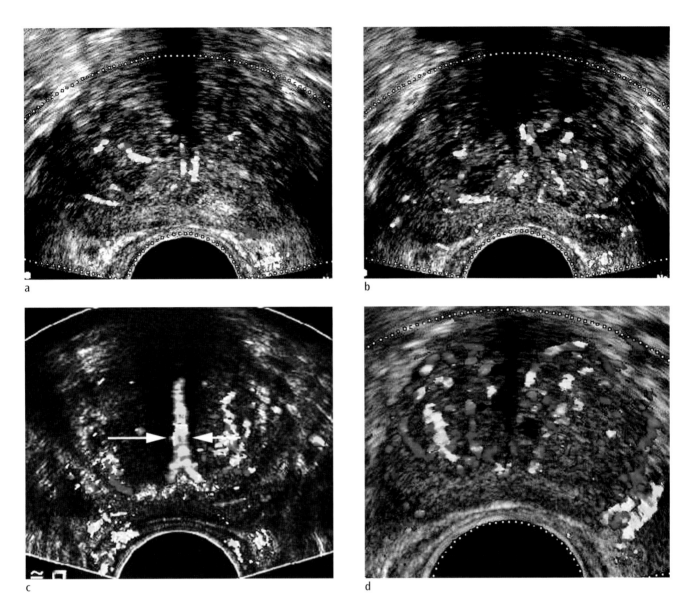

a b c d

Figure 4.15
Color Doppler images of prostate glands with BPH. (a,b) Distortion of the normal radial flow pattern. (c) The classic Eiffel tower appearance of flow between the two enlarged transition zone nodules (arrows). (d) Bilobed enlargement of the transition zone in BPH with increased flow.

vesicle are rare, and should be distinguished from the more common ductal ectasia of the seminal vesicles (Figure 4.17). Examination of the upper urinary tracts is suggested whenever a congenital anomaly of a seminal vesicle is found.

Ejaculatory duct cysts are common acquired cysts that arise along the course of the ejaculatory ducts on either side of the midline, but may appear to lie in the midline. Cysts of the ejaculatory duct are often associated with ejaculatory duct obstruction, although it is unclear whether these cysts are the cause or result of the obstruction (Figure

4.18). The association with ejaculatory duct obstruction cannot definitely discriminate between a Müllerian and ejaculatory duct cyst. However, aspiration of an ejaculatory duct cyst should demonstrate the presence of spermatozoa. Sperm is not present in a Müllerian cyst. The distinction between these two entities is rarely of clinical importance. Nonetheless, it is important to recognize these common cystic entities.

The prostatic utricle, a tiny pouch situated within the verumontanum, arises from the Müllerian tubercle. A utricular cyst may be defined as dilatation of the prostatic

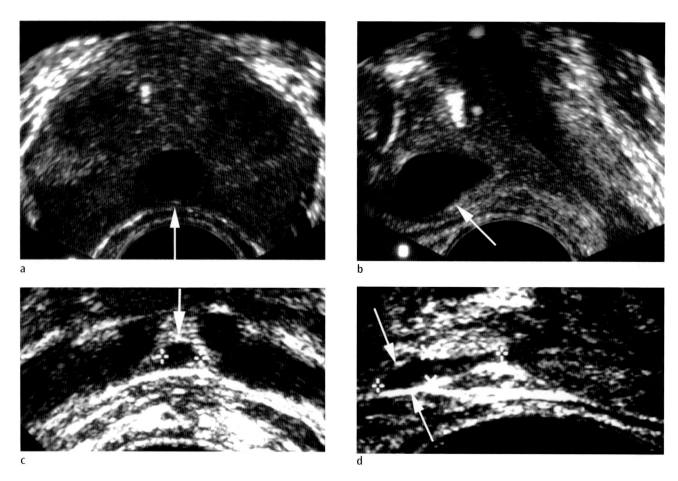

a

b

c

d

Figure 4.16
Müllerian duct cyst. (a) Transverse and (b) sagittal images of the prostate demonstrate a midline cystic structure at the base (arrow). This cyst is indistinguishable from an ejaculatory duct cyst by ultrasound criteria. (c) Transverse and (d) sagittal images above the prostate demonstrates a Müllerian duct cyst between the seminal vesicles (arrow).

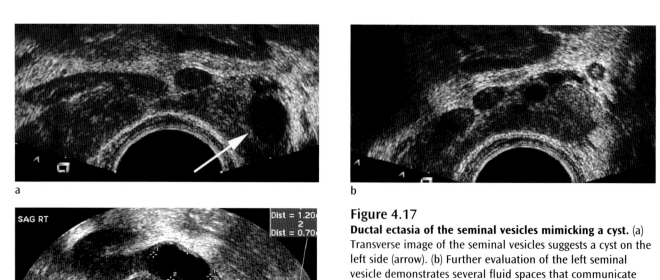

a

b

c

Figure 4.17
Ductal ectasia of the seminal vesicles mimicking a cyst. (a) Transverse image of the seminal vesicles suggests a cyst on the left side (arrow). (b) Further evaluation of the left seminal vesicle demonstrates several fluid spaces that communicate and represent ductal ectasia. (c) Focal area of ductal dilatation within a right seminal vesicle mimicks a cyst.

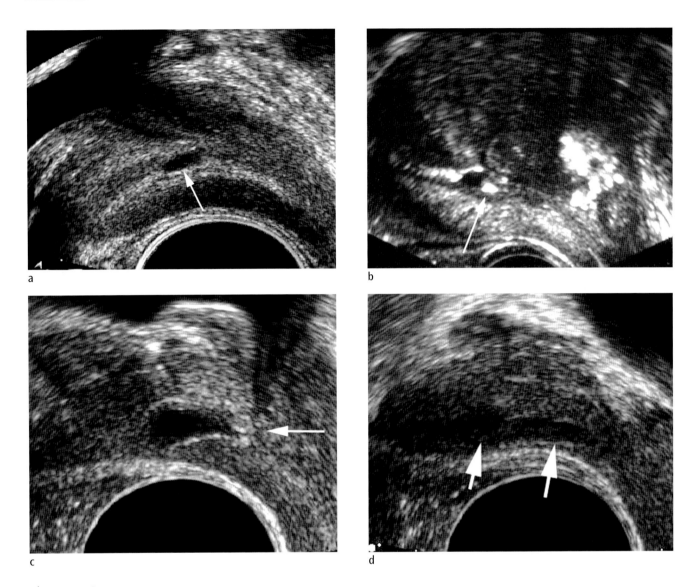

Figure 4.18

Ejaculatory duct cysts. (a) Sagittal image of the prostate demonstrates a cyst along the course of the ejaculatory duct (arrow). The junction of the ejaculatory duct with the verumontanum is a common site for an ejaculatory duct cyst. (b) Sagittal image in another patient demonstrates an ejaculatory duct cyst with an associated calcification (arrow). The sonographer should always evaluate for the presence of calcification associated with the cyst. Sagittal images in a third patient demonstrating (c) an ejaculatory duct cyst just posterior to the verumontanum (arrow) and (d) associated ductal ectasia of the left seminal vesicle (arrows).

utricle to larger than 4 mm with loss of epithelial papillations. Utricular cysts communicate with the urethra and may result in post-void dribbling.[13] Utricular cysts are associated with other anomalies of the genitourinary system, including hypospadias, incomplete testicular descent and renal agenesis.[14] In contrast to Müllerian duct cysts, which are most commonly noted near the base of the prostate in the midline, utricular cysts should be located closer to the verumontanum.

Infection and prostatitis

The most common benign causes of a painful prostate are classified into three categories: (1) acute and chronic bacterial prostatitis, (2) non-bacterial prostatitis and (3) prostatodynia.[15] Bacterial prostatitis is usually associated with infection of the urinary tract. Acute bacterial prostatitis is a highly symptomatic febrile illness, often with an abrupt onset. Chronic bacterial prostatitis presents a more

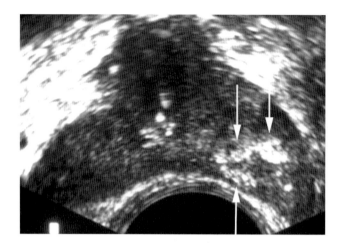

Figure 4.19
Calcifications associated with prostatitis. Dystrophic calcifications (arrows) result from prostatitis, but can also serve as a nidus for infection that is difficult to irradicate.

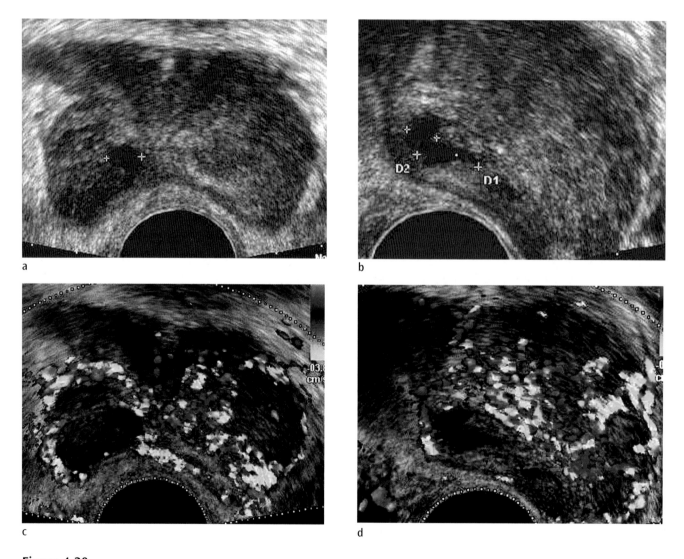

Figure 4.20
Prostatic abscess with increased surrounding Doppler flow. (a) Transverse and (b) sagittal gray-scale images demonstrate a fluid collection, representing an abscess. (c) Transverse and (d) sagittal Doppler images demonstrate increased flow around the abscess.

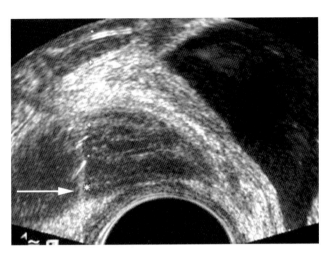

Figure 4.21
Ultrasound-guided drainage procedure for a prostatic abscess. The drainage needle is visualized as it enters the abscess cavity (arrow).

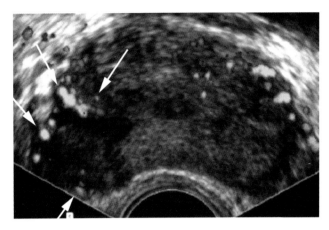

Figure 4.22
Transverse power Doppler image of the prostate in a patient with focal prostatitis. The gray-scale appearance is heterogeneous at the site of infection, with increased surrounding flow (arrows).

indolent course of recurrent urinary tract infection, often refractory to antibiotic therapy. Non-bacterial prostatitis presents with inflammatory cells in prostatic secretions, but no organism is isolated. Prostatodynia presents with symptoms of pelviperineal pain, but with negative cultures and normal prostatic secretions. The distinction among these clinical entities can pose a difficult clinical problem. Symptoms often include low back pain, fever, dysuria and perineal pain. Rectal examination may reveal a tender prostate.

For the sonographer, two important findings in prostatitis are calcifications and fluid collections. The presence of calcification is non-specific, since calcifications are often associated with benign prostatic hyperplasia. However, prostatic calcifications can certainly act as a nidus for infection and may complicate the treatment of prostatitis (Figure 4.19). In the setting of prostatitis, a fluid collection within the prostate should suggest the possibility of an abscess. Internal echoes within a prostatic abscess may make it difficult to distinguish an abscess with debris from a solid mass. The presence of increased Doppler flow around a fluid collection lends further support to the diagnosis of an abscess (Figure 4.20).

Treatment of a prostatic abscess is complicated by the relatively poor penetration of many antibiotics into the prostate. Ultrasound-guided aspiration of an abscess or placement of a drainage catheter, combined with appropriate antibiotics, is a very effective form of treatment. Ultrasound-guided drainage of a prostatic abscess is generally performed with the same transrectal approach used for ultrasound-guided biopsy (Figure 4.21). A needle is introduced into the prostate under direct ultrasound visualization, and a wire is threaded into the abscess through the needle. Once the position of the wire is confirmed sono-

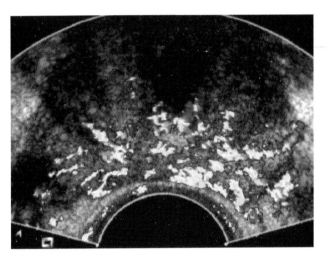

Figure 4.23
Transverse color Doppler image of diffuse prostatitis. There is a heterogeneous appearance to the gland with diffusely increased color flow.

graphically, the needle and ultrasound probe are usually exchanged for a drainage catheter, which may be introduced under sonographic or fluoroscopic visualization.

Other ultrasound findings that have been described with prostatitis include a sonolucent halo around the periurethral tissue, diminished echogenicity within the peripheral zone associated with indistinctness of the capsule, and increased sonolucency of the gland.[16] Unfortunately, these signs are non-specific, and not very sensitive. Prostatitis may present as a focal area of gray-scale and Doppler abnormality (Figure 4.22) or as a diffuse abnormality (Figure 4.23). Both the gray-scale and Doppler findings

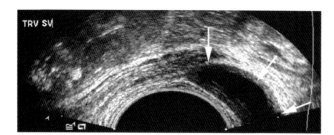

Figure 4.24
Transverse image of the seminal vesicles in a patient with infertility. The left seminal vesicle is obstructed (arrow). The right seminal vesicle is absent.

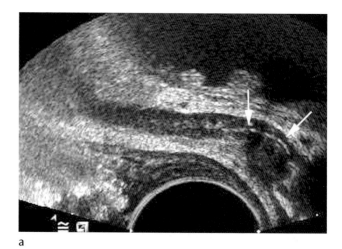

a

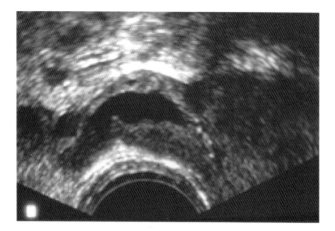

Figure 4.25
Obstructed right seminal vesicle in a patient with infertility.

associated with prostatitis may be indistinguishable from the appearance associated with infiltrating cancer.

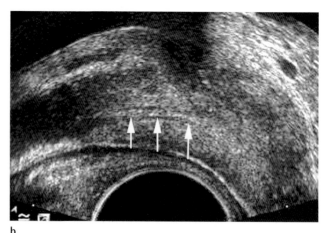

b

Figure 4.26
Inspissated secretions within the ejaculatory system often demonstrate an echogenic appearance in subjects with infertility. (a) Inspissated secretions within the right vas deferens appear as an echogenic line (arrows). (b) Inspissated secretions along the course of a normal-caliber ejaculatory duct produce a linear echogenic appearance (arrows).

Infertility

Ultrasound of the prostate is often requested as part of the evaluation of male infertility. Since congenital anomalies may result in infertility, ultrasound assessment should document the presence of two seminal vesicles, two vasa deferentia and two ejaculatory ducts (Figure 4.24). Seminal vesicles and ejaculatory ducts should be evaluated for obstruction (Figure 4.25). A low semen volume is often associated with inspissated echogenic material within the vasa deferentia and/or ejaculatory ducts (Figure 4.26). The congenital cystic lesions described in the subsection above may cause secondary obstruction and infertility. Benign prostatic hyperplasia may distort the normal course of the ejaculatory ducts and urethra, and can result in inadequate or retrograde ejaculation.

Prostate cancer

The number of new cases of prostate cancer that will be diagnosed in the United States for 2005 is estimated at 232 090, with 30 350 deaths.[17] The upsurge in newly diagnosed cases of prostate cancer in the past 20 years is related to an exponential increase in prostate-specific antigen (PSA) testing and an associated increase in the number of needle biopsy procedures. Between 1986 and 1991 the rate of prostate needle biopsy in men over 65 years of age increased from 685 to 2600 per 100 000.[18] Since the proportion of prostate biopsies positive for cancer is slightly under one-third, the number of prostate biopsies performed annually in the United States in 2004 was probably greater than 700 000.

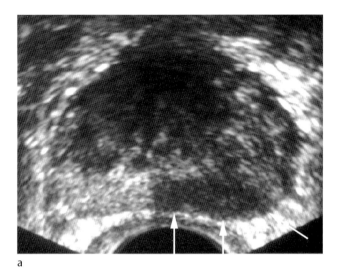

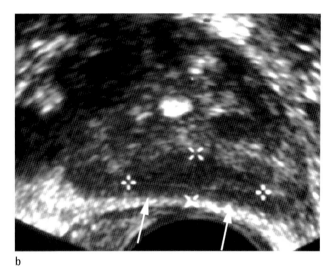

a

b

Figure 4.27
Gleason 7 cancer in the left mid-gland. The cancer appears hypoechoic on (a) transverse and (b) sagittal gray-scale imaging (arrows).

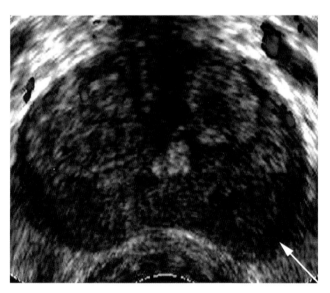

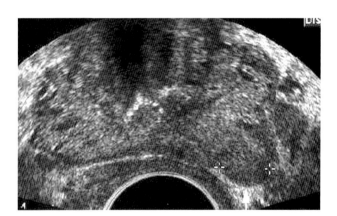

Figure 4.29
Gleason 8 cancer in the left mid-gland (between the two cross-hairs) presents as a palpable nodule with a corresponding focal bulge on the transverse sonographic image.

Figure 4.28
Gleason 6 cancer in the left mid-gland (arrow). In comparison to the right side of the prostate, the left mid-gland appears slightly more hypoechoic on gray-scale, but does not demonstrate increased Doppler flow.

Adenocarcinoma of the prostate arises most frequently in the outer gland.[19–21] Early reports of sonographic detection of prostate cancer suggested that most cancers were echogenic.[22–25] Subsequent studies demonstrated that most cancers were either isoechoic or hypoechoic on gray-scale sonography,[26–28] and that there is a great overlap in the sonographic appearance of benign and malignant lesions.[29] It is now generally accepted that cancer of the prostate

appears hypoechoic on sonography (Figure 4.27). Unfortunately, only about half of all cancers within the prostate are sonographically visible. This may be related, in part, to the growth pattern of adenocarcinoma of the prostate. Prostate cancer infrequently presents as a solitary round mass. Rather, prostate cancer tends to be multifocal with infiltrative growth along a path that is parallel to the capsule of the gland. The growth pattern tends to respect both the surgical capsule and the prostatic capsule as barriers to spread. Although many cancers of the prostate are not visible, a recent study suggests that sonographically visible tumor on gray-scale imaging is more likely to be hypervascular on Doppler imaging, and to have a significantly higher Gleason score.[30]

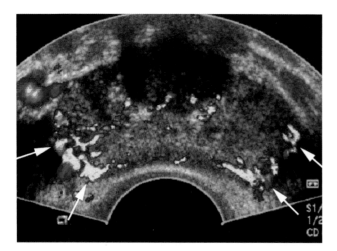

Figure 4.30
Normal prostate flow pattern. Doppler image demonstrates capsular arteries (arrows) with a radial pattern of branches extending toward the center of the prostate.

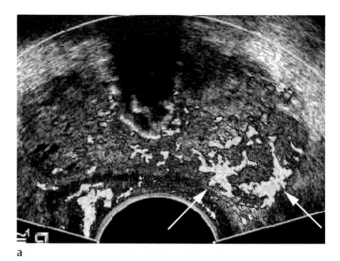

a

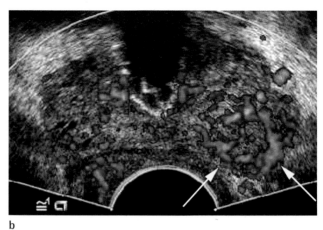

b

Figure 4.31
Gleason 8 cancer in left mid-gland (same patient as Figure 4.29) with increased blood flow on (a) color and (b) power Doppler imaging (arrows).

The hypoechoic nature of prostate cancer is best appreciated on transverse images, which allow a side-to-side comparison of the prostatic parenchyma (Figure 4.28). Whenever possible, a hypoechoic mass seen on gray-scale evaluation should be confirmed in two orthogonal planes to verify findings. Other sonographic features include a focal bulge of the prostate contour, or an irregularity of the margin of the gland (Figure 4.29). The thin fibromuscular stroma surrounding the prostate is responsible for the smooth appearance of the margin of the gland. When this capsule is invaded by tumor, the smooth contour of the gland is lost and the margin may appear irregular. The prostatic capsule invaginates around the ejaculatory ducts, and is incomplete in the region of the prostatic apex. These two areas are relative weak points for extracapsular spread of prostate cancer. Spread of cancer to a seminal vesicle may be visualized as asymmetry of the seminal vesicles or as loss of the normal tapered appearance of the medial aspect of a seminal vesicle.

Color Doppler evaluation of the normal prostate gland demonstrates the presence of blood flow in a symmetric radial pattern that extends from the capsule toward the urethra (Figure 4.30).[31] Capsular vessels and periurethral flow are normal findings. The normal peripheral zone demonstrates relatively little parenchymal flow, although the amount of visible flow varies considerably based upon the sensitivity of different ultrasound systems. Cancer may be associated with focal areas of increased parenchymal flow (Figure 4.31).[32–34] Recent studies suggest that power Doppler offers an extended dynamic range,[35] and may be even more sensitive than color Doppler for the detection of prostate cancer (Figure 4.32).[36–38] Although Doppler evaluation may improve the detection of prostate cancer, neither gray-scale nor Doppler techniques are sufficiently accurate to provide a diagnosis of prostate cancer or benign tissue without biopsy confirmation.[39,40] The author's personal experience suggests that focal areas with increased color or power Doppler flow are more likely to contain cancer than adjacent areas without flow, but that the absence of flow with conventional color and power Doppler imaging is not sufficiently sensitive to exclude a patient from biopsy.[41]

Biopsy techniques

Ultrasound-guided biopsy of the prostate may be obtained from a transperineal or a transrectal approach. Transperineal biopsy is performed with the patient in the lithotomy position. Using a standard sterile technique, the

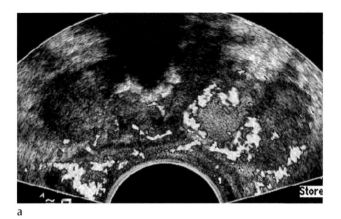
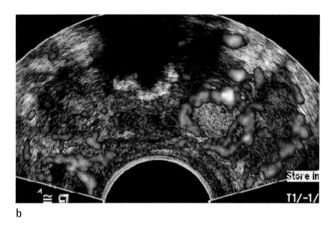

a

b

Figure 4.32
Gleason 9 cancer in the left base demonstrates increased flow in a complex mass with both echogenic and hypoechoic components. (a) Color Doppler demonstrates a ring of flow around the echogenic component. (b) Power Doppler demonstrates the ring of flow around the echogenic component, and demonstrates additional flow around the more laterally placed hypoechoic component.

perineum is prepped and draped. Transperineal imaging and biopsy may be performed with an end-fire transducer operating at 5–7 MHz (Figure 4.33). The transrectal biopsy approach is generally preferred, because it provides better visualization of the prostate and a shorter needle path for the biopsy procedure (Figure 4.34). Transrectal ultrasound may be performed with an end-fire, side-fire or combination end-fire and side-fire probe operating at a frequency of 5–10 MHz. Although transrectal biopsy may be performed with the subject in either the lithotomy or decubitus position, the lithotomy position is preferred for Doppler evaluation.[42]

For any biopsy procedure of the prostate, anticoagulants – including aspirin, nonsteroidal anti-inflammatory drugs and some herbal medications (*Ginkgo biloba*) – should be stopped 1 week prior to biopsy. Such medications may be restarted 24–48 hours after the biopsy procedure, provided the patient is not experiencing urinary or rectal bleeding. Many, although not all, centers instruct the patient to take a cleansing enema prior to the biopsy procedure. The use of an enema reduces the amount of fecal contents within the rectum. A clean rectum provides a superior acoustic window for imaging the prostate, and may reduce the risk of infection.

In contrast to transperineal biopsy, which is performed under sterile conditions, transrectal biopsy of the prostate requires antibiotic prophylaxis. Without antibiotic prophylaxis, the rate of bacteriuria after transrectal needle biopsy of the prostate may be as high as 8%, with a clinical rate of urinary tract infections of 5% and a hospitalization rate of 2%.[43] Antibiotic prophylaxis should be given to all patients prior to transrectal biopsy in order to reduce the risk of

subsequent infection.[44,45] Antibiotics are not needed for transperineal biopsy. For standard transrectal ultrasound-guided biopsy, most centers prefer an oral fluoroquinolone, although there is considerable variability among physicians in the choice of antibiotics for prophylaxis.[46] Ideally, the antibiotic should be administered at least 30–60 minutes before biopsy in order to have adequate serum levels at the time of biopsy.

Although there are no randomized, controlled human trials to definitively establish that antibiotic prophylaxis provides protection against endocarditis, intravenous antibiotic prophylaxis is recommended during biopsy of the prostate for patients in the moderate- or high-risk AHA (American Heart Association) categories.[47] The high-risk category includes patients with bio-prosthetic and homograft heart valves, a prior history of endocarditis, complex congenital heart disease, or surgically constructed systemic pulmonary shunts. The moderate-risk category includes those patients with other congenital cardiac malformations, acquired valve dysfunction (e.g. rheumatic heart disease), hypertrophic cardiomyopathy, or mitral valve prolapse with regurgitation or thickened leaflets.

Biopsy of the prostate is an invasive procedure with potentially serious risks. Life-threatening complications, including severe hemorrhage[48,49] and sepsis, occur in less than 1% of patients, but pain and mild complications are common.[50] Spread of tumor into the biopsy track has been reported after both transrectal[51] and transperineal[52] biopsy, although the clinical significance is uncertain. Hematuria and hematospermia after prostate biopsy are reported at rates of 23.6% and 45.3%, respectively.[53] In one study, 19% of subjects complained of significant complications, the

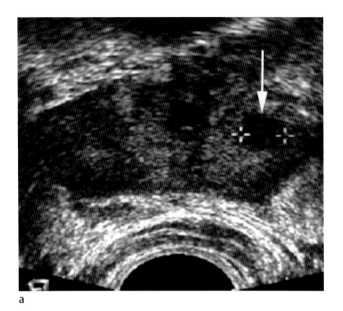

a

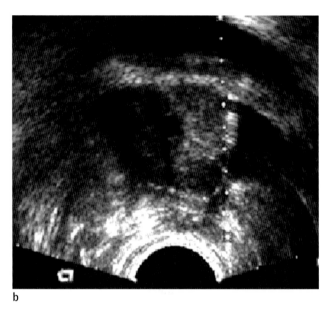

b

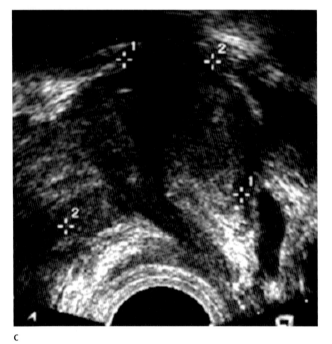

c

Figure 4.33
Transperineal imaging and biopsy of the prostate. (a) Coronal image of the prostate obtained from the transperineal approach demonstrates a focal hypoechoic nodule (arrow). (b) Transperineal biopsy of this nodule demonstrated a Gleason 7 cancer. (c) Sagittal transperineal image of the prostate with measurements.

most common being painful or difficult voiding (13%) and hematuria (11%).[54] Although clinically significant morbidity from prostate biopsy is rare, each biopsy core does require an additional needle pass with the potential to introduce infection and hemorrhage.

Prostate biopsy is an uncomfortable procedure, but need not be painful. Almost all patients can be managed with topical or local anesthesia.[55] Patients with anal strictures may be more difficult to manage. General anesthesia should be reserved only for those patients who cannot

tolerate the physical or emotional stress of biopsy while awake.

Transperineal biopsy should be preceded by local anesthesia with 1% or 2% lidocaine. A 25-gauge needle is used to anesthetize the skin and subcutaneous tissues of the perineum. Deeper anesthesia is obtained under ultrasound guidance by injecting lidocaine along the expected biopsy tract with a spinal needle. It is useful to infiltrate local anesthetic into the tissues down to the level of the prostate. A total of 10–20 ml of local anesthetic agent may be used.

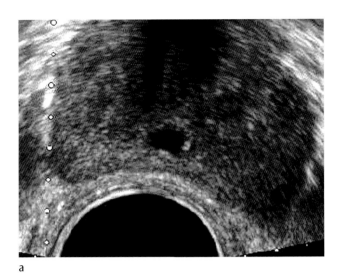 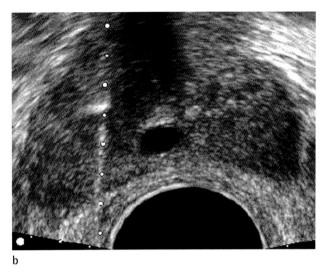

a   b

Figure 4.34
Transrectal biopsy of the right mid-gland in a transverse orientation. The transducer is immediately adjacent to the portion of the prostate to be sampled. (a) Laterally directed biopsy along the margin of the prostate (white dots) targets the expected growth pattern of prostate cancer along the capsule. (b) Traditional parasagittal biopsy location, as described in the original sextant biopsy approach. The projected needle course is more medially directed (white dots). The transrectal biopsy approach provides the shortest needle path for prostate biopsy.

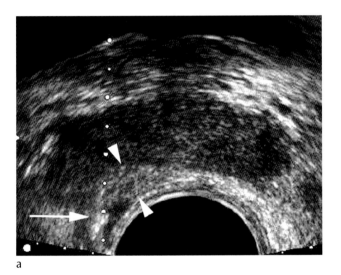 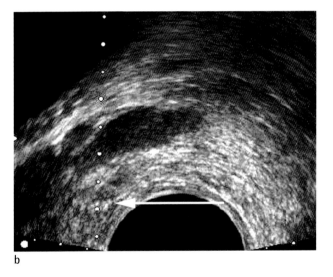

a   b

Figure 4.35
Transrectal injection of local anesthetic into the neurovascular bundle. (a) Transverse image at the base of the prostate demonstrates needle positioning (arrow) and flow of the anesthetic agent into the plane between the rectum and the base of the prostate (arrowheads). (b) Transverse image, rotated to the left, at the level of the seminal vesicles demonstrates needle positioning (arrow) for injection of anesthetic into the left-sided neurovascular bundle.

Transrectal biopsy may be preceded by injection of lidocaine into the region of the neurovascular bundles.[56] Injection of anesthetic is performed under direct sonographic visualization. Anesthetic is injected bilaterally at or just above the base of the prostate (Figure 4.35). In order to achieve adequate anesthesia and to minimize the risk of systemic side effects, it is important to avoid injection into the periprostatic vessels. Anesthetic is readily visualized by sonography when it is properly injected into the plane between the prostate and the rectum. A total of

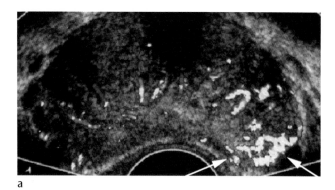
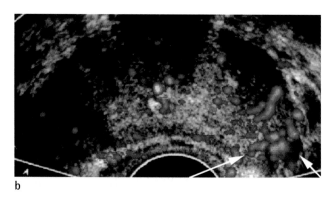

a

b

Figure 4.36
Transverse Doppler images of the base of the prostate during infusion of the microbubble contrast agent Imagent. Increased flow is demonstrated at a site of Gleason 6 cancer in the left base. (a) Contrast-enhanced color Doppler. (b) Contrast-enhanced power Doppler.

10 ml of local anesthetic is generally sufficient for transrectal biopsy.

A full discussion of prostate biopsy strategies is beyond the scope of this chapter. Although most clinicians use ultrasound to guide needle placement, only 20% of clinicians rely upon ultrasound to target specific biopsy sites.[57] The utility of targeted biopsy is limited by the difficulty of identifying prostate cancer with ultrasound. For this reason, many centers use systematic, spatially distributed biopsy strategies.

The sextant biopsy technique for the prostate is a systematic, spatially distributed set of six parasagittal biopsy cores first described in 1989.[58] Although the sextant biopsy strategy was the standard of care for over a decade, a significant minority of cancers are not detected with this technique.[59] One group demonstrated a 19% positive biopsy rate after a second sextant biopsy.[60] One study using two consecutive sets of sextant biopsies increased the positive biopsy rate by 37%,[61] while a second similar study increased the positive biopsy rate by only 8%.[62] Approximately 35% of positive lesions detected by a five-region biopsy approach are not found with the standard sextant.[63] In one PSA-screened population, the sextant biopsy approach missed 36% of cancers in glands under 30 ml in volume, and 64% of cancers in larger glands.[64]

Recent studies have suggested that an optimal systematic approach might require 8–10 biopsy cores,[65,66] and up to 12–14 cores for larger glands.[67] Some groups advocate a 'saturation biopsy' approach.[68] Because prostate cancers often grow along the capsule of the gland, laterally directed biopsy cores may be more sensitive than conventional parasagittal sextant cores.[69] Needless to say, the optimal number and location of systematic biopsy cores remain a matter of controversy.

Clinical application of a limited biopsy approach with conventional gray-scale-guided biopsy of focal lesions has fallen into disfavor because of the diverse appearance of prostate cancer. Color Doppler imaging with targeted biopsy has been proposed to supplement conventional gray-scale imaging in order to increase overall sensitivity.[70–72] In addition to improved cancer detection with color Doppler imaging, increased color Doppler signal correlates positively with both prostate tumor stage and grade, as well as with the risk of recurrence after treatment.[73] Several small studies have suggested that power Doppler may be even more useful in the detection of prostate cancer.[74,75] Nonetheless, the sensitivity of gray-scale and Doppler ultrasound-guided targeted biopsy is not sufficient to eliminate the need for systematic biopsy.[76–79]

Brachytherapy

The application of transrectal ultrasound to guide transperineal placement of radioactive seeds into the prostate has greatly advanced the field of brachytherapy. A special needle guidance template is placed against the perineum to allow accurate placement of radioactive sources into the prostate without fluoroscopic guidance. Seeds are introduced within a long cannula that is positioned in the prostate under ultrasound guidance. The ultrasound system is used in real time to verify the position of the seeds as they are released from the cannula.

Advanced imaging techniques for prostate cancer

Contrast-enhanced sonography

The vascular supply to malignant prostate tissue differs from the vascular anatomy of normal prostate tissue.

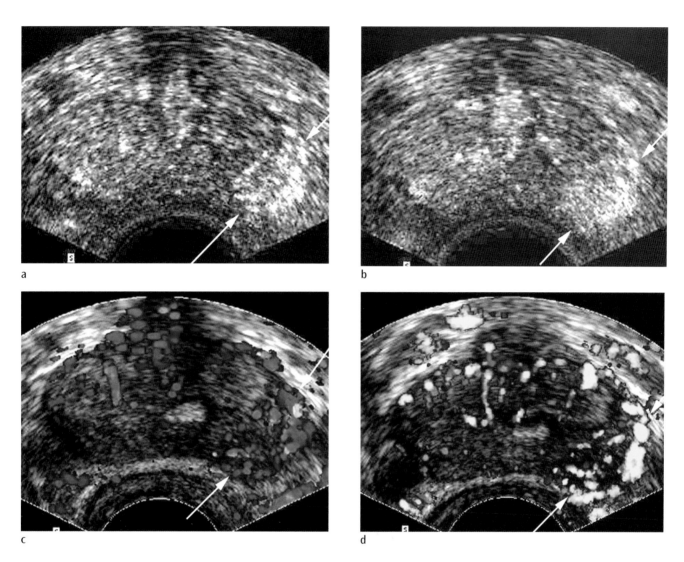

a   b   c   d

Figure 4.37

Contrast-enhanced imaging of a Gleason 6 cancer in the left mid-gland. The baseline gray-scale image in Figure 4.11b demonstrates a subtle hypoechoic area in the left mid-gland. (a) Continuous harmonic imaging and (b) intermittent harmonic imaging demonstrate gray-scale enhancement of the cancer. Contrast-enhanced (c) color Doppler and (d) power Doppler also demonstrate focal enhancement of the cancer (arrows).

Studies of microvessel density within the prostate demonstrate a clear association of increased microvessel density with the presence of cancer,[80] with metastases,[81] with the stage of disease[82–84] and disease-specific survival.[85,86] Quantitative assessment of microvascular density may actually provide important data to guide therapeutic decisions.[87] Unfortunately, the microvessels that proliferate around and within prostate cancers are below the limits of the resolution of conventional Doppler ultrasound.

One potential solution to this problem of visualizing microvessels may be found with ultrasound contrast agents. These agents are gas-filled microbubbles that can increase the echogenicity of the intravascular space. An early study with one such agent, Echogen (Sonus

Pharmaceuticals; Bothell, Washington), suggested that enhanced color flow with contrast was associated with the presence of prostate cancer.[88,89] Several additional studies have demonstrated Doppler enhancement of prostate cancer.[90–92] These preliminary studies suggest that contrast agents may be useful in ultrasound evaluation of prostate vascularity and the presence of cancer (Figure 4.36).

Unfortunately, Doppler imaging delivers power levels which are sufficient to destroy contrast microbubbles, especially when using a high mechanical index. Thus, many microbubbles are imaged and destroyed before they reach the neovasculature. One potential solution to this problem is intermittent ultrasound imaging. With intermittent imaging, the transmitted ultrasound pulse is turned off

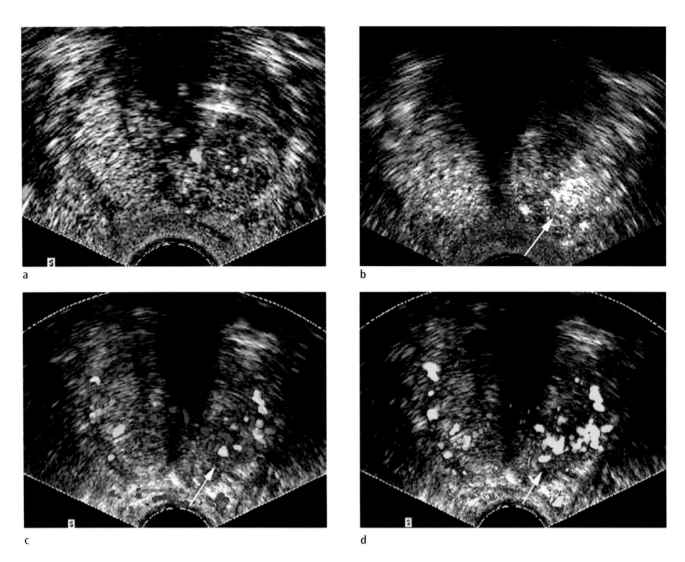

a

b

c

d

Figure 4.38
Contrast-enhanced imaging of a Gleason 6 cancer in the left apex. (a) Baseline color Doppler demonstrates minimal flow in the left apex, but no gray-scale abnormality. (b) Contrast-enhanced harmonic imaging demonstrates gray-scale enhancement of the tumor. Contrast-enhanced (c) color Doppler and (d) power Doppler also demonstrate focal enhancement of the cancer in the left apex (arrows).

between frames, allowing the contrast agent to traverse further into the capillary bed. Intermittent imaging has been shown to increase the enhancement provided by ultrasound contrast agents.[93–95]

Harmonic imaging is a gray-scale technique that allows ultrasound imaging of contrast agents.[96–100] When contrast agents are imaged with ultrasound, the reverberations created by microbubbles may resonate at frequencies which are different to the frequency of insonation. Various harmonics of the insonating frequency are produced by the contrast agent and can be imaged. Since ordinary tissue predominantly reflects ultrasound at the frequency of insonation, most harmonic signals will come from contrast material. Thus, harmonic imaging may be used to improve the imaging of contrast material, and reduce the background signal from surrounding structures.

Harmonic gray-scale imaging utilizes lower energy levels than Doppler imaging, and therefore results in less microbubble destruction. In order to further minimize bubble destruction, gray-scale harmonic imaging may be applied in intermittent mode as described above, or in a low mechanical index mode. Continuous imaging with a low mechanical index of microbubble contrast agents has been used by investigators in various organ systems to improve the enhancement provided by contrast while providing continuous ultrasound imaging.

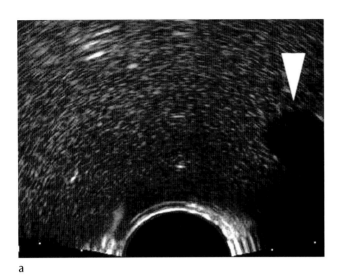

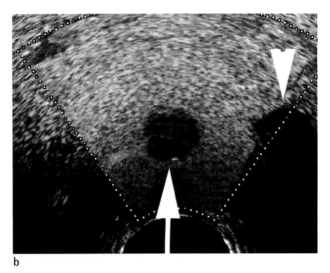

a

b

Figure 4.39

Elastogram of an isoechoic phantom. (a) The round stiff area is isoechoic. (b) It is clearly visualized on the elastogram (arrow). Arrowheads demonstrate a similar-sized hyperechoic round focus within the phantom that is visible with conventional gray-scale imaging.

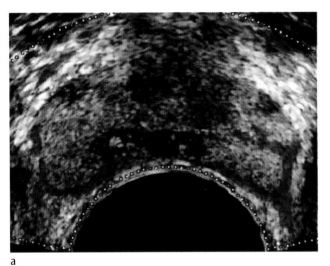

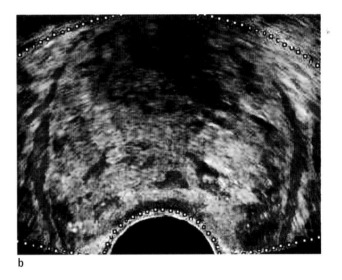

a

b

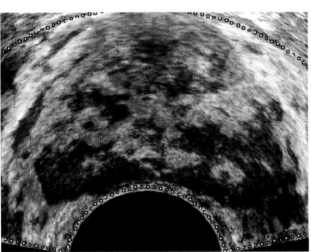

Figure 4.40

(a) Normal prostate elastogram. (b,c) Elastograms from patients with BPH. Note areas of asymmetry within the elastogram in the setting of BPH.

c

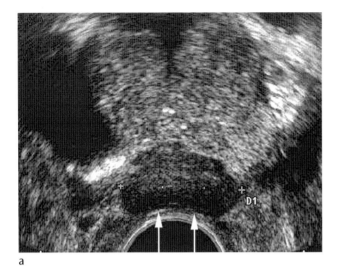

a

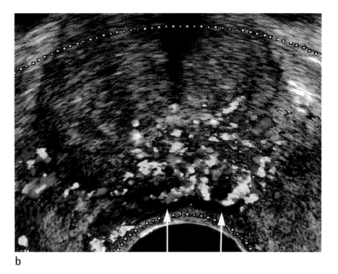

b

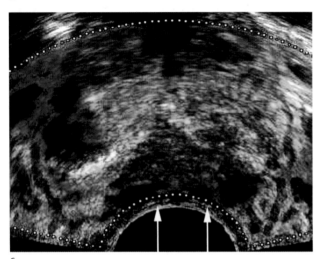

c

Figure 4.41
Gleason 9 cancer in left mid-gland. (a) The cancer is visible as a focal mass on gray-scale imaging. (b) The cancer is hypervascular with color Doppler. (c) The cancer appears stiff on the elastogram.

Both contrast-enhanced color Doppler and harmonic gray-scale imaging have been used successfully by the author to improve imaging of prostate cancer and to guide targeted biopsy for detection of prostate cancer (Figures 4.37 and 4.38).[101–106] In a recent study of subjects evaluated with contrast-enhanced ultrasound, cancer was detected in 363 biopsy cores from 104 of 301 subjects (35%), including 15.5% (175/1133) of targeted cores and 10.4% (188/1806) of sextant cores (p <0.01). Among subjects with cancer, targeted cores were twice as likely to return a positive biopsy (OR = 2.0, p <0.001). Systematic biopsy is the current standard method of obtaining a diagnosis of prostate cancer. Contrast studies may be an alternative. In order to maximize cancer detection and minimize the number of biopsy cores, the author recommends a contrast-enhanced targeted biopsy strategy with additional cores at the apex of the prostate.[107]

Elastography

The application of elastography for imaging of soft tissues was first described in the early 1990s.[108,109] Elastography represents a form of signal processing applied to sonographic radiofrequency (RF) data. The elastogram is a map of tissue stiffness derived from changes in the sonographic RF speckle pattern during the application of external pressure and subsequent relaxation.[110] Intuitively, one would expect less displacement of the speckle pattern in stiffer tissue. Elastography can demonstrate the presence of 'stiff' tissue in the absence of any underlying difference in sonographic echotexture (Figure 4.39).

In-vitro examination of prostate cancer demonstrates that malignant prostate tissue is consistently stiffer than benign tissue.[111] The elastic modulus of normal tissue is lower than that of prostate cancer, whereas the elastic

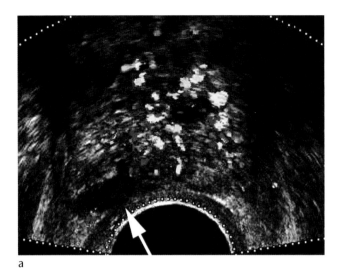
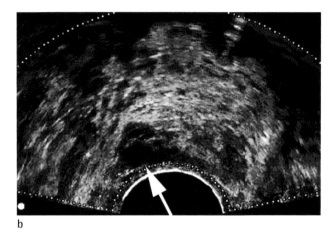

Figure 4.42
Gleason 6 cancer in right apex. (a) The hypoechoic mass does not demonstrate color flow. (b) The cancer does demonstrate increased stiffness on the elastogram.

modulus of tissue with benign prostatic hyperplasia is even lower than that of normal prostate tissue.[112] Although digital rectal examination may detect malignant nodules along the posterior surface of the prostate, elastography has the potential to detect stiff tissue located deep within the gland. Elastography of prostate specimens provides precise anatomical detail throughout the gland (Figure 4.40).[113] A small study comparing conventional sonography to sono-elasticity imaging in prostatectomy specimens suggests that elastography may be more sensitive than gray-scale sonography for detection of prostate cancer in vitro.[114]

In the last few years, several commercial ultrasound systems have introduced real-time elastography for in-vivo imaging. The feasibility of in-vivo elastography has been demonstrated.[115,116] Compression of the prostate may be achieved by inflation of a balloon at the tip of the probe,[117] or by direct manual compression of the prostate. In-vivo elastography can identify cancer within the prostate, based upon its reduced elasticity relative to surrounding tissues (Figures 4.41 and 4.42). Nonetheless, our clinical experience suggests that in-vivo elastography is operator-dependent, and that there may be substantial inter-observer and intra-observer variation in the elastogram image, based upon the individual technique used to apply compression. These findings suggest a need for development of a more reproducible in-vivo compression technique.

Conclusion

Familiarity with the gross anatomy of the prostate as well as the zonal anatomy is essential for proper ultrasound

evaluation. Ultrasound is useful for evaluation of benign diseases, including infection and infertility, and may be used to guide treatment of a prostatic abscess. With respect to malignant disease, anatomical considerations often predict the growth pattern of prostate cancer and determine the optimal distribution of biopsy cores and radiation therapy seeds. New ultrasound techniques, including contrast-enhanced imaging and elastography, represent the next frontier for ultrasound detection and therapy of prostate cancer.

References

1. Fornage BD. Normal US anatomy of the prostate. Ultrasound Med Biol 1986; 12: 1011–21.
2. Watanabe H, Igari D, Tanahashi Y, et al. Measurements of size and weight of prostate by means of transrectal ultrasonography. Tohoku J Exp Med 1974; 114: 277–85.
3. Lee F, Torp-Pederson ST, Siders DB, et al. Transrectal ultrasound in the diagnosis and staging of prostatic carcinoma. Radiology 1989; 170: 609–15.
4. Aboul-Azm TE. Anatomy of the human seminal vesicles and ejaculatory ducts. Arch Androl 1979; 3: 287–92.
5. Villers A, Terris MK, NcNeal JE, Stamey TA. Ultrasound anatomy of the prostate: the normal gland and anatomical variations. J Urol 1990; 143: 732–8.
6. Villers A, McNeal JE, Redwine EA, et al. The role of perineural space invasion in the local spread of prostatic adenocarcinoma. J Urol 1989; 142: 763–8.
7. McNeal JE. The zonal anatomy of the prostate. Prostate 1981; 2: 35–49.
8. McNeal JE. Normal and pathologic anatomy of prostate. Urology 1981; 17(Suppl): 11–16.

9. Glynn RJ, Campion EW, Bouchard GR, Silbert JE. The development of benign prostatic hyperplasia among volunteers of the Normative Aging Study. Am J Epidemiol 1985; 121: 78–90.

10. McNeil JE. Origin and evolution of benign prostatic enlargement. Invest Urol 1978; 15: 340–5.

11. Halpern EJ, Hirsch IH. Sonographically guided transurethral laser incision of a Müllerian duct cyst for treatment of ejaculatory duct obstruction. AJR Am J Roentgenol 2000; 175: 777–8.

12. Heaney JA, Pfister RC, Meares EM. Giant cyst of the seminal vesicle with renal agenesis. AJR Am J Roentgenol 1987; 149: 139–40.

13. Shabsigh R, Lerner S, Fishman IJ, Kadmon D. The role of ultrasonography in the diagnosis and management of prostatic and seminal vesicle cysts. J Urol 1989; 141: 1206–9.

14. Nghiem HT, Kellman GM, Sandberg SA, Craig BM. Cystic lesions of the prostate. Radiographics 1990; 10: 635–50.

15. Drach GW, Fair WR, Meares EM Jr, Stamey TA. Classification of benign diseases associated with prostatic pain: prostatitis or prostatodynia? J Urol 1978; 120: 266.

16. Griffiths GJ, Crooks AJR, Roberts EE, et al, Ultrasonic appearance associated with prostatic inflammation: preliminary study. Clin Radiol 1984; 35: 343–5.

17. Jemal A, Murray T, Ward E, et al. Cancer Statistics, 2005. CA Cancer J Clin 2005; 55: 10–30.

18. Potosky AL, Miller BA, Albertsen PC, Kramer BS. The role of increasing detection in the rising incidence of prostate cancer. JAMA 1995; 273: 548–52.

19. McNeal JE. Origin and development of carcinoma in the prostate. Cancer 1969; 23: 24–33.

20. McNeal JE, Price HM, Redwine EA, Freiha FS, Stamey TA. Stage A versus stage B carcinoma of the prostate: morphologic comparison and biologic significance. J Urol 1988; 139: 61–5.

21. McNeal JE, Redwine EA, Freiha FS, Stamey TA. Zonal distribution of prostatic adenocarcinoma. Correlation with histologic pattern and direction of spread. Am J Surg Pathol 1988; 12(12): 897–906.

22. Resnick MI, Willard JW, Boyce WH. Ultrasonic evaluation of prostatic nodule. J Urol 1978; 120: 86–9.

23. Rifkin MD, Kurtz AB, Choi HY, Goldberg BB. Endoscopic ultrasonic evaluation of the prostate using a transrectal probe: prospective evaluation and acoustic characterization. Radiology 1983; 149(1): 265–71.

24. Fritzsche PJ, Axford PD, Ching VC, et al. Correlation of transrectal sonographic findings in patients with suspected and unsuspected prostatic disease. J Urol 1983; 130: 272–4.

25. Abu-Yousef MM, Narayana AS. Prostatic carcinoma: detection and staging using suprapubic US. Radiology 1985; 156(1): 175–80.

26. Lee F, Gray JM, McLeary RD, et al. Transrectal ultrasound in the diagnosis of prostate cancer: location, echogenicity, histopathology and staging. Prostate 1985; 7: 117–29.

27. Dahnert WF, Hamper UM, Eggleston JC, et al. Prostatic evaluation by transrectal sonography with histopathologic correlation: the echopenic appearance of early carcinoma. Radiology 1986; 158: 97–102.

28. Lee F, Gray JM, McLeary RD, et al. Prostatic evaluation by transrectal sonography: criteria for diagnosis of early carcinoma. Radiology 1986; 158: 91–5.

29. Rifkin MD, Friedland GW, Shortliffe L. Prostatic evaluation by transrectal endosonography: detection of carcinoma. Radiology 1986; 158: 85–90.

30. Cornud F, Hamida K, Flam T, et al. Endorectal color doppler sonography and endorectal MR imaging features of nonpalpable prostate cancer: correlation with radical prostatectomy findings. AJR Am J Roentgenol 2000; 175(4): 1161–8.

31. Neumaier CE, Martinoli C, Derchi LE, Silvestri E, Rosenberg I. Normal prostate gland: examination with color Doppler US. Radiology 1995; 196: 453–7.

32. Lavoipierre AM, Snow RM, Frydenberg M, et al. Prostatic cancer: role of Doppler imaging in transrectal sonography. Am J Radiol 1998; 171: 205–10.

33. Shigeno K, Igawa H, Shiina H, Wada H, Yoneda T. The role of color Doppler ultrasonography in detecting prostate cancer. BJU Int 2000; 86: 229–33.

34. Newman JS, Brea RL, Rubin JM. Prostate cancer: diagnosis with color Doppler sonography with histologic correlation of each biopsy site. Radiology 1995; 195: 86–90.

35. Rubin JM, Bude RO, Carson PL, Bree RL, Adler RS. Power Doppler US: a potentially useful alternative to mean frequency-based color Doppler US. Radiology 1994; 190: 853–6.

36. Downey DB, Fenster A. Three-dimensional power Doppler detection of prostate cancer. AJR Am J Roentgenol 1995; 165: 741.

37. Sakarya ME, Arslan H, Unal O, Atilla MK, Aydin S. The role of power Doppler ultrasonography in the diagnosis of prostate cancer: a preliminary study. Br J Urol 1998; 82: 386–8.

38. Okihara K, Kojima M, Nakanouchi T, Okada K, Midi T. Transrectal power Doppler imaging in the detection of prostate cancer. BJU Int 2000; 85: 1053–7.

39. Cornud F, Belin X, Piron D, et al. Color Doppler-guided prostate biopsies in 591 patients with an elevated serum PSA level: impact on gleason score for nonpalpable lesions. Urology 1997; 49: 709–15.

40. Bree RL. The role of color Doppler and staging biopsies in prostate cancer detection. Urology 1997; 49(Suppl 3A): 31–4.

41. Halpern EJ, Strup SE. Using gray-scale and color and power Doppler sonography to detect prostatic cancer. AJR Am J Roentgenol 2000; 174: 623–7.

42. Halpern EJ, Frauscher F, Forsberg F, et al. High frequency Doppler imaging of the prostate: effect of patient position. Radiology 2002; 222: 634–9.

43. Kapoor DA, Klimberg IW, Malek GH, et al. Single-dose oral ciprofloxacin versus placebo for prophylaxis during transrectal prostate biopsy. Urology 1998; 52(4): 552–8.

44. Taylor HM, Bingham JB. Antibiotic prophylaxis for transrectal prostate biopsy. J Antimicro Chemother 1997; 39: 115–17.

45. Aron M, Rajeev TP, Gupta NP. Antibiotic prophylaxis for transrectal needle biopsy of the prostate: a randomized controlled study. BJU Int 2000; 85(6): 682–5.

46. Shandera KC, Thibault GP, Deshon GE Jr. Variability in patient preparation for prostate biopsy among American urologists. Urology 1998; 52(4): 644–6.

47. Dajani AS, Taubert KA, Wilson W, et al. Prevention of bacterial endocarditis. Recommendations by the American Heart Association. JAMA 1997; 277(22): 1794–801.

48. Gatling RR. Massive retropubic hemorrhage after needle biopsy of the prostate. South Med J 1988; 81(9): 1188–9.

49. Brullet E, Guevara MC, Campo R, et al. Massive rectal bleeding following transrectal ultrasound-guided prostate biopsy. Endoscopy 2000; 32(10): 792–5.

50. Collins GN, Lloyd SN, Hehir M, McKelvie GB. Multiple transrectal ultrasound-guided prostatic biopsies-true morbidity and patient acceptance. Br J Urol 1993; 71(4): 460–3.

51. Bastacky SS, Walsh PC, Epstein JI. Needle biopsy associated tumor tracking of adenocarcinoma of the prostate. J Urol 1991; 145(5): 1003–7.

52. Ryan PG, Peeling WB. Perineal prostatic tumor seedling after 'Tru-Cut' needle biopsy: case report and review of the literature. Eur Urol 1990; 17(2): 189–92.

53. Rietbergen JB, Kruger AE, Kranse R, Schroder FH. Complications of transrectal ultrasound-guided systematic sextant biopsies of the prostate: evaluation of complication rates and risk factors within a population-based screening program. Urology 1997; 49: 875–80.

54. Crundwell MC, Cooke PW, Wallace DM. Patients' tolerance of transrectal ultrasound-guided prostatic biopsy: an audit of 104 cases. Br J Urol Int 1999; 83: 792–5.

55. Pareek G, Armenakas NA, Fracchia JA. Periprostatic nerve blockade for transrectal ultrasound guided biopsy of the prostate: a randomized, double-blind, placebo controlled study. J Urol 2001; 166: 894–7.

56. Berger AP, Frauscher F, Halpern EJ, et al. Periprostatic administration of local anesthesia during transrectal ultrasound-guided biopsy of the prostate: a randomized, double-blind, placebo-controlled study. Urology 2003; 61: 585–8.

57. Plawker MW, Fleisher JM, Vapnek EM, Macchia RJ. Current trends in prostate cancer diagnosis and staging among United States urologists. J Urol 1997; 158(5): 1853–8.

58. Hodge KK, McNeal JE, Terris MK, Stamey TA. Random systematic versus directed ultrasound guided transrectal core biopsies of the prostate. J Urol 1989; 142: 71.

59. Terris MK. Sensitivity and specificity of sextant biopsies in the detection of prostate cancer: preliminary report. Urology 1999; 54: 486–9.

60. Keetch DW, Catalona WJ, Smith DS. Serial prostatic biopsies in men with persistently elevated serum prostate specific antigen values. J Urol 1994; 151(6): 1571–4.

61. Levine MA, Ittman M, Melamed J, Lepor H. Two consecutive sets of transrectal ultrasound guided sextant biopsies of the prostate for the detection of prostate cancer. J Urol 1998; 159: 471–5.

62. O'Connell MJ, Smith CS, Fitzpatrick PE, et al. Transrectal ultrasound-guided biopsy of the prostate gland: value of 12 versus 6 cores. Abdom Imaging 2004; 29(1): 132–6.

63. Eskew LA, Bare RL, McCullough DL. Systematic 5 region prostate biopsy is superior to sextant method for diagnosing carcinoma of the prostate. J Urol 1997; 157: 199–202.

64. Naughton CK, Smith DS, Humphrey PA, Catalona WJ, Koetch DW. Clinical and pathologic tumor characteristics of prostate cancer as a function of the number of biopsy cores: a retrospective study. Urology 1998; 52: 808–13.

65. Presti JC Jr, Chang JJ, Bhargava V, Shinohara K. The optimal systematic prostate biopsy scheme should include 8 rather than 6 biopsy cores: results of a prospective clinical trial. J Urol 2000; 163: 163–6.

66. Gore JL, Shariat SF, Miles BJ, et al. Optimal combinations of systematic sextant and laterally directed biopsies for the detection of prostate cancer. J Urol 2001; 165: 1554–9.

67. Mariappan P, Chong WL, Sundram M, Mohamed SR. Increasing prostate biopsy cores based on volume vs the sextant biopsy: a prospective randomized controlled clinical study on cancer detection rates and morbidity. Br J Urol Int 2004; 94(3): 307–10.

68. Stewart CS, Leibovich BC, Weaver AL, Lieber MM. Prostate cancer diagnosis using a saturation needle biopsy technique after previous negative sextant biopsies. J Urol 2001; 166(1): 86–92.

69. Stamey TA. Making the most out of six systematic sextant biopsies. Urology 1995; 45(1): 2–12.

70. Rifkin MD, Sudakoff GS, Alexander AA. Prostate: techniques, results and potential applications of color Doppler US scanning. Radiology 1993; 186: 509–13.

71. Sudakoff GS, Smith R, Vogelzang NJ, Steinberg G, Brendler CB. Color Doppler imaging and transrectal sonography of the prostate fossa after radical prostatectomy: Early experience. AJR Am j Roentgenol 1996; 167: 883–8.

72. Kravchick S, Cytron S, Peled R, Altshuler A, Ben-Dor D. Using grayscale and two different techniques of color Doppler sonography to detect prostate cancer. Urology 2003; 61(5): 977–81.

73. Ismail M, Petersen RO, Alexander AA, Newschaffer C, Comella LG. Color Doppler imaging in predicting the biologic behavior of prostate cancer: correlation with disease-free survival. Urology 1997; 50: 906–12.

74. Cho JY, Kim SH, Lee SE. Diffuse prostatic lesions: role of color Doppler and power Doppler ultrasonography. J Ultrasound Med 1998; 17(5): 283–7.

75. Okihara K, Kojima M, Naya Y, et al. Ultrasonic power Doppler imaging for prostatic cancer: A preliminary report. Tohoku J Exp Med 1997; 182(4): 277–81.

76. Kelly IMG, Lees WR, Rickards D. Prostate cancer and the role of color Doppler US. Radiology 1993; 189: 153–6.

77. Newman JS, Bree RL, Rubin JM. Prostate cancer: diagnosis with color Doppler sonography with histologic correlation of each biopsy site. Radiology 1995; 195: 86–90.

78. Cornud F, Belin X, Piron D, et al. Color Doppler-guided prostate biopsies in 591 patients with an elevated serum PSA level: impact on Gleason score for non-palpable lesions. Urology 1997; 49: 709–15.

79. Halpern EJ, Frauscher F, Strup SE, et al. Prostate: high frequency Doppler US imaging for cancer detection. Radiology 2002; 225: 71–7.

80. Bigler SA, Deering RE, Brawer MK. Comparison of microscopic vascularity in benign and malignant prostate tissue. Hum Pathol 1993; 24: 220–6.

81. Weidner N, Carroll PR, Flax J, Blumenfeld W, Foldman J. Tumor angiogenesis correlates with metastasis in invasive prostate carcinoma. Am J Pathol 1993; 143: 401–9.

82. Fregene TA, Khanuja PS, Noto AC, et al. Tumor-associated angiogenesis in prostate cancer. Anticancer Res 1993; 13: 2377–82.

83. Brawer MK, Deering RE, Brown M, Preston SD, Bigler S. Predictors of pathologic stage in prostate carcinoma. The role of neovascularity. Cancer 1994; 73: 678–87.

84. Bostwick DG, Wheeler TM, Blute M, et al. Optimized microvessel density analysis improves prediction of cancer stage from prostate needle biopsies. Urology 1996; 48: 47–57.

85. Lissbrant IF, Stattin P, Damber JE, Bergh A. Vascular density is a predictor of cancer-specific survival in prostatic carcinoma. Prostate 1997; 33: 38–45.

86. Borre M, Offersen BV, Nerstrom B, Overgaard J. Microvessel density predicts survival in prostate cancer patients subjected to watchful waiting. Br J Cancer 1998; 78: 940–4.

87. Brawer MK. Quantitative microvessel density. A staging and prognostic marker for human prostatic carcinoma. Cancer 1996; 78: 345–9.

88. Ragde H, Kenny GM, Murphy GP, Landin K. Transrectal ultrasound microbubble contrast angiography of the prostate. Prostate 1997; 32: 279–83.

89. Rifkin MD, Tublin ME, Cheruvu SK, Li S, Ross J. Ultrasound contrast enhanced color Doppler: initial results in the evaluation of the prostate. Radiology 1997; 205(P): 280.

90. Blomley MJ, Cosgrove DO, Jayaram V, et al. Quantitation of enhanced transrectal ultrasound of the prostate: work in progress using the echo-enhancing agent Br1. Radiology 1997; 205(P): 280–1.

91. Eckersley RJ, Butler-Barnes JA, Blomley MJ, DeSouza NM, Cosgrove DO. Quantitative microbubble enhanced transrectal ultrasound (TRUS) as a tool for monitoring anti-androgen therapy in prostate carcinoma: work in progress. Radiology 1998; 209(P): 280.

92. Bogers HA, Sedelaar JPM, Beerlage HP, et al. Contrast-enhanced three-dimensional power Doppler angiography of the human prostate: correlation with biopsy outcome. Urology 1999; 54: 97–104.

93. Porter TR, Xie F. Transient myocardial contrast after initial exposure to diagnostic ultrasound pressures with minute doses of intravenously injected microbubbles. Circulation 1995; 92: 2391–5.

94. Colon PJ, Richards DR, Moreno CA, Murgo JP, Cheirif J. Benefits of reducing the cardiac cycle-triggering frequency of ultrasound imaging to increase myocardial opacification with FS069 during fundamental and second harmonic imaging. J Am Soc Echocardiogr 1997; 10: 602–7.

95. Broillet A, Puginier J, Ventrone R, Schneider M. Assessment of myocardial perfusion by intermittent harmonic power Doppler using SonoVue, a new ultrasound contrast agent. Invest Radiol 1998; 33: 209.

96. Schrope BA, Newhouse VL, Uhlendorf V. Simulated capillary blood flow measurement using a nonlinear ultrasonic contrast agent. Ultrason Imaging 1992; 14: 134–58.

97. Schrope BA, Newhouse VL. Second harmonic ultrasound blood perfusion measurement. Ultrasound Med Biol 1993; 19: 567–79.

98. de Jong N, Cornet R, Lancee CT. Higher harmonics of vibrating gas-filled microspheres. Part one: simulations. Ultrasonics 1994; 32: 447–53.

99. de Jong N, Cornet R, Lancee CT. Higher harmonics of vibrating gas-filled microspheres. Part two: measurements. Ultrasonics 1994; 32: 455–9.

100. Forsberg F, Goldberg BB, Liu JB, Merton DA, Rawool NM. On the feasibility of real-time, in vivo harmonic imaging with proteinaceous microspheres. J Ultrasound Med 1996; 15: 853–60.

101. Halpern EJ, Verkh L, Forsberg F, et al. Initial clinical experience with contrast-enhanced sonography of the prostate. AJR Am J Roentgenol 2000; 174: 1575–80.

102. Frauscher F, Klauser A, Halpern EJ, Horninger W, Bartsch G. Detection of prostate cancer with a microbubble ultrasound contrast agent. Lancet 2001; 357: 1849–50.

103. Halpern EJ, Rosenberg M, Gomella LG. Prostate cancer: contrast-enhanced US for detection. Radiology 2001; 219: 219–25.

104. Halpern EJ, McCue PA, Aksnes AK, et al. Contrast enhanced sonography of the prostate with sonazoid: comparison with whole mount prostatectomy specimens in twelve patients. Radiology 2002; 222: 361–6.

105. Frauscher F, Klauser A, Volgger H, et al. Comparison of contrast-enhanced color Doppler targeted biopsy to conventional systematic biopsy: impact on prostate cancer detection. J Urol 2002; 167: 1648–52.

106. Halpern EJ, Frauscher F, Rosenberg M, Gomella LG. Directed biopsy during contrast enhanced sonography of the prostate. AJR Am J Roentgenol 2002; 178: 915 19.

107. Halpern EJ, Frauscher F, Strup SE, Ramey JR, Gomella LG. Comparison of contrast-enhanced targeted biopsy of the prostate to modified sextant biopsy. Proceedings of the annual meeting of the Radiological Society of North America, November 2004, 268.

108. Yamakoshi Y, Sato J, Sato T. Ultrasonic imaging of internal vibration of soft tissue under forced vibration. IEEE Trans Ultrason Ferroelectr Freq Control 1990; 37: 45.

109. Ophir J, Cespedes I, Ponnekanti H, Yazdi Y, Li X. Elastography, a quantitative method for imaging the elasticity of biological tissues. Ultrason Imaging 1991; 13: 111.

110. Taylor LS, Porter BC, Rubens DJ, Parker KJ. Three-dimensional sonoelastography: principles and practices. Phys Med Biol 2000; 45: 1477–94.

111. Lee F, Bronson JP, Lerner RM, et al. Sonoelasticity imaging: results in in vitro tissue specimens. Radiology 1991; 181: 237–9.

112. Krouskop TA, Wheeler TM, Kallel F, Garra BS, Hall T. Elastic moduli of breast and prostate tissues under compression. Ultrason Imaging 1998; 20: 260–74.

113. Kallel F, Price RE, Konofagou E, Ophir J. Elastographic imaging of the normal canine prostate in vitro. Ultrason Imaging 1999; 21(3): 201–15.

114. Rubens DJ, Hadley MA, Alam SK, et al. Sonoelasticity imaging of prostate cancer: in vitro results. Radiology 1995; 195: 379–83.

115. Ophir J, Garra B, Kallel F, et al. Elastographic imaging. Ultrasound Med Biol 2000; 26(Suppl 1): S23–9.

116. Sommerfeld HJ, Garcia-Schurmann JM, Schewe J, et al. Prostate cancer diagnosis using ultrasound elastography. Introduction of a novel technique and first clinical results. Urologe (Ausg A) 2003; 42(7): 941–5.

117. Souchon R, Soualmi L, Bertrand M, et al. Ultrasonic elastography using sector scan imaging and a radial compression. Ultrasonics 2002; 40(1–8): 867–71.

5

The scrotum

Dennis Ll Cochlin

GENERAL CONSIDERATIONS

Introduction

With improvements in small parts ultrasound imaging, it is increasingly possible to study in great detail almost the whole spectrum of scrotal pathology. As a result, requests for scrotal ultrasound have increased to the extent that they constitute a very large workload. Another consequence is that it is now impossible to include a comprehensive discussion on scrotal ultrasound in a reasonably sized chapter. This chapter, therefore, employs a pragmatic approach, concentrating on those aspects of scrotal ultrasound that influence management.

Imaging strategies

With the increasing tendency to investigate – some would say over-investigate – all symptoms and signs, it has become common practice for referring clinicians to request an ultrasound study on patients with almost any scrotal symptoms or signs.

Perhaps this is inevitable and is a permanent situation. Healthcare resources, however, are being stretched beyond their capacity, even in the richest countries. Professionals are beginning to look at ways of limiting unnecessary investigations. It is, therefore, relevant to discuss possible ways in which scrotal imaging may or may not be limited without unacceptable risk.

There are some who will take the view that any risk, however small, is unacceptable, and that one should not deny any patient a scan. Others are more pragmatic, and take the view that scrotal imaging changes management in so few patients, that a large number of studies are a waste of resources. What follows is, I hope, a balanced argument from which individual practitioners or centers must make their own decisions.

The main consideration of whether the scan affects management will be considered for different symptoms and presentations.

Testicular masses

Testicular tumors may present with a palpable intratesticular mass, in which case an ultrasound scan is definitely indicated. The scan is necessary not only to confirm a tumor, but also to prevent unnecessary surgery on benign tumors, such as tunical granulomas, testicular cysts, adrenal rest tumors and focal orchitis, or to enable testis-preserving surgery in simple cysts or epidermoid cysts.

Extratesticular masses

Extratesticular scrotal masses are, in the large majority of cases, benign lesions – cysts, granulomas or benign epididymal ademomatoid tumors. There are, of course, exceptions. Sarcomas and mesotheliomas are malignant extratesticular tumors. They are both exceedingly rare. Reviews of the admittedly sparse literature on the subject reveal descriptions of large (certainly more than 1 cm) craggy tumors that give a high clinical suspicion of malignancy at the time of clinical presentation, quite unlike the vast majority of small smooth benign extratesticular lesions. Of course, all large tumors must have a period during their development when they are small. In practice, however, it would seem that a policy of not scanning all masses that are definitely clinically extratesticular and less than 1 cm would not miss any malignant tumors. As a safeguard, however, patients should be advised to re-present if there is any change in the mass.

Secondary tumors also occur in the epididymis and tunical membranes. In practice, however, they occur late in the malignant disease process, and rarely, if ever, are the presenting symptom. There is a strong argument, therefore, that a policy of not scanning clinically extratesticular masses would present minimal risk.

Dull ache

Testicular tumors may be impalpable at the time of diagnosis. They may present with dull pain, or hydrocele, or may be incidentally found when asymptomatic (when the patient is scanned for other reasons, e.g. epididymal cyst). It is this group that presents a potential problem. Dull testicular ache is an extremely common symptom, and only a minute proportion of such patients have impalpable testicular tumors. Indeed, it is likely that many of those that are found are incidental findings and not the cause of the ache, which is due to the very common condition labeled idiopathic orchalgia. Is it, therefore, necessary to scan this group of patients?

Acute pain

Very severe acute testicular pain or swelling with a sudden onset may present a differential diagnosis of epididymo-orchitis or testicular torsion, torsion of the testicular or epididymal appendix in boys, or a series of other uncommon causes. Such cases are true emergencies and require urgent investigation, either by ultrasound imaging or direct surgical exploration. The majority of cases of severe pain, however, do not fall into this clinical category. In many, torsion is not clinically indicated and the likely diagnosis is epididymo-orchitis.

The painful swelling associated with acute epididymo-orchitis may admittedly be mimicked by testicular tumor. Epididymo-orchitis is, however, far more common than testicular tumor, and a policy of scanning all patients with suspected epididymo-orchitis in order to exclude tumor results in a high workload for a very low positivity rate. Furthermore, scanning patients in the acute phase of severe epididymo-orchitis may reveal areas of altered echo density, or even masses in the testis due to focal orchitis. It is often not possible to distinguish these from tumor with certainty without a repeat scan following treatment.

A possible alternative policy, therefore, adapted by many clinicians, is to request an ultrasound study only in those patients who, after a reasonable course of treatment, still have symptoms or a palpable mass. Although a substantial proportion of patients with true epididymo-orchitis do not respond totally to the first course of treatment, such a policy significantly reduces workload, without risk.

Hydrocele

Testicular tumors undoubtedly cause hydroceles. However, they invariably cause small hydroceles – not the tense, large chronic hydroceles that make the testis impalpable.

Also, it is questionable whether tumors that are too small to be clinically palpable may cause hydroceles: the answer is probably no. It would be difficult not to scan a truly acute, tense, hydrocele but, this apart, it is questionable whether a policy of not scanning hydroceles will miss tumors. Very tense hydroceles may be difficult to distinguish from a large testicular mass. These clearly need to be scanned.

Any policy of selectively scanning patients with scrotal lesions relies strongly on a good clinical history and physical examination. There is also the need for confident reassurance of the patient by the clinician who in an individual case decides not to request a scan. There has been an unfortunate tendency in recent years to replace clinical skills and patient interaction with the (perhaps) easier option of requesting an ultrasound study.

SCROTAL ANATOMY (Figure 5.1)

The scrotum comprises a sac with several layers, divided into two compartments by the median raphe. Each sac contains a testis and an epididymis with a small volume of fluid. The spermatic cord carries the arteries and veins and the vas deferens. It passes through the inguinal canal to enter the scrotum (Figure 5.1).

Testicular anatomy

The testes are ovoid structures measuring approximately 4 × 3 × 3 cm, but varying from 3–5 cm in length, 2–3 cm in width and 2–3 cm in anteroposterior diameter, with average measurements at 3.8, 3 and 2.8 cm; both sides are normally of similar size. The testis is enclosed in a tough fibrous membrane, the tunica albuginea, which is infolded at the mediastinum testis to form a linear or sail-shaped intratesticular structure visible on ultrasound scans (Figure 5.2).

The tunica albuginea itself is usually poorly seen on an ultrasound scan, although it may be more clearly seen when the fluid of a hydrocele surrounds the testis. It is seen as a line of slightly higher echodensity than the testicular parenchyma where the testicular surface is at a right angle to the ultrasound beam. As the tunical layers curve around the testis to lie at a more shallow angle to the ultrasound beam, they appear to be lifted off the testis. This is an artifact caused by beam splitting. As the angle decreases further, the image of the tunica is lost (Figure 5.3).

Fibrous septae divide the testis into segments centered on the hilum. These are seen as fine linear structures on high-resolution scans (Figure 5.4). The rete testis is a

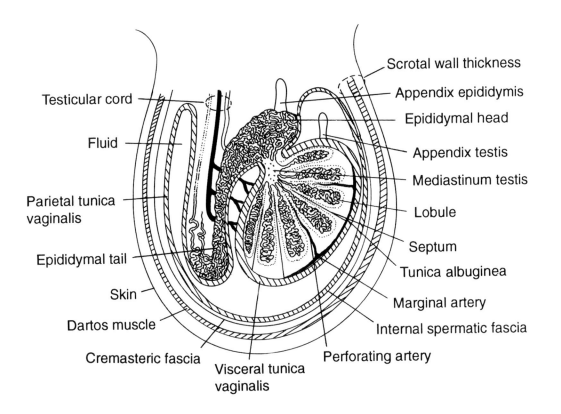

Figure 5.1
Scrotal anatomy.
(Derived with permission of the editors from *Gray's Anatomy*.)

Scrotal wall thickness

Appendix epididymis

Epididymal head

Appendix testis

Mediastinum testis

Lobule

Septum

Tunica albuginea

Marginal artery

Internal spermatic fascia

Perforating artery

Testicular cord

Fluid

Parietal tunica vaginalis

Epididymal tail

Skin

Dartos muscle

Cremasteric fascia

Visceral tunica vaginalis

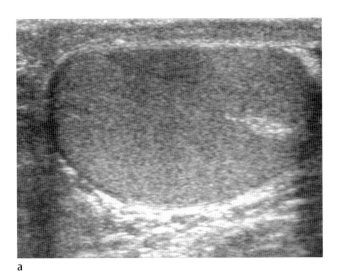

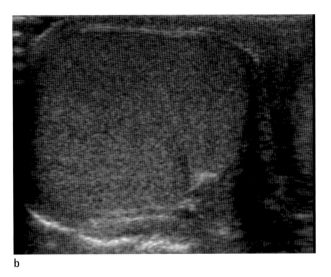

a

b

Figure 5.2
Normal testicular hilum. The hyperechoic linear density (a) represents the testicular hilum. As the scan plane changes, the linear opacity changes to a hyperechoic dot (b).

structure formed by the seminiferous tubules massing together at the testicular hilum before entering the epididymis. It may be seen ultrasonically as an ill-defined echo-poor region at the testicular hilum, sometimes with arboriform projections into the parenchyma (Figure 5.5).

A small pedunculated appendage, the appendix testis extends from the superior surface of the testis in about 30% of individuals. It may occasionally be seen if surrounded by the fluid of a hydrocele (Figure 5.6). A similar appendage may extend from the epididymis. This is called

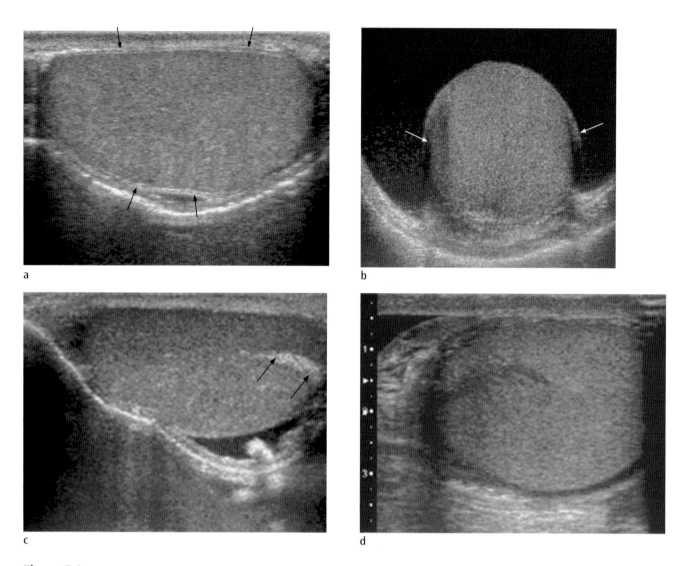

a

b

c

d

Figure 5.3
Tunical layers. (a) The white line (arrow) represents the tunica albuginea and the visceral layer of the tunica vaginalis. (b) The tunica appears to lift off the testis (arrow). This is a beam-splitting artifact. (c) The invagination of the tunica into the testis at the hilum causes an echogenic structure of varying width. In this case it has a narrow sail shape (arrows). (d) At some angles the hilum appears hypoechoic.

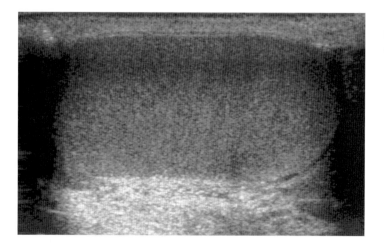

Figure 5.4
Fibrous septae. The fibrous septae are seen as fine black curved lines.

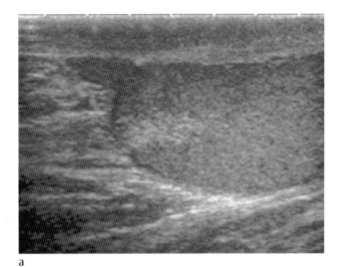

a

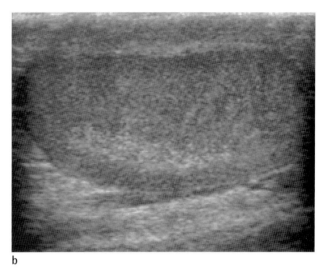

b

Figure 5.5
The rete testis. (a, b) Typical appearance of closely packed echogenic lines forming a discrete structure. (c) A case with anechoic lines between the echogenic lines. These are the lumenae of the tubules. This case is regarded as normal. There is, however, a range of appearances between normal and tubular ectasia (see Figures 5.60 and 5.61).

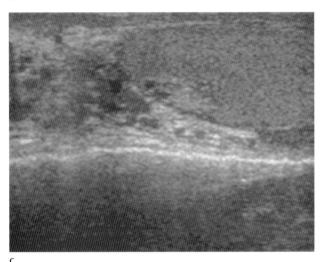

c

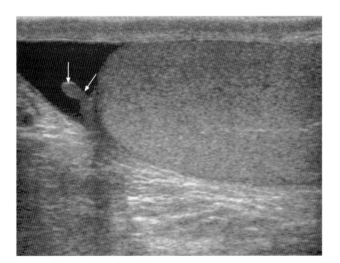

Figure 5.6
Testicular appendix. The testicular appendix is present in 30% of men. It is only seen on ultrasound when surrounded by fluid (arrows).

the appendix epididymis. It sometimes contains a cyst-like remnant of the Müllerian duct lumen termed a hydatid of Morgagni (Figure 5.7). There are two other embryologic appendages (the vas aberrans and the paradidymis), but the appendices testis and epididymis are the only ones commonly seen on ultrasound and the only ones that are clinically important, because the hydatid of Morgagni, and the testicular appendix may tort.

Vascular anatomy

The scrotum and its contents are supplied by three arteries passing through the inguinal canal (Figure 5.8). The larger testicular artery arising from the aorta supplies the testis and epididymis. The small cremasteric artery, arising from the vesical artery, provides part of the blood supply to the scrotal wall and extratesticular structures, and the deferential artery, arising from the inferior epigastric artery, supplies the vas deferens. The three arteries have

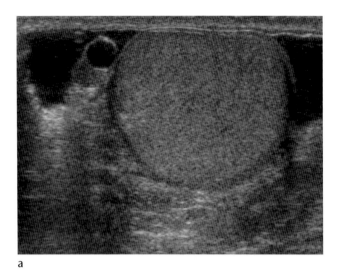

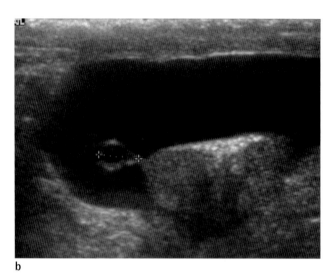

a

b

Figure 5.7
Hydatid of Morgagni. (a, b) The cyst-like hydatid is seen in the epididymal appendix (see also Figure 5.92). ((a) Courtesy of Dr Richard Winter, Royal Glamorgan Hospital.)

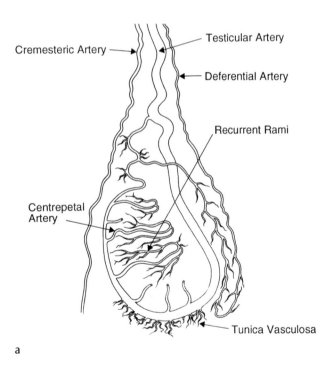

Cremesteric Artery

Testicular Artery

Deferential Artery

Recurrent Rami

Centrepetal Artery

Tunica Vasculosa

a

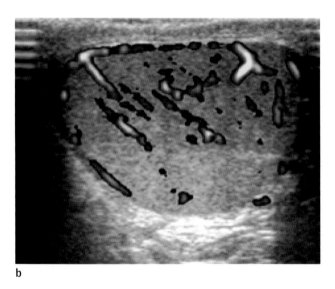

b

Figure 5.8
The arterial supply of the scrotum. (a) Diagram. (b) A typical power Doppler study showing sections of marginal, penetrating and recurrent vessels.

small anastomoses with each other at the level of the cord and the scrotal fascia, but there are no known anastomoses at the intratesticular level. The scrotal wall is also supplied by branches of the internal and external pudendal arteries, which also contribute to the blood supply of the spermatic cord epididymis and, occasionally, the lower pole of the testis. The testicular artery penetrates the tunica albuginea at the cephaloposterior part of the testis and branches into

two or more capsular arteries that course around the testis, giving off branches to form the tunica vasculosa, a network of blood vessels (marginal vessels) and loose areolar tissue that surrounds the testis, deep to the tunica albuginea and accompanies the septae.

Centripetal terminal branches penetrate the testis, running towards the mediastinum. Some recurrent rami pass back in the opposite direction. In 10–20% of men, a large

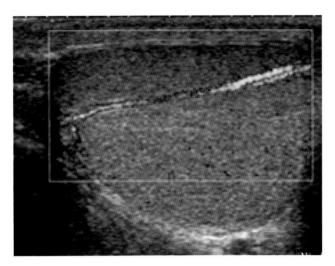

Figure 5.9
Transmediastinal artery. In 10–20% of men, a large branch of the testicular artery (the transmediastinal artery), often accompanied by a vein, crosses the testis to form capsular branches on the other side. This artery is visible on the gray-scale image as a hypoechoic band.

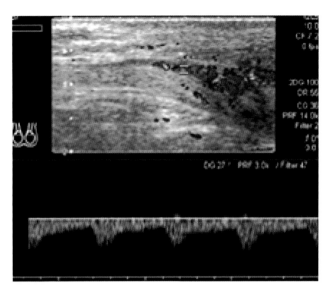

Figure 5.10
The testicular artery in the spermatic cord. Several vessels are seen within the cord. The artery studied is identified as the testicular artery by its low resistive waveform.

branch of the testicular artery enters at the mediastinum and runs across the testis to form capsular branches on the opposite side (Figure 5.9). This is termed the transmediastinal artery. It often has an accompanying vein.

The testicular veins run in similar planes to the arteries, and emerge from the back of the testis where they are joined by branches from the epididymis and form a loose plexus, the pampiniform plexus. This passes, as part of the spermatic cord, through the inguinal canal.

Knowledge of the vascular supply of the scrotum is important for an understanding of the mechanism of testicular torsion. The detailed vascular anatomy is, however, only demonstrated in part on an ultrasound study. The supplying arteries in the spermatic cord may be identified, and the testicular artery may be distinguished as it has a low resistive biphasic waveform, whereas the other arteries have a high resistive triphasic waveform (Figure 5.10). The marginal testicular arteries and the larger of the penetrating arteries are seen on a color Doppler scan. Only short segments are seen in a single scan plane, as the vessels are tortuous. If there is hyperemia, or if ultrasound contrast agents are used, the penetrating arteries may be more clearly seen, and their spiral configuration may be appreciated. The transmediastinal artery and vein, if present, are clearly seen.

The intratesticular veins are also seen in short segments only. The extratesticular veins constituting the pampiniform plexus are clearly seen (Figure 5.11). The clarity with which these veins are seen on high-resolution scanners both on gray-scale and color Doppler, has led to a tendency to over-diagnose varicoceles.

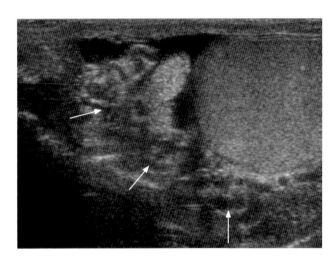

Figure 5.11
The Pampiniform plexus. In this case the plexus (arrow) may be seen separately from the epididymis and on other scan planes could be followed to the inguinal ring. Often, the body of the epididymis and the pampiniform plexus cannot be seen as clearly separate structures.

Epididymal anatomy

The epididymis is described as having three segments, the head (globus major), the body (corpus epididymis) and the tail (globus minor). The tail drains into the vas deferens,

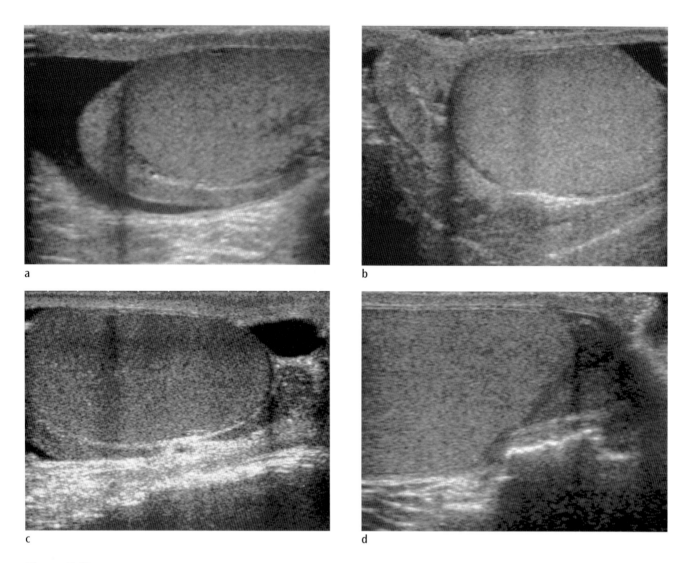

a   b

c   d

Figure 5.12
Epididymis. (a) The head of the epididymis is seen closely adherent to the upper pole of the testis. The body is clearly seen alongside the testis; it is not always so clearly demarcated. (b) The epididymal head is large. There is considerable variation in the size and this is considered normal. (c) The epididymal tail in this case is well circumscribed. (d) The epididymal tail in this case is a loose incoherent structure. This is the more common appearance.

which courses up the scrotum with the pampiniform plexus of veins, arteries, nerves and lymphatics to pass through the inguinal ring as the spermatic cord. In normal patients, the epididymal head may be identified closely adherent to the posterosuperior surface of the testis. Parts of the body and tail are seen, but are poorly shown as discrete structures and are often not clearly distinguished from the pampiniform plexus (Figure 5.12). The spermatic cord, however, may often be identified as a large structure running posterior to the testis (Figure 5.13). In patients with a hydrocele, the extratesticular structures may be seen more clearly, although the body and tail of the epididymis are usually loose structures with no discrete shape.

The pampiniform plexus is a plexus of veins draining the testis and running posterior to the testis. They may sometimes be distinguished in part from the epididymis (see Figure 5.11), but the two structures usually form an inseparable complex.

The testis and epididymis are loosely covered by a serous membrane, the tunica vaginalis, which is reflected at the spermatic cord to cover the inner surface of the scrotal wall. Between the two layers lies a small, but variable volume of fluid. In some cases the volume of fluid is too small to see, whereas in others fluid may be seen in some part of the scrotum, often around the upper pole of the testis and head of epididymis. An increased volume of fluid

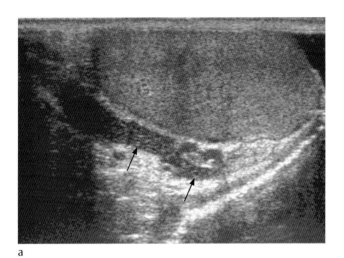
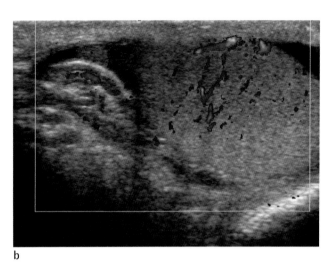

a   b

Figure 5.13
Spermatic cord. (a, b) The spermatic cord (arrows).

constitutes a hydrocele. What constitutes a normal volume of fluid, and what a hydrocele, is largely subjective but, if fluid is seen completely surrounding the testis, this is definitely a hydrocele. A patent processus vaginalis is an anomaly in which the layers of the tunica vaginalis retain continuity with the peritoneum, allowing ascitic or other peritoneal fluid to pass into the scrotum, causing a hydrocele.

The scrotal wall is a structure of even thickness of about 3–6 mm. Three layers may barely be visualized, representing the skin, dartos layer and tunica.

ULTRASOUND TECHNIQUE[1–7]

The scrotum may be supported by a folded sheet placed beneath it with the patient's legs together. The penis is displaced over the pubis and another sheet placed over it. The patient may hold the penis in place. If the examination is intended to investigate scrotal masses, it is good practice to palpate the scrotum first. Small epididymal masses may be difficult to find, in which case the patient may be asked to demonstrate where they lie. If the scrotum is very tender, however, palpation is best avoided.

The scrotum is best examined with a high-frequency (typically 7–12 MHz) high-resolution linear transducer. Such devices are usually of fairly short length so that the whole of the scrotum, sometimes even the whole of one testis, may not be displayed on a single image. It is therefore sometimes desirable, particularly if the scrotum is enlarged, to supplement the high-resolution images with images produced by a larger, usually lower-frequency linear or curved linear transducer. This produces an image of the whole scrotum, both sides being displayed in the transverse plane and the whole length of the hemiscrotum in the longitudinal plane.

Views of the body and tail of the epididymis require oblique and lateral views. The epididymis lies posteromedial to the testis during scanning, although the medial position is variable and may be altered by placing the scrotum on the supporting sheet. The epididymal body and tail are best examined either from the lateral or medial oblique approach or from the lateral approach using the opposite testis as a 'window'. The scrotal contents are, however, mobile and vary in position. Ultrasound planes should therefore also be varied to produce the ideal image.

Small epididymal masses may be isolated between two fingers, or a finger placed under them from the posterior aspect of the scrotum. This ensures that what is seen on the screen is indeed the mass being investigated.

Water bath techniques have been tried and, despite obvious advantages, have been largely abandoned in adults because of their relative inconvenience. In young children, however, the technique is less inconvenient and has definite advantages. A warm bath, with a few bath toys, will usually keep small children happy. The water produces an ideal standoff, as the distance between transducer and scrotum may be varied, and the tendency for young boys' testes to retract is diminished in a warm bath.

Examinations of suspected varicoceles are initially performed with the patient supine. This is adequate in the majority of cases. If, however, the examination is negative, and clinical suspicion is strong, the examination should be repeated with the patient standing. The patient should stand for some time before scanning, as varicoceles often empty when the patient lies down and do not refill for some time. The operator's left hand is placed behind the scrotum for support and a second operator manipulates the machine controls. Technical problems are often encountered when scanning the scrotum. Adequate immobilization of the testes in a good position is the most common problem. If difficulty is experienced, using the technique of supporting the scrotum with the left hand is usually successful.

Retractile testes are a problem usually found in children, but occasionally encountered in adults. In young children, scanning in a warm bath is usually successful. In older children or adults, one has to wait for the testes to descend, and then place a finger over the external ring to prevent retraction. Even then, scanning may be difficult.

The sheet supporting the scrotum may easily indent the posterior wall, causing a characteristic artifact. This is easily remedied by adjusting the sheet.

TESTICULAR TUMORS

General considerations[8–12]

Testicular tumors constitute only 1% of all malignant tumors in the male, but in the 15–34 age group they account for 8.8% of all cancer deaths, and their incidence appears to be increasing. They are more common in the northern countries and are 6–10 times more common in white than in colored populations. Most are, however, curable if detected early. Orchidectomy is often curative, followed as necessary with radiotherapy or chemotherapy. Seminoma metastases are very radiosensitive, and non-seminomatous metastases respond well to chemotherapy regimens. Early detection is therefore important. Ultrasound may detect impalpable lesions and can therefore contribute to the early detection of testicular cancer. Most testicular tumors, however, present as a palpable mass. Some give a dull ache or pain. Others are detected when scanning the scrotum for other reasons or when screening high-risk patients. A minority present as secondary deposits.

Screening high-risk patients

Patients at increased risk of testicular carcinoma include those with cryptorchidism, who have a risk 2.5–8.8% greater than that of a normal population. The increased risk still remains after orchidopexy and there is also an increased risk of developing malignancy in the opposite non-cryptorchid testis. Those who have had an orchidec-tomy for cancer have a 1–3% chance of developing cancer in the other testis which may be present at the time of presentation or may present up to 20 years later. Mumps orchitis, recurrent bacterial orchitis, testicular dysfunction, abnormal endocrine function or infertility are all described as risk factors, but increase risk less than cryptorchidism or contralateral cancer. Testicular microcalcification gives a probably quite small increased risk. It is discussed later in this chapter. Screening of high-risk populations for testicular carcinoma varies greatly between different centers. Most patients treated for testicular cancer are offered screening of the opposite testis, whereas only a few centers screen cryptorchids. The other risk factors are deemed to be too small to justify screening. There is no set routine for such screening, but in those centers that offer it, annual screening is common.

Ultrasound is the screening method of choice. It will detect early tumors which have not changed the testicular outline and are thus not clinically palpable. Detection of lesions as small as 4 mm is possible. Sensitivity has been assessed as 80–90%. This figure is quite old. Increased resolution of ultrasound systems has probably resulted in a significantly higher sensitivity.

Presentation as secondary deposits

Some patients with testicular cancer present with evidence of secondary disease and no palpable primary. A figure of 10% has been quoted, but the true figure may be lower. Ultrasound is the method of choice in these patients for the detection of small occult primary testicular tumors.

Classification of testicular tumors[13]

Testicular tumors may be primary or non-primary. The most common non-primary tumors are lymphoma and leukemia, other secondary tumors being rare. There are also benign cysts and granulomas.

The first classification of primary testicular tumors is into germ cell tumors and non-germ cell tumors. Germ cell tumors constitute 93% of testicular tumors, and are malignant. Non-germ cell tumors constitute 7% of testicular tumors, and 90% are benign. Tumors may be further classified – the main division of germ cell tumors is into seminoma and non-seminoma. The non-seminoma group is a rather heterogeneous group comprising embryonal carcinoma with differentiation, embryonal carcinoma per se, teratoma, chorion carcinoma and yolk sac tumor, with various combinations of these types.

Table 5.1 *Classification of testicular tumors*

Germ cell tumors
Tumors of one histologic type:
    Seminoma
    Spermatocystic seminoma
    Embryonal cell carcinoma
    Yolk sac tumor (infantile embryonal carcinoma)
    Choriocarcinoma
    Teratoma
        Mature
        Immature
        Teratoma with malignant transformation
Tumors of more than one histologic type:
    Embryonal cell carcinoma and teratoma (teratocarcinoma)
    Choriocarcinoma and any other type
    Other combinations

Gonadoblastoma (elements of both germ cell and non-germ cell tumors)

Non-germ cell tumors
Leydig cell tumor
Sertoli cell tumor
Undifferentiated tumors
Connective tissue tumors
Lymphoma
Leukemia
Other secondary deposits (rare)
Adrenal rest tumors
Sarcoid
Benign cysts – (testicular, tunical and epidermoid) and
    granulomas

The main division into seminoma and non-seminoma is of clinical relevance, as seminomas are very radiosensitive and are primarily treated by radical orchidectomy and radiotherapy, whereas non-seminomatous tumors are treated by radical orchidectomy, lymphadenectomy and/or chemotherapy. Seminomas and the various forms of non-seminomatous tumors also have some broad differences in ultrasonic appearance. In practice, however, the initial treatment for any malignant testicular tumor is orchidectomy, and the histology is determined subsequently. A classification of testicular tumors, taken from the World Health Organization classification of Germ Cell Tumors 1977, with a classification of non-germ cell tumors added, is included in Table 5.1.

Testicular masses – differentiation of benign from malignant

By far the most valuable role of ultrasound in evaluating scrotal masses is to distinguish intratesticular from extra-testicular masses. Extratesticular masses are usually clearly benign cystic lesions but, even when solid, are so rarely malignant that a conservative approach is usually adopted.

The large majority of intratesticular masses are malignant. About 10 years ago the teaching was that distinction of these from the few benign masses was not possible, at least with any accuracy. Virtually all intratesticular masses were therefore treated by radical orchidectomy. However, it is now possible to accurately identify some benign lesions which may need no treatment or, in other cases may be treated by local excision, thus conserving the testis.

Increased resolution of ultrasound systems and the tendency to scan more patients has led to the detection of a small but steady stream of incidentally found tumors. Some of these are very small and cannot be categorized. Some, after discussion with the patient, are treated by active surveillance.

It is often not the ultrasound appearances alone that make the diagnosis. An accurate clinical history and physical examination are vital. This information is not always available to the sonologist at the time of the ultrasound study. In relevant cases, however, it must be obtained before the final report is issued.

As far as the ultrasound report is concerned, unless a lesion is unequivocally benign, the possibility of malignancy should be strongly stated. It is still a good aphorism that any intratesticular lesion should be assumed malignant until proven benign.

Serum tumor markers – human chorionic gonadotropin (HCG) and alfa-fetoprotein (AFP) – should be measured in all cases of solid testicular lesions. A positive result indicates a germ cell tumor. A negative result does not, however, exclude one. Percutaneous biopsy is not an option because of the risk of seeding the tumor to the inguinal lymphatic field. Biopsy of the lesion after delivering the testis through an inguinal incision as the first part of an operation and proceeding to radical orchidectomy or wedge excision depending on frozen section histology is possible. This may be an ultrasound-guided procedure if the tumor is impalpable.

Ultrasonic features of malignancy and benignity

Intratesticular masses may be malignant or benign. Malignant intratesticular tumors are usually hypoechoic and focal, although their appearance is variable.

With malignant tumors, however, large areas of normal testicular tissue invariably remain (Figure 5.14). By contrast, in non-malignant conditions such as orchitis or hematoma, no normal testis is usually visible (Figure 5.15). Even in cases of focal orchitis or localized hematoma, the rest of the testis is usually edematous in the acute stage.

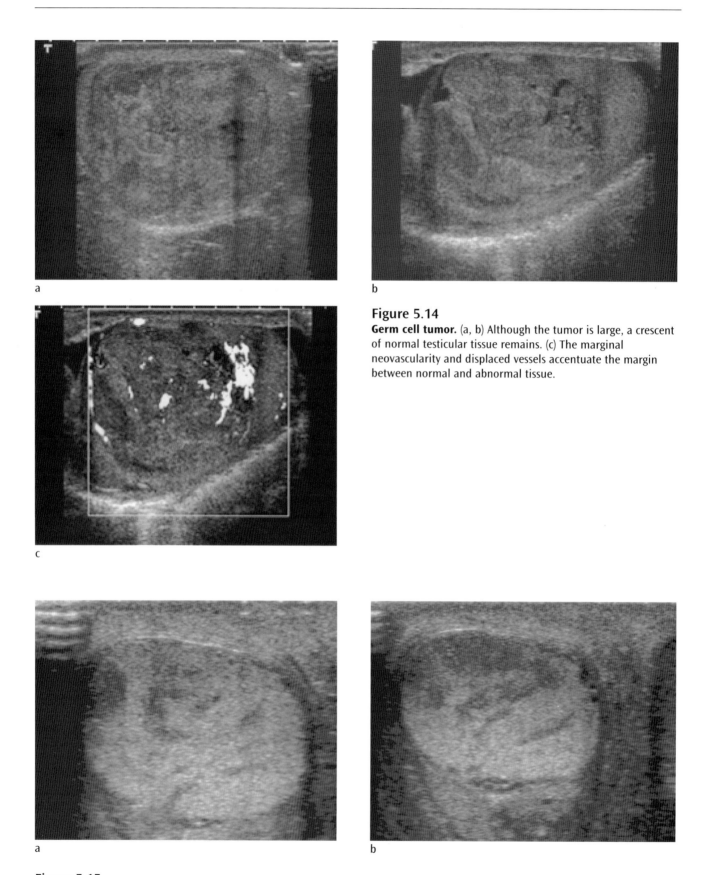

Figure 5.14
Germ cell tumor. (a, b) Although the tumor is large, a crescent of normal testicular tissue remains. (c) The marginal neovascularity and displaced vessels accentuate the margin between normal and abnormal tissue.

Figure 5.15
Focal orchitis. (a) There are focal hypoechoic lesions simulating tumor. (a, b) However, the whole testis is abnormal. There is also marked epididymal swelling.

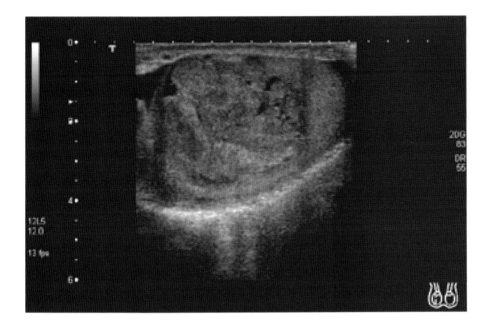

Figure 5.16
Irregular testicular surface: germ cell tumor. The tumor is causing irregularity of the anterior surface of the testis.

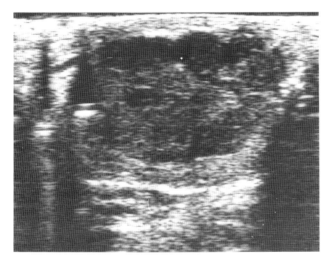

Figure 5.17
Testicular abscess. There is an abscess bulging the outline of the testis. Unlike cases of testicular tumor, the whole of the testis is abnormal and edematous.

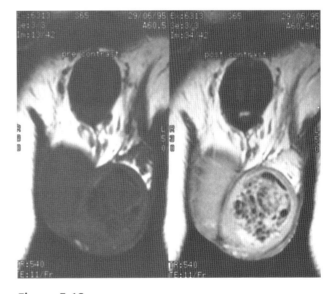

Figure 5.18
MRI of teratoma. The patient presented with clinical signs of epididymo-orchitis. Ultrasound study suggested a tumor, but no normal testicular tissue was seen, and testicular abscess was not excluded. The MRI study shows a teratoma, with a rim of normal tissue.

An irregularly shaped testis is highly indicative of malignancy (Figure 5.16), as benign lesions tend to enlarge the testis in an even manner, the exception being severe orchitis with intratesticular abscess (Figure 5.17). Extratesticular features may also help in the differentiation of benign from malignant. Epididymal swelling suggests epididymitis and, together with an appropriate history, suggests that an intratesticular mass is due to orchitis (see Figure 5.15). Scrotal wall swelling also suggests focal orchitis or hematoma. It is not a feature of testicular cancer. Large hydroceles also suggest a benign condition. Small hydro-celes are a common feature of testicular cancer, but large hydroceles do not occur. Doppler studies are usually unhelpful. In general, small tumors are hypovascular, large ones hypervascular. Ultrasound contrast studies are new and are largely untried in this field. Magnetic resonance imaging (MRI) rarely adds anything to the diagnosis, although it has a place as an occasional problem-solving tool (Figure 5.18).

Thus, an intratesticular mass which changes the outline of the testes, or which is focal with normal testicular tissue visible, and with no history of either trauma or orchitis, must be considered a tumor, either primary or secondary. A mass associated with testicular and scrotal wall edema or with a large hydrocele, or with a good history of epididymitis or severe trauma, may be considered benign, but must be followed up. Intermediate cases require the full gamut of studies, including tumor markers and MRI studies. A chest X-ray for secondary deposits and a computed tomography (CT) or MRI for enlarged nodes are carried out in malignant or intermediate cases, and may detect secondary nodal metastases, evidence of lymphoma or leukemia. Finally, in the case of secondary deposits of possible or biopsy-proven testicular origin, a thorough examination and appropriate radiology may detect the primary tumor.

Although there are differences between the 'typical' appearances of different testicular tumors, overlap of appearances are such that ultrasound may not usually distinguish between different histologic types of primary tumor, or between primary and secondary tumors. Without the help of a clinical history, the differentiation between tumor and hematoma, orchitis, abscess or infections may be impossible.

Typical appearances of different tumors are, however, described and included here for the sake of completeness.

Virtually all testicular tumors are hypoechoic compared with the normal testicular tissue: about 80% are completely hypoechoic, and 20% are mainly hypoechoic with hyperechoic areas.

The section that follows is an attempt to describe how a useful interpretation of the ultrasound study may be achieved. The illustrated examples are meant to show differences that aid diagnosis rather than provide a complete atlas of all possible tumors.

Solid intratesticular masses with no relevant history

First we must define 'relevant history' in this context. Any testicular tumor may present as a palpable mass or as a dull ache. For the purpose of this section, however, 'no relevant history' means no history of severe trauma, severe pain, fever or symptoms suggesting other systemic disease or known disease.

In the absence of such history, the majority of solid testicular masses in young or middle-aged men are germ cell tumors. In older men, lymphoma is the most common tumor. The histologic classification of these is complex, with classical, non-classical and mixed forms. For the purpose of ultrasound diagnosis, however, we may consider them divided into seminoma and teratoma. For clinical purposes, distinction is not important at this stage of the ultrasound study, but as their appearances differ (although with some overlap), we have to consider them separately.

Seminomas[14]

Seminomas typically occur in middle-aged men, although they may occur at any age after puberty. They are, however, rare in men over 60 years of age. They are typically hypoechoic, round or lobulated tumors with a smooth well-demarcated outline (Figure 5.19). They are occasionally

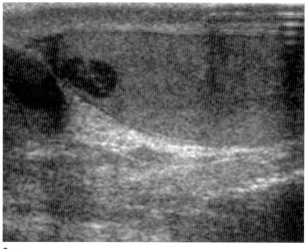
a

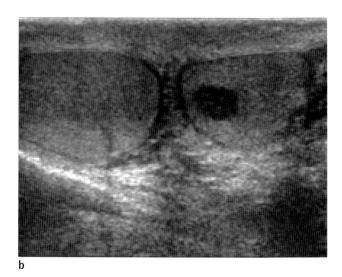
b

Figure 5.19
Seminoma. (a,b) A typical small, round, fairly evenly hypoechoic seminoma.

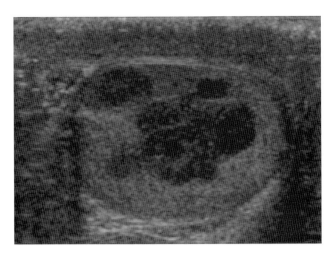

Figure 5.20
Multifocal seminoma. There are several separate foci of hypoechoic tumor.

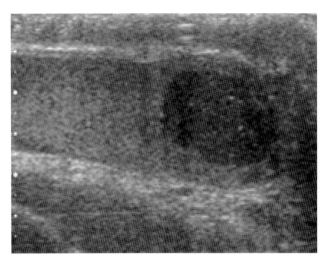

Figure 5.22
Cystic seminoma. There are anechoic foci. At excision, these were hemorrhagic cyst-like spaces.

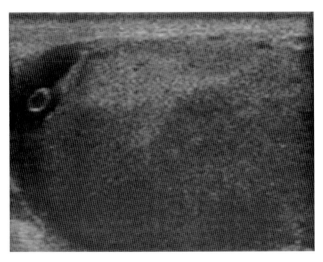

Figure 5.21
Infiltrating seminoma. A relatively hypoechoic infiltrative tumor. Most infiltrating tumors look similar. Histology showed a seminoma.

multifocal (Figure 5.20). Some have a more infiltrating pattern (Figure 5.21) and others have a mixed pattern with hyperechoic areas, often due to hemorrhage and cystic areas (Figure 5.22). It is this group that resembles the common appearance of teratoma.

Teratomas typically occur on younger men. Children are discussed later in the book, but it is worth stating that teratomas in prepubescent boys are always benign (Figure 5.23). Although orchidectomy is necessary, it is curative without any other treatment.

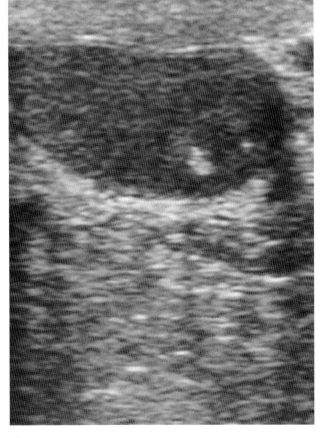

Figure 5.23
Childhood teratoma. This tumor in a 9-year-old boy was a benign teratoma. Below the age of puberty, testicular teratomas are benign.

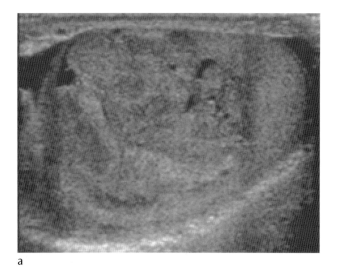

a

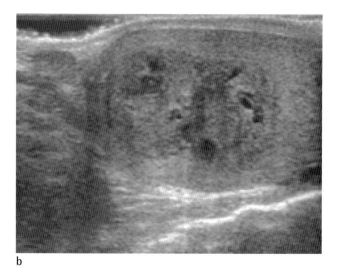

b

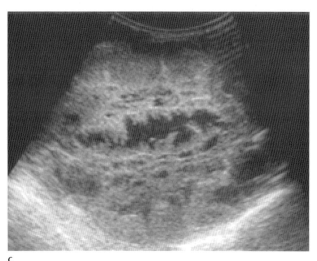

c

Figure 5.24
Teratoma. (a) The tumor is quite heterogeneous in pattern. This is typical of a teratoma. (b) A teratoma with marked cystic elements. (c) The bizarre bowel-like pattern in this tumor reflects the very heterogeneous elements that comprise a teratoma.

Teratomas[14]

Teratomas typically contain mixed tissue, and this is reflected in their ultrasound (and MRI) appearances. Embryonal carcinomas and mixed germ cell tumors have similar appearances, and cannot be distinguished from teratomas.

Teratomas appear on ultrasound as rounded or lobulated masses. They are usually predominantly hypoechoic, but contain mixed areas of hyperechoic or cystic nature (Figure 5.24). They may be predominantly cystic, but unlike simple cysts, they always contain some solid elements (Figure 5.25).

Lymphoma[15–17]

Lymphoma is the most common tumor in older men. It may be secondary or primary, the appearance being

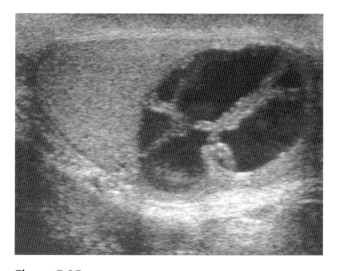

Figure 5.25
Cystic teratoma. The tumor is predominantly cystic but there are also marked solid elements.

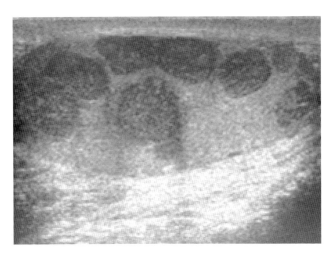

Figure 5.26
Lymphoma – multifocal pattern. The multiple rounded focal homogeneous echo-poor tumors are the most common pattern for testicular lymphoma.

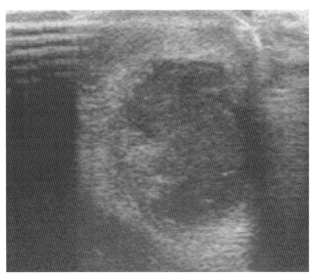

a

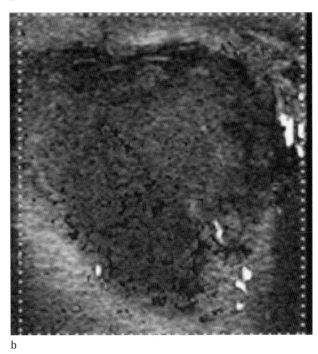

b

Figure 5.27
Lymphoma – infiltrative pattern. (a) The hypoechoic infiltrative tumor almost fills the testis. (b) Color Doppler shows tortuous feeding vessels, but the tumor parenchyma shows few vessels, as the tumor vessels in lymphoma are often very small in diameter.

identical. There is usually, although not invariably, other evidence of disease, usually enlarged lymph nodes.

Ultrasound appearance of testicular involvement is of hypoechoic rounded lesions, usually multiple, often bilateral (Figure 5.26) or a hypoechoic infiltrative pattern (Figure 5.27).

Small tumors

Small solid tumors, often impalpable and found incidentally when scanning for other reasons, are a difficult problem. Many are small germ cell tumors that require orchidectomy. A significant proportion, however, turn out to be non-germ cell tumors. When tumors are small, they rarely have any distinguishing features on ultrasound (Figure 5.28). Positive tumor markers are helpful, but very small germ cell tumors most often do not secrete significant tumor markers. A good thorough clinical history and physical examination is vital. Perhaps the most relevant finding is gynecomastia or symptoms and signs that suggest change in hormone status. Evidence of these would lead to a presumptive diagnosis of non-germ cell or stromal tumor (Leydig or Sertoli cell tumor), with the options of simple excision. Although these tumors 'classically' present with symptoms and signs of altered hormonal status, most have no such history. They are described in the following section.

In cases without significant clinical findings, the safe option is orchidectomy. Patients must be advised, however, that these small tumors may not be malignant, and that the other options are frozen section or active surveillance, with repeat ultrasound scans, typically initially in 2 weeks, then monthly for 3 months, then 6 monthly. Lack of growth may probably be taken to indicate a benign lesion. Any increase in size must indicate excision.

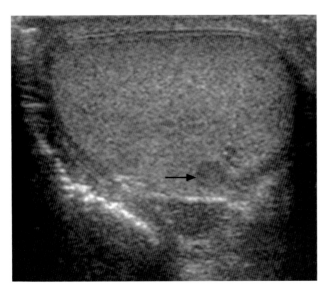

Figure 5.28
Small testicular tumor. This small round tumor lying posterior in the testis (arrow) was found incidentally when scanning for an epididymal cyst in the opposite testis. Tumor markers were negative. After discussion with the patient, it was decided to carry out orchidectomy. Histology revealed a Leydig cell tumor.

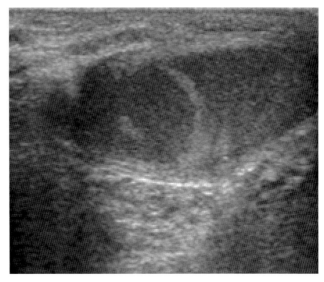

Figure 5.29
Ischemic atrophy. The patient had felt a hard lump in the upper pole of the testis. He had undergone a herniorrhaphy 6 months previously. He had not noticed the testis getting smaller in the postoperative period. Nevertheless, ultrasound revealed a significantly atrophic testis, probably secondary to ischemia, secondary to herniorrhaphy. The upper pole felt clinically hard. On the ultrasound image it is slightly lobulated, with the impression of a mass, but not a definite tumor. Follow-up in 1 year revealed no change.

Postinflammatory and post-traumatic change simulating tumor

Postinflammatory and post-traumatic change may produce transient or often permanent changes in the testis that may simulate tumor. These are discussed later.

Atrophy simulating tumor

Atrophy may produce similar changes, with hypoechoic areas simulating tumor (Figure 5.29). The small, heterogeneous testis suggests the diagnosis. The problem is, however, that dysplastic testes have a similar appearance, and are of increased risk of developing germ cell tumor. A history of the testis becoming smaller is useful. If this is not forthcoming, then close follow-up is mandatory.

Epidermoid cysts[18–20]

Epidermoid cysts often, although not invariably, have a characteristic appearance. Although they are cysts, they are filled with keratin, and so appear solid. They are rounded lesions, hypoechoic to the testis, although characteristically not as hypoechoic as seminoma. The characteristic pattern is that of concentric rings, indicating layers of keratin. This feature is seen on ultrasound but more elegantly shown on MRI, which may be used to confirm equivocal cases (Figure 5.30). Epidermoid cysts sometimes have a more speckled appearance (Figure 5.31). On Doppler imaging, vascularity is seen around the wall, but the center is totally avascular. An anechoic capsule may be visible. Any vascularity within the lesion excludes the diagnosis. A firm diagnosis of an epidermoid cyst enables simple testis-preserving excision. A minority have atypical appearances, and these cannot be distinguished from germ cell tumors.

Tunical granuloma[21]

Tunical granulomas (and small cysts) usually present as small, hard protrusions from the surface of the testis. They have a fairly characteristic feel on palpation as a hard lump, usually only the size of a grain of rice, on the surface of the testis. The worry is, however, that one is feeling the

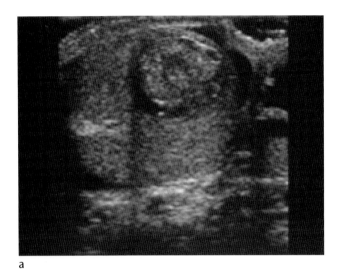
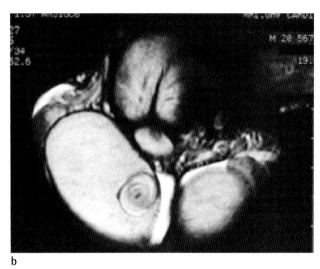

a

b

Figure 5.30
Epidermoid cyst. (a) A definitive pattern of concentric rings, representing concentric spheres of keratin. (b) The T2-weighted MRI study also clearly shows the concentric rings.

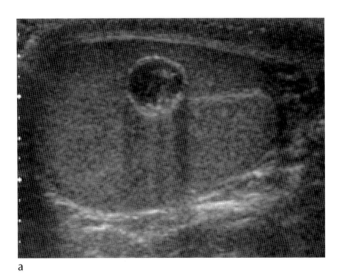
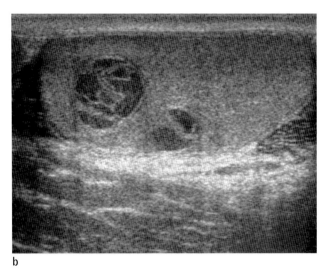

a

b

Figure 5.31
Epidermoid cyst. (a) In this case, there are no concentric rings, but there is an outer high-echodensity rim with speckled high-density internal foci, causing shadowing; this pattern is also pathognomonic. (b) Two cysts: a less-typical appearance, but the anechoic capsules are clearly seen.

edge of a larger intratesticular tumor. They must, therefore, be ultrasonically scanned. They are often surprisingly difficult to find, and may often only be seen by palpating with a finger, then scanning while using the palpating finger to indicate the position of the lesion. Granulomas are small, hypoechoic ovoid lesions in the tunica (Figure 5.32).

Occasionally, they may be larger and multiple (Figure 5.33). This condition is sometimes termed granulomatous

periorchitis. They are of no pathologic significance and require no treatment or follow-up.

Embryonal cell carcinomas[22]

These are typically only slightly hypoechoic compared with normal testicular tissue. They are less inhomogeneous than teratomas and commonly cause lobulation of the testis, an

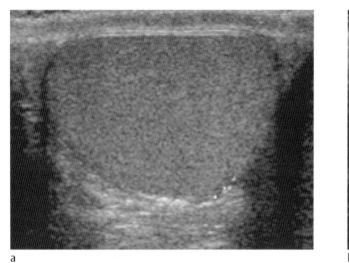
a

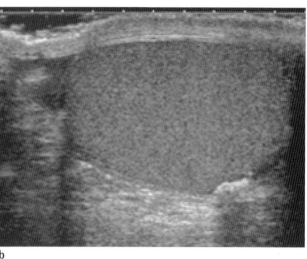
b

Figure 5.32
Tunical granuloma. (a,b) Two different patients with hard lumps on the surface of the testis. (a) A typical hypoechoic tunical granuloma with a small fleck of calcification; (b) shows a calcified granuloma.

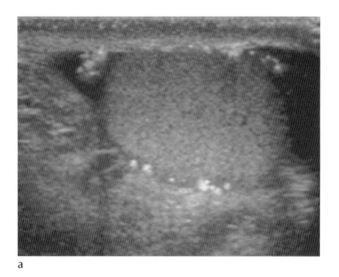
a

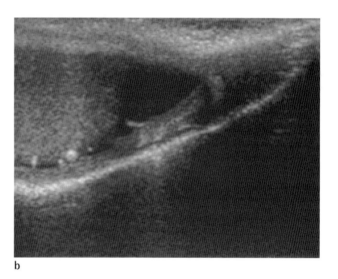
b

Figure 5.33
Granulomatous periorchitis. (a) There are multiple calcified tunical granulomas. (b) In another plane there are also anechoic fibrous granulomas.

appearance that does not necessarily indicate capsular invasion. Because their echodensity is close to that of normal testicular tissue, tumors may be missed until they distort the testicular outline (Figure 5.34).

Choriocarcinoma[23]

Pure choriocarcinoma is rare, most cases forming elements of mixed tumors. Their ultrasound appearances are variable.

Yolk sac carcinoma[24] (Figure 5.35)

This is a rare tumor in its pure form, virtually always occurring in children under the age of 5 years, although it may form an element of mixed tumors in adults. The ultrasound appearances in childhood have only been described in a few patients and descriptions vary between heterogeneous, homogeneous and mixed echodensity with anechoic areas. The age of the patient suggests the diagnosis especially with pulmonary metastases, which are the usual method of spread.

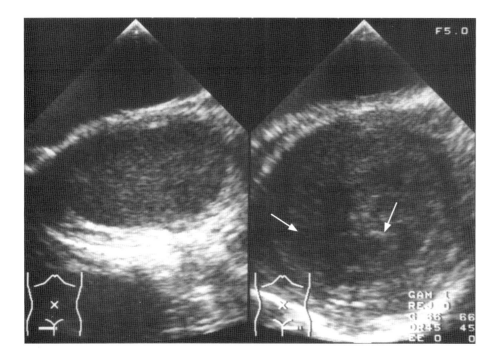

Figure 5.34
Embryonal cell carcinoma. The tumor (arrows) is only slightly hypoechoic compared with the normal testis. It is enlarging the testis. The right testis is imaged at the same magnification. (Courtesy of Dr Richard Winter, Royal Glamorgan Hospital, Mid-Glamorgan, UK.)

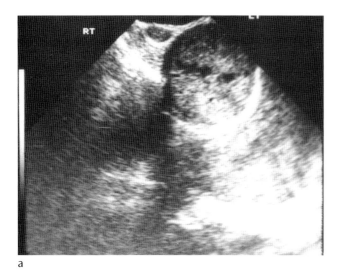

a

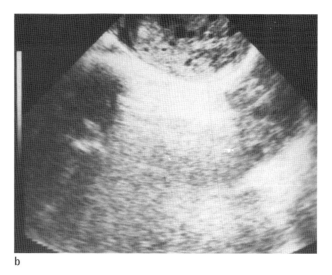

b

Figure 5.35
Yolk sac tumor. (a,b) In this child the testis is markedly enlarged by a mixed echodensity tumor containing multiple anechoic foci. (Courtesy of Dr Juliet Egginton, City General Hospital, Stoke-on-Trent, UK; reproduced by kind permission of the British Journal of Radiology.)

Primary extragonadal germ cell tumors[25,26]

These tumors arise in rests of primitive germ cells or pleuripotential cells left from the embryonic migration of the testis at early somatic development. They occur in the mediastinum or retroperitoneum, and rarely in the sacrococcygeal region or the pineal gland. Careful histologic examination of the testis in such cases has shown that these are truly primary tumors, not secondary deposits from a testicular primary. It has also been shown, however, that in a proportion of tumors initially diagnosed as primary retroperitoneal germ cell tumors, with clinically normal testes, ultrasound reveals an occult primary lesion. Careful ultrasound scans of the testes should therefore be performed in all cases of presumed primary extragonadal germ cell tumor (Figure 5.36). The tumors are histologically the same range of tumors that occur in the testis. Because of their site, mediastinal and retroperitoneal

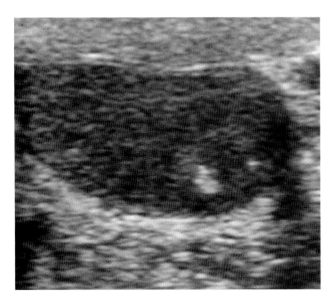

Figure 5.36
Testicular primary presenting with retroperitoneal mass.
This 15-year-old boy presented with a retroperitoneal mass.
Biopsy showed a seminoma. The scrotum felt normal on
examination. The ultrasound image shows a small primary
seminoma.

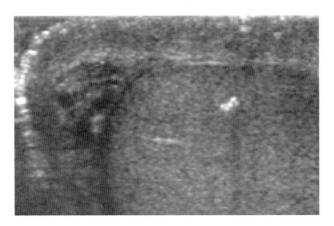

Figure 5.37
Hyperechoic testicular lesion. Small hyperechoic lesions like
this are usually benign and non-progressive.

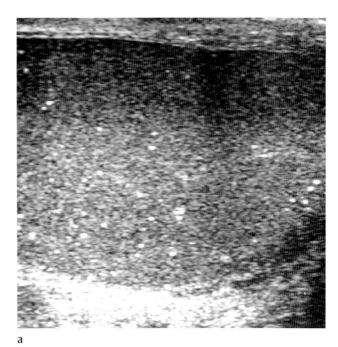

a

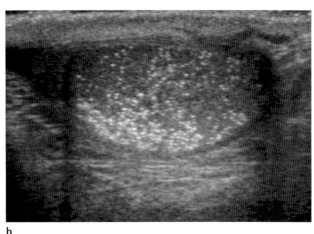

b

Figure 5.38
Testicular microcalcification. (a) This is a classic pattern of
microcalcification. (b) A slightly coarser but also typical pattern.

tumors may grow to a large size before presentation, and
often invade surrounding tissue. The diagnosis is made by
biopsy.

Hyperechoic testicular lesions

Small hyperechoic lesions are sometimes seen in the testis
(Figure 5.37). If they are not associated with more complex
lesions, they are assumed to be benign and most often his-

tology is not obtained. Where histology has been obtained
for such lesions, they have been shown to represent scar tissue, old hematoma and adenomatoid tumor. Smaller
hyperechoic lesions are more likely to be due to testicular
microlithiasis, small calcified collagen nodules of no
apparent clinical significance, although possibly more frequent in previously cryptorchid testes.

Testicular microcalcification[27–34]

It is appropriate to discuss testicular microcalcification
in this section on testicular tumors. Testicular

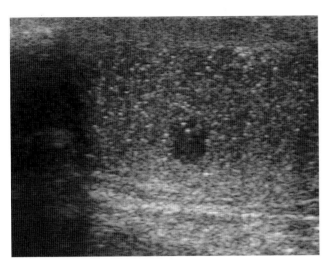

Figure 5.39
Microcalcification with a tumor. The patient, who was being monitored by ultrasound, developed the hypoechoic seminoma shown.

microcalcifications are multiple fine, less than 2 mm, calcific deposits in the seminiferous tubules (Figure 5.38). Their etiology is unknown, but it is known that they are more common in Klinefelter's syndrome, and possibly in previously undescended testes. The majority are idiopathic and they are more common in patients with oligospermia. Men with testicular microcalcification are at increased risk of developing germ cell tumors (Figure 5.39). The severity of the risk is, however, not clearly defined. It appears to be greater with larger numbers of microcalcifications and with few, perhaps less than five per single ultrasound slice, the increased risk is probably negligible. With larger numbers, early papers showed a large increase in risk. It has subsequently been shown that these papers were flawed and the risk is relatively small, although not clearly quantified. Currently, some centers offer 6-monthly ultrasound screening. With increasing evidence of a relatively small risk, many centers advocate counseling and regular self-examination.

Solid intratesticular masses with a relevant history

These constitute true tumors when the history helps to categorize the tumor, scrotal tumors that are a part of a multisystem disease and 'pseudotumors' such as hematoma, focal orchitis, post-inflammatory change, atrophy or dysplasia.

Lymphoma[15–17]

Testicular lymphoma usually, although not always, occurs in patients with established disease. It is discussed in the previous section.

Leukemia[15]

The testes are an immunologically privileged sanctuary site in leukemia and are thus a common site for involvement in the acute phase and a common site for relapse during remission. There are three patterns of involvement. There are most frequently multiple circumscribed hypoechoic masses varying in size from a few millimeters to about 1 cm. The nodules are frequently irregular and tend to follow the lines of the septae (Figure 5.40). Another pattern is infiltration by hypoechoic tumor along the septae (Figure 5.41). The third pattern is a mass infiltrative pattern, occupying a large part of the testis. Occasionally, the whole testis is involved, when it is enlarged and hypoechoic compared with the contralateral testis (Figure 5.42). Testicular leukemia is frequently extremely hypervascular.

Stromal tumors[35,36]

Stromal tumors arise from Leydig cells or Sertoli cells or are undifferentiated. Mixed forms also exist. They comprise about 5% of testicular tumors, and Leydig cell tumors are the most common. Descriptions of Sertoli cell tumors are few, but all types appear to be tumors of mixed echodensity, ultrasonographically indistinguishable from the germ cell group of tumors (Figures 5.43 and 5.44). About one-third of patients have endocrine symptoms of gynecomastia and impotence in adults or precocious puberty in prepubertal boys. In the other two-thirds, the histologic diagnosis is only appreciated after orchidectomy. Leydig cell and Sertoli cell tumors are usually benign. There is a spectrum between hyperplastic foci of cells and tumors. In patients with gynecomastia or altered hormone status, however, the diagnosis is likely, and simple excision is possible.

Gonadoblastoma

This is a rare tumor containing elements of gonadal stroma and germ cell tumor. It is exclusively found in patients with gonadal dysgenesis. Descriptions are few but it does not appear to have any distinguishing features on ultrasound.

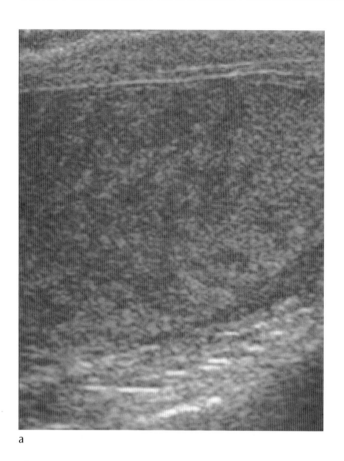

a

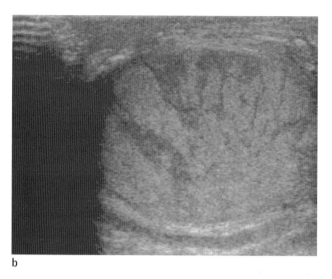

b

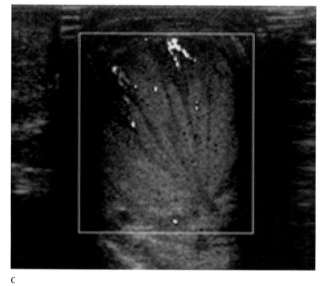

c

Figure 5.40

Leukemia – multiple focal pattern. (a) Fine irregular nodular deposits are seen throughout the testis. (b) A larger irregular nodular pattern. The nodules tend to follow the line of the septae. (c) The same case as (b), showing typical hypervascularity.

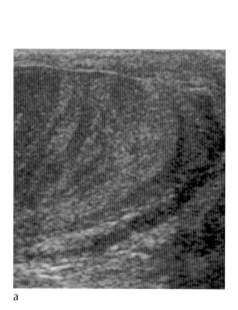

a

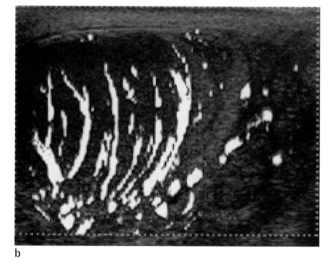

b

Figure 5.41

Leukemia. (a) The tumor is infiltrating along the septae. (b) Shows the hypervascularity of the lesions.

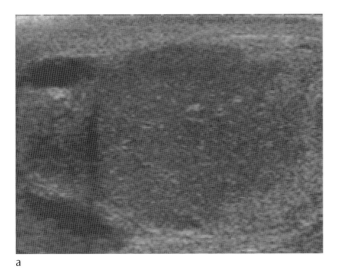
a

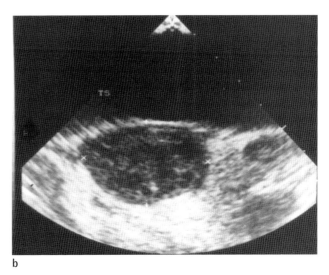
b

Figure 5.42
Leukemia – mass infiltration pattern. (a) A hypoechoic tumor nearly fills the testis. (b) The whole testis is involved with hypoechoic, slightly inhomogeneous leukemic tissue. (Courtesy of Dr Richard Winter, Royal Glamorgan Hospital, Mid-Glamorgan, UK.)

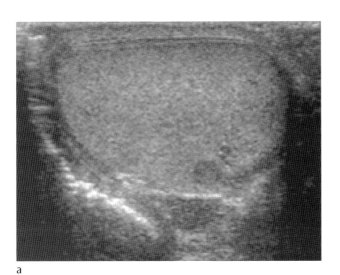
a

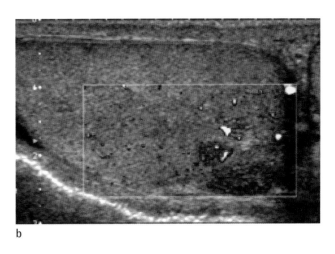
b

Figure 5.43
Leydig cell tumor. (a) A small tumor found incidentally. The patient has no hormonal problems. It was initially thought that this may be a small epidermoid cyst, but color Doppler studies (b) discounted this by showing that the tumor was vascular. (The center of epidermoid cysts is entirely avascular.) The diagnosis was made histologically at orchidectomy.

Adrenal rest tumors[37–41]

Adrenal rest tumors are benign proliferations of ectopic adrenal tissue in patients with adrenal hypoplasia, particularly in those that are poorly compliant with their hormone replacement therapy. They appear as multiple hypoechoic lesions, near the hilum, and are usually bilateral (Figure 5.45). The history of adrenal hypoplasia makes the diagnosis likely. Excision or biopsy is not necessary. Confirmatory evidence is the partial regression of the lesions when good hormone replacement is restored.

Sarcoidosis[42]

Sarcoidosis may cause multiple rounded hypoechoic deposits in the testes (Figure 5.46). Knowledge that the patient has sarcoidosis is vital to the diagnosis.

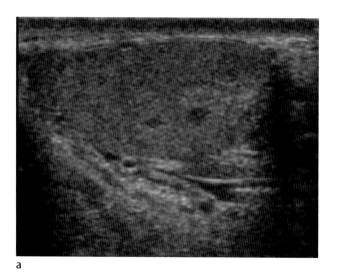
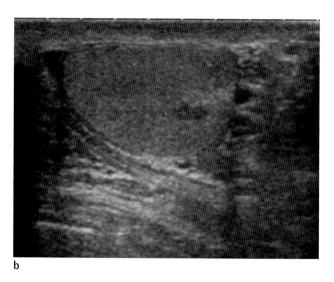

a   b

Figure 5.44
Leydig cell hyperplasia. There are small tumors in both testes: (a) right, (b) left. These were histologically Leydig cell hyperplasia rather than tumor.

Orchitis simulating tumor

Epididymo-orchitis has a significant effect on the testis in only a small proportion of severe cases. In some of these, however, focal change may occur within the testis, simulating tumor (Figure 5.47). The history and clinical signs of epididymo-orchitis will be evident in these cases. However, we have seen several cases of coexisting epididymo-orchitis and germ cell tumor that may occur by chance, although there is some evidence that testicular tumors may cause orchitis by obstructing the seminiferous tubules.

Such cases should, therefore, be carefully followed until there is resolution of the changes. In some cases the testis is permanently scarred, with hypoechoic and, less often, hyperechoic areas. The appearances are usually more altered texture than discrete mass (Figure 5.48). Nevertheless, it may be difficult to exclude tumors. Follow-up scans are indicated, looking for progression. Any increase in size or conspicuity of the lesion indicates that orchidectomy should be considered.

Trauma: hematoma

Severe trauma may produce an acute hematoma and long-term changes similar to post-inflammatory change (Figure 5.49), and similar follow-up is indicated. Testicular tumors may present after a misleading history of trauma. An intratesticular mass, even if it appears to be a hematoma, must therefore be carefully followed and tumor markers

measured. Scrotal trauma is more fully considered later in this chapter.

Atrophy simulating tumor

Atrophic testes may be caused by ischemia, either due to atheroma, or post surgical, typically herniorrhaphy. These testes are also often inhomogeneous and may simulate tumor (Figure 5.50).

The history of a testis that has become smaller provides the diagnosis. Testes that are atrophic in young men, either from previous maldescent or idiopathic, are different as they are often dysplastic histologically, with an increased risk of developing a germ cell tumor. Ultrasonically, however, they are less inhomogeneous (Figure 5.51). As they are at increased risk of developing malignant change, any focal areas of altered echo density in these testes must be closely followed.

Infarcts[43–45]

Infarcts of the testis may occur in patients with hypercoagulability states, notably sickle cell disease. They may also be postinfective or idiopathic. They present with pain of varying intensity. Most cases have geographic or wedge-shaped hypoechoic area within the testis (Figure 5.52). Some have more rounded areas that may simulate tumor (Figure 5.53).

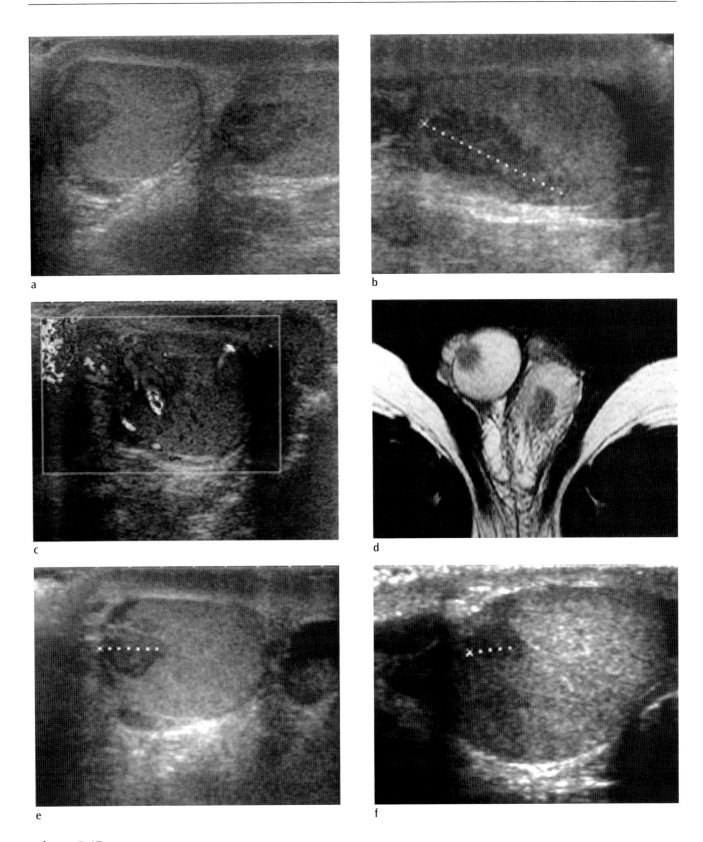

Figure 5.45

Adrenal rest tumors. This 17-year-old boy presented with a bilateral palpable testicular mass. Ultrasound revealed bilateral tumors (a, b), initially thought to be germ cell tumors. (c) Doppler study revealed highly vascular tumors, which is typical. (d) An MRI scan showed the tumor but did not add any useful information. During discussion of the case, it became evident that the boy had adrenal hypoplasia, and was non-compliant with his replacement therapy. Repeat studies after correcting his replacement therapy showed regression in the tumor: (e) right (f) left.

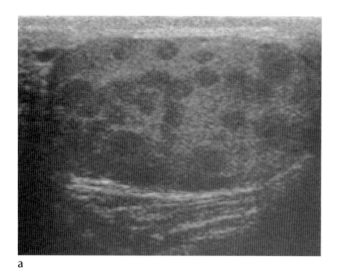
a

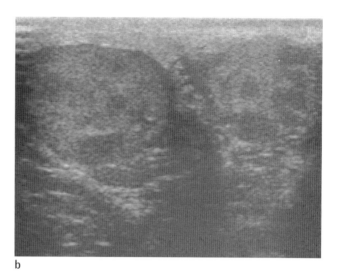
b

Figure 5.46
Sarcoidosis. (a,b) Multiple bilateral hypoechoic lesions in both testes. There is a wide differential diagnosis, although this pattern is compatible with sarcoidosis. The diagnosis was only made with the knowledge that the patient had sarcoidosis.

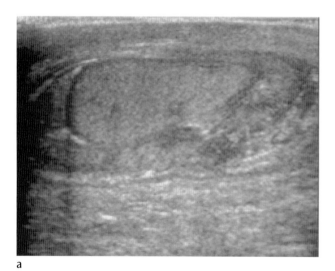
a

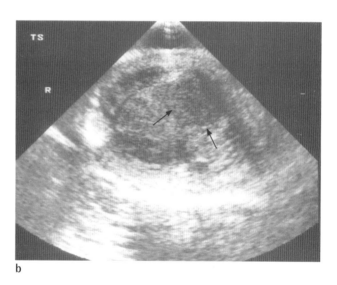
b

Figure 5.47
Focal orchitis. (a) The upper pole of the testes is enlarged and a little inhomogeneous. The very swollen epididymis, however, makes it most likely that this is focal orchitis. (b) A case of granulomatous orchitis. There is an area of focal orchitis (arrow), which is bulging the outline of the testis. The rest of the testis is edematous, which renders some of the fibrous septae just visible.

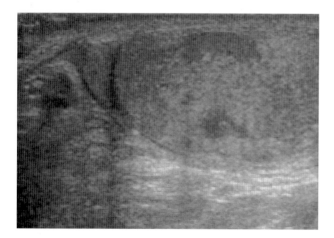

Figure 5.48
Postinflammatory change. There are several irregular hypoechoic area in the testis. The patient had has a recent episode of severe epididymo-orchitis. Follow-up showed partial, although not complete, resolution.

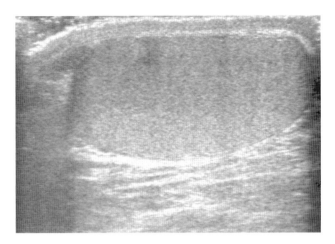

Figure 5.49

Post-traumatic change. Six months after severe scrotal trauma, a hypoechoic area remains anteriorly in the testis.

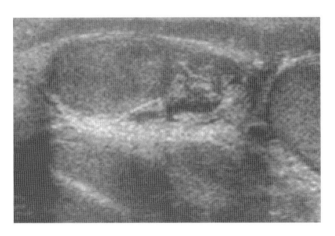

Figure 5.50

Atrophy simulating tumor. The atrophic testis due to ischemia has a very inhomogeneous texture. It was hard on palpation, which is often the case. It is difficult to exclude a tumor. Follow-up showed no progress.

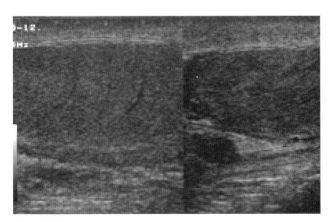

Figure 5.51

Atrophy from previous undescent. The left testis is atrophic. It is less inhomogenous than the ischemic testis in Figure 5.50, but is likely to be histologically dysplastic.

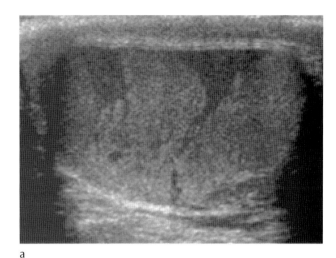

a

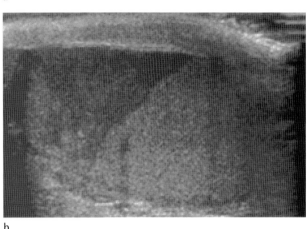

b

Figure 5.52

Testicular infarcts. (a) There are two wedge-shaped hypoechoic lesions. (b) Another case with a larger but also wedge-shaped lesion. In these cases, the shape of the lesions strongly suggests infarcts. (Reproduced with permission from Cochlin D Ll. Acute testicular pain. Imaging 2005; 17: 1–10.)

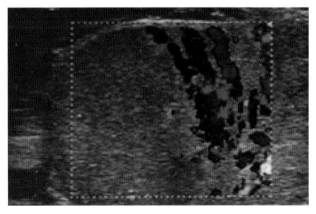

Figure 5.53

Testicular infarct. This large infarct has a rounded appearance and the gray-scale appearances simulate a tumor. Color Doppler shows absent flow within the lesion, suggesting an infarct. A tumor of this size would usually be hypervascular. (Reproduced with permission from Cochlin D Ll. Acute testicular pain. Imaging 2005; 17: 1–10.)

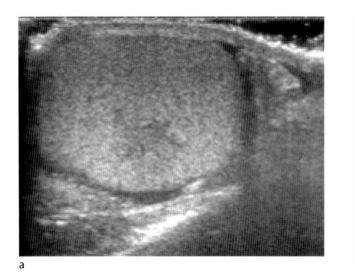

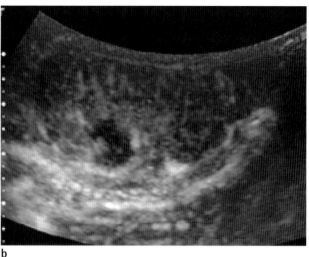

a   b

Figure 5.54

Testicular infarct with contrast study. (a) This poorly defined, irregular, somewhat rounded hypoechoic lesion would be difficult to categorize on the gray-scale image. (b) A contrast ultrasound study (Sonovue with low MI images) clearly shows an avascular infarct. (Reproduced with permission from Cochlin D Ll. Acute testicular pain. Imaging 2005; 17: 1–10.)

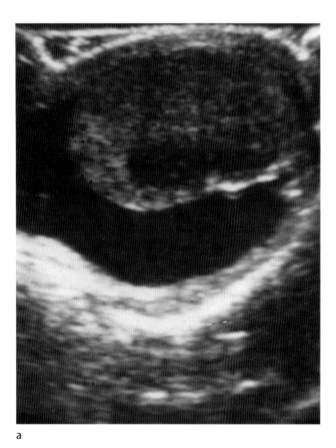

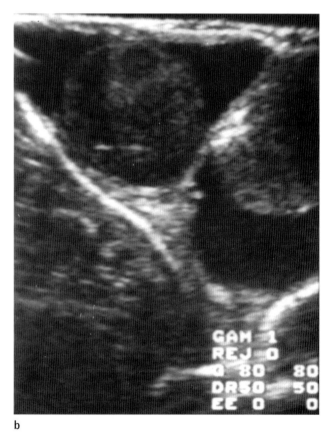

a   b

Figure 5.55

Melanoma metastases. (a,b) There are multiple slightly hypoechoic lesions in the left testis. The apparent multiplicity of the lesions suggests secondary deposits, leukemia or lymphoma. The patient had a previously excised ocular melanoma. The bilateral fairly large hydroceles are atypical of malignant disease and may just be incidental findings. (Courtesy of Dr Richard Winter, East Glamorgan Hospital, Mid-Glamorgan, UK.)

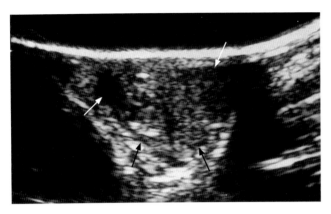

Figure 5.56
Secondary deposits from a colonic carcinoma. Four lesions
are seen in the testis (arrows). Three have a hypoechoic rim
with iso- and hypoechoic centers, and the other is hypoechoic.
This accentuates the variability that may occur in the
sonographic appearances of secondary deposits.

It would seem logical that Doppler studies would help in
the differential diagnosis. Large infarcts may indeed show
avascularity (Figure 5.53). In most small infarcts, however,
they appear to be of normal or often increased vascularity.
This is difficult to explain. Presumably, hypervascularity of
the tissues adjacent to the infarct mask the avascular area.
Contrast ultrasound studies show fine vasculature in great
detail and show promise in this field (Figure 5.54), but the
cases that have been studied are too few to make any definite statement about usefulness at the time of writing.

Metastatic deposits[45]

These are rare. They may arise from prostate, lung, gastrointestinal tract, kidney or melanoma. They have variable
appearances and are indistinguishable from primary testicular tumors on ultrasound appearances when solitary
(Figures 5.55 and 5.56).

Primary adenocarcinoma of the rete testis[46]

This is a rare tumor occurring in middle age, most often
presenting with hematospermia. Sonographically, it
appears as a multicystic lesion in the rete testis with nodular septations and an associated hydrocele (Figure 5.57). It
should not be confused with cystic dilatation of the rete
testis, which is an innocent condition with tubular dilatation or cysts but no nodules, septation, hydrocele or
hematospermia (Figures 5.60 and 5.61).

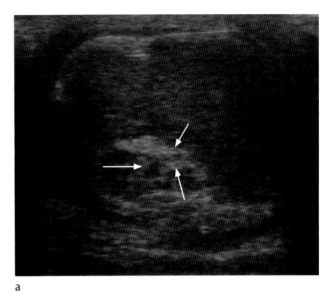

a

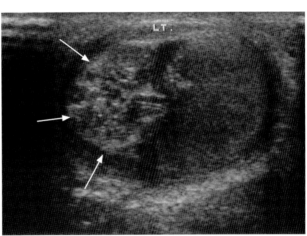

b

Figure 5.57
Papillary adenocarcinoma of the rete testis. (a) A
multiloculated cystic lesion is seen at the rete testis. Small solid
areas are seen which may represent papillary elements (arrow).
The demonstration of papillary elements is important in
making this diagnosis. (b) In this case, the solid elements
predominate. Some appear nodular (arrows).

Intratesticular cysts[47–49]

Simple cysts in the testes are either testicular cysts that tend
to occur close to the hilum (Figure 5.58), or tunical cysts
that may bulge into the testis or out into the peritesticular
space. Both are usually small, although may occasionally
reach a large size (Figure 5.59). As with simple cysts elsewhere, simple intratesticular cysts are thin-walled with no
solid elements. If they fulfill these criteria, the patient may
be reassured. They require no treatment or follow-up.

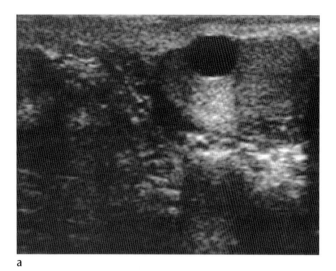

a

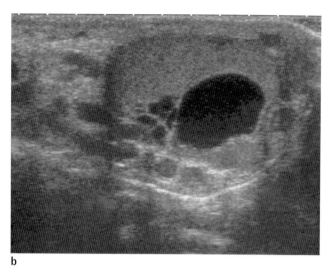

b

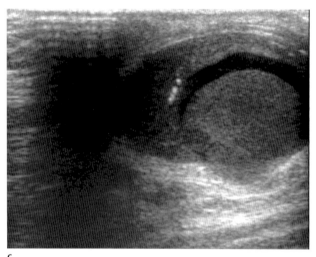

c

Figure 5.58
Testicular cysts. (a) A cyst within the testes. It fulfills the criteria of any simple cyst: smooth wall, no solid elements, anechoic center and enhanced through transmission. (b) Multiple cysts of the rete testis. The large cyst is irregular in shape but thin-walled with no solid elements. It is therefore a benign simple cyst. (c) A cystic teratoma. The testicular cyst contains a hematoma. At first glance, it appears to be a simple cyst. However, the calcification in the wall is not compatible with a simple cyst.

Epidermoid cysts are filled with keratin and so appear solid on an ultrasound study. They are therefore discussed with solid tumors.

Germ cell tumors often contain cystic areas, but the solid tumor elements are usually obvious. Teratoma may be predominantly cystic: there are, however, always some solid elements. Many embryonal cell carcinomas and teratomas may contain cystic areas, but are usually predominantly solid (see Figure 5.25).

Liquefying hematoma and abscess may contain fluid-filled spaces.

Ectasia of the rete testis[50–52]

Ectasia of the rete testis may superficially simulate tumor, although, with high-resolution systems, the tubular or cystic nature of the lesion is obvious (Figure 5.60). Most cases

appear as multiple tubular structures representing the dilated tubules. In some there is cystic change. Any associated solid elements, however, should raise the suspicion of the rare tumor, adenocarcinoma of the rete testis (see Figure 5.57), particularly if the patient has hematospermia. Tubular ectasia of the rete testis is, in most cases, an asymptomatic innocent condition found in older men. In young men, it suggests obstruction of the sperm transport mechanism. This is particularly likely if it is associated with multiple epididymal cysts (Figure 5.61).

ACUTE, SEVERE SCROTAL PAIN

Acute, severe scrotal pain, swelling and tenderness denote, with a few uncommon exceptions, epididymo-orchitis or torsion of the testis in the adult or torsion of the testis,

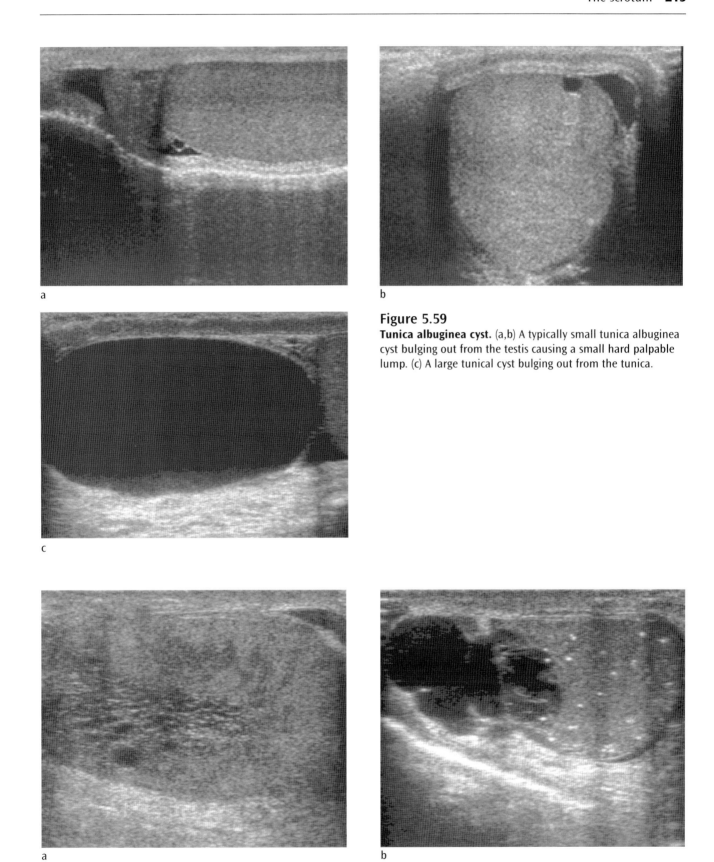

a

b

Figure 5.59
Tunica albuginea cyst. (a,b) A typically small tunica albuginea cyst bulging out from the testis causing a small hard palpable lump. (c) A large tunical cyst bulging out from the tunica.

c

a

b

Figure 5.60
Ectasia of the rete testis. (a) The tubules at the rete testis are dilated. (b) There is gross dilatation of the rete testis. It is not clear whether the testicular calcification is associated with the ectasia.

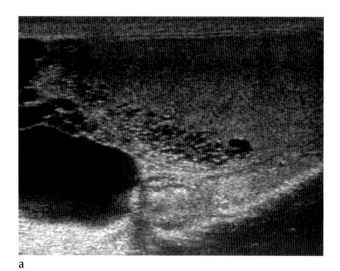

a

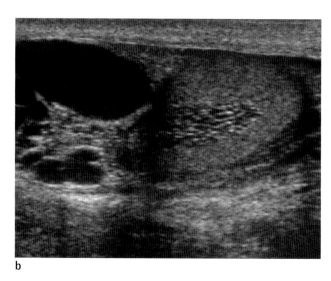

b

Figure 5.61
Tubular ectasia of the rete testis. A 32-year-old man with oligospermia. There is ectasia of the rete testis, with large epididymal cysts on both sides, indicating obstruction of the sperm transport mechanism: (a) right, (b) left.

hydatid of Morgagni or testicular appendix in boys. These conditions will be considered first. The uncommon causes, including testicular infarcts, Henoch–Schönlein purpura and childhood appendicitis, will be discussed later.

Epididymo-orchitis

The term epididymo-orchitis is in some respects misleading, as in the majority of cases only the epididymis is affected. In young men the most common cause is sexually transmitted disease, *Chlamydia* being the most common organism. In older men, urinary tract infections are a more common cause. Urethral catheterization is a common predisposing cause. Tuberculous epididymo-orchitis is sometimes encountered and BCG (bacille Calmette–Guérin) bladder instillation as a treatment for bladder cancer may give identical appearances (BCG-itis). Syphilis is now rarely seen. The mumps virus causes orchitis without epididymitis. Parasitic epididymo-orchitis occurs in some parts of the world. Chemical or sterile epididymo-orchitis is due to retrograde reflux of urine, or an ectopic ureter opening into the vas deferens. Repetitive mild trauma, typically cycle riding, is the most common cause in young boys.

Epididymitis[53–57]

The epididymal changes are described first, as in most cases only the epididymis is involved and in all cases (except mumps) is predominantly involved.

Appearances vary greatly with the severity of the disease. The principal change is swelling and hyperemia of the epididymis. The tail is the part most often affected, the head and body less often. In most severe cases, the whole epididymis is affected (Figure 5.62). There is a variable reactive hydrocele, often echogenic due to blood and inflammatory debris (Figure 5.63).

In severe cases, and those that are not responsive to antibiotic treatment, abscesses may occur within the epididymis. These start as focal areas of altered echo density, often with a low echodensity center (Figure 5.64). They may rupture into the scrotal sac, causing a pyocele (Figure 5.65) or through the scrotal wall (Figure 5.66).

Marked swelling and hyperemia resolve rapidly with response to antibiotics, as do the symptoms of severe pain. Some swelling and focal echogenic areas in the epididymis, however, often remain after infection has been eradicated.

Hard areas may be found within the epididymis, particularly the tail, for long periods and often permanently following epididymitis. They are easily palpable but difficult to see on ultrasound studies. Subtle differences in echo texture may be seen when moving the epididymis with a palpating finger while scanning.

Funiculitis

The spermatic cord is often involved in the inflammatory process: this is termed funiculitis. The ultrasonic signs are swelling and hyperemia of the cord. Involvement of the cord is usually less marked than in the epididymis, but occasionally the funiculitis is the most marked element

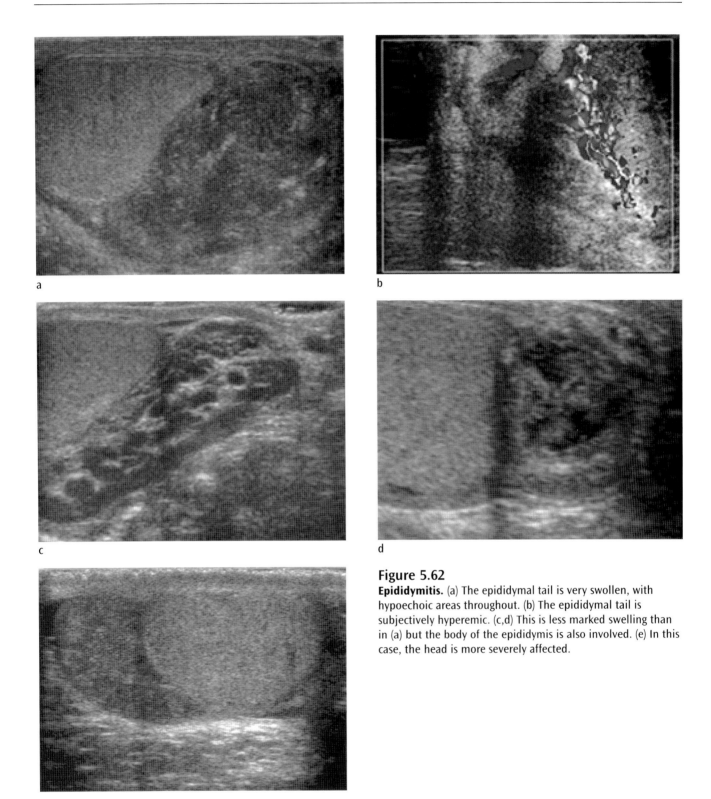

Figure 5.62
Epididymitis. (a) The epididymal tail is very swollen, with hypoechoic areas throughout. (b) The epididymal tail is subjectively hyperemic. (c,d) This is less marked swelling than in (a) but the body of the epididymis is also involved. (e) In this case, the head is more severely affected.

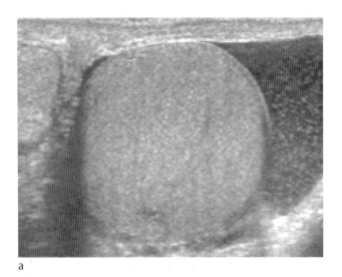

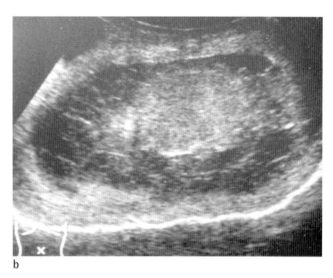

a

b

Figure 5.63
Inflammatory hydrocele. (a) The hydrocele has echogenic inflammatory debris. (b) In the more chronic cases, there are marked adhesions.

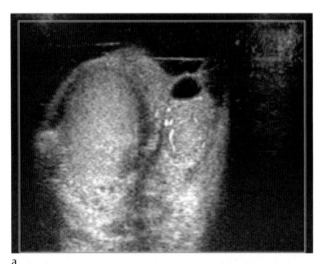

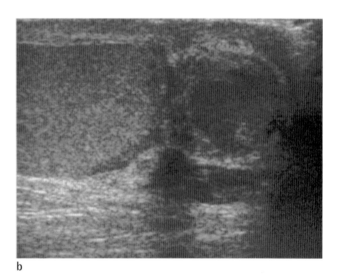

a

b

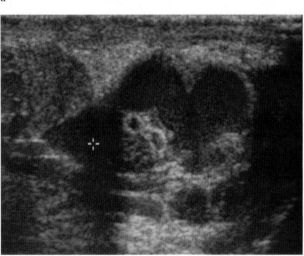

c

Figure 5.64
Epididymal abscess. (a) There is an inflammatory mass within the epididymis containing an abscess with a fluid level. (b,c) A larger epididymal abscess.

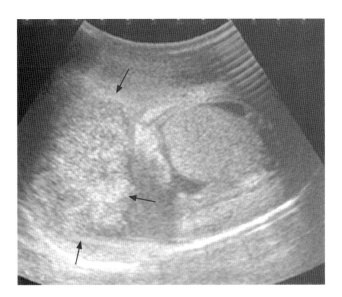

Figure 5.65
Pyocele. There is a large collection of echogenic pus in the scrotal sac (arrows).

(Figure 5.67). Severe funiculitis may rarely cause compression of the cord vessels within the inguinal canal, with resultant testicular ischemia.

Orchitis

Clinical considerations

The testis is relatively protected against infection because of its rich blood supply and lymphatic drainage. Isolated orchitis is therefore rare. The vast majority of cases of orchitis are metastatic via the epididymis, bloodstream or lymphatics. Almost any infection may metastasize to the testis, but the majority are secondary to epididymitis (epididymo-orchitis). Orchitis may be pyogenic, viral, spirochetal, mycotic or parasitic. Traumatic orchitis (or epididymitis) may occur after trauma, vas ligation or surgical manipulation and is usually considered to be a pyogenic infection resulting from a lowered resistance of the damaged tissues, although a granulomatous reaction caused by protein released from sperm may be responsible.

Thus, although many organisms may in theory cause orchitis, with the exception of mumps, orchitis in the absence of epididymitis is rare.

Orchitis as part of epididymo-orchitis

The involvement of the testis in the inflammatory process is less frequent than the common usage of the term

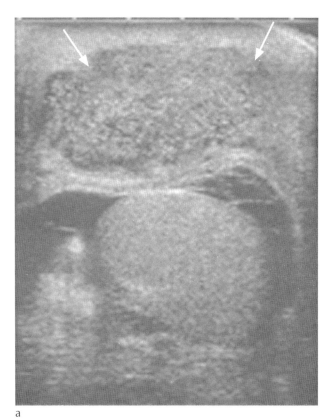

a

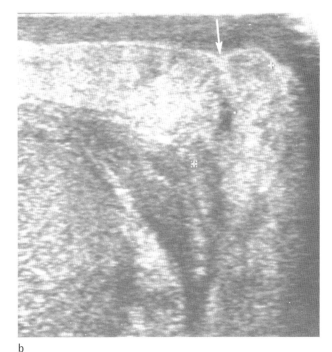

b

Figure 5.66
Scrotal wall abscess. (a) A scrotal wall abscess due to extension of an epididymal abscess into the scrotal wall (arrows). (b) Fistula through the scrotal wall (arrow marks the fistula). (Reproduced with permission from Rifkin MD, Cochlin DL. Imaging of the scrotum and penis. London: Martin Dunitz; 2002.)

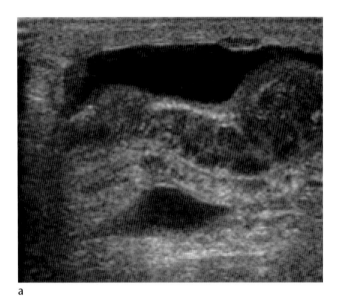

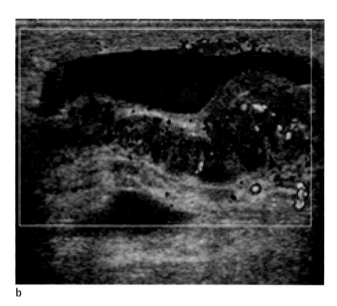

a

b

Figure 5.67
Funiculitis. (a) The spermatic cord is swollen. (b) It is hyperaemic. In this case, there is clearly no vascular compression.

epididymo-orchitis implies. It usually takes the form of diffuse orchitis, which may progress to focal orchitis and abscess formation, sometimes necessitating orchidectomy. It seems that in some cases the orchitis is focal de novo.

Diffuse orchitis appears as mild to moderate enlargement of the testis, classically with a fairly even hypoechoic texture. This is easiest to appreciate by comparison with the other testis if the disease is unilateral, although it should be remembered that a surrounding hydrocele or scrotal wall edema will modify the ultrasound beam on the affected side and this must be allowed for (Figure 5.68).

Although an enlarged hypoechoic testis is typical of diffuse orchitis, in practice one sees cases that are hypoechoic but not enlarged, hyperechoic and mixed (Figure 5.69). Orchitis must be distinguished from tumor, which usually causes irregular enlargement with loss of the normal ovoid shape and greater variations in echodensity in different parts of the testis. Ischemia is more difficult to differentiate. The appearance of the testis may be identical, but Doppler may be helpful.

Focal orchitis is less common and usually more severe. It appears as an area of mixed echodensity in the testis (Figure 5.70). This is often indistinguishable from tumor on ultrasound appearances, and a judgment must be made on clinical grounds. There is most often, but not always, a reactive hydrocele.

Abscess formation is really a progression of severe focal orchitis, and the two entities merge. Full abscesses of the testis are rare. The presence of very hypoechoic spaces, sometimes with thick walls, suggests full-blown abscess formation (Figure 5.71). Rupture of a testicular abscess

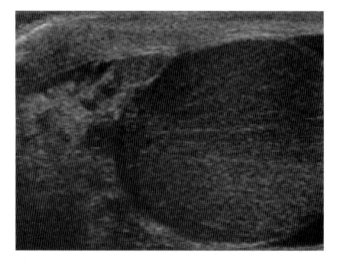

Figure 5.68
Orchitis. The testis is enlarged and uniformly hypoechoic. This makes the septae more prominent than usual.

into a surrounding hydrocele causes a pyocele, which, as with a ruptured epididymal abscess, may have a fluid–fluid level.

Mumps orchitis[58,59]

This causes a diffuse uniform or patchy hypoechoic pattern (Figure 5.72). It does not cause focal orchitis. The diagnosis

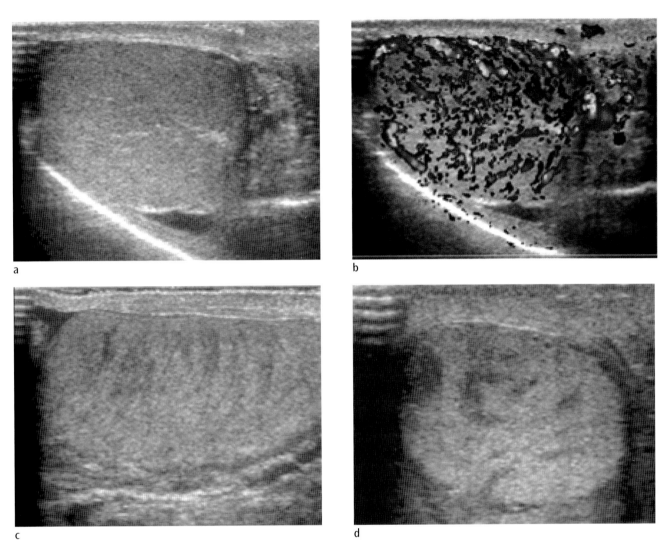

a

b

c

d

Figure 5.69

Orchitis – varying patterns. (a) The testis appears normal but in the same case (b) shows marked hyperemia. (c) The testis is hyperechoic, causing prominence of the septae and major vessels. (d) The testis is of very mixed echo density but predominantly hyperechoic. There are also areas of focal orchitis.

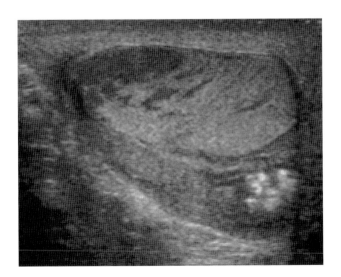

Figure 5.70

Focal orchitis. There are several areas of focal orchitis in the upper pole of the testis. Note that there is epididymal calcification, although the cause was chlamydial orchitis, not TB as the calcification may suggest. (See also Figure 5.69d.)

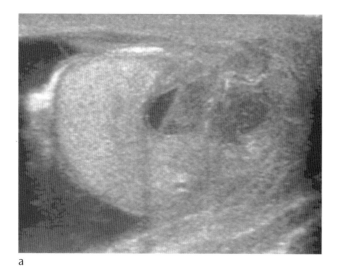

a

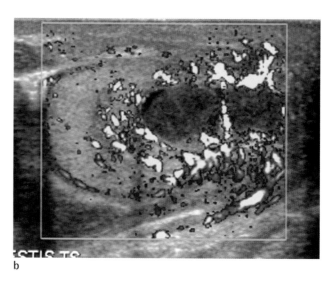

b

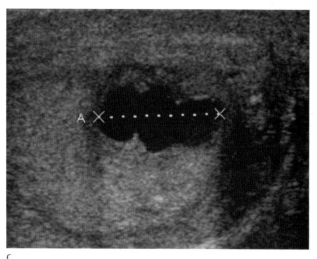

c

Figure 5.71
Testicular abscess. (a,b) A testicular abscess. (c) Progression after 4 weeks with liquefaction of the contents.

is usually clear clinically, although the diagnosis may be very difficult in the occasional case where orchitis occurs without parotitis. Infarcts may occur during the acute episode. Atrophy is a common long-term complication.

Doppler studies in epididymo-orchitis

Doppler studies should always be obtained, most importantly to exclude torsion. If the testis is involved in the epididymo-orchitis, then it is often hyperemic. It is assessed as a subjective increase in vascularity over that in the opposite, unaffected testis, or above what is normally seen with the particular ultrasound system and settings used. It is usual to see more vessels and a greater length of vessels than in normal testis (Figure 5.73). The epididymis is usually also subjectively hyperemic (Figure 5.74). Absence of

hyperemia does not exclude epididymo-orchitis, and often disappears rapidly with antibiotic treatment.

Testicular ischemia has been reported in cases of very severe epididymo-orchitis, when swelling of the cord within the confines of the inguinal canal obstructs the venous return. In these cases, Doppler studies show reduced or absent flow, and spectral Doppler of any artery that may be seen may show reversed diastolic flow. This is, however, a very rare complication and is only seen in the most severe cases. Surgery, usually with epididymectomy, is required to restore the blood flow if testicular function is to be preserved.

Spectral Doppler patterns are, in general, unhelpful. The inflammation causes arteriolar dilatation and a low resistance arterial waveform. Swelling of the testis within the relatively inelastic tunica causes venous compression and a high-resistance arterial waveform. In practice, therefore, any waveform may be found depending on which element predominates. Reversed diastolic flow, however, suggests

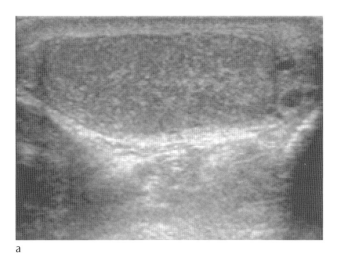

a

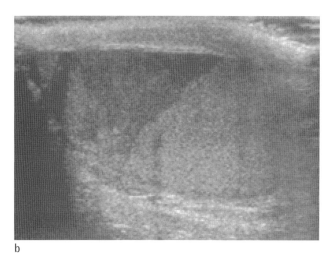

b

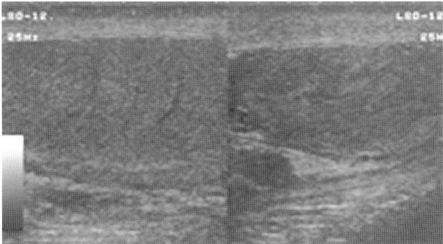

c

Figure 5.72
Mumps orchitis. (a) The left testis has a patchy hyperechoic pattern, without significant enlargement. (b) At 2 weeks, there is a wedge-shaped infarct. (c) At 3 months, there is atrophy. The testis is small and patchily hypoechoic.

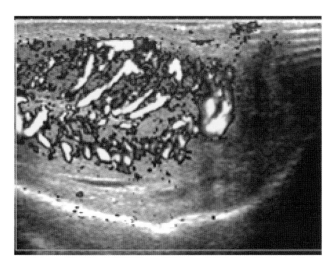

Figure 5.73
Orchitis – Doppler study. This testis is intensely hyperemic. The vessels are enlarged, and a greater number and length of vessels are seen than in the normal testis.

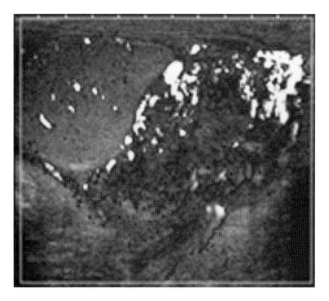

Figure 5.74
Epididymitis – Doppler study. The epididymal tail is swollen and intensely hyperemic.

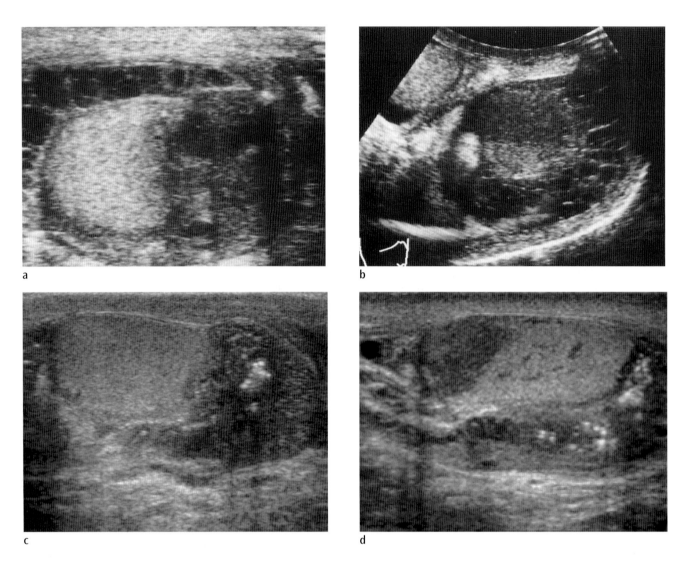

Figure 5.75
Tuberculous epididymo-orchitis. (a) The inferior testicular pole is swollen and hypoechoic. There are characteristically thick adhesions around the testis. (b) The adhesions are so marked that the differentiation of the testis and epididymis is lost. (c,d) There is marked calcification of the enlarged epididymis. The epididymis is typically adherent to the testis. (Parts (a) and (b) are reproduced with permission from Rifkin MD, Cochlin DL. Imaging of the scrotum and penis. London: Martin Dunitz; 2002.)

the rare complication of testicular ischemia. Peak systolic velocities are generally increased.

Tuberculous and BCG epididymo-orchitis[60–62]

Tuberculous epididymo-orchitis is occasionally encountered. One of the treatments for bladder tumor is bladder instillation with a solution containing BCG bacillus. This may cause infections almost identical to tuberculosis, including renal and scrotal infections. Symptoms differ from those in pyogenic epididymo-orchitis, there being little or no pain. The main symptom is scrotal swelling. The

pattern of change seen on the ultrasound scan also differs from pyogenic infection. Both the epididymis and testis are often equally involved, with adhesions between them. They often fuse on the ultrasound study into one complex mass in which it is difficult to distinguish the two (Figure 5.75). MRI is better at distinguishing testis and epididymis than ultrasound (Figure 5.76). Calcifications within the epididymis sometimes occur (Figure 5.77).

Fournier gangrene[63]

Fournier gangrene is an anaerobic infection that causes a necrotizing fasciitis of the perineum and scrotum. It most

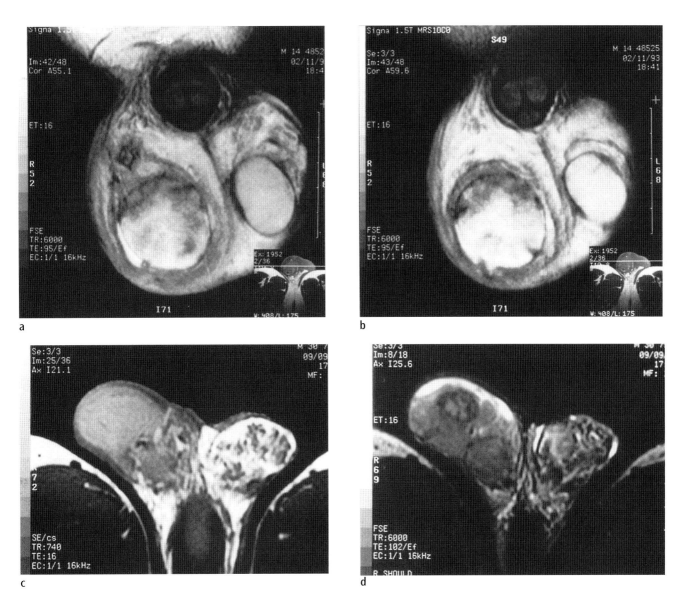

Figure 5.76
MRI of tuberculous epididymo-orchitis. (a,b) T2-weighted studies. The testis and epididymis are both very abnormal, with marked adhesions. Unlike an ultrasound study, however, testis and epididymis are clearly distinguished as separate structures. (c,d) In this case, the adhesions are more marked. (Reproduced with permission from Rifkin MD, Cochlin DL. Imaging of the scrotum and penis. London: Martin Dunitz; 2002.)

often affects older men and neonates. Diagnosis is usually clinical, but the first sign may be seen on an ultrasound study as gas in the soft tissues or the epididymis causing dense shadows (Figure 5.78).

Testicular torsion[64–70]

Torsion of the spermatic cord occurs most commonly in preadolescence and adolescence and in the perinatal peri-

od. It may, however, occur at any age, including old age. It presents with acute unilateral scrotal pain, frequently associated with nausea and vomiting. The diagnosis is usually obvious from the history and clinical examination and, because of the importance of early surgery (within the first 24 hours if infarction is to be avoided), patients are usually taken directly to the operating theater with no imaging investigations. In some cases the diagnosis is less clear, the differential diagnosis being acute epididymo-orchitis or, in boys, torsion of the appendix testis or appendix epididymis. In these cases, confirmation of the diagnosis is

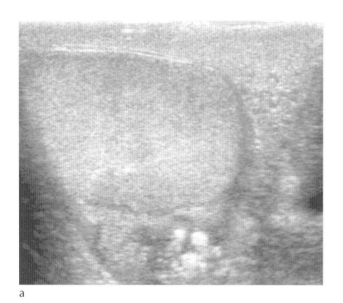

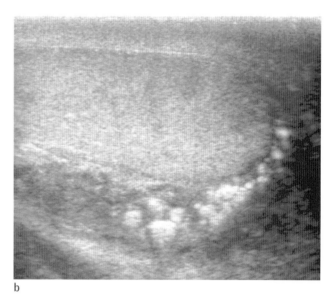

a

b

Figure 5.77
Tuberculous epididymo-orchitis. There is extensive epididymal calcification.

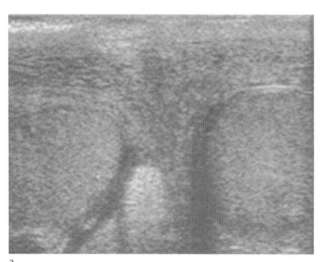

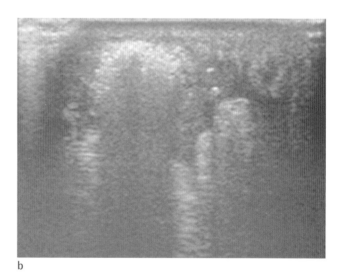

a

b

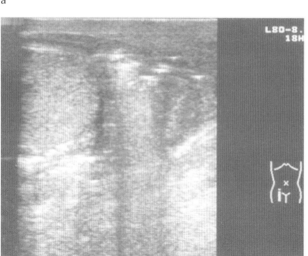

c

Figure 5.78
Fournier gangrene. (a) There is marked edema of the scrotal wall. There is a suspicious sonodense area with weak shadowing. (b) A scan of the perineum shows definite soft tissue gas with shadowing. (c) A different case study showing gas in the epididymis.

desirable to prevent unnecessary surgery, provided that it does not lead to unacceptable delay in treatment.

With clinical assessment it is important to avoid a false-negative diagnosis. Some patients that are operated upon have a high clinical probability of torsion; others have a lower probability, but it is felt that torsion cannot be excluded. Consequently, in most centers, about two-thirds of patients operated upon for suspected torsion have no torsion found. It is, therefore, increasingly common for those patients presenting within normal working hours to request an immediate ultrasound and Doppler study: this is, undoubtedly, a progressive step. However, there is one potential drawback. In cases of torsion and spontaneous detorsion, the testis develops rebound hyperemia and, on ultrasound and Doppler study, resembles orchitis. Many of these patients will later progress to an episode of full torsion.

Doppler studies

The appropriate imaging test is an ultrasound scan with a Doppler study. Isotope studies have been used in the past but are no longer used. It is important that a high-resolution ultrasound system is used, with high-sensitivity Doppler. This is particularly important in prepubertal boys when the testicular vessels are small. Indeed, even with modern equipment, there are still a proportion of young boys with vessels too small to detect by Doppler. The proportion is decreasing as equipment improves but, even so, failure to detect Doppler flow in prepubescent boys does not necessarily indicate torsion. If there are gray-scale

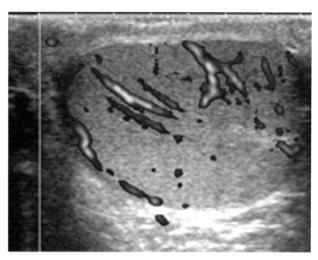

Figure 5.79
Normal testicular Doppler flow. The number and length of the intratesticular vessels seen on a Doppler study is very variable. This example is average. In other cases, significantly more or fewer vessels are seen.

changes compatible with torsion and a history that fits, the diagnosis becomes more probable. Failure to show vessels in the contralateral normal testis should, however, suggest a technical failure, and renders the Doppler test non-diagnostic. In cases of doubt, intravenous microbubble ultrasound contrast agents may be used. They are more sensitive in demonstrating blood perfusion or non-perfusion than Doppler studies, but their use is only occasionally necessary in cases of doubt and they are at present not licensed for use in children, the group most likely to benefit.

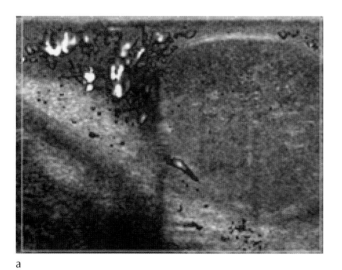

a

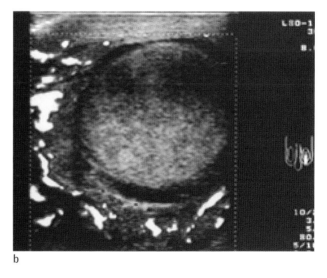

b

Figure 5.80
Testicular torsion – Doppler studies. (a) An early case (4 hours) shows flow in the epididymis, but no flow in the testis. (b) A later case (8 hours) shows hyperemia of the paratesticular tissue, and an avascular testis.

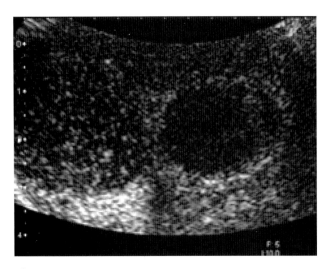

Figure 5.81

Testicular torsion – contrast study. In this case of missed torsion, the patient wanted a confirmation of the diagnosis. The contrast study (Sonovue with low MI technique) shows a non-perfused left testis. The right testis shows a normal perfusion pattern. (See also Figure 5.82b.). (Reproduced with permission from Cochlin D Ll. Acute testicular pain. Imaging 2005; 17: 1–10.)

The demonstration of a normal pattern of arterial and venous intratesticular flow virtually excludes the diagnosis of torsion (although not torsion with spontaneous detorsion) (Figure 5.79). It is important to realize that torsion of the cord may occlude the veins, but not the artery. Initially, therefore, there may be arterial flow as far as the testicular hilum, although there is little or no flow in the parenchyma (Figures 5.80 and 5.81). With the use of high-resolution equipment, it is now clear that some cases of torsion retain flow in a few intratesticular arteries, particularly in the lower pole. This is because some collateral flow to the testis may exist. The conventional teaching that there are no collaterals is not strictly true. It is, however, practically true, as the collateral supply to the testis is small and insufficient to prevent infarction. It does mean that the old statement that there is no intratesticular blood flow in torsion is not necessarily true. The statement has to be modified to absent or extremely reduced flow. In a few cases, torsion may be incomplete, and in these cases there may be a little intratesticular flow. There are often arteries seen at the hilum but with reversed diastolic flow due to impaired venous return. The epididymis retains some blood flow, and enlarged vessels in the scrotal wall may be shown (Figure 5.82).

Following detorsion, either surgical or spontaneous, the testicular flow may return to normal, but there is often increased flow with enhanced diastolic flow for a short time.

The extratesticular scrotal tissue, the epididymis and scrotal wall have more than one blood supply; following torsion, they develop a reactive hyperemia (Figure 5.83).

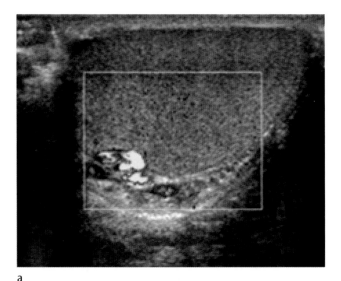

a

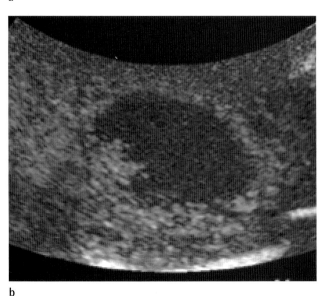

b

Figure 5.82

Incomplete torsion. (a) In the case of incomplete (less than 360°) torsion of less than 5 hours duration, flow is seen at the testicular hilum, but none in the rest of the testis. (b) A contrast Doppler study (Sonovue and low MI imaging) shows perfusion of the hilum, but none of the rest of the testis.

This hyperemia occurs within a few hours and it accentuates the avascularity of the testis.

The twisted vessels within the cord may be seen, the appearances being described as the torsion knot (Figure 5.84). This usually lies high in the scrotum, and is not usually immediately visible, but may be found in a proportion of patients, if looked for. It is not, therefore, important in the primary diagnosis of torsion, although it provides additional confirmation if seen.

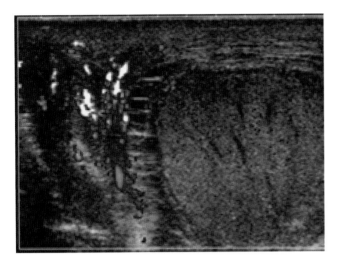

Figure 5.83
Testicular torsion – epididymal flow. In this case of torsion of 6 hours' duration, the epididymis is hyperemic due to an attempt at collateral formation. The testis is avascular, swollen and inhomogeneous.

Torsion with spontaneous detorsion, as previously stated, may be a diagnostic problem in which the Doppler study may give misleading information. There is transient rebound hyperemia of the testis followed by normal flow. The testis is often swollen. There is often, although not invariably, a reactive hydrocele. This may be useful as it may delineate a narrow testicular pedicle (bell-clapper deformity) (Figure 5.85). This is the anatomical variant that predisposes to testicular torsion and, if seen in this context, suggests torsion and detorsion. It is, however, only visible if delineated by a hydrocele. The diagnosis of torsion with spontaneous detorsion is, therefore, a clinical diagnosis in most cases.

Whereas the Doppler study is the definitive test for torsion, the gray-scale appearances are also important. This is particularly so in incomplete torsion where there is some testicular blood flow. In these cases the gray-scale findings may increase confidence in the diagnosis. The gray-scale findings are particularly important in suspected spontaneous detorsion.

Gray-scale appearance

Although the Doppler study is the main diagnostic test for torsion, the gray-scale appearances are also important to consider, particularly where Doppler studies are equivocal. This typically occurs in young boys, in incomplete torsion or spontaneous detorsion. The coexistence of appropriate

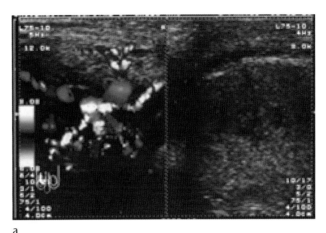

a

Figure 5.84
Torsion knot. (a,b) Two separate examples of the stellate vascular pattern of a torsion knot. (Reproduced with permission from Cochlin D Ll. Acute testicular pain. Imaging 2005; 17: 1–10.)

gray-scale findings in such cases may make the diagnoses more likely. Torsion and spontaneous detorsion is a very difficult diagnosis to make. The presence of gray-scale changes of acute torsion, however, in the presence of normal or hyperemic testicular blood flow suggests the diagnosis. In such cases, careful ultrasound and clinical study is necessary to detect a bell-clapper abnormality (see Figure 5.85). Finally, the testicular scan may be performed for atypical pain, and torsion may not be the suspected

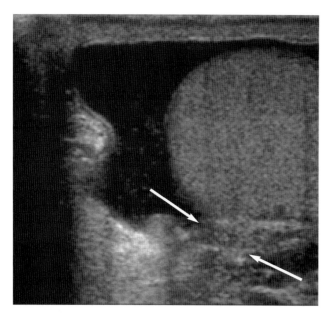

Figure 5.85
Bell-clapper deformity in spontaneous detorsion. The patient had symptoms of torsion. The Doppler study showed normal testicular flow, but the testis is swollen, slightly inhomogeneous. The hydrocele outlines a narrow pedicle (arrows), indicating likely spontaneous detorsion.

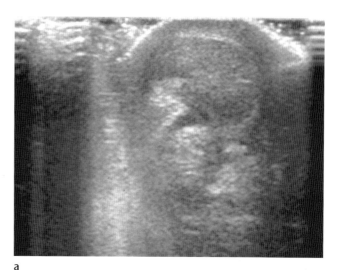

a

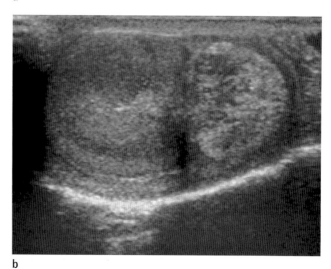

b

Figure 5.86
Testicular torsion: hyperechoic epididymis. (a,b) In the case of torsion of 6 hours' duration, the epididymis is markedly hyperechoic. The testis is also inhomogeneous.

diagnosis. In some cases, the gray-scale changes may alert the sonographer to the possibility of torsions, and prompt a Doppler study. It is, however, good practice to do a Doppler study on all cases of scrotal pain.

The appearances of the gray-scale ultrasound scan in torsion may be characteristic. Within the first few hours, the testis is enlarged and hypoechoic. The epididymis is swollen, but usually predominantly hyperechoic (Figure 5.86), as opposed to epididymitis, when it is predominantly hypoechoic with a few hyperechoic areas. The appearances are due to epididymal hemorrhage. There is often a small reactive hydrocele and a thickened scrotal wall (Figure 5.87). After about 24 hours the testicular appearance changes to mixed echodensity with areas of high and low echodensity, indicating areas of infarction and hemorrhage (Figure 5.88).

The most characteristic sign is the hyperechoic epididymis, but this is not always present or easy to appreciate.

Late appearances

A 'missed' torsion is a term used to denote a torsion that has not been diagnosed or treated for 48 hours or more. The ultrasound appearances are of an enlarged testis, either homogeneously hypoechoic or of mixed echodensity due to areas of hemorrhage, often with a characteristic hyper-

echoic rim around the periphery of the testis (Figure 5.89). The epididymis, by this stage, is enlarged and of mixed echodensity. There is a small reactive hydrocele or hematocele and a thickened scrotal wall. The reason for the characteristic echodense rim around the testis is not understood, but it clearly resembles the photon-rich ring described in isotope studies.

Long-term changes are variable. Successful detorsion may result in a normal testicular appearance, although hypoechoic areas due to infarction may remain, and there may be some atrophy. Such appearances do not denote failed treatment, as function may be preserved, and vascular flow in the ultrasonically normal portions of the testis can be shown to be normal. Non-treatment, or

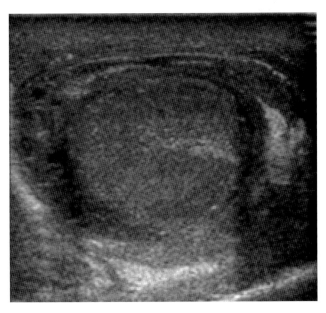

Figure 5.87
Testicular torsion: reactive hydrocele and hyperechoic epididymis.

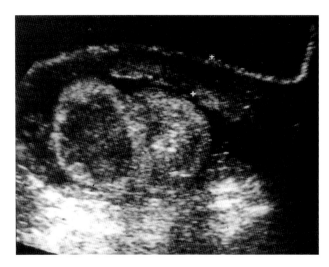

Figure 5.89
Testicular torsion: Hyperechoic testicular rim. Missed torsion of 4 days' duration. The testis is hypoechoic but with a marked hyperechoic rim.

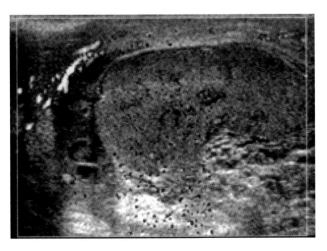

Figure 5.88
Testicular torsion: inhomogeneous testis. Torsion of 9 hours' duration shows an inhomogeneous testis.

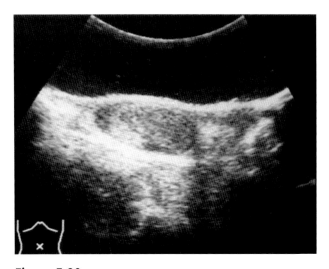

Figure 5.90
Mixed torsion: late appearance. The testis is atrophied (3 cm length), with no demonstrable blood flow on Doppler study. There are hyperechoic areas in the epididymis.

insufficiently early treatment, leads to a small atrophic testis, lacking in function (Figure 5.90).

Torsion of the hydatid of Morgagni, epididymal or testicular appendix[71–74]

The testis and epididymis have four appendices – small projections of tissue. In the context of torsion, only two of these are important, the testicular and epididymal appendices. The testicular appendix is a remnant of the Wolffian duct. It is a projection of tissue, often worm-like, from the upper pole of the testis. The epididymal appendix is a remnant of the Müllerian duct, and is a worm-like projection from the head of the epididymis. Sometimes a remnant of the duct lumen remains, causing a cyst within the stricture. This is called a cyst or hydatid of Morgagni. (Cysts of the Wolffian duct may also occur in the female, when they lie adjacent to the ovary. They may also tort, and are also called cysts or hydatids of

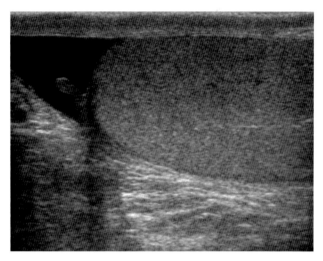

Figure 5.91
Testicular appendix. A testicular appendix is seen surrounded by fluid. It is a worm-like structure attached to the upper pole of the testis.

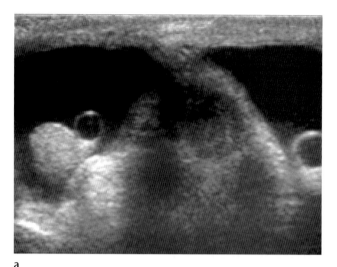

a

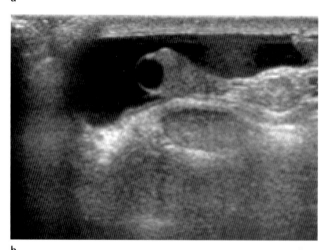

b

Figure 5.92
Hydatid of Morgagni. (a) Bilateral cysts, found incidentally. (b) Oblique planes (right) lie within epididymal appendices and are hydatid of Morgagni.

Morgagni. This is mentioned here as it sometimes causes confusion.)

Either appendix may tort. It is probable that the hydatid of Morgagni is more likely to tort than the appendix testis. Torsion of an appendix is the most common cause of acute scrotal pain in boys, accounting for 50–70% of cases. The diagnosis is often firmly made on clinical grounds. The condition resolves with no treatment and no sequelae. The differential diagnosis is testicular torsion or epididymo-orchitis. In cases of doubt, therefore, surgical exploration is indicated, but if immediate ultrasound examination is available this may avoid unnecessary surgery.

It has been thought that the torted appendix eventually calcifies and becomes a scrotolith; a free rounded calcified body lying in the scrotal sac. There is, however, no evidence for this, and the torted tissue is probably resorbed. Scrotoliths probably have a different, unknown etiology.

The normal appendices are usually only seen if there is sufficient fluid surrounding them (Figure 5.91). Hydatids of Morgagni may be seen as cystic structures within an epididymal appendix (Figure 5.92), although some are probably misdiagnosed as epididymal cysts. Torsion of the hydatid of Morgagni typically causes a rounded mass above the testis with a cystic center, often containing some medium echoic material, probably blood clot, and a thick wall (Figure 5.93). Other cases, probably torsions of appendices without hydatids, appear more solid (Figure 5.94). Surrounding tissues, including the head of the epididymis are edematous and hyperemic. There is a reactive hydrocele, also often with echogenic contents representing blood. The testis shows hyperemic or normal Doppler flow.

Less common causes of acute scrotal pain

In children, less common causes of scrotal pain include Henoch–Schönlein purpura and acute appendicitis; in adults and children, testicular infarcts and a bleed into a tumor. Henoch–Schönlein purpura causes a hemorrhagic orchitis. On ultrasound study, the testis is hyperemic but otherwise normal. There is a hydrocele and a thickened scrotal wall. There is usually little epididymal swelling. The diagnosis is made by the knowledge that the patient is suffering from Henoch–Schönlein purpura. Appendicitis may cause right-sided epididymitis by the tracking or

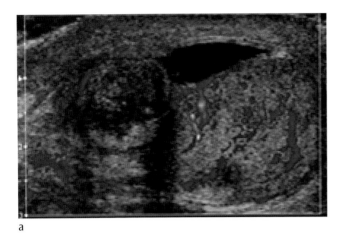
a

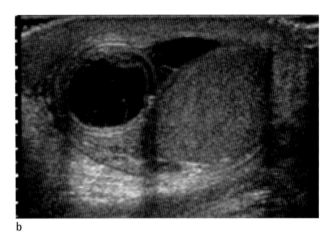
b

Figure 5.93
Torted hydatid of Morgagni. A 14-year-old boy with acute pain of 5 hours' duration. (a) The rounded torted hydatid is seen. The testis shows normal vascularity. (b) A different plane, showing the cystic nature of the lesion. (Reproduced with permission from Cochlin D Ll. Acute testicular pain. Imaging 2005; 17: 1–10.)

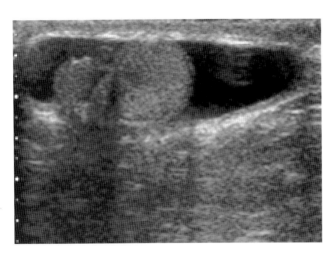

Figure 5.94
Torted testicular appendix. An 8-year-old boy with acute pain of about 6 hours' duration. The round swollen torted appendix is seen. This is a hydrocele. Doppler imaging showed normal testicular blood flow.

inflammation through the patent processus vaginalis. Usually, the right iliac fossa pain predominates. Occasionally, patients present with scrotal pain. There is, however, always right iliac fossa tenderness. The diagnosis is easily made provided the possibility is considered. Ultrasound or the lower abdomen is a good modality for the detection of acute appendicitis in children.

Testicular infarcts and hemorrhage into a tumor are both discussed earlier in this chapter.

OTHER SCROTAL LESIONS

Extratesticular cysts, tumors and masses[75–77]

General considerations

A large majority of extratesticular scrotal masses, unlike intratesticular masses, are benign. Cysts and small dense, rounded granulomas need no treatment unless symptomatic. Larger solid lesions are usually excised because of the small risk of malignancy and because they often cause discomfort. Smaller lesions of undetermined etiology are often monitored.

Cysts[78]

Cystic lesions may be epididymal cysts, spermatoceles or, occasionally, a loculated hydrocele. Spermatoceles may have slightly higher echodensity contents than epididymal cysts, always occur in the head of the epididymis and tend to be larger than epididymal cysts, which are usually small and anechoic. In most cases, however, a definitive distinction cannot be made. As they are all benign and are only treated if symptomatic, differentiation is not important.

Cysts or spermatoceles are almost always thin-walled, smooth regular structures with anechoic or slightly speckled low-echodensity contents (Figures 5.95 and 5.96) Very occasionally, however, they have echogenic contents,

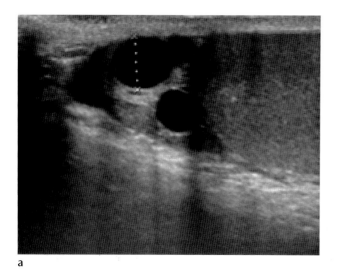
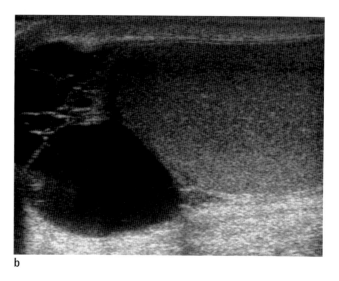

a

b

Figure 5.95
Epididymal cyst. (a) There are two cysts in the head of the epididymis. (b) Multiple epididymal cyst.

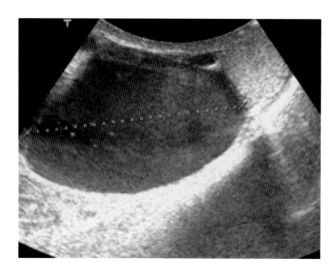

Figure 5.96
Spermatocele. A typically large echogenic spermatocele.

presumably due to hemorrhage, possibly infection (Figure 5.97). Torsion with hemorrhage has been described. Occasionally, they are irregular. Unlike cysts in other parts of the body, however, they are never malignant, so such changes are of no practical importance.

Small cysts may be surprisingly difficult to find. If this is so, the best approach is to ask the patient to locate the lesion, and then to hold it between finger and thumb while scanning from the other side of the testis. This will readily locate the lesion on the scan. Palpable lesions must be found and categorized. Failure to find a lesion leads to a loss of confidence in the patient. The demonstration that

such a lesion is a cyst or other benign lesion is very reassuring to the patient.

A large cyst may simulate a hydrocele, but, unlike a hydrocele, there is no fluid anterior to the testis.

Multiple cysts or spermatoceles are sometimes seen. They are often associated with tubular or cystic ectasia of the rete testis (Figure 5.98). This is presumed to be due to obstruction of the sperm transport mechanism.

Cysts of the tunica albuginea are less common. They are described in the section on testicular cysts, but they are included here as they sometimes project out into the extratesticular space. It is usually clear that the tunica surrounds them (Figure 5.99).

Tubular ectasia of the epididymis[79]

Tubular ectasia of the epididymis is a condition that occurs usually as a long-term sequel to vasectomy, occasionally idiopathic. It presents clinically as a bulky epididymis or sometimes as a focal mass. With high-resolution systems, normal epididymal tubules are often seen. The dilated tubules of tubular ectasia are clearly seen, but there is a range of sizes between normal and ectasia (Figure 5.100).

Solid extratesticular masses[80–88]

The swollen epididymis of acute epididymitis, chronic epididymitis or postinflammatory change may present as a palpable mass (see section on epididymo-orchitis).

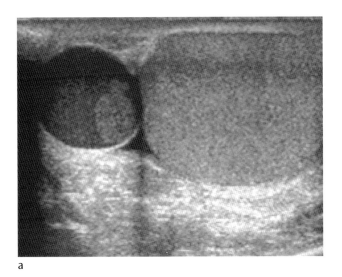

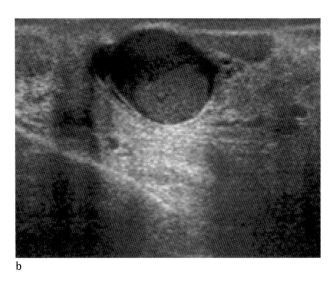

a

b

Figure 5.97
Echogenic cyst. (a,b) A rounded echogenic intracystic mass. This is presumably due to hemorrhage. On follow-up scans, the echogenic contents had disappeared.

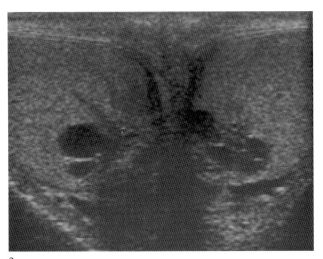

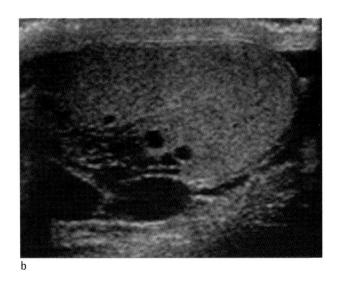

a

b

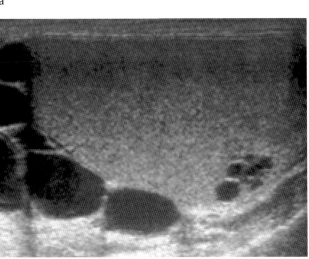

c

Figure 5.98
Obstruction of the sperm transport mechanism. (a,b) A 34-year-old man with oligospermic infertility. There are multiple epididymal cysts and cystic ectasia of the rete testes. (c) Another case with more marked epididymal cysts.

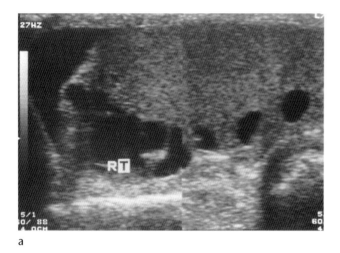

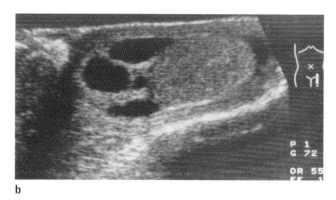

Figure 5.99
Tunica albuginea cyst. (a,b) Multiple tunica albuginea cysts in two separate patients. (Reproduced with permission from Rifkin MD, Cochlin DL. Imaging of the scrotum and penis. London: Martin Dunitz; 2002.)

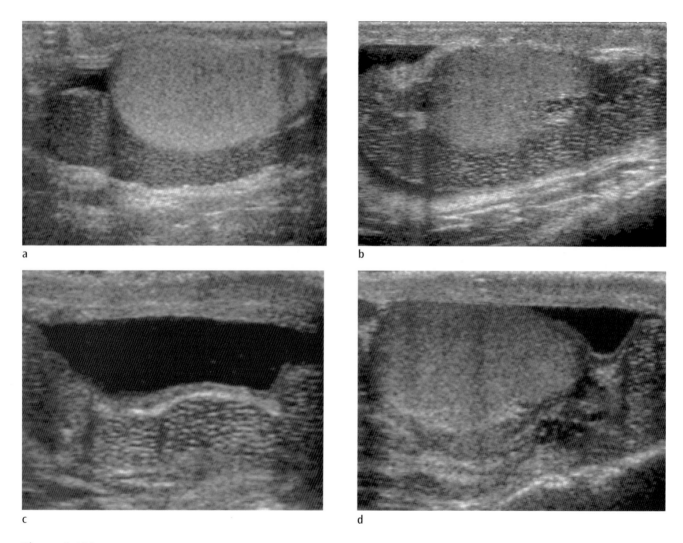

Figure 5.100
Tubular ectasia of the epididymis. (a) There is enlargement of the epididymal head and body. The ectatic tubules are readily seen. (b) A case affecting the whole epididymis and the rete testis. (c,d) Cases of ectasia affecting principally the epididymal body and tail.

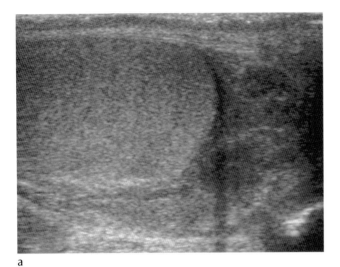

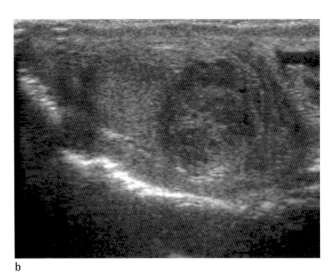

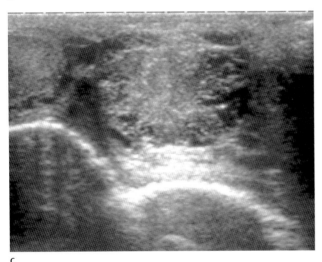

Figure 5.101
Postinflammatory epididymal mass. Three cases of postinflammatory masses in the epididymal tail. (a) The epididymal tail remains swollen after an episode of epididymitis. (b) There is a more circumscribed mass. (c) This mass is more echoic than usual. This case was presumed to be postinflammatory. The patient wanted excision. Histology showed non-specific fibrous and inflammatory changes.

Postinflammatory change has a range of ultrasonic appearances (Figure 5.101). The majority of masses are easily palpable but almost isoechoic with the epididymis, and thus poorly seen on ultrasound study. Others masses are more or less well-circumscribed and hypoechoic. Some of these masses are probably granulomas. However, few are excised, so the diagnosis is usually presumed from the history of previous epididymitis. It is certainly clear that these lesions do not progress: some apparently regress completely; some partially regress, but in some cases a smaller hard mass remains; and some, particularly the circumscribed hypoechoic lesions, remain unchanged.

Other solid masses represent a range of pathologic lesions, few of which may be distinguished by ultrasound. Perhaps the most common mass is a small mass, typically 5–10 mm, which often, though not invariably, presents some years after a vasectomy (Figure 5.102). Such masses are assumed to be sperm granulomas. They are smooth round lesions, almost isoechoic with the epididymis.

They are often only seen as the epididymis moves around them while scanning with palpation. Also common, are similar but larger lesions, that are usually situated in the tail of the epididymis (Figure 5.103). These are presumed to be benign adenomatoid tumors. The diagnosis is usually presumed as few of these lesions are excised. Other very rare lesions include cystadenoma, rhabdomyosarcoma, mesothelioma, lipoma, liposarcoma, leiomyoma, fibrosarcoma and myxochondrosarcoma (Figure 5.104). The usual policy is to assume that small, less than 20 mm lesions are benign, but to advise the patient to present for a rescan if they change. For rapidly growing lesions, lesions that are irregular or more than 20 mm, excision is advised, although even in this group the majority are benign.

The juvenile form of rhabdomyosarcoma is an exception. It grows to a large size. A large extratesticular tumor occurring in children may thus be assumed to be a rhabdomyosarcoma (Figure 5.105).

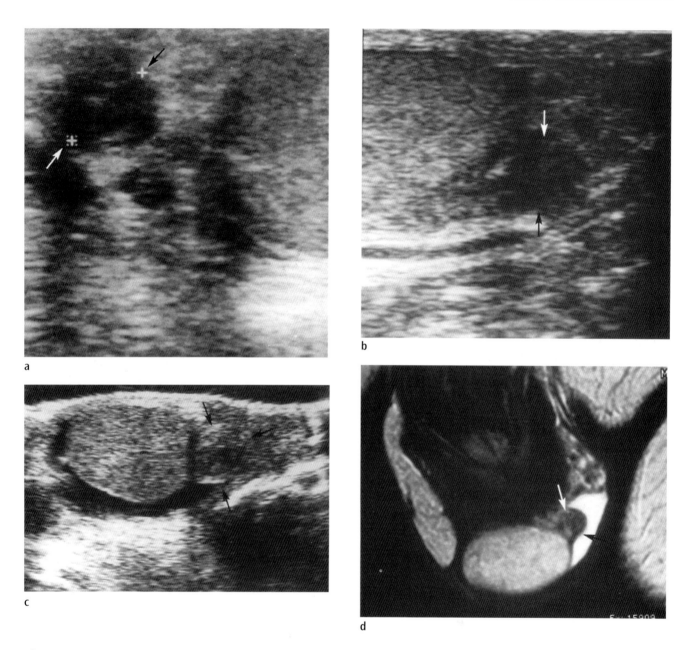

Figure 5.102
Sperm granuloma. (a–c) Ultrasound scans of sperm granulomas, demonstrating well-defined generally slightly hypoechoic lesions within the epididymis (arrows). (d) A T2-weighted MRI study shows a low-signal-intensity lesion. (Reproduced with permission from Rifkin MD, Cochlin DL. Imaging of the scrotum and penis. London: Martin Dunitz; 2002.)

Secondary deposits are rare in the scrotum. Epididymal metastases occasionally occur from the prostate, kidney and the gastrointestinal tract. They are indistinguishable from primary tumors (Figure 5.106).

Scrotoliths, scrotal 'pearls' or calculi, are freely mobile small round calcified masses that lie free and mobile in the scrotal cavity. The history is of a painless freely mobile palpable lesion. Many are incidental findings. They can be readily shown to move on ultrasound (Figure 5.107). They

were thought to be due to previously torted testicular appendices, but this is unlikely. Their etiology is unknown, but they are entirely innocuous.

Inguinal hernias

Inguinal hernias present as scrotal masses. In the vast majority of cases, the diagnosis is obvious on clinical

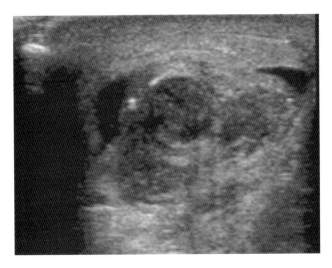

Figure 5.103
Adenomatoid tumor. Transverse view of the epididymal tail, showing a rounded, predominantly hypoechoic mass. The patient opted for excision, and histology showed a benign adenomatoid tumor.

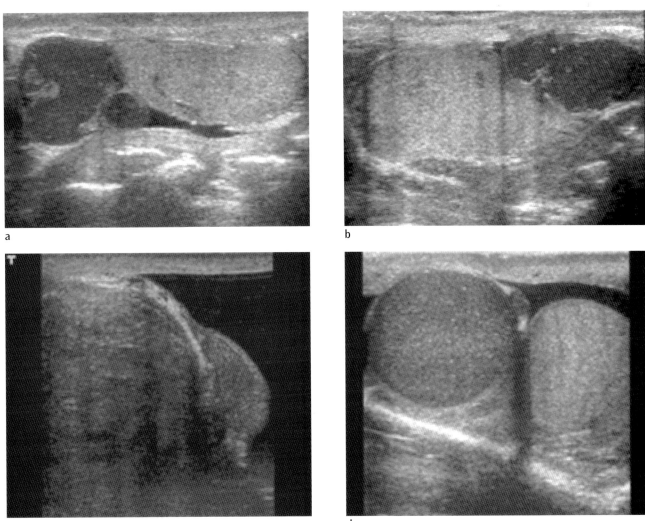

Figure 5.104
Large epididymal tumors. A selection of epididymal tumors, which, because of their size, were excised, with one exception: (d), the diagnosis was only made histologically after excision. (a) A very large tumor adherent to an atrophied testis very vascular on Doppler. This was a benign angioleiomyoma: (b) a sarcoma, (c) mesothelioma, (d) lipoma. In this case, the diagnosis was suggested pre-excision by the even shape and even hypoechoic echo pattern.

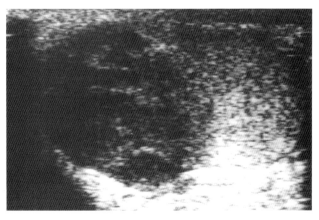

Figure 5.105
Juvenile rhabdomyosarcoma. This 5-year-old boy presented with scrotal mass. Excision revealed a rhabdomyosarcoma. These are often much larger than this at presentation.

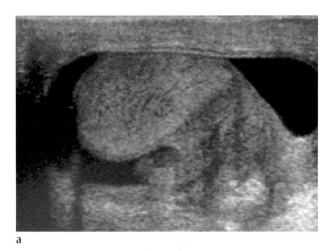

a

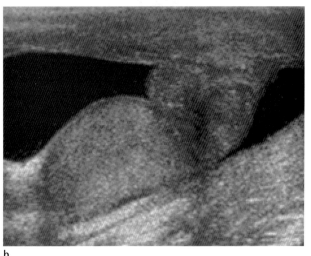

b

Figure 5.106
Secondary deposits. (a,b) A non-specific epididymal mass. The patient had known advanced prostate cancer. Excision revealed secondary deposits.

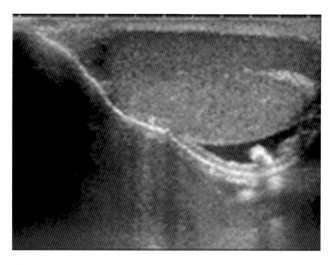

Figure 5.107
Scrotolith. There is a typical sonodense shadowing lesion lying posterior to the testis. This was mobile. It is typical of a scrotolith (also called scrotal pearls or scrotal calculi).

examination, but a minority may prove a diagnostic problem and be referred for ultrasound. The ultrasound picture is that of a confusing mass of mixed echodensity. If loops of bowel are present, they may be recognized by their pattern on the ultrasound image. Peristalsis may be seen. Otherwise, the position of the mass extending down from the inguinal ring is a clue. The ultrasonic picture may, however, be surprisingly difficult to interpret. The diagnosis must always be considered in a high complex mass (Figure 5.108).

Hydrocele

A hydrocele is an abnormally large volume of fluid between the tunical layers. A small amount of fluid is normally present and where the line is drawn between normal fluid and a hydrocele is subjective.

Clinically, hydroceles are divided into simple, containing fluid with no cells, and complicated, containing inflammatory cells or blood. Simple hydroceles may be idiopathic or secondary to testicular cancer, whereas complicated hydroceles may be due to inflammation or trauma. The distinction has little relevance to ultrasound, as both types initially have similar appearances, although complicated hydroceles may be more echogenic and later may develop fibrous septae.

In Western countries the majority of hydroceles are idiopathic, whereas a minority are secondary to tumor, inflammation or trauma. In some parts of the world the majority are due to parasitic infection. The role of ultrasound is to

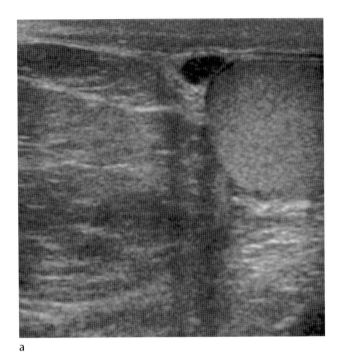

a

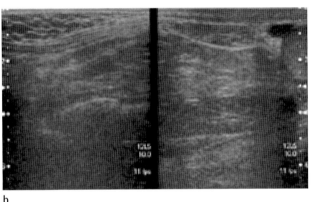

b

Figure 5.108
Inguinal hernia containing omentum. (a) The hernia with the scrotal sac. (b) Hernia passing through the inguinal canal.

confirm the diagnosis in cases of clinical doubt and to exclude underlying pathology, principally testicular tumor.

Testicular cancer normally, however, causes relatively small hydroceles. A large hydrocele is more suggestive of an idiopathic hydrocele or an inflammatory cause.

Ultrasonic appearances

Acute hydroceles are usually described as echo-free collections of fluid. With high-resolution systems, however, very fine swirling echoes, representing crystals, are seen (Figure 5.109). In certain parts of the world, bilharzia (*Schistosoma*

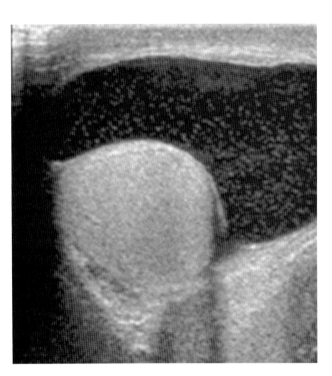

Figure 5.109
Simple hydrocele. There is excessive fluid, representing a simple hydrocele. The fine echoes are due to crystals.

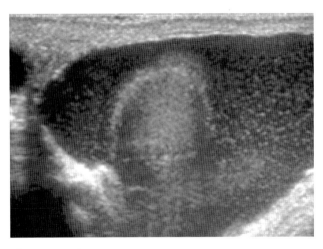

Figure 5.110
Schistosomiasis. There are coarse echoes due to ova.

haematobium) is the most common cause of hydrocele. In these cases, the hydrocele contains multiple slightly coarser echoes due to masses of eggs (Figure 5.110). Late cases are usually associated with calcification of the tunica and large masses in the spermatic cord. Filariasis is also a common cause of hydrocele in some parts of the world, associated with an epididymitis and often elephantiasis of the scrotal wall. In these cases the hydrocele is echo-free.

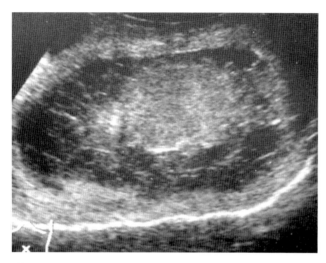

Figure 5.111
Inflammatory hydrocele. There is a heavily stranded
inflammatory hydrocele.

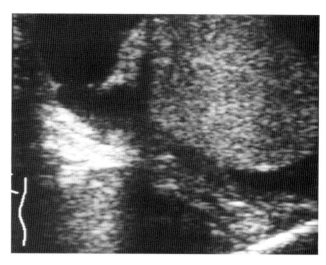

Figure 5.113
Recurrent postoperative hydrocele. This hydrocele recurred
after hydrocele surgery (Lord's procedure).The thick septae are
typical of a postoperative recurrence.

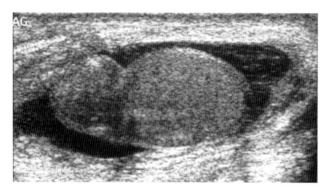

Figure 5.112
Chronic hydrocele. There are multiple septae adherent to the
tunica. The tunical layers are also thickened. These
appearances occur in a chronic or inflammatory hydrocele.

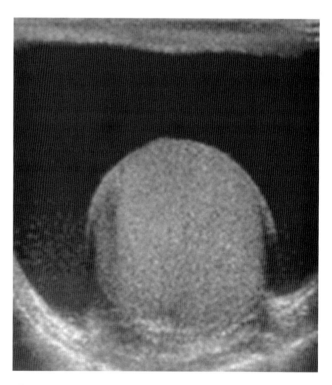

Figure 5.114
Simple hydrocele. The testis is seen lying in the most common
posterior position, attached to the scrotal wall.

Hydroceles secondary to epididymo-orchitis often contain echogenic material representing an inflammatory exu-
date (see Figure 5.63a). This may result, later, in echogenic
fibrous strands crossing the hydrocele fluid (see Figure
5.63b). Large amounts of echogenic material, however,
particularly if there is also a fluid–fluid level, suggest an
infected hydrocele (Figure 5.111).

Some chronic hydroceles have multiple septae (Figure
5.112), which are thought by some to occur due to chronicity; others believe that they represent previous infection or
inflammation.

Recurrent hydroceles occurring after surgery to prevent
hydrocele commonly have multiple coarse septae (Figure
5.113).

The testis is seen to lie at the posterior scrotal wall, where
the tunica is deficient (Figure 5.114).

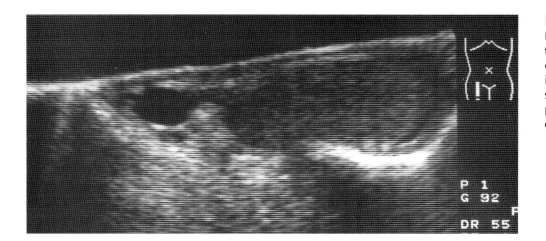

Loculated hydrocele

This term refers to cyst-like fluid collections occurring along the path of the processus vaginalis, representing part of the original lumen that remains patent (Figure 5.115). The diagnosis is suggested by the high position, although they cannot be distinguished from cysts of the cord. The distinction is in any case of no clinical importance.

Varicocele[89–96]

A varicocele is a dilatation of the pampiniform venous plexus with slow flow. The majority are due to incompetent valves in the testicular veins, whilst a minority result from obstruction of the spermatic vein, due to renal vein thrombosis or renal tumor extension on the left, or more rarely, involvement of the testicular vein by retroperitoneal tumor. The 'nutcracker' effect of compression of the left renal vein by the superior mesenteric artery is a contentious cause. An acute varicocele in an older man suggests one of these causes. Arteriovenous malformations of the scrotal vessels are rare. They cause a so-called high-flow varicocele.

A varicocele may present as a palpable mass, sometimes causing a 'dragging' pain on standing and after exercise. In these cases, clinical examination confirms the diagnosis. Emptying of the varicocele in the supine position distinguishes a varicocele due to reflux from one due to obstruction. If there is any clinical doubt about the diagnosis or the cause, however, imaging may be requested.

The other possible presenting symptom of varicoceles is infertility. Varicoceles may be associated with a decreased sperm count and/or decreased testicular volume, and bilateral varicoceles may cause infertility. Clinically, unilateral varicoceles may also do so, although some such cases are really bilateral with impalpable varicoceles on the opposite side. Hypospermia and decreased testicular size appear to be unrelated to the size of the varicocele, which is often clinically impalpable. In these cases, ultrasound with color flow Doppler is far more sensitive than clinical examination. Although the exact relationship between varicocele and infertility is poorly understood, it is clear that the general incidence of varicocele is 10% in all men, most on the left, 1% bilateral, whereas in infertile men the incidence is 40% on the left and 4% bilateral. These figures are based mainly on clinical examination, and the true incidence may be far higher. It is likely, in any case, that in young men varicocele is the most common cause of a low sperm count.

Technique of ultrasound examination

Varicoceles are usually readily demonstrated on a standard ultrasound examination. They may be confirmed by color Doppler examination. Most refluxing varicoceles show little spontaneous flow on color Doppler, because blood flow is very slow and below the threshold of the Doppler system. A Valsalva maneuver or a cough will cause retrograde flow in a refluxing varicocele, which fills with color. This is all that is necessary in the majority of patients.

A varicocele due to reflux will enlarge with the patient standing or sitting upright, and partially empty in the supine position. The usual technique is to carry out the ultrasound scan with the patient supine. Repeat with the patient standing or sitting is only infrequently used, and only if necessary. Some workers, however, argue that, once emptied, a varicocele may take up to 20 minutes to refill. They therefore examine the patient standing or sitting without first placing them supine. This seems to be logical, although in our practice we rarely do any more than a

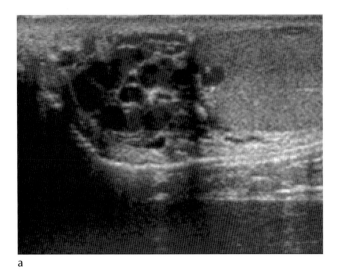

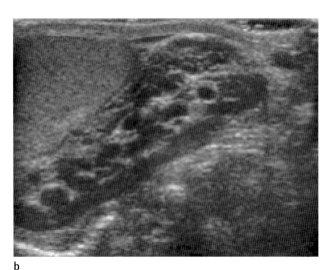

a   b

Figure 5.116
Varicocele. There is a large varicocele (a) above (b) posterior to the testis shown on gray-scale imaging.

supine scan with Valsalva. A Valsalva maneuver in the supine position enlarges a varicocele, but rarely as much as standing the patient.

If an obstructive varicocele is suspected, ultrasound examination of the left kidney and retroperitoneum is performed. Some would advocate scanning the left kidney in all cases. This is a safe approach. Others will only scan the kidney in cases of older men who think the varicocele is of recent onset, or if the Doppler study suggests an obstructive varicocele by demonstrating little reflux flow.

Ultrasound appearances

Large varicoceles appear as serpiginous lesions (Figure 5.116). Smaller ones may not show their serpiginous nature, but appear as multiple close-packed tubular structures.

Normal values for the size of pampiniform veins vary, but it is generally considered that veins measuring more than 2 mm in the supine position or 2.5 mm standing or with a Valsalva are abnormal. Using this criterion alone, however, small varicoceles will be missed. Enlargement of the normal veins on standing or with Valsalva should be minimal and less than 1 mm. Greater distension than this denotes a varicocele (Table 5.2).

Doppler examination should always be used, as it improves sensitivity and specificity. Small varicoceles may often only be demonstrated by color Doppler. The vast majority of varicoceles are refluxing varicoceles, and these are described first. One of the features of a varicocele is very slow venous flow. Little or no passive flow may be

Table 5.2 *Maximal diameter of the lumen of pampiniform plexus veins. Values above these indicate a varicocele*

Supine	Standing	Increase in size with Valsalva or cough
2 mm	2.5 mm	1 mm

demonstrated with Doppler imaging. Typically, at the most sensitive settings, a few segments of vein show color filling during quiet respiration. A Valsalva maneuver or a cough will cause a brief period of retrograde flow in cases of refluxing varicoceles (Figure 5.117). Standing a patient

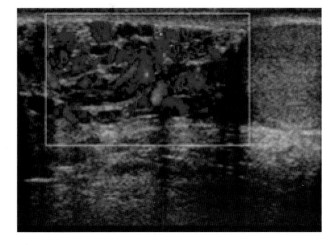

Figure 5.117
Varicocele. Colour Doppler image during a maneuver showing retrograde filling of the varicocele.

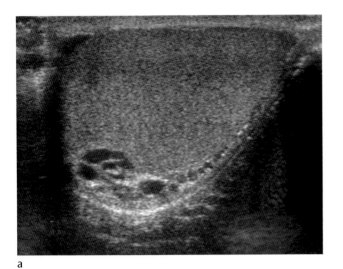

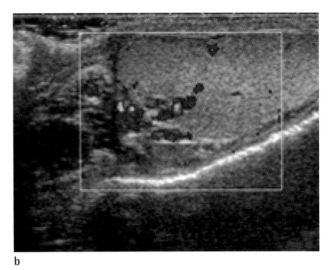

a   b

Figure 5.118
Intratesticular varicocele. (a) Cyst-like lesions in the testis. There was also a varicocele. (b) Doppler during a Valsalva maneuver shows extension of the varicocele into the testis.

after a period in the supine position often causes marked increase in flow due to rapid filling of the distending veins. This lasts for a variable period. In normal patients, minimal transient reversed flow may be seen during these maneuvers, but this is readily distinguished from retrograde flow through incompetent valves, which is greater and more prolonged. Some workers have reported reflux flow in normal subjects' pampiniform plexes, and suggest that this may not be distinguished from reflux in varicoceles but, in our experience, only minimal very transient reflux is seen in normal subjects.

The degree of reflux may be graded depending on whether less than one-third, between one-third and two-thirds or more than two-thirds of the veins in the field of view fill with color. The value of such grading is debatable, however. It probably depends on the velocity of the reflux stream. A low velocity will only register in those veins lying at a shallow angle to the Doppler beam. As the velocity increases, flow is registered in veins with greater angles to the Doppler beam.

Rarely, varicoceles extend into the testis. These have cyst-like structures at the testicular hilum, extending a variable depth into the testis. Their nature is readily demonstrated by Doppler study (Figure 5.118).

Obstructive varicoceles do not demonstrate significant reversed flow. In such cases it is important to extend the ultrasound study to the left kidney and retroperitoneum to look for a causative tumor.

A minority of varicoceles show high passive flow due to the formation of large collateral veins to epigastric, hypogastric, scrotal or the opposite gonadal veins (Figure 5.119). These cases tend not to respond well to embolization of the testicular vein alone, and may also require surgery to ligate collaterals.

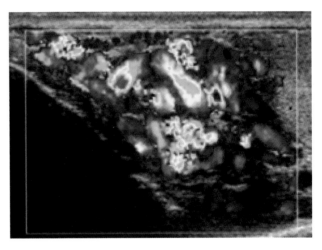

Figure 5.119
High-flow varicocele. Doppler study without a Valsalva shows high spontaneous flow.

The rare arteriovenous malformation of the scrotum shows increased arterial and often high pulsatile venous flow, quite different from a varicocele (Figure 5.120).

Follow-up after treatment

Varicoceles may be treated by catheter embolization of the testicular vein, percutaneous sclerotherapy or vascular surgery. Successful treatment leads to reduction in the size of the varicocele, cure of symptoms, arrest of testicular

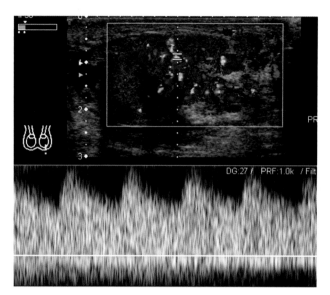

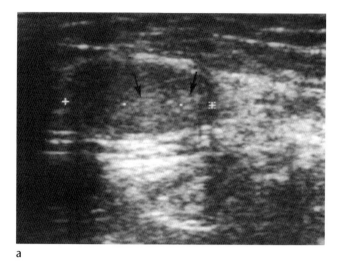

a

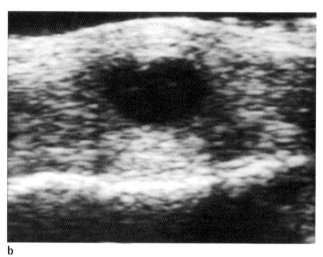

b

Figure 5.120
Arteriovenous malformation. Enlarged veins similar to a varicocele. Spectral Doppler shows very low resistance arterialized flow, indicating that the lesion is an arteriovenous malformation.

Figure 5.121
Undescended testis in the inguinal canal. (a) An undescended testis in the inguinal canal of a 30-year-old man. The testis is small but otherwise normal. Note the hilum (arrows). (b) An undescended testis in the inguinal canal in a 26-year-old man. In this case, the testis is irregular and hypoechoic, indicating fibrosis. (Reproduced with permission from Rifkin MD, Cochlin DL. Imaging of the scrotum and penis. London: Martin Dunitz; 2002.)

atrophy and, in cases of hypospermia, increase in sperm count, unless there is severe testicular atrophy.

Follow-up ultrasound will show any decrease in size of the varicocele and, in the longer term, will exclude continuing testicular atrophy. Reflux flow detected on Doppler examination may, however, persist despite successful treatment.

Undescended testes (cryptorchidism)[97,98]

Cryptorchidism is a term usually used as synonymous with undescended testis. Strictly, however, cryptorchidism describes abdominal testes, whereas those in the inguinal canal should be termed incompletely descended. Those found in any other position, such as the thigh, are termed ectopic. It is probably best to classify undescended testes as ectopic, totally undescended or incompletely descended, and to state the position. Often, however, the position, at least initially, is unknown and the general term 'undescended' must be used.

Approximately 3% of term male infants and up to 20% of premature male infants have undescended testes. The incidence at birth is, however, unimportant as 80% descend by 1 year, the incidence at this stage being 1%. Only a small minority are bilateral.

If orchidopexy is not performed probably below the age of 5, certainly below the age of puberty, the undescended

testis is usually sterile or hypospermic and atrophic. The incidence of malignancy (usually seminoma) is increased in the undescended testis (2.5–8.8% increased risk); 15–20% of tumors in cryptorchidism, however, occur in the contralateral (scrotal) testis. This suggests a common causative factor, possibly hormonal. Undescended testes are often histologically abnormal, although they may revert to a normal structure following orchidopexy. An abdominal testis may rarely produce sperm, but will always produce androgens. Because of the increased risk of malignancy, however, undescended testes in the postpubescent

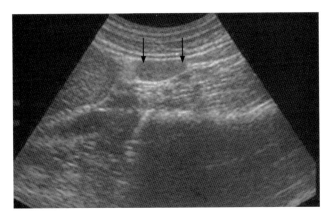

Figure 5.122
Undescended testis in the abdomen. The testis (arrowed) is lying anterior to the psoas muscle just below the inferior pole of the kidney. Detection of an abdominal testis by ultrasound study is exceptional.

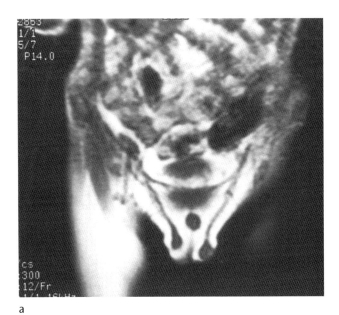

a

b

Figure 5.123
MRI study of undescended testis. MRI study in a child showing the right undescended testis at the internal ring and a normally descended left testis. (a) T1-weighted study. (b) Fat suppression study. (Reproduced with permission from Rifkin MD, Cochlin DL. Imaging of the scrotum and penis. London: Martin Dunitz; 2002.)

patient under 35 years of age are usually removed, if they can be found. Above the age of 35 it has been estimated that the risk of surgery is greater than the risk of leaving the testis in situ. The evidence is, however, weak.

Ultrasound may be requested to search for the undescended testis preorchidopexy or preorchidectomy. If a mass can be felt clinically in the inguinal canal, then ultrasound may determine whether this is the undescended testis. Rosenfield et al stress that the structure of the testis, particularly the mediastinum testis, should be positively identified, as otherwise the bulbous termination of the gubernaculum (the pars infravaginalis gubernaculi) may be mistakenly identified as the testis.[98a] The undescended testis usually appears as a smaller version of the normal testis. It sometimes has an inhomogeneous texture, probably indicating dysplasia.

About half of undescended testes lie in the inguinal canal or below the external ring, and these are easily seen on ultrasound (Figure 5.121). Half are situated intra-abdominally, anywhere between the inguinal canal and the renal hilum. For these, ultrasound is rarely helpful (Figures 5.122 and 5.123), and other forms of imaging should be used. The best modality to search for the testis is laparoscopy, followed by laparoscopic surgery for its excision. MRI is the best non-invasive modality, and has largely replaced CT. Arteriography and venography have also been used. A proportion of undescended testes may be very atrophic, due either to primary atrophy or torsion, and these will not be found by any imaging modality. A small minority of testes lie in ectopic sites (Figure 5.124). These are often clinically palpable. The sonologist should be aware of these potential sites when performing the ultrasound study.

Ultrasound may be requested postorchidopexy to assess the viability of the testis. In these cases, Doppler studies

may be performed. Some prepubescent testes, however, have very small vessels. It has been stated that up to 50% may not be detectable on Doppler studies, less in atrophic testes. With the marked improvement in current ultrasound systems, however, the figure is probably far lower. The demonstration of flow therefore indicates viability, but

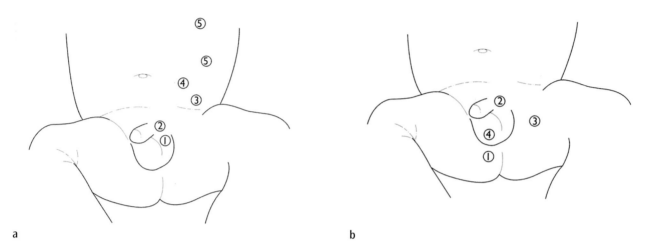

a

b

Figure 5.124
(a,b) Diagram of sites of ectopic testes. (Reproduced with permission from Rifkin MD, Cochlin DL. Imaging of the scrotum and penis. London: Martin Dunitz; 2002.)

failure to demonstrate flow does not necessarily indicate non-viability. In cases where no flow is shown, isotope studies are necessary to assess viability. Ultrasound contrast studies may be utilized in the future, but currently available agents are not licensed for use in children.

Because of the increased risk of malignancy in the undescended testis even after orchidopexy and in the contralateral testis, it would be logical to use ultrasound as a screening test for this but, to the author's knowledge, this is performed in few if any centers.

Differential diagnosis

The differential diagnoses are congenital absence of testis and retractile testes. Congenital absence is, however, rare, and if a testis is absent from the scrotal sac, undescended testes must always be assumed as by far the more common anomaly. Retractile testes, sometimes called pseudocryptorchidism, may usually be distinguished from true undescended testes by a good clinician. Although difficult to see ultrasonically, they will be detected with good technique.

Pseudocryptorchidism

This is a condition usually occurring in young children in whom contraction of the cremaster muscle causes a normal scrotal testis to retract into the inguinal canal or even

into the abdomen, thus simulating true cryptorchidism. The distinction can usually be made by a skilled clinician. Occasionally, however, the condition may persist in older children or even adults, rendering ultrasonic examination impossible if retraction has occurred. Such retraction usually occurs after the examination has commenced. It then has to be temporarily abandoned, but may be recommenced later. This time, a finger placed over the external inguinal ring will prevent ascent of the testis. Scanning infants in a bath of warm water often prevents retraction.

Congenital absence of the testis

Congenital absence of one or both testes is relatively rare, occurring in about 30/100 000 males. It accounts, however, for about 4% of cases of apparent undescended testes. In cases of an empty hemiscrotum, if an undescended testis is not detected, the differentiation between an absent testis and an undetected undescended or ectopic testis is very difficult. Undescended testes above the inguinal canal or ectopic testes are rarely shown by ultrasound, more often by CT or MRI, but failure to detect a testis by any of the methods does not prove its absence. At venography, an absent gonadal vein suggests an absent testis, although in 30% of such cases a testis is present. If no testis is found at laparoscopy, absence is assumed. Although undescended testis may be associated with other congenital anomalies, congenital absence is usually an isolated anomaly.

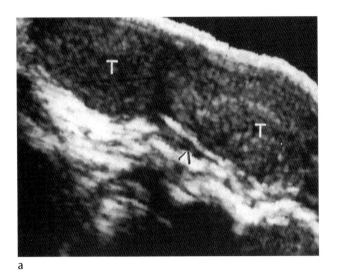
a

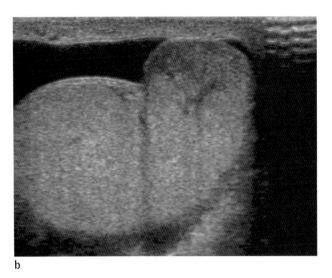
b

Figure 5.125
Polyorchidism. (a) A bifid testis with separate moieties (T). There is a single epididymis (arrowhead). (Reproduced with permission from Rifkin MD, Kurtz AB, Pasto MB, Goldberg BB. Polyorchidism diagnosed preoperatively by ultrasound. J Ultrasound Med 1983; 2: 93–94.) (b) A double testis with both moieties joined.

Other congenital conditions

Polyorchidism[99–102]

This is a rare congenital anomaly not associated with any other abnormality. It is usually unilateral, but occasionally bilateral. The testis may be bifid, or the duplicated testis may have two completely separate moieties. They usually share a common tunica albuginea epididymis and vas deferens, but may rarely be totally duplicated with separate epididymes and vas. Spermatogenesis is normal, and the condition is usually regarded as innocent, although an increased incidence of malignancy has been reported.

The diagnosis may come to light at any age when a scrotal mass is noted either by the patient or incidentally during medical examination. The diagnosis may be confirmed by ultrasound, when the duplicated moieties have the same appearance as the normal testis (Figure 5.125). MRI is increasingly being used, normal testicular tissue giving a uniformly high signal on T2-weighted images. Imaging is usually sufficient to confirm the diagnosis and surgery is unnecessary. If there is any doubt, however, either on imaging or clinically, open biopsy is advisable, particularly in view of the small but definite increase in malignancy in duplicated testes.

Splenogonadal fusion syndrome[103–105]

This rare condition is a form of accessory spleen in which the splenic tissue is fused, to a greater or lesser degree, to

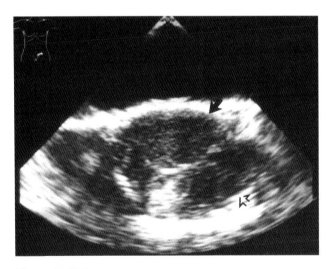

Figure 5.126
Splenogonadal fusion. A mass (closed arrow) is seen above the testis (open arrow). Open biopsy revealed normal splenic tissue. (Reproduced with permission of Dr R G Henderson and the editors Clinical Radiology.)

the upper pole of the left testis. It may be associated with inguinal hernia and cryptorchidism. The ultrasound appearances have only been described in a few cases, but appearances are of a hypoechoic testicular mass, indistinguishable from testicular tumor or lymphoma (Figure 5.126). The diagnosis may be suspected if the testicular mass presents in childhood, especially if there are other congenital anomalies. If the diagnosis is suspected, isotope scanning with technetium sulfur-colloid will confirm the diagnosis by showing uptake in the lesion.

Testicular size: macro-orchidism, hypogonadism and atrophy

Measurement[106,107]

Testes are traditionally measured by subjective clinical palpation or by calipers through the scrotal wall. Ultrasound provides a far more accurate method of measurement, if such accuracy is required. Accurate measurements are only required in the treatment of hypogonadism with gonadotropin-releasing hormone, where serial measurements are necessary to evaluate the efficacy of the treatment.

The simplest and most reproducible method of ultrasonic measurement is to make linear measurements in the long axis and two short axes. These measurements may be used alone, or may be used to calculate a volume by assuming a regular ovoid shape. The three measurements are multiplied together, and the product multiplied by 0.523.

Another method of measuring volume is to take multiple transverse scans of the testis at known length increments and calculate the volume from the multiple areas so obtained. Although methods for doing this have been devised, in practice the inability to completely immobilize the testis, and to accurately scan at the small length increments involved, makes it less accurate than the simpler three-linear method.

Normal adult testicular measurements are given at the beginning of the chapter.

Anomalies in size

Clinical considerations

Macro-orchidism is rare. It occurs in the fragile X syndrome in association with macrogenitosomia, and in this condition the cause is obvious. Idiopathic macro-orchidism has also been described in which the testes exceed normal values for linear measurements and volume, but otherwise appear normal.

Decrease in testicular size is more common, occurring in cryptorchidism, in association with varicocele and a low sperm count, and in ischemia due to previous herniorrhaphy, atheroma, diabetes, trauma, torsion, severe orchitis or mumps orchitis. Hypogonadotrophism is a less common cause.

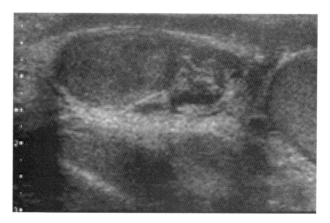

Figure 5.127
Ischemic atrophy. The right testis is atrophied and inhomogeneous with hypoechoic foci.

Ultrasound appearances

As well as being small, an atrophic testis due to ischemia or mumps may appear normal, be hypoechoic or of mixed normoechoic and hypoechoic pattern (Figure 5.127). This is due to variously sized infarcts in the testis, which cause hypoechoic areas in part or the whole of the testis and hyperechoic areas presumably due to scarring. Atrophy from other causes may also cause inhomogeneous testis, but usually less marked. The appreciation of this is important so as not to confuse the changes with tumor. A tumor would normally have enlarged a testis by the time of presentation. Tumors do, however, occur in small previously undescended and dysplastic testes. If there is any doubt, close ultrasonic follow-up is necessary.

Scrotal trauma[108]

Blunt trauma to the scrotum often results in a swollen, tender scrotum, rendering clinical examination unhelpful. The reason for imaging is to avoid unnecessary surgery. Early surgical intervention is necessary in cases of testicular rupture to preserve testicular function, whereas intra-testicular hematoma, hematoma of the scrotal layers or hematocele with a normal testis may be treated conservatively. Although it is not possible to definitely distinguish between these in all cases, in most the distinction may be made. In cases of a testicular lesion presumed to be hematoma, the possibility of trauma revealing a pre-existing testicular tumor must also be considered.

Ultrasound appearances

The common features of scrotal trauma are swelling of the testis or scrotal wall, hematoma in the testis, epididymis or

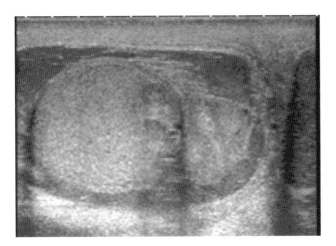

Figure 5.128
Scrotal trauma. There is a hematocele and an intratesticular hematoma. The epididymis is enlarged, presumably due to traumatic epididymitis.

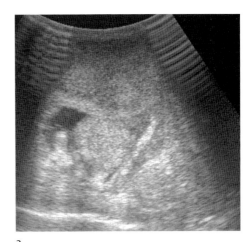

a

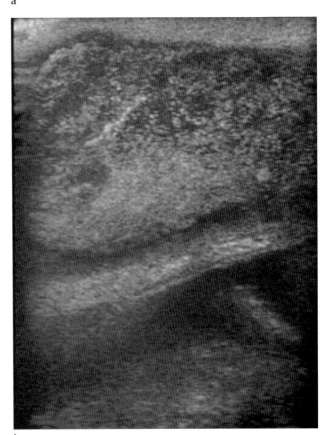

b

Figure 5.129
Scrotal wall hematoma. (a) A few hours after the trauma, there is a large scrotal wall hematoma. The testis is intact. (b) 4 days later, and the hematoma is becoming more hypoechoic.

scrotal wall, and hematocele (blood in the scrotal cavity) (Figure 5.128).

None of these normally require intervention. The importance of ultrasonic examinations is to detect or exclude rupture of the tunica albuginea (fractured testis) and to detect or exclude pre-existing testicular tumor, the latter particularly if the symptoms and signs appear to be greater than expected from the severity of the traumatic incident.

Analysis of rather small series produces conflicting results, varying from very high to very low sensitivities and specificities. It seems clear, however, that the majority of blunt scrotal trauma cases show a picture of swelling of the testis and scrotal wall, but with a homogeneous testis. There may also be a hematocele or reactive hydrocele (these cannot be distinguished from each other in the early stages). Such cases can be reassured and need no surgical intervention.

Hematomas of the scrotal wall may be indistinguishable from edema, or may be more discrete hypoechoic or hyperechoic areas, depending on chronicity (Figure 5.129). Hematoceles are hypoechoic in the early stages and indistinguishable from a hydrocele. Like hematomas elsewhere, they solidify and become echoic, and then undergo patchy liquefaction and eventually resorb, but often leaving a residual hydrocele with fibrous strands across it (Figure 5.130).

Testicular hematomas are a more difficult problem. It is never possible, on a single scan, to distinguish between a hematoma and a tumor (Figure 5.131). In cases where there are no associated features of testicular rupture, ultrasonic follow-up is indicated. The typical temporal changes of a hematoma, or absence of these changes, will give a probability of hematoma or tumor on which treatment may be based.

Cases of testicular hematoma with associated scrotal cavity fluid are difficult. These are the cases that lead in

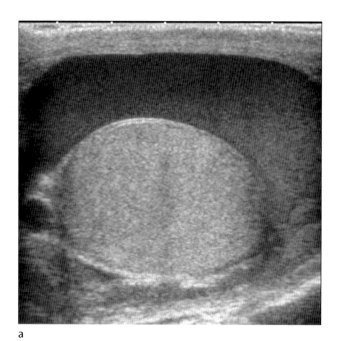

a

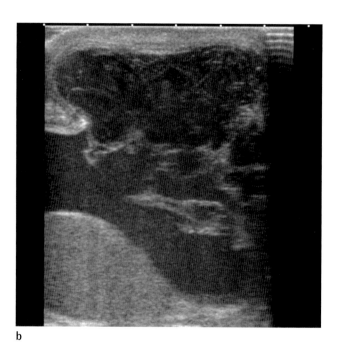

b

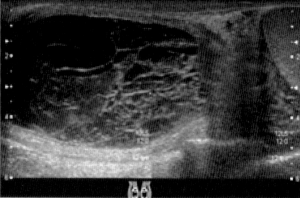

c

Figure 5.130
Hematocele: stages in development. (a) Acute hematocele 2 hours after trauma. The blood is echogenic but still liquid. (b) Three weeks after injury, the hematocele is of mixed liquid and semi-solid appearance. (c) Six weeks later, there is a typical liquefied hematoma with fibrous strands.

some series to poor prediction of testicular rupture. Such cases must be regarded as possible ruptured testis and treated accordingly, even without obvious ultrasound appearances of rupture of the tunica albuginea. Although a fairly high proportion of these will be found to be 'false-positive' diagnoses at surgery, the alternative is to accept false negatives with resultant loss of the testis.

Finally, a minority of cases will show an obvious irregular area at the surface of the testis. The testicular tubules spilling out through the tunical rupture may resemble the bristles of an old toothbrush. Together with fluid in the scrotal cavity, this appearance is diagnostic of a fractured testis (Figure 5.132).

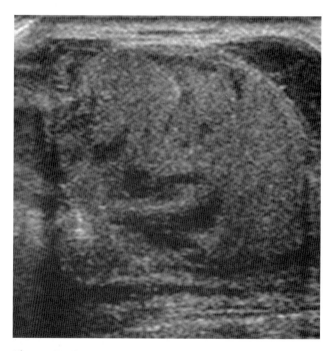

Figure 5.131
Intratesticular hematoma. Hypoechoic areas in the testis, representing hematomas.

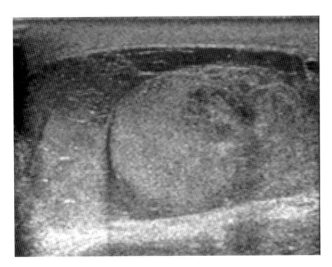

Figure 5.132
Testicular rupture. Intratesticular hematomas and a hematocele. The line of the tunica albuginea is irregular and broken anteriorly due to testicular fracture.

References

1. Blaivas M, Brannam L. Testicular ultrasound. Emerg Medicine Clin North Am 2004; 22(3): 723–48, xi.
2. Oyen RH. Scrotal ultrasound. Eur Radiol 2002; 12(1): 19–34.
3. Horstman WG. Scrotal imaging. Urol Clin North Am 1997; 24(3): 653–71.
4. Black JA, Patel A. Sonography of the normal extratesticular space. AJR Am J Roentgenol 1996; 167(2): 503–6.
5. Dogra VS, Gottlieb RH, Oka M, Rubens DJ. Sonography of the scrotum. Radiology 2003; 227(1): 18–36.
6. Bree RL, Hoang DT. Scrotal ultrasound. Radiol Clin North Am 1996; 34(6): 1183–205.
7. Keener TS, Winter TC, Nghiem HV, Schmiedl UP. Normal adult epididymis: evaluation with color Doppler US. Radiology 1997; 202(3): 712–4.
8. Dieckmann KP, Pichlmeier U. Clinical epidemiology of testicular germ cell tumors. World J Urol 2004; 22(1): 2–14.
9. Carmignani L, Gadda F, Gazzano G, et al. High incidence of benign testicular neoplasms diagnosed by ultrasound. J Urol 2003; 170(5): 1783–6.
10. Hindley RG, Chandra A, Saunders A, O'Brien TS. Impalpable testis cancer. BJU Int 2003; 92(6): 572–4.
11. Browne RF, Jeffers M, McDermott T, et al. Technical report. Intraoperative ultrasound-guided needle localization for impalpable testicular lesions. Clin Radiol 2003; 58(7): 566–9.
12. Passarella M, Usta MF, Bivalacqua TJ, Hellstrom WJ, Davis R. Testicular-sparing surgery: a reasonable option in selected patients with testicular lesions. BJU Int 2003; 91(4): 337–40.
13. Mostafi FK, Sisterhenn IA. Histologic typing of testis tumors, 2nd edn. Berlin: Springer-Verlag, 1998.
14. Grantham JG, Charboneau JW, James EM, et al. Testicular neoplasms: 29 tumors studied by high-resolution US. Radiology 1985; 157: 775–80.
15. Mazzu D, Jeffrey RB Jr, Ralls PW. Lymphoma and leukemia involving the testicles: findings on gray-scale and color Doppler sonography. AJR Am J Roentgenol 1995; 164(3): 645–7.
16. Eskey CJ, Whitman GJ, Chew FS. Malignant lymphoma of the testis. AJR Am J Roentgenol 1997; 169(3): 822.
17. Moorjani V, Mashankar A, Goel S, et al. Sonographic appearance of primary testicular lymphoma. AJR Am J Roentgenol 1991; 157(6): 1225–6.
18. Cho JH, Chang JC, Park BH, Lee JG, Son CH. Sonographic and MR imaging findings of testicular epidermoid cysts. AJR Am J Roentgenol 2002; 178(3): 743–8.
19. Atchley JT, Dewbury KC. Ultrasound appearances of testicular epidermoid cysts. Clin Radiol 2000; 55(7): 493–502.
20. Moghe PK, Brady AP. Ultrasound of testicular epidermoid cysts. Br J Radiol 1999; 72(862): 942–5.
21. Lowenthal SB, Goldstein AM, Terry R. Cholesterol granuloma of tunica vaginalis simulating testicular tumor. Urology 1981; 18(1): 89–90.
22. Schwerk WB, Schwerk WN, Rodeck G. Testicular tumors: prospective analysis of real-time US patterns and abdominal staging. Radiology 1987; 164: 369–74.
23. Fraley EE, Lange PH, Kennedy BJ. Germ-cell testicular cancer in adults. N Engl J Med 1979; 301: 1371–7.
24. Thava V, Cooper N, Egginton JA. Yolk sac tumor of the testis in childhood. Br J Radiol 1992; 65: 1142–6.
25. Comiter CV, Renshaw AA, Benson CB, Loughlin KR. Burned-out primary testicular cancer: sonographic and pathological characteristics. J Urol 1996; 156(1): 85–8.
26. Tasu JP, Faye N, Eschwege P, Rocher L, Blery M. Imaging of burned-out testis tumor: five new cases and review of the literature. J Ultrasound Med 2003; 22(5): 515–21.
27. Derogee M, Bevers RF, Prins HJ, et al. Testicular microlithiasis, a premalignant condition: prevalence, histopathologic findings, and relation to testicular tumor. Urology 2001; 57(6): 1133–7.
28. Miller RL, Wissman R, White S, Ragosin R. Testicular microlithiasis: a benign condition with a malignant association. J Clin Ultrasound 1996; 24(4): 197–202.
29. Bach AM, Hann LE, Shi W, et al. Is there an increased incidence of contralateral testicular cancer in patients with intratesticular microlithiasis? AJR Am J Roentgenol 2003; 180(2): 497–500.
30. Middleton WD, Teefey SA, Santillan CS. Testicular microlithiasis: prospective analysis of prevalence and associated tumor. Radiology 2002; 224(2): 425–8.
31. Leenen AS, Riebel TW. Testicular microlithiasis in children: sonographic features and clinical implications. Pediatr Radiol 2002; 32(8): 575–9.
32. Bushby LH, Miller FN, Rosairo S, Clarke JL, Sidhu PS. Scrotal calcification: ultrasound appearances, distribution and aetiology. Br J Radiol 2002; 75(891): 283–8.
33. Ganem JP. Testicular microlithiasis. Curr Opin Urol 2000; 10(2): 99–103.
34. Golash A, Parker J, Ennis O, Jenkins BJ. The interval of development of testicular carcinoma in a patient with previously demonstrated testicular microlithiasis. J Urol 2000; 163(1): 239.
35. Drevelengas A, Kalaitzoglou I, Destouni E, Skordalaki A, Dimitriadis A. Bilateral Sertoli cell tumor of the testis: MRI and sonographic appearance. Eur Radiol 1999; 9(9): 1934.
36. Maizlin ZV, Belenky A, Kunichezky M, Sandbank J, Strauss S. Leydig cell tumors of the testis: gray scale and color Doppler sonographic appearance. J Ultrasound Med 2004; 23(7): 959–64.
37. Avila NA, Shawker TS, Jones JV, Cutler GB Jr, Merke DP. Testicular adrenal rest tissue in congenital adrenal hyperplasia: serial sonographic and clinical findings. AJR Am J Roentgenol 1999; 172(5): 1235–8.
38. Dogra V, Nathan J, Bhatt S. Sonographic appearance of testicular adrenal rest tissue in congenital adrenal hyperplasia. J Ultrasound Med 2004; 23(7): 979–81.
39. Stikkelbroeck NM, Suliman HM, Otten BJ, et al. Testicular adrenal rest tumors in postpubertal males with congenital adrenal hyperplasia: sonographic and MR features. Eur Radiol 2003; 13(7): 1597–603.

40. Stikkelbroeck NM, Otten BJ, Pasic A, et al. High prevalence of testicular adrenal rest tumors, impaired spermatogenesis, and Leydig cell failure in adolescent and adult males with congenital adrenal hyperplasia. J Clin Endocrinol Metab 2001; 86(12): 5721–8.

41. Proto G, Di Donna A, Grimaldi F, et al. Bilateral testicular adrenal rest tissue in congenital adrenal hyperplasia: US and MR features. J Endocrinol Invest 2001; 24(7): 529–31.

41a. Eraso CE, Vrachliotis TG, Cunningham JJ. Sonographic findings in testicular sarcoidosis simulating malignant nodule. J Clin Ultrasound 1999; 27(2): 81–3.

42. Flanagan JJ, Fowler RC. Testicular infarction mimicking tumor on scrotal ultrasound–a potential pitfall. Clin Radiol 1995; 50(1): 49–50.

43. Sriprasad S, Kooiman GG, Muir GH, Sidhu PS. Acute segmental testicular infarction: differentiation from tumor using high frequency color Doppler ultrasound. Br J Radiol 2001; 74(886): 965–7.

44. Lee FT Jr. Sonographic diagnosis of superior hemispheric testicular infarction. AJR Am J Roentgenol 2002; 179: 775–6.

45. Piekos EJ, Jablokow VR. Secondary testicular tumors. Cancer 1972; 30: 481–5.

46. Glazier DB, Vates TS, Cummings KB, Antoun S. Adenocarcinoma of the rete testis. World J Urol 1996; 14(6): 397–400.

47. Chou SJ, Liu HY, Fu YT, Shyu JS, Sun GH. Cysts of the tunica albuginea. Arch Androl 2004; 50(2): 89–92.

48. Dogra VS, Gottlieb RH, Rubens DJ, Liao L. Benign intratesticular cystic lesions: US features. Radiographics 2001; 21 Spec No: S273–81.

49. Martinez-Berganza MT, Sarria L, Cozcolluela R, et al. Cysts of the tunica albuginea: sonographic appearance. AJR Am J Roentgenol 1998; 170(1): 183–5.

50. Weingarten BJ, Kellman GM, Middleton WD, Gross ML. Tubular ectasia within the mediastinum testis. J Ultrasound Med 1992; 11(7): 349–53.

51. Older RA, Watson LR. Tubular ectasia of the rete testis: a benign condition with a sonographic appearance that may be misinterpreted as malignant. J Urol 1994; 152(2 Pt 1): 477–8.

52. Tartar VM, Trambert MA, Balsara ZN, Mattrey RF. Tubular ectasia of the testicle: sonographic and MR imaging appearance. AJR Am J Roentgenol 1993; 160(3): 539–42.

53. Siegel MJ. The acute scrotum. Radiol Clin North Am 1997; 35(4): 959–76.

54. Black JA, Patel A. Sonography of the abnormal extratesticular space. AJR Am J Roentgenol 1996; 167(2): 507–11.

55. Dogra V, Bhatt S. Acute painful scrotum. Radiol Clin North Am 2004; 42(2): 349–63.

56. See WA, Mack LA, Krieger JM. Scrotal ultrasonography: a predictor of complicated epididymitis requiring orchidectomy. J Urol 1988; 139: 55–9.

57. Cook JL, Dewbury K. The changes seen on high-resolution ultrasound in orchitis. Clin Radiol 2000; 55: 13–18.

58. Basekim CC, Kizilkaya E, Pekkafali Z, et al. Mumps epididymo-orchitis: sonography and color Doppler sonographic findings. Abdom Imaging 2000; 25(3): 322–5.

59. Tarantino L, Giorgio A, de Stefano G, Farella N. Echo color Doppler findings in postpubertal mumps epididymo-orchitis. J Ultrasound Med 2001; 20: 1189–95.

60. Yang DM, Yoon MH, Kim HS, et al. Comparison of tuberculous and pyogenic epididymal abscesses: clinical, gray-scale sonographic, and color Doppler sonographic features. AJR Am J Roentgenol 2001; 177: 1131–5.

61. Turkvatan A, Kelahmet E, Yazgan C, Olcer T. Sonographic findings in tuberculous epididymo-orchitis. J Clin Ultrasound 2004; 32(6): 302–5.

62. Muttarak M, Peh WC, Lojanapiwat B, Chaiwun B. Tuberculous epididymitis and epididymo-orchitis: sonographic appearances. AJR Am J Roentgenol 2001; 176: 1459–66.

63. Begley MG, Shawker TH, Robertson CN, et al. Fournier gangrene: diagnosis with scrotal US. Radiology 1988; 169: 387–9.

64. Sidhu PS. Clinical and imaging features of testicular torsion: role of ultrasound. Clin Radiol 1999; 54: 343–52.

65. Mernagh JR, Caco C, De Maria J. Testicular torsion revisited. Curr Probl Diagn Radiol 2004; 33(2): 60–73.

66. Jequier S, Patriquin H, Filiatrault D, et al. Duplex Doppler sonographic examination of the testis in prepubescent boys. J Ultrasound Med 1993; 12: 317–22.

67. O'Regan S, Robitaille P. Orchitis mimicking testicular torsion in Henoch–Schönlein's purpura. J Urol 1981; 126: 834–5.

68. Ben-Sira L, Laor T. Severe scrotal pain in boys with Henoch–Schönlein purpura: incidence and sonography. Pediatr Radiol 2000; 30: 125–8.

69. Albrecht T, Lotzof K, Hussain HK, et al. Power Doppler US of the normal prepubertal testis: does it live up to its promises? Radiology 1997; 203(1): 227–31.

70. Dogra V, Bhatt S. Acute painful scrotum. Radiol Clin North Am 2004; 42: 349–63.

71. Sellars ME, Sidhu PS. Ultrasound appearances of the testicular appendages: pictorial review. Eur Radiol 2003; 13(1): 127–35.

72. Strauss S, Faingold R, Manor H. Torsion of the testicular appendages: sonographic appearance. J Ultrasound Med 1997; 16(3): 189–92; quiz 193–4.

73. Johnson KA, Dewbury KC. Ultrasound imaging of the appendix testis and appendix epididymis. Clin Radiol 1996; 51(5): 335–7.

74. Hesser U, Rosenborg M, Gierup J, et al. Gray-scale sonography in torsion of the testicular appendages. Pediatr Radiol 1993; 23(7): 529–32.

75. Black JA, Patel A. Sonography of the abnormal extratesticular space. AJR Am J Roentgenol 1996; 167(2): 507–11.

76. Yang DM, Kim SH, Kim HN, et al. Differential diagnosis of focal epididymal lesions with gray scale sonographic, color Doppler sonographic, and clinical features. J Ultrasound Med 2003; 22(2): 135–42; quiz 143–4.

77. Tessler FN, Tublin ME, Rifkin MD. Ultrasound assessment of testicular and paratesticular masses. J Clin Ultrasound 1996; 24(8): 423–36.

78. Rifkin MD, Kurtz AB, Goldberg BB. Epididymis examined by ultrasound. Radiology 1984; 151: 187–90.

79. Reddy NM, Gerscovich EO, Jain KA, Le-Petross HT, Brock JM. Vasectomy-related changes on sonographic examination of the scrotum. J Clin Ultrasound 2004; 32(8): 394–8.

80. El-Beheiry AH, El-Akhras AI, El-Sayed AI, Soliman A. Epididymal sperm granuloma. Arch Androl 1982; 8(1): 65–7.

81. Goodson JM, Fruchtman B. Spermatic granulomas of epididymis. Urology 1975; 5(2): 278–80.

82. Rovinescu I, Reid RG. The granulomatous lesions of the testicle and epididymis. Urol Int 1966; 21(6): 564–73.

83. Makarainen HP, Tammela TL, Karttunen TJ, et al. Intrascrotal adenomatoid tumors and their ultrasound findings. J Clin Ultrasound 1993; 21(1): 33–7.

84. Wood A, Dewbury KC. Case report: paratesticular rhabdomyosarcoma – color Doppler appearances. Clin Radiol 1995; 50(2): 130–1.

85. Mak CW, Tzeng WS, Chou CK, et al. Leiomyoma arising from the tunica albuginea of the testis: sonographic findings. J Clin Ultrasound 2004; 32(6): 309–11.

86. Bruno C, Minniti S, Procacci C. Diagnosis of malignant mesothelioma of the tunica vaginalis testis by ultrasound-guided fine-needle aspiration. J Clin Ultrasound 2002; 30(3): 181–3.

87. Fujisaki M, Tokuda Y, Sato S, et al. Case of mesothelioma of the tunica vaginalis testis with characteristic findings on ultrasonography and magnetic resonance imaging. Int J Urol 2000; 7(11): 427–30.

88. Kassis A. Testicular adenomatoid tumors: clinical and ultrasonographic characteristics. BJU Int 2000; 85(3): 302–4.

89. Mihmanli I, Kurugoglu S, Cantasdemir M, et al. Color Doppler

ultrasound in subclinical varicocele: an attempt to determine new criteria. Eur J Ultrasound 2000; 12(1): 43–8.

90. Ozcan H, Aytac S, Yagci C, et al. Color Doppler ultrasonographic findings in intratesticular varicocele. J Clin Ultrasound 1997; 25(6): 325–9.

91. Arslan H, Sakarya ME, Atilla MK. Clinical value of power Doppler sonography in the diagnosis of varicocele. J Clin Ultrasound 1998; 26(4): 229.

92. Pourbagher MA, Guvel S, Pourbagher A, Kilinc F. Intratesticular varicocele: report of two cases. Int J Urol 2003; 10(4): 231–2.

93. Atasoy C, Fitoz S. Gray-scale and color Doppler sonographic findings in intratesticular varicocele. J Clin Ultrasound 2001; 29(7): 369–73.

94. Kocakoc E, Serhatlioglu S, Kiris A, et al. Color Doppler sonographic evaluation of inter-relations between diameter, reflux and flow volume of testicular veins in varicocele. Eur J Radiol 2003; 47(3): 251–6.

95. Kocakoc E, Kiris A, Orhan I, et al. Incidence and importance of reflux in testicular veins of healthy men evaluated with color duplex sonography. J Clin Ultrasound 2002; 30(5): 282–7.

96. Tasci AI, Resim S, Caskurlu T, et al. Color doppler ultrasonography and spectral analysis of venous flow in diagnosis of varicocele. Eur Urol 2001; 39(3): 316–21.

97. Nguyen HT, Coakley F, Hricak H. Cryptorchidism: strategies in detection. Eur Radiol 1999; 9(2): 336–43.

98. Vijjan VK, Malik VK, Agarwal PN. The role of laparoscopy in the localization and management of adult impalpable testes. J Soc Laparoendosc Surg 2004; 8(1): 43–6.

98a. Rosenfield AT, Blair DN, McCarthy S, et al. The pars infravaginalis gubernaculi and associated structures: an imaging pitfall in the identification of the undescended testis (abstract). Society of Uroradiology Members' Scientific Program. Uroradiology, 1988.

99. Kao EY, Gerscovich EO. Benign testicular lobulation: sonographic findings. J Ultrasound Med 2003; 22(3): 299–301.

100. Amodio JB, Maybody M, Slowotsky C, Fried K, Foresto C. Polyorchidism: report of 3 cases and review of the literature. J Ultrasound Med 2004; 23(7): 951–7.

101. Chung TJ, Yao WJ. Sonographic features of polyorchidism. J Clin Ultrasound 2002; 30(2): 106–8.

102. Berger AP, Steiner H, Hoeltl L, Bartsch G, Hobisch A. Occurrence of polyorchidism in a young man. Urology 2002; 60(5): 911.

103. Stewart VR, Sellars ME, Somers S, Muir GH, Sidha PS. Splenogonadal fusion: B-mode and color Doppler sonographic appearances. J Ultrasound Med 2004; 23(8): 1087–90.

104. Kalomenopoulou M, Katsimba D, Arvaniti M, et al. Male splenic-gonadal fusion of the continuous type: sonographic findings. Eur Radiol 2002; 12(2): 374–7.

105. Nimkin K, Kleinman PK, Chappell JS. Abdominal ultrasonography of splenogonadal fusion. J Ultrasound Med 2000; 19(5): 345–7.

106. Taskinen S, Taavitsainen M, Wikstrom S. Measurement of testicular volume: comparison of 3 different methods. J Urol 1996; 155(3): 930–3.

107. Schiff JD, Li PS, Goldstein M. Correlation of ultrasonographic and orchidometer measurements of testis volume in adults. BJU Int 2004; 93(7): 1015–7.

108. Micallef M, Ahmad I, Ramesh N, Hurley M, McInerney D. Ultrasound features of blunt testicular injury. Injury 2001; 32(1): 23–6.

6

Ultrasound of the male anterior urethra

Laurence Berman

Introduction

The indications for urethral ultrasound are similar to those for the more familiar ascending contrast urethrogram. In the author's practice, referrals comprise two main groups:

- patients with suspected urethral strictures, referred by urologic surgeons
- patients with refractory or recurrent urethritis, who have attended the genitourinary medicine clinic.

In the former group, presenting symptoms may be a poor urine stream in a patient unlikely to have another cause such as prostatic hypertrophy, or patients with postmicturition dribbling, suspected to originate from a sump of urine proximal to a urethral stricture.

Referrals from the genitourinary medicine clinic are frequently under investigation both for a cause of their urethritis, such as a stricture or papilloma, as well as a urethral abnormality such as scarring that may be the result of recurrent infection. Rarer indications for referral may be for the demonstration of the pre- or postoperative urethra in patients with hypospadias.

Whether urethral ultrasound is adopted in any institution will depend on the attitudes of referring clinicians, as much as the aptitude and repertoire of the radiologist.

Classically, the urethra is divided into the anterior urethra, consisting of the penile and bulbar regions, and the posterior urethra, comprising the membranous and prostatic urethra. Some clinicians may consider a urethral investigation incomplete unless the entire urethra, anterior and posterior, has been defined by ascending and voiding contrast urethrography. This is an extremely conservative approach, as the symptoms and etiology of posterior urethral abnormalities are generally distinct from those involving the anterior urethra. Other clinicians confine their requests for imaging to the anterior urethra, whether by contrast study or ultrasound. Urethral ultrasound has little to offer clinicians who insist on voiding views of the posterior urethra.

Advantages of ultrasound over contrast urethrography

The ascending contrast urethrogram results in the distal urethra or fossa navicularis being occluded by a catheter or Knutson clamp, and therefore this region of the distal urethra cannot be imaged. Both these techniques of catheter anchorage are unsuitable for use in some patients with an abnormal urethral meatus such as in epispadias or hypospadias. Scrupulous technique is required to avoid both the introduction of infection and bubbles in the contrast medium, which may be misinterpreted as small filling defects or mucosal tags. Conversely, urethral ultrasound studies can, by the use of voiding images, demonstrate the fossa navicularis.

Whereas contrast studies only demonstrate the urethral lumen, urethrosonography demonstrates the periurethral soft tissue structures. The echo pattern of strictures and periurethral tissues may be useful in distinguishing strictures that may be treated by urethrotomy, from those requiring urethroplasty.

Subtle filling defects that are undetectable on contrast studies can be shown.

By definition, even in the most radiation-aware hands, contrast urethrography frequently necessitates gonadal irradiation.

Urethral ultrasound can be regarded as intrusive and embarrassing for the patient, but it is relatively private and discreet in comparison with the several operators usually present for the contrast urethrographic technique. Finally, although high-resolution ultrasound machines are a major investment, they are considerably more practicable for installation in a urologic outpatient clinic or office practice than fluorographic equipment.

Ultrasound technique

The normal anterior urethra is a collapsed structure when not voiding. Urethral ultrasound requires fluid distension

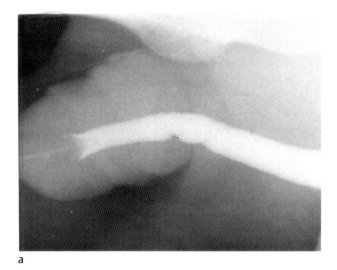

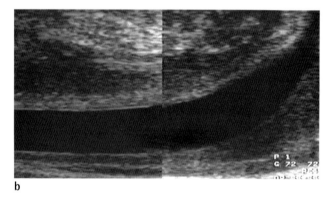

a   b

Figure 6.1
(a,b) Ascending contrast urethrograms demonstrating normal penile and bulbar urethra.

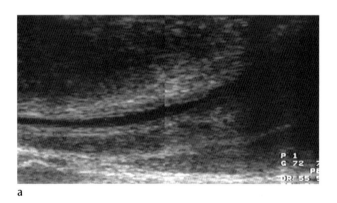

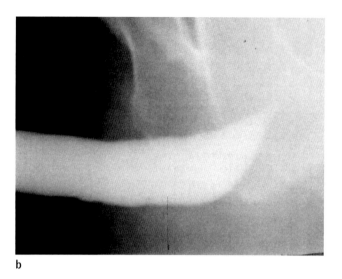

a   b

Figure 6.2
Normal bulbar urethra demonstrated by descending sonographic technique. (a) Under-distension due to poor stream. (b) Same patient demonstrates normal lumen, obtained a few seconds later.

of the lumen for the demonstration of strictures and filling defects unlike other penile ultrasound techniques, e.g. the demonstration of soft tissue abnormalities of Peyronie's disease or the Doppler studies of erectile dysfunction. Our initial sonographic experience involved scanning the penis and perineum during an ascending contrast urethrogram. The results of this early work convinced us that sonography demonstrated most abnormalities of the anterior urethral lumen with superior definition than the contrast study.[2] This confirmed the reports of other workers.[3–7]

Two different approaches have been described regarding the method of fluid distension required for urethral ultrasound and some authors have combined the techniques. The first involves retrograde injection, usually of saline but

occasionally of sterile gel, to achieve distension analogous to the contrast study. The disadvantages are patient discomfort and inability to demonstrate the fossa navicularis.[4–6,8] The alternative approach utilizes the patient's urine for urethral distension by the application of a clamp proximal to the corona of the glans during voiding.[3,9] The technique does not permit the demonstration of the fossa navicularis, but Gluck et al combined this with a limited ascending study with local anesthetic gel to achieve distension.[3] Both the ascending and descending sonographic techniques demonstrate the anterior urethra in a sagittal plane analogous to the contrast urethrogram (Figures 6.1 and 6.2). In addition, transverse views, which have no contrast urethrographic equivalent, but actually correspond to the view

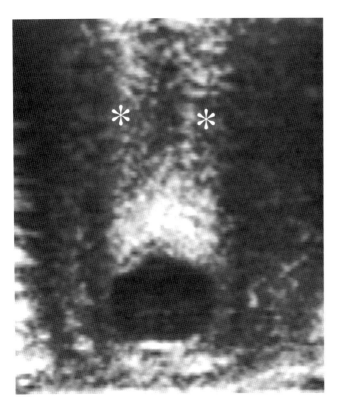

Figure 6.3
Transverse view of normal penile urethra. The corpora cavernosa are marked with asterisks.

down a urethroscope, may be obtained with both sonographic techniques (Figure 6.3). We have found that a further disadvantage of the voiding technique is that it requires a sufficient urine flow rate prior to clamping the glans, to achieve adequate distension and is therefore inappropriate where severe prostatism coexists with a stricture or indeed is the primary pathology.

We have modified the descending technique to achieve a method that appears to be more acceptable to patients, and has the advantage of demonstrating the fossa navicularis, in those patients where distal pathology is suspected. The same technique is invaluable in the assessment of hypospadias. Satisfactory studies have been performed in over 500 studies.

The patient attends with a full bladder. An initial conventional ultrasound study of the kidneys and bladder is only performed if specifically requested by the referring physician. The patient then stands adjacent to the ultrasound machine. Before voiding, the foreskin is retracted and the patient holds his penis at the level of the corona of the glans between thumb and forefinger. Voiding is attempted into an appropriate receptacle, such as a child's potty, placed on a stool of appropriate height for the patient. The patient is instructed to clamp the tip of the penis between thumb and forefinger once a steady flow of urine has been achieved.

Once the patient is applying this manual pressure, they are instructed to relax and not to continue to attempt to void. Penile, subscrotal and perineal views are obtained from a ventral approach. In contrast to the practice of other authors, we recommend inverting all images of the penile and bulbar urethra on the monitor to correspond to the familiar orientation of the contrast urethrogram.

A high-frequency linear array transducer is essential, and this should preferably be a variable-frequency transducer under the control of the operator. We find 7.5 MHz or even higher frequencies with direct skin contact suitable for the penile or subscrotal views, although other groups have achieved satisfactory images with a 5 MHz transducer and a dorsal approach to the penile urethra.[3,4] There is an extremely variable amount of subcutaneous fat in the normal male perineum. The bulbar urethra is often better demonstrated with a 5 MHz transducer, since it is deep to the thicker tissues of the perineum; therefore, the ability to rapidly switch between high and low frequencies may be extremely helpful. It is also an advantage to video the study, as this considerably shortens the study compared with trying to obtain excellent 'still' images from a frozen frame.

It is advisable to discuss an approach to probe sterility with the local microbiological department and infection control officer. Proprietary transducer condoms are available, while an alternative less-expensive approach is to protect the transducer face with transparent kitchen film, liberally coated with ultrasound gel.

It is our convention, for no good reason, to orientate all sagittal images with the tip of the penis directed to the left of the monitor. To image the fossa navicularis, the penile tip is scanned from a dorsal approach while the patient voids as vigorously as possible (Figure 6.4). The images for this part of the study are displayed conventionally and not inverted, once again to correspond to the position of the patient and conventional contrast urethrographic orientation.

In our experience, most patients after one false start are able to cooperate and coordinate for the descending study. Our failures have occurred in elderly subjects, patients with poor flow due to prostatism and the rare individual who is too inhibited to void in the presence of the ultrasonologist. In addition, patients with any motor handicap such as previous stroke or multiple sclerosis are unsuitable for the 'self-pinching' technique. For local convenience, we proceed to contrast urethrography in these 5% of subjects, but an ascending sonographic study would be an alternative. Children as young as 11 have been successfully evaluated using this self-clamping technique and studies on even younger children have been performed with the parent gently compressing the glans at the appropriate moment. As the descending ultrasound technique at our institute is no longer accompanied by a contrast study, our confidence

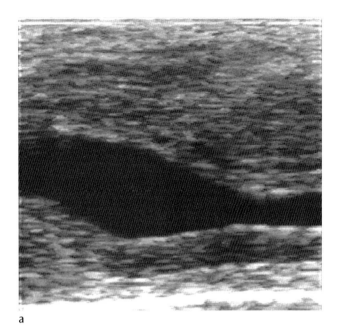

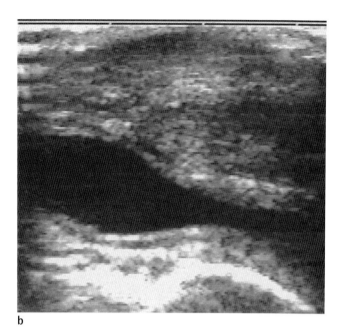

a   b

Figure 6.4
(a,b) Normal fossa navicularis. Images obtained during voiding.

with this approach is based on extensive clinical, urethro-scopic and surgical follow-up.

We recommend that, when commencing urethral ultrasound, the beginner undertakes the first few studies in conjunction with an ascending contrast urethrogram using the contrast medium as the distending medium. This enables the operator to become familiar with the anatomy and correlate the sonographic features with the more familiar contrast study appearances. The comparative images are also extremely helpful for securing the confidence and cooperation of the referring physician. Subsequently, either the ascending saline-distension technique or the descending urine-distension technique may be attempted.

Where it is intended to adopt the ascending technique using the instillation of saline as the standard method, we have noted that it is helpful to amputate the catheter tip distal to the balloon, as this obscures a further centimeter of lumen proximal to the fossa navicularis if it is not removed[2] (Figure 6.5).

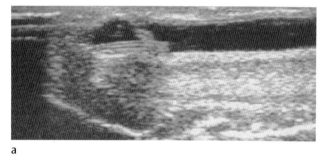

a

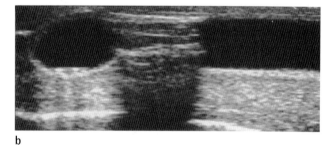

b

Figure 6.5
Montage of two studies performed by the ascending sonographic technique. (a) The catheter trimmed beyond the balloon. (b) Excess catheter obscuring the lumen.

The normal urethra

The normal urethra is demonstrated as a parallel-walled anechoic tube limited by the thin echogenic line of the mucosa. The bulbar urethra curves cephalad and tapers in the same configuration as the contrast study. Observation

of this curve is important to avoid one of the pitfalls described below. The fossa navicularis, an unfamiliar landmark to practitioners of contrast urethrography, is a focal dilatation of the distal penile urethra, identical to

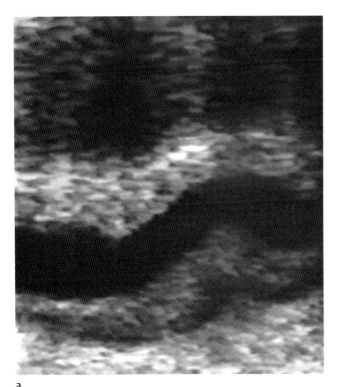

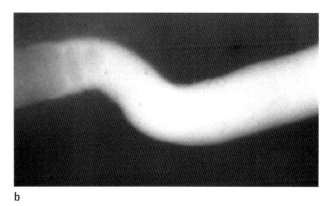

b

Figure 6.6
Normal kink at peno-scrotal junction. (a) This should not be misinterpreted as pathology. The analogous contrast study (b) is demonstrated.

a

illustrations in anatomy texts, which can be successfully demonstrated in the majority of normal subjects.

Care must be taken to ensure that the patient is voiding with sufficient flow before he occludes his stream with thumb and forefinger. Figure 6.2 demonstrates an apparently narrowed urethra, which appears normal on more forceful voiding a few seconds later.

In transverse view, the urethra appears as an anechoic circular structure in the center of the corpus spongiosum, with the two corpora cavernosa superiorly (see Figure 6.3). Contraction of the bulbospongiosus and elevation of the urogenital diaphragm can be seen in real time as the patient contracts his pelvic floor. A kink at the peno-scrotal junction is a normal finding, corresponding to the

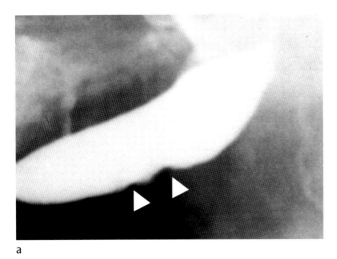

a

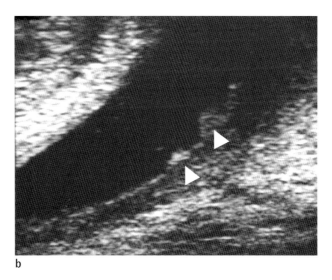

b

Figure 6.7
Subtle mucosal irregularities. (a) Subtle irregularities on the posterior aspect of the bulbar urethra are demonstrated on the descending sonographic study and (b) these correlate with ascending contrast study. Arrowheads demonstrate corresponding soft tissue abnormality.

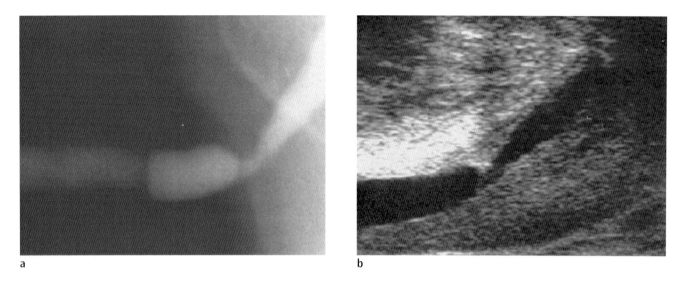

a   b

Figure 6.8
Mid-bulbar stricture. (a) A mid-bulbar stricture performed by voiding technique. (b) Corresponding ascending contrast urethrogram.

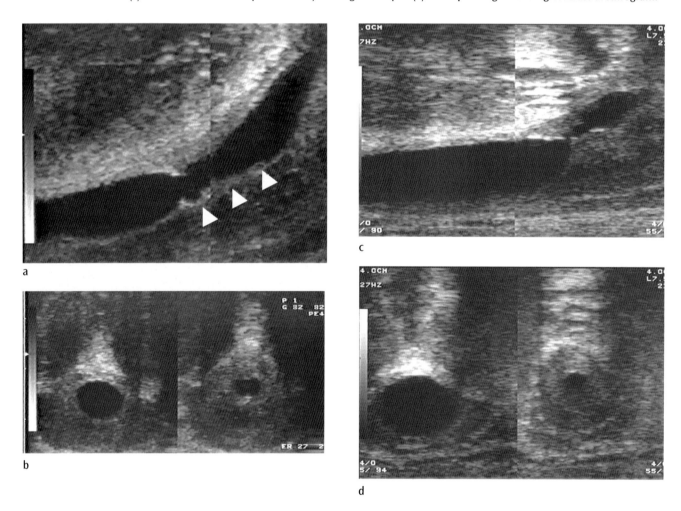

Figure 6.9
Bulbar stricture. (a) Bulbar stricture demonstrating echogenic periurethral fibrosis (arrowheads). (b) Transverse views of same patient through normal area (left) and through the stricture (right). Sagittal (c) and transverse (d) views of a further short mid-bulbar stricture associated with periurethral fibrosis.

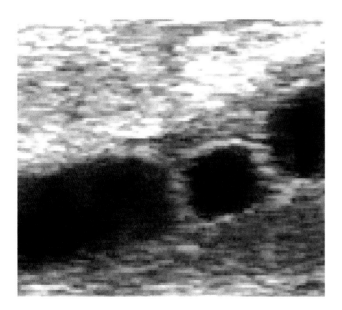

Figure 6.10
Web-like stricture in mid-bulbar urethra.

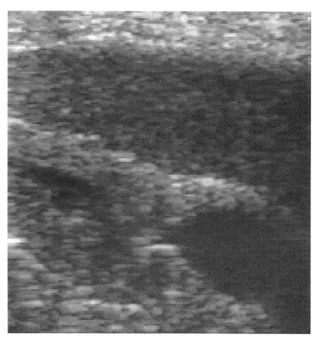

Figure 6.11
Images obtained during voiding demonstrate a stricture in the fossa navicularis. This would be a challenging diagnosis using an ascending technique.

contrast study, and should not be misinterpreted as a stricture (Figure 6.6). The glands and ducts of Cowper and Littre, which are sometimes seen on normal ascending contrast urethrography, are not demonstrable sonographically.

Abnormal findings

Strictures and focal mucosal irregularity

These occur at any site in the anterior urethra but are most frequently found in the bulbar urethra. They produce sonographic findings that correspond closely to their contrast urethrographic counterpart. Subtle focal mucosal irregularities (Figure 6.7) can be shown in addition to obvious strictures (Figures 6.8–6.11). Strictures in the fossa navicularis (Figure 6.11) are rare, but may be shown on the voiding study. We have noticed two interesting features of these distal strictures. First, the patients are usually able to indicate that they feel an obstruction at the tip of their penis when micturating. Second, the distension of the penile urethra proximal to the stricture can usually be demonstrated sonographically during voiding, in the pres-

ence of a distal stricture. In contrast, the normal fossa navicularis and distal penile urethra usually distends minimally, or not at all, during the normal voiding study of the tip of the penis.

In the presence of a stricture, it is important to demonstrate and comment on the adjacent periurethral soft tissues. Whereas some strictures merely consist of mucosal abnormalities, others are surrounded by echogenic soft tissue. This cuffing is more than an incidental interesting observation. Several excellent studies have correlated this finding with biopsy-proven fibrosis of the spongiosus. McAninch's group, who devised a classification of strictures based on the degree of periurethral fibrosis,[4] also noticed in a subsequent study that the degree of fibrosis is underestimated by the ultrasound study compared with full-thickness surgical biopsy.[8] A further interesting observation of McAninch's group is that sonography and contrast urethrography provide equal and accurate estimates of stricture length in the penile urethra, but sonography is more accurate in the bulbar urethra where retrograde urethrography frequently underestimates stricture length. The relationship of these findings to surgical planning is discussed in detail.[8,10]

An alternative classification based on periurethral cuffing and stricture length was suggested by Chiou et al. They also offered a novel approach to the estimation of fibrosis using color Doppler ultrasound, where an absence of signal in the periurethral corpus spongiosum has been claimed to

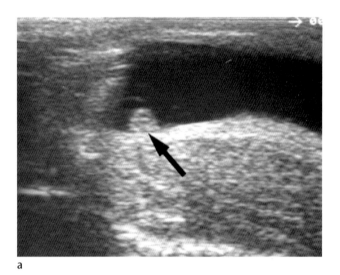

a

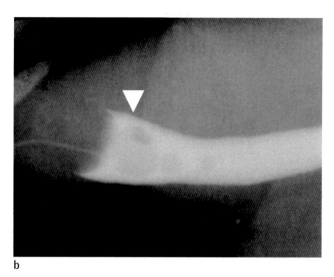

b

Figure 6.12
Filling defects. (a) Viral papilloma (arrow) in distal urethra on ascending sonogram. (b) Ascending contrast study of same patient, where the filling defect (arrowhead) was overlooked because of a superimposed bubble.

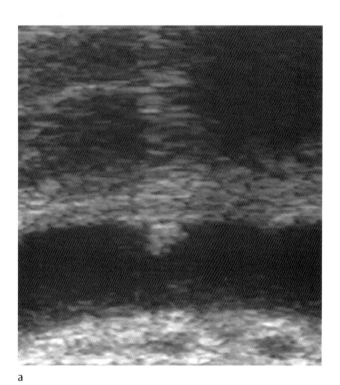

a

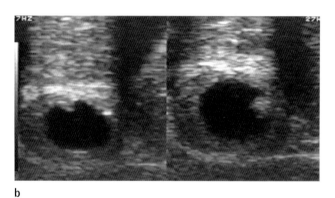

b

Figure 6.13
Filling defects. Sagittal (a) and transverse (b) views of viral papillomas in a different patient.

correspond to fibrosis.[5] In a prospective study, Merkle and Wagner[11] found that the degree of periurethral scarring correlated with a poor prognosis for urethrotomy, suggesting that open urethroplasty would be a more appropriate approach.

Filling defects

Our group has found the accurate demonstration of intraurethral filling defects one of the major uses and advantages of urethrosonography, yet this aspect of the study has largely been ignored in the literature, which has

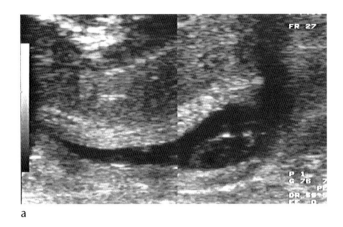
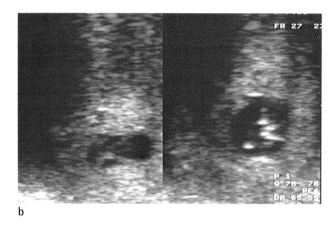

a

b

Figure 6.14
Filling defects. Sagittal (a) and transverse (b) views of filling defects within bulbar urethra due to desquamated skin and hair from previous urethroplasty.

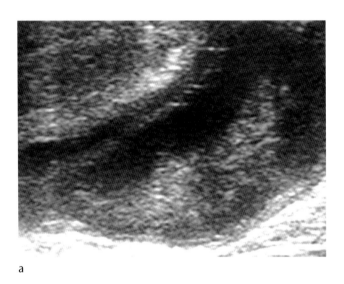
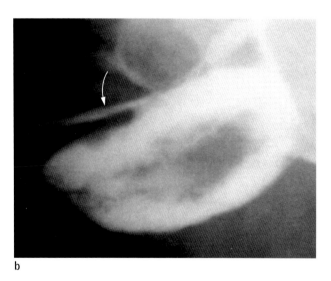

a

b

Figure 6.15
Filling defects. Debris in a perineal diverticulum on (a) ascending sonographic study and (b) ascending contrast urethrogram. The curved arrow demonstrates lumen of urethra. The neck of the diverticulum has not been defined.

emphasized the demonstration of urethral strictures. In a series of 17 strictures, Gluck et al[3] comment on the incidental finding of a urethral clot. We mentioned this topic specifically in a previous study,[2] where five intraluminal filling defects were defined, of which only two were demonstrated convincingly on contrast urethrogram. Examples of these in our practice include intraluminal viral papillomas, desquamated hair and epithelium following scrotal skin urethroplasty, mucosal tags or webs and debris within diverticula (Figures 6.12–6.16). We have also demonstrated transverse urethral webs, where the contrast study has been apparently normal. This was found in several cases to be due to lack of a perfect lateral view on

the contrast study, the web being concealed by projectional superimposition.

Calculi have been successfully identified in the urethra,[12] as well as in urethral diverticula.[8] We have demonstrated iatrogenic false passages, as have other authors.[8]

Diverticula

Although there is no difficulty in demonstrating diverticula sonographically, it is sometimes difficult to define the neck precisely[13] (see Figure 6.15). The contents of the diverticulum, however, are easily demonstrated.

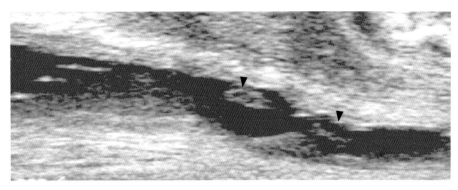

a

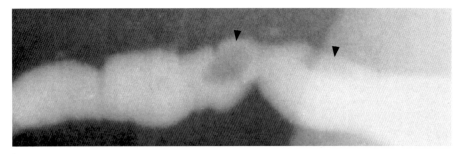

b

Figure 6.16
Filling defects. Complex urethral stricture with mucosal tags. Arrowheads demonstrate corresponding filling defects. (a) The ascending sonogram and (b) the corresponding ascending contrast study.

Hypospadias

The urethra in the setting of hypospadias has been largely neglected by the contrast urethrographic literature, mainly because the technique is intricate or impossible in this group of patients. These examinations may be complicated by the site of urethral meatus, which may not be easily accessible to the clamping required in a descending study. We regularly perform studies of the native or post-reconstruction urethra, as well as studying subjects where there is a mild degree of hypospadias and surgery has not been contemplated.[14] It may be necessary to consider using either the ascending or the descending sonographic approaches, and we have used both techniques in a single patient where appropriate. The symptoms in most of these cases are often unhelpful, with vague complaints such as penile discomfort on voiding. The relationship of native to neourethra may be demonstrated and, occasionally, bizarre unexpected patterns are encountered which would not be obvious on contrast study (Figure 6.17). Distal strictures may be successfully demonstrated using the 'fossa navicularis' voiding technique, scanning from a dorsal approach while the patient micturates (Figures 6.18 and 6.19).

Limitations and pitfalls

Undoubtedly, some subjects are unable to coordinate the manual clamping required for the descending technique.

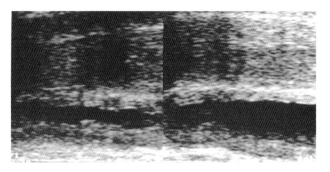

Figure 6.17
Long penile urethral stricture following prolonged catheterization.

They would still be suitable subjects for an alternative descending study using a mechanical clamp.[9] Inadequate urine flow due to prostatism or inhibition has already been mentioned. There are indirect contrast urethrographic features of urethral inflammation of questionable diagnostic importance, such as reflux into prostatic and Cowper's ducts, or intravasation of contrast, and these contrast study signs have no sonographic equivalent. Generalized long strictures involving all or much of the anterior urethra may be demonstrated on ascending contrast urethrograms as generalized lack of distensibility in the absence of mucosal irregularity (see Figure 6.17). In our practice, these are usually the result of prolonged catheterization. As the

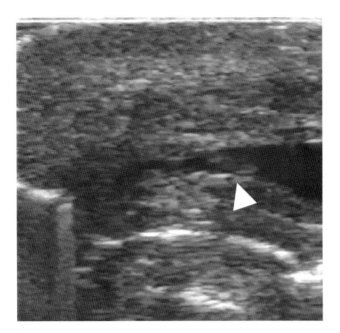

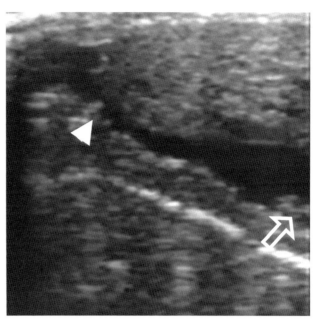

Figure 6.18
Distal stricture in micturating study of corrected hypospadias. A soft tissue intraluminal filling defect (arrowhead) is demonstrated.

Figure 6.19
Micturating study of corrected hypospadias, demonstrating stricture (arrowhead) and filling defect (open arrow).

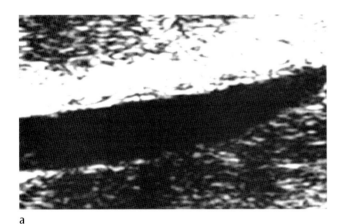

a

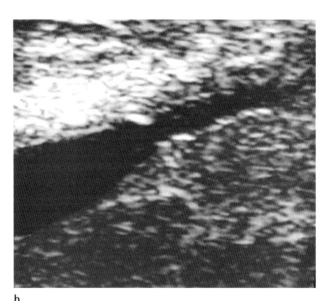

b

Figure 6.20
Bulbar stricture. (a) On this descending study, the slightly underfilled bulbar urethra was considered normal. (b) On scanning during micturition, a tight bulbar stricture was identified beyond what had been considered the proximal extent of the bulbar urethra. (c) A montage of the two images demonstrates the relationship of the stricture to the bulbar urethra.

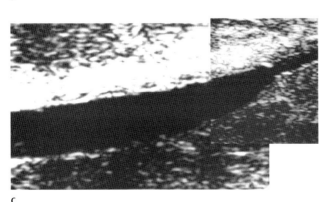

c

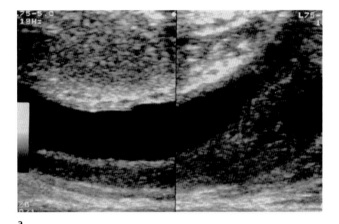

a

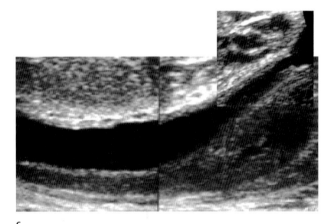

c

b

Figure 6.21
Bulbar stricture. (a) On the initial voiding study, the extent of the proximal bulbar stricture was not appreciated. (b) However, the micturating study demonstrated a tight bulbar stricture. (c) A montage of the two images indicates the anatomy of the stricture.

distension achieved in the voiding technique is variable, and depends on the patient's coordination and flow rate, it is theoretically possible to dismiss a non-distensible urethra with no focal stricture as an example of inadequate technique. Conversely, an underfilled urethra due to inadequate flow should not be misinterpreted as a long stricture (see Figure 6.2).

In the description of normal anatomy, we emphasized the importance of demonstrating the characteristic cephalad tapering curve of the proximal bulbar urethra (see Figure 6.2). We have encountered several examples where the bulbar urethra was considered normal apart from loss of this curve (Figures 6.20 and 6.21). This departure from the normal contour alerted the operator to the possibility that the entire bulbar urethra was not being demonstrated. The patient's perineum was scanned during voiding and this maneuver, which is not part of our routine study, revealed a proximal bulbar stricture in all cases. The importance of this normal contour cannot be overstressed; if there is the slightest suspicion of an abnormal configuration to the bulbar urethra, this area should be insonated during micturition.

Vascular malformations, which are sometimes post-traumatic, may masquerade as diverticula. Figure 6.22 demonstrates a hypoechoic structure adjacent to the bulbar urethra. This study was performed shortly after the patient's urethrotomy had to be abandoned due to severe urethral bleeding. Initially considered to be a diverticulum, its vascular nature was defined on color flow imaging. The abnormality was undetectable a week later, presumably due to spontaneous thrombosis.

Summary

Both ascending and descending sonographic techniques are suitable for the demonstration of the anterior urethra. Ascending studies have several of the drawbacks of contrast urethrography, such as the discomfort of catheterization, but are useful when acquiring experience of urethrosonography. The descending technique may be performed with an external clamp or with the patient compressing his own urethra manually. We have chosen to

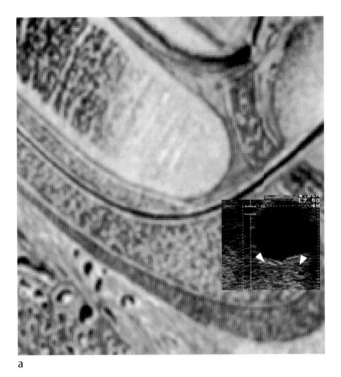
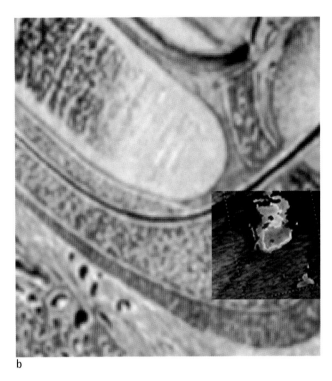

a   b

Figure 6.22
A well-defined hypoechoic structure is shown on this montaged sagittal view. Originally misinterpreted as a diverticulum, (b) color Doppler studies indicate turbulent flow within the structure. A week after an attempt at urethrotomy the cystic structure was no longer detectable.

develop the latter approach, with excellent results and patient acceptance. Initially, our local urologists accepted a normal study but were reluctant to operate on the basis of an abnormal ultrasound study. As their confidence in the accuracy of the sonographic technique increased, contrast urethrography was abandoned as a routine procedure in this institution and is now reserved for those patients where sonography has been or is likely to be unsuccessful. Contrast studies still provide our routine image in the setting of acute urethral trauma.

Urethral ultrasound continues to lack widespread acceptance even though there are several advantages to the technique, which include the avoidance of ionizing radiation, relatively accessible and inexpensive equipment, and a single operator, which make it suitable for office practice and regular follow-up studies. In addition, practitioners of the technique believe it to be superior to contrast urethrography, particularly with regard to the definition of the periurethral soft tissues and more accurate estimation of the length of bulbar stricture and the demonstration of filling defects.

It is interesting to speculate why the technique has not gained acceptance despite numerous studies demonstrating its merits. Undoubtedly, considerable skill is required

in the practice of small-parts sonography, but this has not stopped musculoskeletal ultrasound from flourishing. I must reluctantly conclude that many radiologists are prudish about what they perceive is the hands-on, intrusive nature of this study. In our department, in common with testicular ultrasound, most female radiologists and sonographers have been reluctant to learn the technique. There is obviously the need for a forum for debate about these aspects of the study that are essentially social rather than clinical, particularly if a valuable study is to be rejected because of the inhibitions of medical practitioners. I would, nevertheless, encourage those readers who wish to consider acquiring the technique that several sonographic studies performed in conjunction with ascending contrast urethrography will convince them of the merits and the ease of this application of small-parts sonography.

References

1. McCullum RW. The adult male urethra: normal anatomy, pathology and method urethrography. Radiol Clin North Am 1979; 17: 227–31.

2. Bearcroft PW, Berman LH. Sonography in the evaluation of the male anterior urethra. Clin Radiol 1994; 49: 621–6.

3. Gluck CD, Bundy AL, Fine C, Loughlin KR, Richie JP. Sonographic urethrogram: comparison to Roentgenographic techniques in 22 patients. J Urol 1988; 140: 1404–8.

4. McAninch JW, Laing FC, Jeffrey RB Jr. Sonourethrography in the evaluation of urethral strictures: a preliminary report. J Urol 1988; 139: 294–7.

5. Chiou RK, Anderson JC, Tran T, et al. Evaluation of urethral strictures and associated abnormalities using high-resolution and color Doppler ultrasound. Urology 1996; 47: 102–7.

6. Heidenreich A, Derschum W, Bonfig R, Wilbert DM. Ultrasound in the evaluation of urethral stricture disease: a prospective study in 175 patients. Br J Urol 1994; 74: 93–8.

7. Gupta S, Majumdar B, Tiwari A, et al. Sonourethrography in the evaluation of anterior urethral strictures: correlation with radiographic urethrography. J Clin Ultrasound 1993; 21: 231–9.

8. Morey AF, McAninch JW. Ultrasound evaluation of the male urethra for assessment of urethral stricture. J Clin Ultrasound 1996; 24: 473–9.

9. Merkle W, Wagner W. Sonography of the distal male urethra – a new diagnostic procedure for urethral strictures: results of a retrospective study. J Urol 1988; 140: 1409–11.

10. Nash PA, McAninch JW, Bruce JE, Hanks DK. Sono-urethrography in the evaluation of anterior urethral strictures. J Urol 1995; 154: 72–6.

11. Merkle W, Wagner W. Risk of recurrent stricture following internal urethrotomy. Prospective ultrasound study of distal male urethra. Br J Urol 1990; 65: 618–20.

12. Kessler A, Rosenberg HK, Smoyer WE, Blyth B. Urethral stones: US for identification in boys with hematuria and dysuria. Radiology 1992; 185: 767–8.

13. Benson CB, Doubilet PM, Richie JP. Sonography of the male genital tract. AJR Am J Roentgenol 1989; 153: 705–13.

14. Toms AP, Bullock KN, Berman LH. Descending urethral ultrasound of the native and reconstructed urethra in patients with hypospadias. Br J Radiol 2003; 76: 260–3.

7

The penis

Dennis Ll Cochlin

Applications

Requests for imaging of the penis are uncommon, but there are a few important applications. General applications may be seen from the subheadings in this chapter.

Erectile dysfunction was, at one time, extensively investigated by a combination of pharmacologically stimulated penile arterial and venous Doppler studies and contrast cavernosography. As new algorithms have been developed for the assessment of erectile dysfunction, however, most patients are studied and treated without Doppler studies. Despite this trend, Doppler studies are still used in some centers on selected patients, and so they are included in this chapter.

Sonourethrography is an important advance in the study of urethral pathology, and is included in Chapter 6.

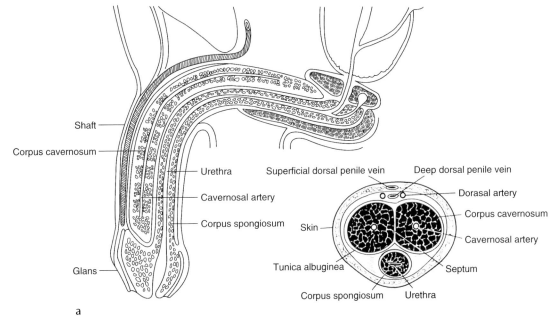

a

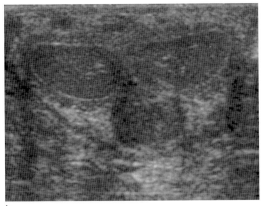

b

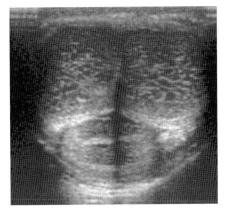

c

Figure 7.1
Penile anatomy. (a) Diagrammatic transverse section. (b) Transverse scan of the penile shaft corresponding to (a). (c) Transverse section of the erect penile shaft. The venous spaces of the corpora are engorged.

Anatomy (Figure 7.1)

The body of the penis contains three elongated masses of erectile tissue. The two corpora cavernosa lie dorsally alongside each other. They are separated by a fibrous septum, which contains multiple fenestrations allowing free communication of the venous sinusoids on both sides. Ventral to these lies the corpus spongiosum, through the center of which runs the urethra. The corpora cavernosa and the spongiosum are each surrounded by the tunica albuginea, a fibrous sheath some 2 mm thick in the case of the corpora cavernosa, somewhat thinner around the corpus spongiosum. Outside these are two fascial layers, the deep Buck's fascia and the superficial Colles fascia.

Through the centers of each corpus cavernosum run the right and left cavernosal arteries, which provide the primary blood source for erection. Along the dorsum of the penis run the dorsal penile veins and, lateral to these, the dorsal arteries. These arteries supply blood to the glans penis. The separate blood supply to the corpora cavernosa and the glans is important to recognize, as pathology in the dorsal arteries may cause a flaccid glans in the presence of a normal shaft erection.

The structure of the penis is readily demonstrated by high-resolution (10–12 MHz) ultrasound. A linear transducer is most appropriate. Transverse views of the shaft may be obtained from the dorsal or ventral shaft, thus avoiding the poorer resolution of the near field (Figure 7.1). Standoff gel may be used. Images may be obtained in transverse planes and any appropriate longitudinal plane. The root of the penis is demonstrated by scanning through the perineum or angling posteriorly from the base of the

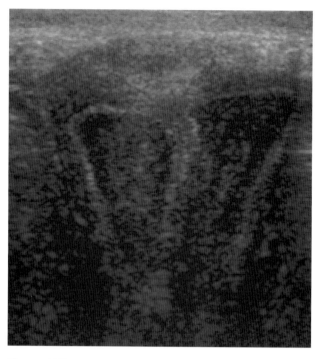

Figure 7.2
Penile root. The corpora are seen to diverge as they pass posteriorly along the perineum.

penis in the transverse plane (Figure 7.2). The glans penis appears as shown in Figure 7.3.

The cavernosal arteries may be visualized in the same manner via a dorsal or ventral approach (Figure 7.4) and

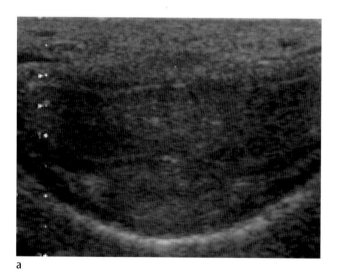

a

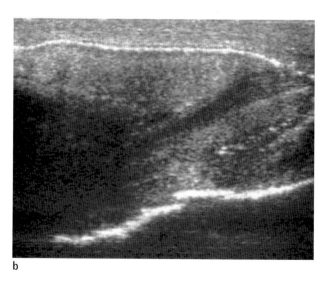

b

Figure 7.3
Transverse and longitudinal sections of the glans penis. (a) In transverse section, the glans has an oval shape with a homogeneous pattern. (b) In longitudinal section, it curves around the ends of the corpora cavernosae.

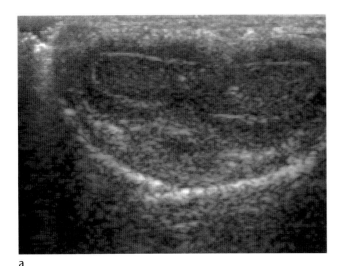

a

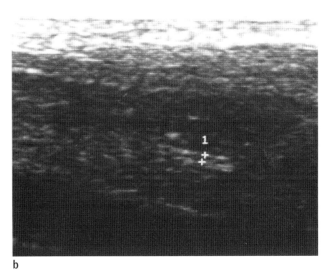

b

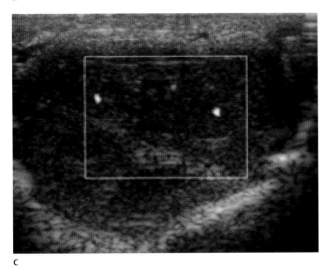

c

Figure 7.4

Cavernosal arteries. (a) In the transverse plane the cavernosal arteries are just visible as small parallel echogenic foci. (b) The cavernosal arteries are more easily seen in the longitudinal plane as parallel lines. (c) Transverse section showing the cavernosal arteries on color Doppler.

their change in diameter in response to attempted erection may be measured. For duplex Doppler measurements, a transducer designed for peripheral vascular studies with an ability to offset the beam is necessary. The arteries, however, are so easily found, that imaging is not strictly necessary, and a simple continuous-wave Doppler device is often used.

The cavernosal and spongiosal veins are visible on Doppler ultrasound, although in the flaccid penis only a few have sufficient flow to register on the color Doppler image. The engorged cavernosal veins are easily seen in Doppler studies in complete or partial penile erection (Figure 7.5).[1]

Peyronie disease[2–6]

Fibrous plaques of the tunica albuginea, usually on the dorsal aspect of the penis, cause bending of the penis towards the lesion during erection, which is sometimes

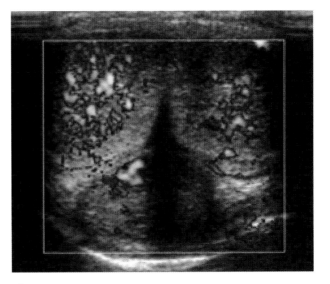

Figure 7.5

Cavernosal veins. The engorged cavernosal veins are seen in a transverse section of the erect penis.

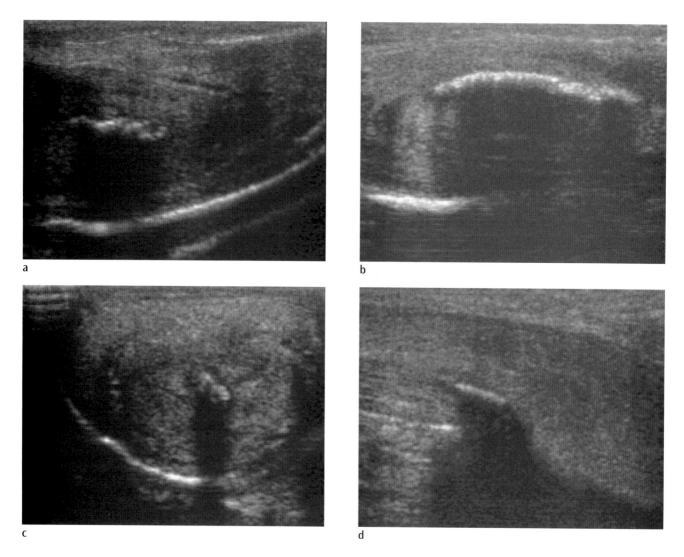

a

b

c

d

Figure 7.6
Calcified Peyronie plaques. (a,b) Typical Peyronie plaques on the dorsal tunica. (c,d) A plaque in a less common position on the medial tunica. Many plaques are not as clearly seen as these.

painful. This condition is known as Peyronie disease. The plaque may calcify. Non-calcified plaques may resolve spontaneously; those that do not may resolve with treatment by systemic or locally injected steroids. Extracorporeal short-wave lithotripsy is a new treatment that is often effective. It may be used for calcified or fibrous plaques, although calcified plaques tend to respond better.

Ultrasound imaging is needed before planning treatment. A plaque needs to be ultrasonically visible to treat with lithotripsy. Plaques may be characterized as calcified or fibrous. Calcified plaques are more likely to respond to lithotripsy. Fibrous plaques may respond to steroids.

Finally, if the treatment fails, surgery with excision of the affected area of tunica may be necessary. Most surgeons require ultrasound imaging to assess the distribution of plaques prior to surgery. Some find assessment of the proximity of the cavernosal artery to the plaque helpful. There is also an increased incidence of mixed arterial and venous abnormality associated with Peyronie's disease that may cause erectile dysfunction. Some would, therefore, advocate full Doppler studies, as for erectile dysfunction. Most, however, treat the Peyronie's plaques first and then assess the patient clinically.

Calcified plaques appear on ultrasound as dense linear shadowing lesions (Figure 7.6). Fibrous plaques are more difficult to demonstrate. They are less echogenic than the normal tunica and are often seen as discontinuities in the dense white line of the tunica (Figure 7.7). In cases of difficulty, plaques are often more conspicuous in the erect penis. Finally, if visualization is difficult, and the

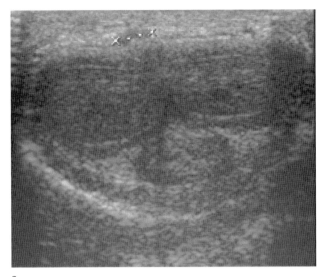

a

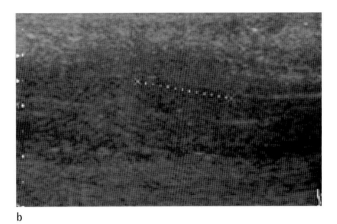

b

Figure 7.7
Fibrous Peyronie's plaque. (a) Transverse and (b) longitudinal sections of a fibrous plaque appearing as a hypoechoic mass interrupting the echogenic line of the tunica.

ultrasound study suboptimal, magnetic resonance imaging (MRI) may be employed. These studies are also often performed on the erect penis. Pharmacologic stimulation with sildenafil (Viagra) maintains an erection for the duration of the study.

Fibrous or even calcified plaques may also occur following treatment of erectile dysfunction by intracavernosal injection, and also following tunica rupture from trauma, particularly if not properly treated by surgery. These plaques appear identical on ultrasound to Peyronie's plaques. In the case of intracavernosal injections, however, it is important not to confuse shadowing from small bubbles, which may be present for a short time post injection, with plaques.

Penile trauma[7]

In the case of blunt trauma to the penis or suspected rupture of the corpora during intercourse, it is important to establish the integrity of the fibrous sheath covering the corpora.

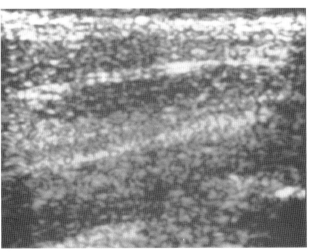

a

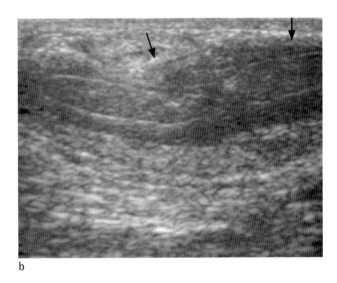

b

Figure 7.8
Tunical rupture. (a) Longitudinal sonogram of left corpus cavernosum demonstrating interruption of the tunica albuginea (calipers) as a result of a fracture or tear of the tunica. (Courtesy of Carol B Benson MD, Brigham and Women's Hospital, Boston, MA, USA.) (b) This case of trauma with clinically suspected tunical rupture shows a hematoma (arrow) but an intact tunica.

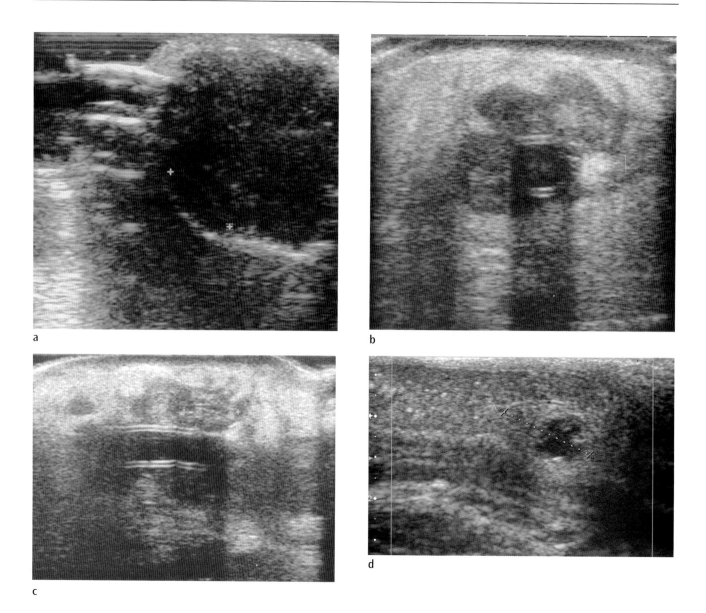

Figure 7.9
Penile cancer. (a) A small cancer in the glans penis (calipers). (b,c) Transverse and longitudinal sections of a cancer in the penile shaft. (d) Another case.

Tunica rupture requires surgical repair. Failure to repair a rupture often results in a fibrous scar, similar in appearance and in effect to Peyronie disease, or continuing venous leak and erectile failure.

The usual method of diagnosing clinically suspected tunica rupture is by contrast cavernosography, when a contrast leak outside the corpora indicates a rupture. The integrity of the corpora may, however, be determined by high-resolution ultrasound and this non-invasive technique may replace cavernosography.

In cases of tunica rupture, the ultrasound study may show hematoma within and outside the tunica at the site of rupture. The actual defect in the tunica may also be seen

and, in some cases (Figure 7.8), Doppler may reveal blood flow through the defect.

Tumors and masses[8–14]

Various malignant tumors and benign masses may occur in the penis. Ultrasound may differentiate between solid tumors and cysts of Cowper's or Littre's glands, and various cutaneous or subcutaneous lesions. Accurate differentiation is, however, usually achieved by physical examination, and ultrasound is rarely necessary.

Squamous carcinoma of the penis usually starts in the glans penis and spreads along the corpora or urethra. In such cases, the extent is usually easy to assess clinically, and imaging is rarely required. If the extent of spread into the shaft is equivocal, however, ultrasound imaging will show the extent of tumor in the glans and the corpora (Figure 7.9). However, MRI is often utilized, as some surgeons find the images easier to interpret when planning surgery (Figure 7.10). Some cases of penile cancer arise primarily within the corpora of the penile shaft. These cause palpable masses that are more difficult to assess clinically. Ultrasound will readily show these as hypoechoic masses (Figure 7.11), although these are indistinguishable from other tumors such as bladder or prostate carcinoma which may involve the penis by direct spread through the perineal membrane to the root of the penis and hence the corpora. These produce palpable masses in the penis, which are seen on ultrasound as hypoechoic masses within the corpora (Figure 7.11).

Penile cancer spreads to the inguinal nodes. Follow-up is by physical examination of the inguinal region, but also

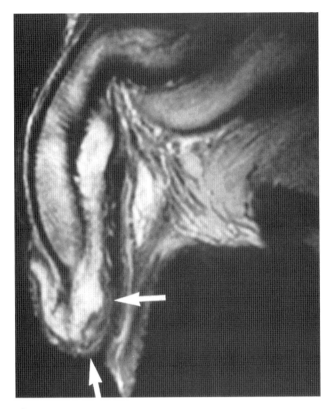

Figure 7.10
Penile cancer – MRI scan. Sagittal view of the penis demonstrating a small cancer (arrows) of the distal penis arising from the skin and invading the glans ventrally. (Courtesy of Carol B Benson MD, Brigham and Women's Hospital, Boston, MA, USA.)

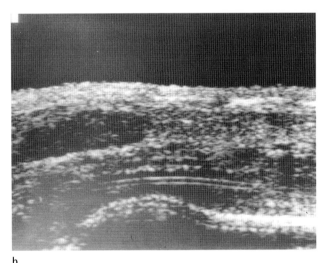

b

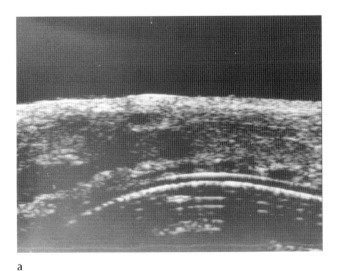

a

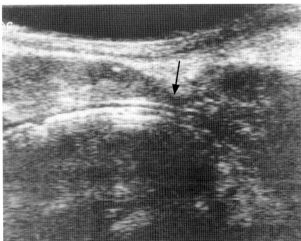

c

Figure 7.11
Prostate cancer spread to the penis. There are hypoechoic masses in the right (a) and left (b) corpora cavernosa. A transrectal scan (c) shows the tumor passing through the perineal membrane (perineal membrane arrowed). The patient is catheterized.

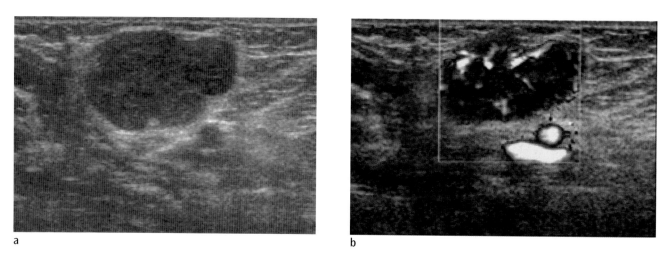

a b

Figure 7.12
Inguinal node involved with penile cancer. (a,b) The node is enlarged, hypoechoic and irregular. Its architecture is destroyed and the normal hilar blood supply has been replaced by peripheral neovascularity.

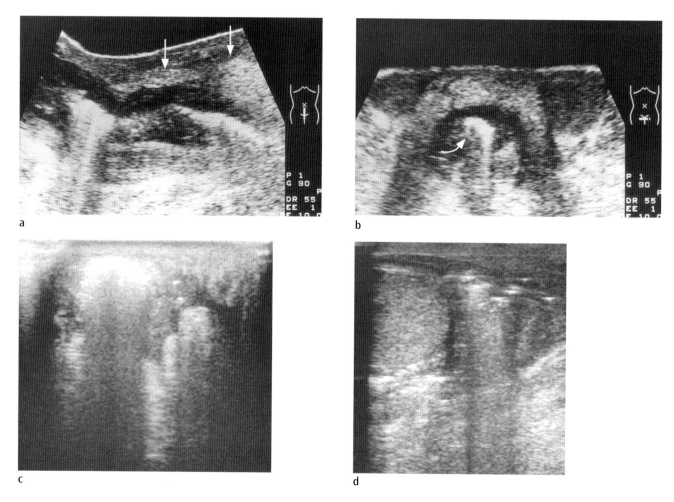

a b

c d

Figure 7.13
Fournier gangrene. (a,b) There is gross thickening of the cutaneous tissues at the root of the penis (straight arrows) with gas in the periurethral tissues (curved arrow). (Courtesy of Dr Guy Sissons, Countess of Chester Hospital, UK.) (c) A more advanced case with extensive soft tissue gas. (d) The same case showing gas in the scrotum.

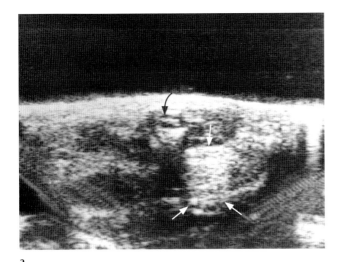

a

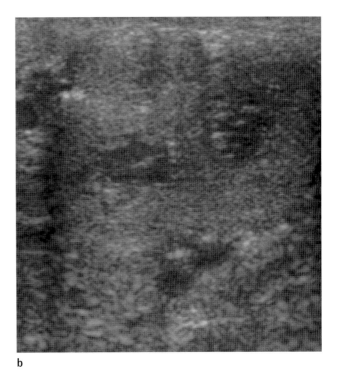

b

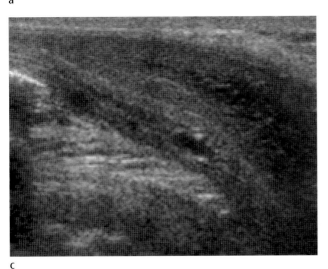

c

Figure 7.14
Priapism. (a) The scan, taken from the ventral surface of the penis, shows echodense thrombus in the left corpus cavernosum (straight arrows). The curved arrow points to the urethra. (b,c) Transverse and longitudinal scans of another case. The venous spaces at the center of the corpora are engorged and the surrounding spaces are thrombosed and echogenic.

imaging. Computed tomography (CT) has been the modality most often used, but ultrasound examination with guided biopsy of any enlarged nodes is being increasingly used (Figure 7.12).

stage, will show the marked edema, and shadowing from periurethral, perineal or scrotal gas (Figure 7.13).

Ultrasound may often establish the diagnosis before it is clinically obvious.

Fournier gangrene[15,16]

Gangrene of the penis may occur as secondary spread from venereal disease, cavernositis of balanitis, but more frequently is the primary idiopathic spontaneous fulminating gangrene described by Fournier. This usually occurs in debilitated or immunocompromised patients and also in newborn babies.

Fournier gangrene starts in the penis, sometimes spreading to the scrotum and perineum. Diagnosis is clinical, with erythema and edema leading, within 24 hours, to exudative moist desquamation. Ultrasound, in the early

Priapism[17–22]

Priapism is a persistent painful erection of the penis. It is broadly classified as low flow (veno-occlusive or ischemic) or high flow (arterial). The low-flow form is more common. It is caused by impaired venous drainage. There is often blood clot in the corpora. It is often idiopathic, but is also often associated with hypercoagulability states, particularly sickle cell trait, spinal cord stenosis or a variety of drugs, including sildenafil (Viagra) and antihypertensives. Malignant tumors, either direct invasion from bladder or prostate, or metastatic may also be a cause. Ultrasound will

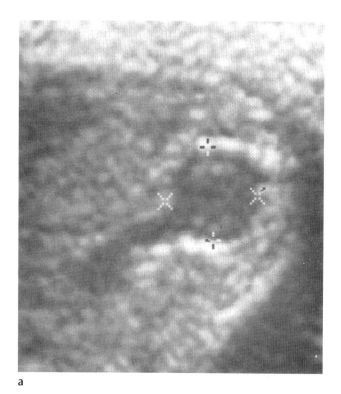

a

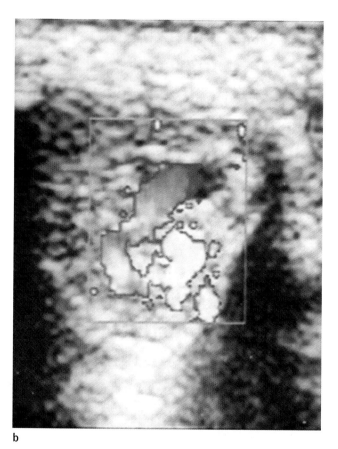

b

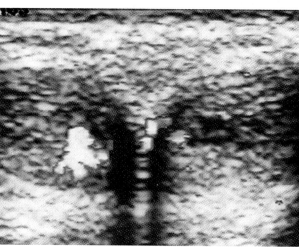

c

Figure 7.15
High-flow priapism. (a) A small rounded hypoechoic lesion within the corpus cavernosum. (b) Blood flow within the lesion indicates an arteriosinusoidal fistula. (c) A different case; the fistula causes a blush of color adjacent to the right cavernosal artery. (Reproduced with permission from Feldstein[22].)

demonstrate distension of a whole or part of the corpora by relatively hyperechoic clot (Figure 7.14). If tumor is the cause, this will be demonstrated. Imaging appearances do not, however, usually influence management of low-flow priapism, and ultrasound is not routinely employed.

High-flow or arterial priapism is caused by increased arterial flow. This is usually due to an arteriovenous fistula caused by trauma or surgery. It may also occur in cocaine abuse. If the high-flow form is suspected, then Doppler studies should be employed to look for an arteriocavernous fistula. Reports in the literature suggest that the fistula may be demonstrated as a high-flow channel, or as a blush,

probably due to tissue vibration adjacent to the cavernosal artery (Figure 7.15). However, large series are not available, and it is likely that not all fistulas are detectable by Doppler study. Contrast arteriography remains the gold standard.

Penile erection devices

Malfunction of these devices usually only occurs in the inflatable types, and is associated with leaks or kinked connection tubes. The devices are usually filled with contrast

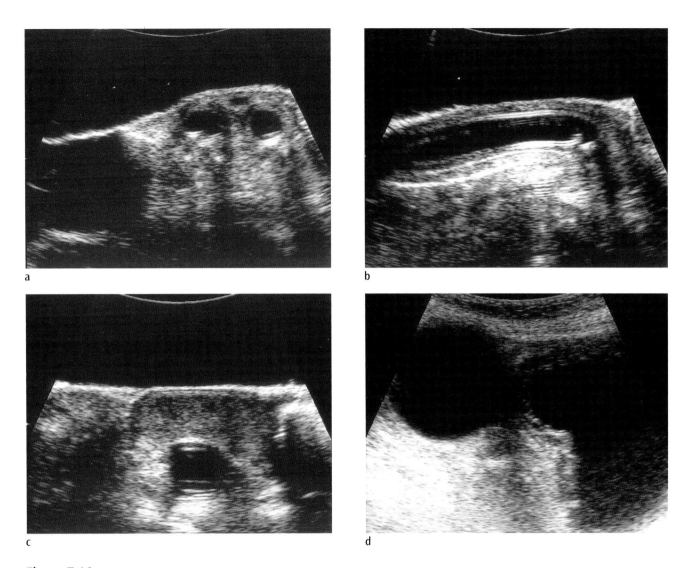

a

b

c

d

Figure 7.16
Inflatable penile erection device. The erectile tubes are seen within the corpora cavernosa in transverse (a) and longitudinal sections (b). The bulb that initiates erection is seen in section (c) and the reservoir is seen behind the bladder (d).

agent, and evaluation of dysfunction is normally by plain film X-ray.

Ultrasound demonstrates the prosthesis well (Figure 7.16), but only has a small place to play in evaluation.

Wrongly positioned catheters

Urethral catheters may be inadvertently positioned wrongly with the inflated balloon in the urethra (Figure 7.17a) or in a false passage (Figure 7.17b). These may drain a little urine but do not empty the bladder. An ultrasound scan of the bladder clearly shows that the catheter tip and balloon do not lie in the bladder and then scanning of the pelvis,

perineum or penis will demonstrate the position of the catheter tip and balloon. Sometimes the catheter may be gently repositioned under real-time ultrasound control. If repositioning is not easy, however, there may be a false passage and the catheter should be removed and a suprapubic catheter inserted.

Urethral spring stents

These devices are sometimes used for the treatment of urethral strictures. They are most often used in strictures of the prostatic urethra. They are, however, occasionally used for strictures of the penile or membranous urethra and

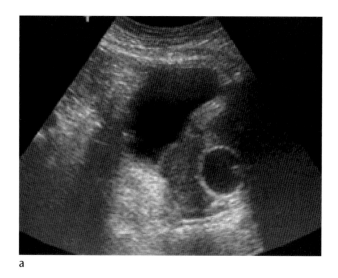

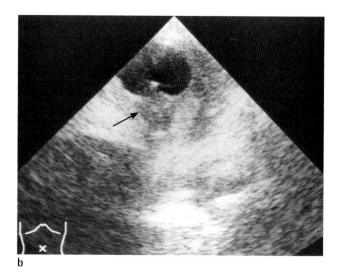

a   b

Figure 7.17

Poorly positioned catheter. (a) The catheter lies in the prostatic urethra. (b) The catheter lies alongside the prostatic urethra (urethra arrowed). A false passage has obviously been produced. The catheter was removed and a suprapubic catheter inserted.

may be imaged by penile ultrasound in these situations, sometimes in combination with ultrasonic urethrography (Figure 7.18).

Urethral strictures

The study of urethral strictures is discussed in Chapter 4. Here we will discuss study of the corpus spongiosum around a stricture. In some cases of urethral stricture, leakage of urine into the corpus spongiosum causes fibrosis. If repair of the stricture is corrected by excision and anastomosis, the area of fibrosis must also be excised. Therefore the presence and, if possible, the extent of the fibrosis should be established preoperatively. Fibrosis is established by the absence of blood flow in the suspected area on Doppler scan, sometimes associated with subtle increase in echodensity (Figure 7.19).

Tunica albuginea defect

Weak areas of the tunica may lead to herniation of the corpora, with a palpable mass and venous leak. The hernia may be demonstrated by ultrasound (Figure 7.20).

Erectile dysfunction[23–28]

Erection of the penis is initiated by neuronal impulses. These cause relaxation of the arterioles, which in turn

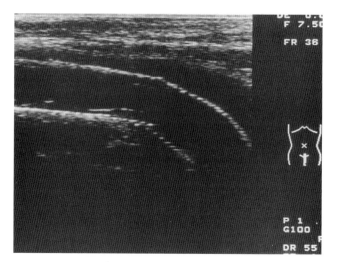

Figure 7.18

Urethral spring stent. These stents are commonly used in the prostatic urethra. They may, however, be used for the treatment of penile or membranous urethral strictures as shown here, and these may be demonstrated on penile scans. The examination may be combined with ultrasonic urethrography.

cause increased blood flow to the corpora cavernosa. These expand and compress the draining veins against the tunica albuginea. This leads to an imbalance between arterial input and venous drainage that causes and maintains turgidity of the corpora, and penile erection. Failure of erection may be due to psychogenic causes, or failure of

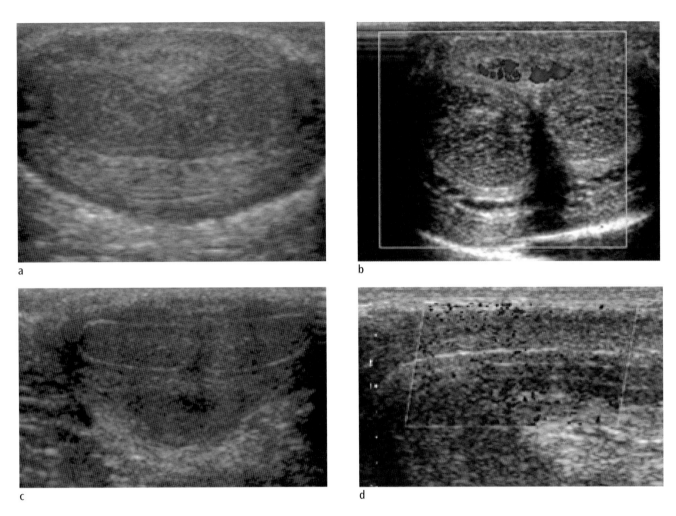

a

b

c

d

Figure 7.19
Urethral stricture. (a) A transverse section of the penis at the level of a urethral stricture. In this case, the corpus spongiosum around the strictured urethra appears normal, with no evidence of thrombosis. (b) Normal vasculature. (c) A case with low echodensity fibrosis around a urethral stricture. (d) A Doppler study showed no demonstrable Doppler vascular flow.

neuronal response, arterial response or the veno-occulsive mechanism. A few cases are due to other causes such as endocrinologic dysfunction. Doppler ultrasound has a role mainly in detecting failure of arterial response, and possibly in veno-occlusive failure.

Erectile dysfunction is, however, an extremely common condition. It would not be practical, nor is it necessary to investigate the majority of patients by Doppler ultrasound. The First International Consultation on Erectile Dysfunction, co-sponsored by the World Health Organization, was held in Paris, France in 1999. Their recommendations for tests are summarized in Table 7.1. This is included here to show how many tests are available, and to show that, in their opinion, Doppler ultrasound studies are specialized tests, to be reserved for a few cases only. They only really have a place when there is a high suspicion of a remediable vascular cause, the patient is suitable for vascular intervention and the surgical expertise is available.

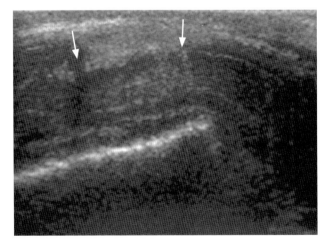

Figure 7.20
Tunica albuginea defect. There is disruption of the tunica albuginea (arrows).

Table 7.1 *World Health Organization recommendations for the diagnostic evaluation of erectile dysfunction (ED)*

I HIGHLY RECOMMENDED EVALUATION AND TESTS
1. Comprehensive sexual, medical and psychosocial history
Medical and sexual history, including erectile insufficiency (onset, duration, progression, severity, nocturnal, self-stimulation and visual erotic-induced erections), altered sexual desire, ejaculation, orgasm, sexually induced genital pain, partner sexual function, lifestyle factors, smoking, chronic medical illnesses, pelvic/perineal/penile trauma and surgery, medications, recreational drug use, pelvic radiotherapy, neurological disease, endocrine disease, psychiatric illness, current psychological state, depression, ED intensity and impact scales, e.g. ED intensity scale, ED impact scale
2. Focused physical examination
Assessment of body habitus and cardiovascular, neurological and genitourinary system, including penile, testicular and rectal examination, blood pressure, heart rate

II RECOMMENDED DIAGNOSTIC TESTS
1. Fasting glucose or glycosylated hemoglobin (Hbalc) and lipid profile
2. Evaluation of the hypothalamic–pituitary–gonadal axis with a testosterone assay

III OPTIONAL DIAGNOSIS TESTS
1. Psychological and/or psychiatric consultation
2. Laboratory investigations: serum prolactin, luteinizing hormone, complete blood count, urinalysis

IV SPECIALIZED EVALUATION AND DIAGNOSTIC TESTS
1. In-depth psychosexual and relationship evaluation
2. Psychiatric evaluation
3. Nocturnal penile tumescence and rigidity assessment
4. Vascular diagnosis (penile injection pharmacocavernosometry and pharmacocavernosography, penile arteriography, computed tomography/magnetic resonance imaging, nuclear imaging)
5. Specialized endocrinological testing (thyroid function studies, hypothalamic–pituitary–gonadal function studies, magnetic resonance imaging of sella turcica)
6. Neurophysiology testing (vibrometry, bulbocavernous reflex latency, cavernosal electromyogram, somatosensory evoked potential testing, pudendal and sphincter electromyogram)

The use of Doppler studies in erectile dysfunction has, for this reason, declined in recent years. Nevertheless, they do still have a place in suitable patients and are used in some specialized centers. When investigation of vasculogenic erectile dysfunction is deemed appropriate, the 'gold standard' test is dynamic infusion, cavernosography and cavernosometry. The full details of this technique are beyond the scope of this book. However, a brief description is appropriate in order to understand the place of ultrasound. Basically, a needle is introduced into one of the corpora cavernosae, through which pharmacologic agents such as papaverine hydrochloride, phentolamine or prostaglandin E_1, are injected. These produce arterial smooth muscle relaxation, and this initiates the process of penile erection. This pharmacologic approach has proved more reliable than psychogenic stimuli.

The initial response to the injection is measured by recording the intracorporeal pressure and the circumference of the penis. These are a measure of the combined arterial and veno-occlusive response. Next, saline is infused into the corpora until a pressure above the systolic pressure is achieved, and the rate of fall-off of pressure is recorded.

This assesses the veno-occlusive response alone. Thirdly, the systolic occlusion pressures of the two dorsal penile arteries are measured, as an indicator of arterial disease. This is achieved by placing a continuous-wave or pulsed-wave duplex Doppler transducer on the dorsal penis near the root, at a suitable angle to the arterial flow, and altering the position until a good arterial signal is produced. The intracorporeal infusion is then adjusted to produce a pressure above the brachial artery systolic pressure. The Doppler signal then disappears. The intracorporeal pressure is allowed to decrease until the systolic Doppler component reappears. This is repeated on both sides. The pressure at which the systolic signal reappears is the maximal systolic penile artery pressure (systolic occlusion pressure). A penile artery systolic occlusion pressure of less than 80 mmHg, or 35 mmHg less than brachial artery pressure, indicates arterial disease of a severity that makes any venous surgery unsuccessful. Finally, radiologic contrast is injected at a pressure of about 90 mmHg, and the presence or absence of draining veins is recorded by fluoroscopy.

While this technique of dynamic infusion cavernoscopy is the gold standard in the investigation of penile erectile dysfunction, it is a time-consuming, expensive test, not without risk. Therefore in those few patients that need such investigation, most centers prefer first to study the penile artery by Doppler ultrasound before and after intracavernosal pavaverine (or alternative pharmaceutical) on the grounds that significant arterial dysfunction shown on this test renders the other tests unnecessary. If the patient achieves an erection following the injection, then it can be assumed that the arterial inflow and veno-occlusive mechanisms are intact. In this case, the examination may be concluded. If there is no erection or an inadequate erection, this may indicate vasculogenic impotence, but does not distinguish arterial from veno-occlusive causes. In these cases the examination proceeds to the next phase. Normal arterial response to the injection gives an increase in diameter of the cavernosal arteries of greater than 75%. A less than 25% increase indicates significant arterial disease. The cavernosal arteries are, however, small, so that diameter measurements are inaccurate. Most centers therefore prefer to rely on changes in the Doppler signal. The Doppler examination is best carried out with a high-frequency near-focused linear array Doppler transducer, preferably with color to facilitate accurate angle correction (Figure 7.21). If this is not available, a simple continuous-wave device with the transducer at a fixed angle to the penile shaft, although less satisfactory, will suffice. A normal response results in a peak systolic velocity of more than 30 cm/s measured between 5 and 15 minutes after the intracavernosal injection (Figure 7.21a). Values below 25 cm/s indicate definite arteriogenic impotence. A slow systolic rise time of less than 110 ms also indicates proximal arterial disease. Measurements are taken in both cavernosal arteries, although an abnormal response in only one may or may not indicate that this is causing the impotence. Some centers average the two values.

Doppler studies are, however, an alternative. As erection is initiated, the resistance in the cavernosal arteries decreases. If the veno-occlusive mechanism is intact, the draining veins are compressed when the erection is achieved and the arterial resistance then increases due to the increased outflow resistance. This causes very reduced or reversed diastolic flow. An end-diastolic velocity, at this stage, of more than 6 cm/s or a resistance index of less than 0.7 appears to indicate failure of the veno-occlusive mechanism (Figure 7.21c).

The integrity of the veno-occlusive mechanism is traditionally measured by cavernosometry and cavernosography, and these remain the gold standard. Some centers measure the flow in the dorsal penile vein 7–10 minutes post-injection. A measurable flow at this time indicates an incompetent veno-occlusive mechanism. In some cases, however, the venous leak occurs into the deeper cavernosal or crural veins. These leaks will not be detected by this method. Study of the arterial spectral waveform is therefore preferable. Some patients will have arterial insufficien-

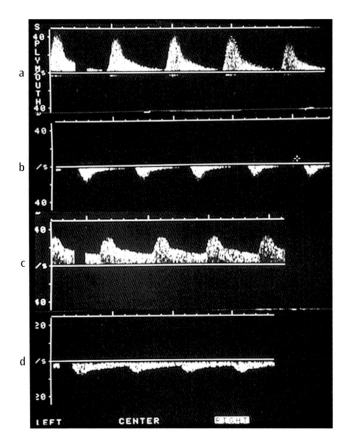

Figure 7.21
(a) **Normal cavernosal artery response to intracorporeal injection.** A Doppler signal from the cavernosal artery 10 minutes after papaverine injection shows a peak systolic velocity of 42 cm/s (normal more than 30 cm/s). The veno-occlusive mechanism is functioning, resulting in a reduction of the diastolic flow to almost zero. (b) **Arterial response to intracorporeal injection: vasculogenic impotence.** Ten minutes after intracorporeal injection of papaverine, peak systolic velocity is only 16.8 cm/s (normal more than 30 cm/s). (c) **Veno-occlusive disease.** Ten minutes after intracorporeal injection of papaverine the peak systolic velocity is normal (35 cm/s) but the end-diastolic velocity is too high at 18 cm/s (normal at this stage less than 6.0 cm/s), giving a resistance index of 0.48 (normal more than 0.7). This indicates failure of the veno-occlusive mechanism. (d) **Arterial insufficiency and possible veno-occlusive failure.** In this case there is high diastolic flow 10 minutes after intracorporeal injection. The systolic flow is, however, below normal. In such cases the arterial inflow may be insufficient to activate the veno-occlusive mechanism so that the high diastolic flow does not necessarily imply veno-occlusive failure.

cy and poor venous occlusion. In these cases the standard Doppler technique cannot be used to assess the venous side as the arterial insufficiency will in any case prevent venous occlusion (Figure 7.21d). In such cases a pressure cuff may be placed at the base of the penis in order to occlude the venous return. An improvement in the Doppler signal after inflating the cuff indicates veno-occlusive failure.

Detection of arterial insufficiency should be followed by arteriography with a view to angioplasty or arterial bypass in suitable cases. Some cases with mild to moderate disease may achieve erection by self-injection or intracorporeal vasoactive agents (papaverine, phentolamine or prostaglandin E_1). These may promote more efficient arteriolar dilatation than the normal neuronal mechanism and thus increase arterial flow sufficiently to compensate for the proximal arterial narrowing. Patients with failure of the veno-occlusive mechanism (venous leak) may respond to venous ligation if the arterial response is normal or there is mild to moderate arterial insufficiency. In severe arterial insufficiency (peak velocity less than 25 cm/s), neither venous ligation, nor arterial bypass nor angioplasty is effective. A prosthetic penile erection device may be considered in these cases.

References

1. Wilkins CJ, Sriprasad S, Sidhu PS. Colour Doppler ultrasound of the penis. Clin Radiol 2003; 58(7): 514–23.
2. Hauck EW, Hackstein N, Vosshenrich R, et al. Diagnostic value of magnetic resonance imaging in Peyronie's disease – a comparison both with palpation and ultrasound in the evaluation of plaque formation. Eur Urol 2003; 43(3): 293–9; 299–300.
3. Bertolotto M, de Stefani S, Martinoli C, Quaia E, Buttazzi L. Color Doppler appearance of penile cavernosal-spongiosal communications in patients with severe Peyronie's disease. Eur Radiol 2002; 12(10): 2525–31.
4. Kadioglu A, Tefekli A, Erol H, Cayan S, Kandirali E. Color Doppler ultrasound assessment of penile vascular system in men with Peyronie's disease Int J Impot Res 2000; 12(5): 263–7.
5. Andresen R, Wegner HE, Miller K, Banzer D. Imaging modalities in Peyronie's disease. An intrapersonal comparison of ultrasound sonography, X-ray in mammography technique, computerized tomography, and nuclear magnetic resonance in 20 patients. Eur Urol 1998; 34(2): 128–34.
6. Ahmed M, Chilton CP, Munson KW, et al. The role of color Doppler imaging in the management of Peyronie's disease. Br J Urol 1998; 81(4): 604–6.
7. Eke N. Fracture of the penis. Br J Surg 2002; 89(5): 555–65.
8. Herbener TE, Seftel AD, Nehra A, Goldstein I. Penile ultrasound. Semin Urol 1994; 12(4): 320–32.
9. Dorak AC, Ozkan GA, Tamac NI, Saray A. Ultrasonography in the recognition of penile cancer. J Clin Ultrasound 1992; 20(9): 624–6.
10. Lont AP, Besnard AP, Gallee MP, van Tinteren H, Horenblas S. A comparison of physical examination and imaging in determining the extent of primary penile carcinoma. BJU Int 2003; 91(6): 493–5.
11. Agrawal A, Pai D, Ananthakrishnan N, Smile R, Ratnaker C. Clinical and sonographic findings in carcinoma of the penis. J Clin Ultrasound 2000; 28(8): 399–406.
12. Nakayama F, Sheth S, Caskey CI, Hamper UM. Penile metastasis from prostate cancer: diagnosis with sonography. J Ultrasound Med 1997; 16(11): 751–3.
13. Andresen R, Wegner HE, Dieberg S. Penile metastasis of sigmoid carcinoma: comparative analysis of different imaging modalities. Br J Urol 1997; 79(3): 477–8.
14. Horenblas S, Kroger R, Gallee MP, Newling DW, van Tinteren H. Ultrasound in squamous cell carcinoma of the penis; a useful addition to clinical staging? A comparison of ultrasound with histopathology. Urology 1994; 43(5): 702–7.
15. Rajan DK, Scharer KA. Radiology of Fournier's gangrene. AJR Am J Roentgenol 1998; 170(1): 163–8.
16. Kane CJ, Nash P, McAninch JW. Ultrasonographic appearance of necrotizing gangrene: aid in early diagnosis. Urology 1996; 48(1): 142–4.
17. Sadeghi-Nejad H, Dogra V, Seftel AD, Mohamed MA. Priapism. Radiol Clin North Am 2004; 42: 427–33.
18. Wilkins CJ, Sriprasad S, Sidhu PS. Colour Doppler ultrasound of the penis. Clin Radiol 2003; 58(7): 514–23.
19. Bertolotto M, Quaia E, Mucelli FP, et al. Color Doppler imaging of posttraumatic priapism before and after selective embolization. Radiographics 2003; 23(2): 495–503.
20. Pegios W, Rausch M, Balzer JO, et al. MRI and color-coded duplex sonography: diagnosis of partial priapism. Eur Radiol 2002; 12(10): 2532–5.
21. Volkmer BG, Nesslauer T, Kuefer R, et al. High-flow priapism: a combined interventional approach with angiography and color Doppler. Ultrasound Med Biol 2002; 28(2): 165–9.
22. Feldstein VA. Posttraumatic 'high-flow' priapism. Evaluation with color flow Doppler sonography. J Ultrasound Med 1993; 12(10): 589–93.
23. Shamloul R, Ghanem HM, Salem A, Kamel II, Mousa AA. The value of penile duplex in the prediction of intracavernous drug-induced priapism. Int J Impot Res 2004; 16(1): 78–9.
24. Wilkins CJ, Sriprasad S, Sidhu PS. Colour Doppler ultrasound of the penis. Clin Radiol 2003; 58(7): 514–23.
25. Speel TG, van Langen H, Wijkstra H, Meuleman EJ. Penile duplex pharmaco-ultrasonography revisited: revalidation of the parameters of the cavernous arterial response. J Urol 2003; 169(1): 216–20.
26. Sakamoto H, Shimada M, Yoshida H. Hemodynamic evaluation of the penile arterial system in patients with erectile dysfunction using power Doppler imaging. Urology 2002; 60(3): 480–4.
27. Arslan D, Esen AA, Secil M, et al. A new method for the evaluation of erectile dysfunction: sildenafil plus Doppler ultrasonography. J Urol 2001; 166(1): 181–4.
28. Mancini M, Bartolini M, Maggi M, et al. Duplex ultrasound evaluation of cavernosal peak systolic velocity and waveform acceleration in the penile flaccid state: clinical significance in the assessment of the arterial supply in patients with erectile dysfunction. Int J Androl 2000; 23(4): 199–204.

8

Pediatric and prenatal urological ultrasound

Rosalie de Bruyn, Lyn S Chitty

Introduction

Whereas the ultrasound examinations of the kidneys and bladder in adults and children are basically very similar, there are some differences in the early renal anatomical appearances and pediatric pathologies encountered.

Ultrasound is ideally suited to prenatal and pediatric diagnosis as it is a reliable, non-invasive method of examining the renal tract without the use of ionizing radiation. It has become the cornerstone on which all further imaging of the pediatric urinary tract is based and has a unique role in that all neonates and children suspected of having urinary tract problems or presenting with an abdominal mass have an ultrasound examination before any other imaging is undertaken.

The presentation of renal disease in the pediatric period has changed significantly as improvements in prenatal imaging have progressed. Few infants now present with an undiagnosed mass and most cases of congenital renal obstruction are diagnosed in the prenatal period. The role of ultrasound in pediatric diagnosis now therefore involves the fetal medicine specialist as well as the pediatric radiologist. Consequently, where the diagnosis of renal abnormality might be expected to be made in utero, we have included such examples in this section. Similarly the pre- and post-

natal appearances will be presented where both might be encountered. Management in the early neonatal period, in particular, has been dramatically changed, with some diagnoses now being almost the exclusive domain of prenatal diagnosis. The unexpected diagnosis of renal agenesis or bilateral multicystic dysplastic disease is now a rarity and the effective management of renal disease now involves the prenatal diagnostician, the pediatric radiologist, the pediatrician and, in many cases, the clinical geneticist.

Prenatal diagnosis of fetal renal abnormalities

Renal abnormalities account for around 17% of all anomalies diagnosed prenatally, but many are not detected until late in the second or into the third trimester of pregnancy (Table 8.1), although many of the severe bilateral abnormalities will be detected around 20 weeks, at the time of the routine anomaly scan. While the prognosis in these severe cases which are associated with oligo- or anhydramnios is usually clear, abnormalities which are clinically silent at birth with uncertain pathologic significance produce a significant management dilemma. It is important to

Table 8.1 *Summary of papers detailing gestational age at diagnosis of renal abnormalities*

	Obstructive uropathy			Renal agenesis			Bilateral renal dysplasia		
	<24	*>24*	*ND*	*<24*	*>24*	*ND*	*<24*	*>24*	*ND*
Levi et al[3]	9	56	18	6	8	5	11	7	3
Levi and Hyjazi[4]	2	32	13	3	3	0	4	5	2
Chitty et al[5]	7	0	0	4	0	0	2	1	0
Crane et al[6]	10	16	1	1	0	0	2	1	0
Smith et al[7]	–	–	–	21	30	14	–	–	–
Total (%)	28 (17)	104 (63)	32 (20)	35 (37)	41 (43)	19 (20)	19 (50)	14 (37)	5 (13)

remember that prenatal sonography can only describe anatomical findings and cannot make a histopathologic diagnosis in low-risk cases; thus, the underlying pathology often has to await the results of postnatal investigations. A team approach, comprising a fetal medicine specialist, urologist, nephrologists and, if possible, a geneticist (as there is a high incidence of renal abnormalities in genetically inherited syndromes)[1,2] is the ideal approach to the prenatal diagnosis of renal abnormalities. In all cases where the pregnancy ends in a perinatal death or termination of pregnancy, detailed postnatal pathologic examination should be encouraged with expert histology in order that the diagnosis can be accurately defined. Finally, the spectrum of renal disease seen in the prenatal period is very different from that seen postnatally and, in many cases, there is an association with aneuploidy. Proper counseling of parents with regard to likelihood of aneuploidy, recurrence risk and for appropriate management in future pregnancies requires detailed information from all investigations.

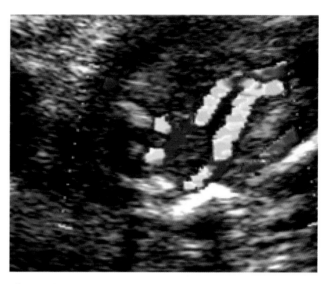

Figure 8.1
Color Doppler showing the paravesical vessels outlining the empty bladder in bilateral renal agenesis.

Sonography of the normal renal tract

Fetal kidneys can be imaged from around 9 weeks' gestation using transvaginal ultrasound, approximately 80% being identified by 11–12 weeks' gestation or from 12–13 weeks' transabdominally. In early pregnancy, the kidneys appear uniformly echogenic. With increasing gestation, corticomedullary differentiation becomes apparent, and by 18–22 weeks, calyceal pattern can be identified. Fetal kidneys continue to grow throughout pregnancy and there are several charts of fetal renal size available.[8]

Fetal urine production begins at around 13 weeks' gestation and, prior to this, amniotic fluid is primarily thought to be a dialysate of fetal blood across the skin. The fetal bladder can be identified transabdominally from 11–12 weeks' postmenstrual age and fetal gender at about the same time.[9] In earlier pregnancy, differentiation between a male and a female can be difficult because of the prominence of the genital tubercle.

Normal fetal ureters are never visualized with ultrasound.

Many renal anomalies do not present until later in pregnancy, reflecting the development of structure and function over time.

Absent kidneys[10]

Failure to identify the kidney(s) in the renal bed can be due either to renal agenesis or to an abnormally positioned kidney.

Renal agenesis

Renal agenesis can be uni- or bilateral and results from early failure of the development of the ureteric bud. Renal agenesis can, however, be mimicked by the end stage of other pathologic process such as multicystic dysplastic kidney disease. The prenatal diagnosis of bilateral renal agenesis is usually made following detailed examination of the fetal urinary tract because of oligohydramnios. It is a difficult diagnosis that should not be made unless there is a persistently empty bladder, which can be defined using color Doppler to outline the umbilical arteries (Figure 8.1), and by the absence of demonstrable kidneys in the renal beds, although this may be complicated because, in the absence of the kidneys, the adrenal glands may take on a globoid or reniform shape within the renal fossa. Failure to demonstrate the renal arteries using color Doppler is a useful adjunct to diagnosis.

Unilateral renal agenesis is less frequently diagnosed prenatally and is often an incidental finding at the time of the detailed scan to examine the fetal anatomy. As with bilateral renal agenesis, the diagnosis can be difficult as the adrenal gland will often occupy the renal bed and give the appearance of a small dysplastic kidney. The use of both color and power Doppler can be a useful aid to diagnosis. In many situations the contralateral normal kidney is enlarged due to compensatory hypertrophy.

Bilateral renal agenesis is a uniformly lethal condition which can occur in isolation but may often be associated with other anomalies, aneuploidy and genetic syndromes. Other abnormalities may be difficult to detect in utero because of the technical difficulties of scanning in the absence of liquor. If the diagnosis is certain, then termination of pregnancy should be discussed and the importance of postnatal pathology stressed. When found as an isolated lesion, the recurrence risk is likely to be small (2–3%). The parents' kidneys should be scanned and if one has a renal abnormality the recurrence risk may be increased.

Pelvic kidney (Figure 8.2)

Failure to identify both kidneys in normal position should stimulate a careful examination of the fetus to exclude location in other sites. Pelvic kidneys are often smaller than expected for the gestational age and may have an abnormal shape. Color Doppler is useful to demonstrate the blood supply to the ectopic kidney which may arise from the lower aorta, common iliac and, rarely, from the middle sacral or inferior mesenteric vessels. Although a pelvic location of the kidneys is most common, they can occasionally be found in other sites such as the chest.

Abnormal kidneys

Abnormal kidneys can be large or small, echogenic or cystic or a combination of both.

Large echogenic kidneys[12]

Large hyperechoic kidneys pose a considerable diagnostic dilemma, particularly in the presence of a normal liquor volume. Some underlying pathologies are shown in Table 8.2. Sonographic detection of large bright kidneys should stimulate a detailed examination of the rest of the fetus, paying particular attention to other measurements. If all measurements lie above the 95th percentile, then an overgrowth syndrome (Beckwith–Wiedemann, Perlman, Simpson–Golabi–Behmel syndromes, etc.) could be considered. If diagnosis of a syndrome can be made, then the prognosis will be that associated with the syndrome. Karyotyping should be discussed, particularly where other malformations are detected.

If, following these investigations, it appears that the fetus has isolated hyperechogenic kidneys and a normal karyotype with no evidence of renal tract obstruction, then the etiology lies between autosomal recessive polycystic kidney disease (ARPCKD), autosomal dominant polycystic kidney disease (ADPCKD), renal dysplasia, nephrocalcinosis or (rarely) a variant of normal. A detailed family history, parental renal scans and a genetic opinion may help in

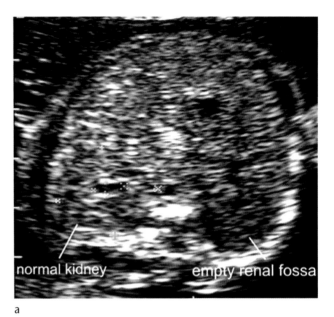

a

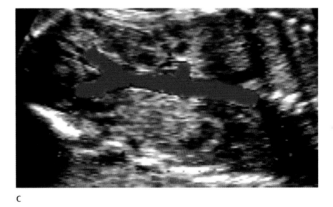

b

c

Figure 8.2
Pelvic kidney. Images showing a pelvic kidney with the empty renal fossa (a), a pelvic kidney located anteriorly and inferiorly to the normal kidney (b) and absence of normal renal artery flow to the pelvic kidey (c). This was subsequently identified as arising from the iliac vessels.

Table 8.2 *Conditions which may be seen in presence of large bright kidneys*

	Liquor	Renal cyst	RPD	Macrosomy	Other anomaly	Gene locus	Inheritance
ARPCKD	N/oligo	–	–	–	–	6p	AR
ADPCKD	N/oligo	(+)	–	–	–	16p, 4q	AD
BWS	N/poly	–	+/–	+	Omphalocele, macroglossia, hemihypertrophy, visceromegaly	11p15	Disomy, sporadic
Perlman	N/oligo	–	+/–	+	Ascites, cardiac, CDH, genital	n/k	AR
SGB	?	?	?	+	Visceromegaly, polydactyly, cardiac, CDH, genital, vertebral	Xq25–27 GPC3	X-linked
Trisomy 13	Oligo	–	+/–	–	Holoprosencephaly, cardiac, polydactyly, IUGR, facial cleft		Sporadic
Meckel–Gruber	Oligo	–	–	–	Encephalocele, CNS, polydactyly, cardiac	17q, 11q, 8q	AR
Obstruction	N/oligo	–	+	–	–	–	Sporadic
Nephrocalcinosis	N	–	–	–	–	–	
Bardet–Biedl	N/poly	–	–	–	Polydactyly, cardiac, genital	3p, 11q, 15q, 16q	AR
Finnish congenital nephrosis	N	–	+/–	–	Very high MSAFP, edema, ascites	NPHS 1	AR

ARPCKD, Autosomal recessive polycystic kidney disease; ADPCKD, autosomal dominant polycystic kidney disease; BWS, Beckwith–Wiedemann syndrome; SGB, Simpson–Golabi–Behmel syndrome; N, normal; RPD, renal pelvic dilatation; AD, autosomal dominant; AR, autosomal recessive; MSAFP, maternal serum alpha fetoprotein; IUGR, intrauterine growth retardation; CDH, coronary heart disease.

identifying the underlying cause; if one of the parents is found to have renal cysts or a history suggestive of adult polycystic kidney disease, the findings may suggest a rare prenatal presentation of this condition.

Alternatively an X-linked pattern of inheritance, together with facial dysmorphisms in the mother, may indicate a diagnosis of the Simpson–Golabi–Behmel syndrome.

In the presence of absent or significantly reduced amniotic fluid, the outcome is likely to be poor, and the pregnancy will frequently end in a neonatal death subsequent to pulmonary hypoplasia as well as renal failure. In these circumstances, if detected before viability, termination of pregnancy is a reasonable option; however, parents should be strongly encouraged to consent to a postmortem examination, as histology will be critical in defining the underlying pathology. In the presence of normal liquor volume, prediction of outcome is more difficult, and serial scanning should be undertaken to monitor the size of the kidneys and liquor volume. Unless there is a positive family history, it will not be possible to define the etiology, which must await the results of postnatal investigations.

Autosomal recessive polycystic kidney disease (Figure 8.3)

ARPCKD is characterized by bilateral symmetrical enlargement of the kidneys, which contain numerous microscopic corticomedullary cysts throughout the kidney. Liver changes, including bile duct proliferation with portal fibrosis, are invariably present, although only detectable histologically. In-utero presentation is variable, although some signs are usually evident by 24 weeks' gestation. Typically, there are enlarged hyperechoic kidneys, with loss of the corticomedullary differentiation in association with oligohydramnios. In some cases, it may be difficult to differentiate the calyceal pattern, but in others this remains defined. The reduction in liquor is usually gradual, and the early manifestation is of enlarged hyperechoic kidneys with normal liquor. Serial scanning will show a gradual reduction in liquor volume to anhydramnios at the varying stages of pregnancy. Many cases diagnosed in utero die after birth or in the neonatal period, as a result of the combination of renal failure and pulmonary hypoplasia due to

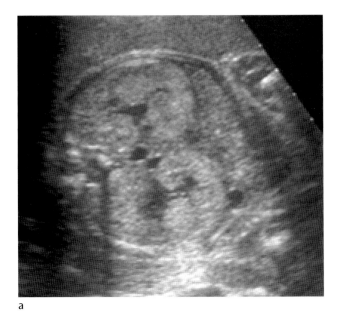
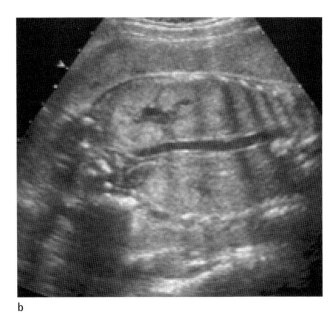

a

b

Figure 8.3

Autosomal recessive polycystic kidney disease. Ultrasound images of enlarged echogenic kidneys seen in the axial (a) and coronal (b) planes and identified histologically after birth as being due to autosomal recessive polycystic kidney disease. Note the absence of amniotic fluid.

severe oligohydramnios. An analysis of the patients surviving the first month of life revealed an actuarial renal survival of 86% at 1 year and 67% at 15 years.[12] Other authors observed that the survival probability at 1 year was 94% for male patients and 82% for female patients ($p < 0.05$).

Autosomal dominant polycystic kidney disease

ADPCKD usually presents in the fourth or fifth decade of life. However, in-utero renal enlargement with cystic change has been reported and the diagnosis should be considered when large bright kidneys are seen in utero in association with normal amounts of amniotic fluid. In most cases of ADPCKD, there will be a positive family history and cystic change should be detectable in one of the parents using ultrasound, as new mutations do not occur frequently. Oligohydramnios is uncommon, as renal function is usually maintained in utero. When presenting prenatally, cystic change is usually present by the second trimester of pregnancy, although late manifestation has been reported. The prognosis for those fetuses with ADPCKD who present in utero is variable, but in the rare cases which present with renal enlargement and severe oligohydramnios perinatal death can ensue. Of 83 cases who presented in utero or during the first few months of life, 43% died before 1 year of age.[13] In two other studies, 16 of 24 survivors developed hypertension in early life and three had end-stage renal failure at a mean age of 3 years. The most useful prenatal prognostic predictors appear to be the presence of oligohydramnios and the outcome of pregnancy of a previously affected sibling.[13] Prenatal diagnosis with ultrasound is not reliable and, in pregnancies at high risk of ADPCKD where linkage has been established in the family, prenatal diagnosis, if requested, should be done using molecular methods.

Enlarged echogenic kidneys and overgrowth syndromes[14]

The presence of large, echogenic kidneys in a fetus with generalized macrosomia and normal or increased liquor points towards the diagnosis of an overgrowth syndrome: all are rare, the most common being Beckwith–Wiedemann syndrome (BWS) and Simpson–Golabi–Behmel (SGB) syndrome (see Table 8.2). Prenatally, differentiation between these syndromes may be extremely difficult unless there is a positive family history, a distinctive pattern of structural abnormalities, or positive molecular or cytogenetic diagnosis.

Beckwith–Wiedemann syndrome

BWS is characterized by overgrowth, macroglossia, visceromegaly (liver, spleen, kidneys, adrenals), abdominal

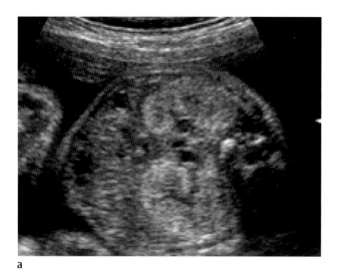

a

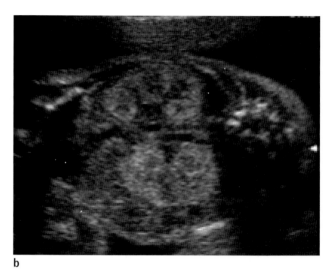

b

Figure 8.4
Beckwith–Wiedemann syndrome. Enlarged echogenic kidneys seen in the axial (a) and coronal (b) planes of a fetus with Beckwith–Wiedemann syndrome. Note the liquor volume.

wall defects (omphalocele and umbilical hernia) and predisposition to embryonal tumors, particularly Wilms' tumor. The features can be very variable, but in all cases of BWS detected prenatally polyhydramnios was reported in association with bilateral enlarged echogenic kidneys (Figure 8.4). Other features reported include hepatomegaly, macroglossia, generalized macrosomia, omphalocele, mild hydronephrosis and placental enlargement, and the condition is associated with a very high beta-human chorionic gonadotropin. If BWS is suspected, cytogenetic analysis can be performed to exclude the possibility of a deletion on 11p15.5 and uniparental disomy of this region, although this is present in only around 20% of cases. The prognosis for BWS is now recognized to be much better than previously thought.[15]

Simpson–Golabi–Behmel syndrome

SGB syndrome is an X-linked overgrowth syndrome which is characterized by a large head with coarse features, hepatosplenomegaly, cryptorchidism and variable degrees of developmental delay, with some cases having normal intelligence. Associated structural abnormalities amenable to prenatal diagnosis include polydactyly, cardiac abnormalities, vertebral anomalies and umbilical hernia. Referral to a clinical geneticist may be of value, as there is often a family history of X-linked problems and female carriers may have distinctive facial features.

Perlman syndrome[16]

Perlman syndrome is a rare overgrowth syndrome inherited in an autosomal recessive fashion, characterized by general organomegaly, facial dysmorphisms and renal hamartomas. Sonographic features include generalized fetal macrosomia and large echogenic kidneys, hydronephrosis and hydroureter, skeletal abnormalities, diaphragmatic hernia and cardiac defects. Polyhydramnios or oligohydramnios have been reported. The prognosis is poor, with neonatal death occurring in many cases often secondary to pulmonary hypoplasia and prematurity. The survivors have a high incidence of developmental delay and Wilms' tumors.

Meckel–Gruber syndrome

Meckel–Gruber syndrome is a lethal genetic syndrome inherited in an autosomal recessive fashion, not associated with overgrowth. Characteristic sonographic features include bilateral large echogenic kidneys (100%) (Figure 8.5a), encephalocele or other major intracranial abnormality (90%) (Figure 8.5b) and post-axial polydactyly (90%) (Figure 8.5c) with severe oligo- or anhydramnios. Polydactyly is not often detected prenatally due to difficulties in examining the fetus with oligohydramnios. Diagnosis early in gestation, between 11 and 14 weeks, may be easier as liquor volume should be normal at this stage. Prenatally, the major differential diagnosis is that of

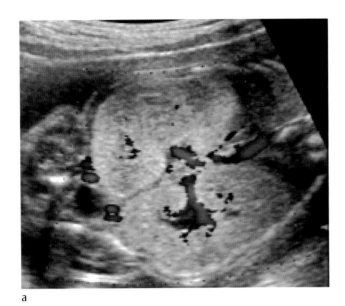

a

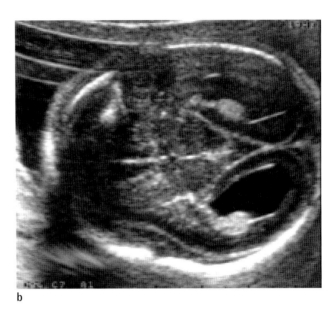

b

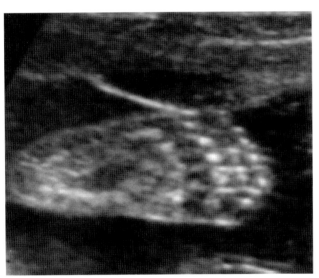

c

Figure 8.5
Meckel–Gruber syndrome. Echogenic kidneys (a), abnormal brain (b) and polydactyly of the toes (c) in a fetus with Meckel–Gruber syndrome.

trisomy 13. The prognosis is awful for a fetus with Meckel–Gruber syndrome, and neonatal death occurs within a few hours of life as a result of renal failure and pulmonary hypoplasia.

Large cystic kidneys[11]

Fetuses with large cystic kidneys usually have multicystic dysplastic kidney (MCDK). MCDK classically presents as a multiloculated mass in the fetal abdomen which consists of the random distribution of multiple thin-walled cysts which cannot be shown to connect with each other or with a renal pelvis (Figure 8.6a,b). Parenchymal tissue between the cysts is often hyperechogenic. Occasionally, cysts can be mainly peripheral (Figure 8.6c). In the unilateral form (76% of cases), liquor volume is usually normal but, when bilateral (24%), oligo- or anhydramnios is usually found. The appearances of the kidney may change during pregnancy – an initially large kidney, which may then start to decrease in size as gestation progresses. In the unilateral presentation, the contralateral kidney is often enlarged, secondary to compensatory hypertrophy, and the bladder is normal, but when bilateral, no fetal bladder is seen. Differential diagnosis includes upper tract dilatation (Figure 8.6d,e) and other intra-abdominal cystic masses. Karyotyping should only be discussed if other anomalies are present or when bilateral, as the incidence of aneuploidy in association with unilateral dysplastic kidneys is very low.

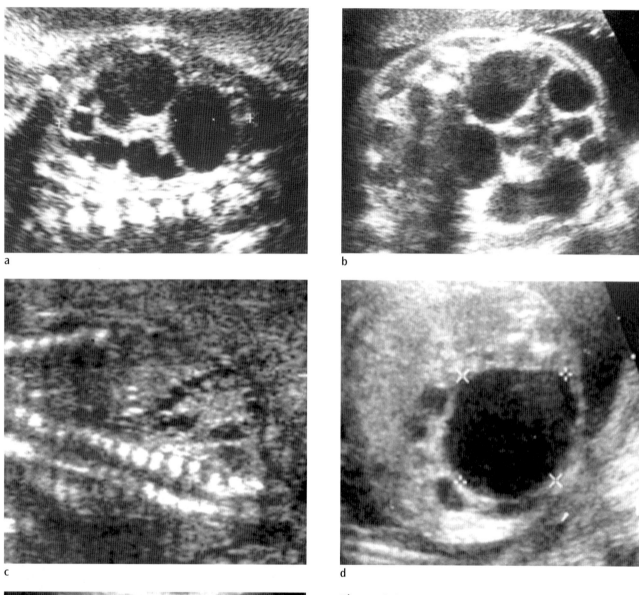

Figure 8.6
Multicystic dysplastic kidney. Sagittal (a) and axial (b) views through the abdomen of a fetus with a typical unilateral multicystic kidney. Note the large irregular cysts, which do not communicate. (c) A sagittal view of a fetus with a multicystic kidney, with cysts confined to the cortical region. The ease with which multicystic kidneys can be confused with upper tract dilatation is demonstrated in the axial (e) and sagittal (d) views of a fetus, where the MCDK had one major cyst and a few scattered smaller ones only visible in the axial view (d).

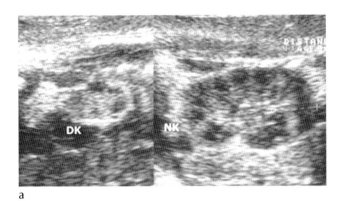

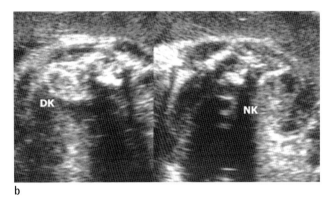

a

b

Figure 8.7
Small echogenic kidneys. Sagittal (a) and axial (b) views of a unilateral small dysplastic kidney (DK) with the normal contralateral kidney (NK) showing compensatory hypertrophy.

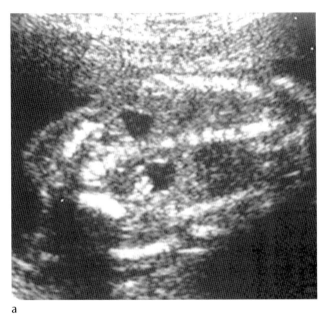

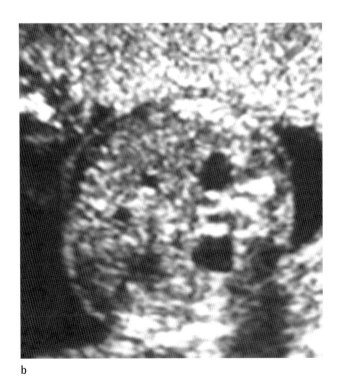

a

b

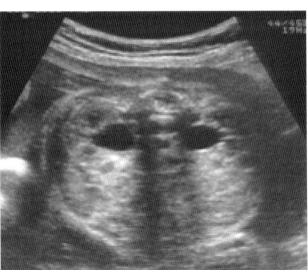

c

Figure 8.8
Renal pelvic dilatation. Mild bilateral renal pelvic dilatation seen in the second trimester in the coronal (a) and axial (b) planes and third (c) trimesters.

Table 8.3 *Etiology of upper tract dilatation*		
Obstructive causes	*Extrarenal obstruction*	*Non-obstructive causes*
Pelviureteric junction obstruction	Sacrococcygeal teratoma	Vesicoureteric reflux
Vesicoureteric junction obstruction	Hydrometrocolpus	Megaureter
Duplex systems	Other pelvic mass (mesenteric, duplication or ovarian cyst)	Megacystis microcolon
Posterior urethral valves		Hypoperistalsis syndrome
Urethral atresia		
Cloacal anomalies		
Ureterocele/ectopic ureters		

Detailed examination of the contralateral kidney is essential, as there is a high incidence of pathology (although this may not be detected until postnatally). Color Doppler assessment may be useful in determining the diagnosis, as in MCDK the renal artery is always small or absent. The prognosis for unilateral isolated MCDK is good. The kidney may involute spontaneously, or remain unchanged, but does not usually require intervention. The prognosis for the bilateral form is universally poor, and neonatal death often ensues secondary to pulmonary hypoplasia and renal failure. Recurrence risks are small, of the order of 2–3%, unless associated with a genetically inherited syndrome.

Small echogenic kidneys

Small echogenic kidneys are seen less frequently than large ones, and the unilateral form is rarely detected in utero unless associated with some renal abnormality, where it may appear as the end stage of some other pathology, e.g. an involuting MCK (Figure 8.7). In the bilateral form it may be difficult to distinguish between renal agenesis and small dysplastic kidneys due to the difficulties performing fetal ultrasound in the presence of oligo- or anhydramnios, and the appearance of the adrenals in renal dysplasias. The prognosis for unilateral cases is good if the contralateral kidney is normal. When bilateral, the prognosis is variable. If there is oligo- or anhydramnios, neonatal death often ensues. Where liquor volume is preserved, renal function may be preserved, but renal replacement is often required in childhood or early adult life.

Urinary tract dilatation

Renal pelvic dilatation

Renal pelvic dilatation (RPD) (Figure 8.8), pyelectasis or hydronephrosis is one of the most common abnormalities

detected on prenatal ultrasound scan and accounts for approximately 50% of all renal lesions detected. It can be due to obstruction at the site of the pelviureteric junction, vesicoureteric junction or bladder outflow tract, but may also occur without any obvious obstruction (Table 8.3). It may represent the in-utero presentation of reflux but often, when mild, it is a normal variant.

Mild renal pelvic dilatation[17]

The anterior/posterior (AP) diameter of the pelvis taken in the axial plane through the kidneys is the most commonly used measurement for the diagnosis of RPD. Much controversy exists over the limit which defines a significant association with postnatal pathology. Most authors take an upper limit of normal of 4–5 mm AP diameter before around 24 weeks' gestation, and up to 10 mm later in pregnancy. Features which are more likely to be associated with a pathologic outcome include progression of dilatation in utero with an AP diameter of ≥10 mm in the third trimester, increased renal cortical echogenicity with or without cysts and lower tract and calyceal dilatation.

Several studies have shown an association between RPD and chromosomal abnormalities: in particular, Down syndrome. However in the presence of mildly dilated renal pelves with no other risk factor present, the prior risk of aneuploidy is only increased slightly, and the risk of miscarriage associated with an invasive procedure will usually exceed this risk.

Fetuses with mild renal pelvic dilatation should be rescanned in the third trimester to look at the extent of the dilatation. If the dilatation has resolved, most authors would consider it unnecessary to perform further scans in the prenatal period, but some would recommend a postnatal scan at around a week or so of life. If the dilatation has progressed and the AP diameter is ≥10 mm, postnatal examination is mandatory, as the risk of significant underlying pathology is increased. Overall, the prognosis for a fetus with mild RPD is good. One large study of low-risk fetuses has shown that around 50% had normal postnatal

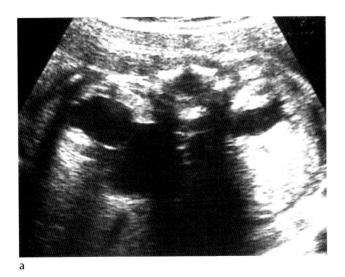

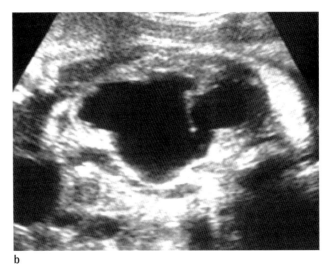

a b

Figure 8.9
Pelviureteric junction obstruction (PUJO). Images of a fetus with bilateral PUJO. Note the asymmetry of the dilatation demonstrated in the axial plane (a). The image taken in the sagittal plane (b) demonstrates the dilatation of the pelvis, which ends abruptly at the junction with the ureters, giving the classical 'micky mouse ears' appearance.

renal ultrasound scans and only 4% of neonates required postnatal surgery.[17]

Pelviureteric junction obstruction (Figure 8.9)[18]

Pelviureteric junction obstruction (PUJO) is a congenital abnormality characterized by obstruction, either functional or anatomical, at the level of the junction between the renal pelvis and the ureter, occurring more commonly in males than females. It is usually unilateral (70%), but, if bilateral, is often asymmetrical. Sonographic diagnosis depends on the demonstration of a moderate or severely dilated renal pelvis in the absence of any dilatation of the ureter or bladder. The overall prognosis for unilateral PUJO is good. Even in bilateral cases, the outcome is often reasonable provided liquor volume is maintained in utero. There is an increased risk of aneuploidy, particularly in the presence of other sonographic findings, and karyotyping should be discussed. Serial scans in pregnancy may be helpful to monitor the evolution of the dilatation.

Vesicoureteric junction obstruction[18]

Vesicoureteric junction obstruction (VUJO) is defined as obstruction at the level of the junction between the ureter and the bladder, leading to dilatation of the ureter. It is

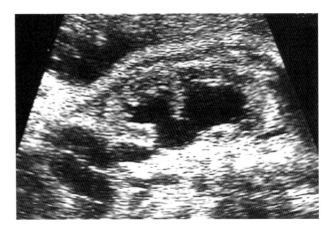

Figure 8.10
Vesicoureteric junction obstruction. Ultrasound image showing the dilated ureter and pelvis in a fetus subsequently found to have vesicoureteric reflux.

bilateral in 13% of cases and 90% of affected fetuses are male. It is often associated with duplex systems and a ureterocele. VUJO should be suspected in the presence of a dilated ureter (Figure 8.10), with or without dilatation of the renal pelvis and calyces. It presents as a serpentine fluid-filled structure that can be mistaken for the fetal bowel, but careful examination will often demonstrate the proximal ureter connecting with the renal pelvis and a distal ureter emptying into the bladder. A fluid-filled ectopic ureterocele (Figure 8.11) may also aid the diagnosis.

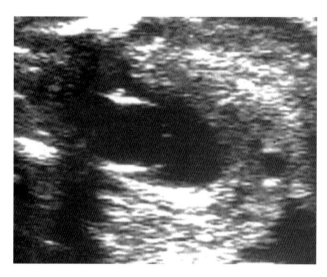

Figure 8.11
Axial view through the bladder demonstrating a ureterocele.

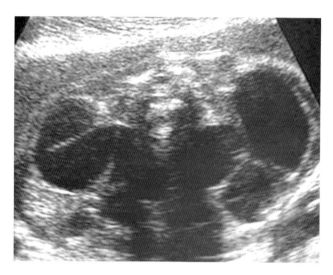

Figure 8.12
Axial view through the abdomen of a fetus with bilateral megaureters.

Megaureter

Megaureter is a dilated ureter with or without dilatation of the renal pelvis and calyces which appears as a hypoechogenic intra-abdominal structure that can be traced back to the renal pelvis. Normal ureters are not visible using ultrasound. The course is often tortuous and a dilated ureter may fill much of the lower abdomen (Figure 8.12).

Duplex systems (Figure 8.13)

Duplex systems are characterized by the presence of a kidney having two pelvic structures with two ureters which may be completely or partially formed. The sonographic diagnosis of a duplex system can be made in the presence of two or more of the following signs:

- two separate renal poles
- dilated pole
- dilated ureter
- ureterocele (see Figure 8.11)

The major differential diagnosis is between a primary megaureter, polycystic kidney, solitary renal cyst or hydronephrosis.[19]

Abnormalities of the bladder

The fetal bladder may be absent, enlarged (megacystis) or exhibit focal abnormality.

Table 8.4 *Etiology of bladder abnormalities*

Absent bladder	*Enlarged bladder (megacystic)*
Renal agenesis	Posterior urethral valves
End-stage outflow obstruction	Vesicoureteric reflux/megaureter
Severe bilateral renal dysplasia	Cloacal anomalies
Bladder exstrophy	Urethral stenosis
Cloacal exstrophy	Megacystis microcolon syndrome
Severe intrauterine growth retardation	Extrarenal obstruction (e.g. hydrometrocolpus, sacrococcygeal teratoma)
Neurological abnormalities:	Twin–twin transfusion syndrome
Generalized neuropathy	
Spinal lesion, e.g. spina bifida, caudal regression	

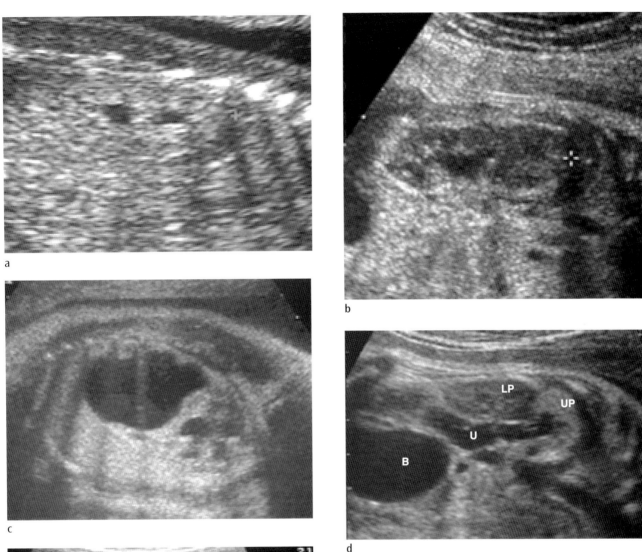

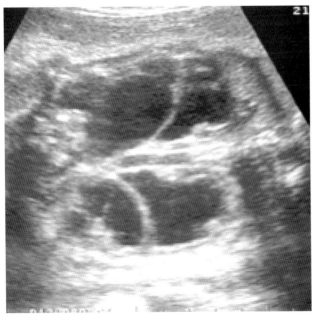

Figure 8.13

Duplex systems. Ultrasound images of duplex systems showing a simple duplex (a), a duplex with one dilated pole at 20 weeks' gestation (b) and with progressive dilatation at 32 weeks (c). A dilated upper pole with a dilated tortuous ureter is shown in (d), and a bilateral duplex system with both poles dilated in (e).

continued overleaf

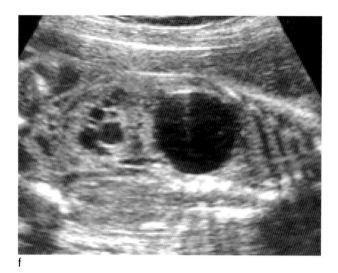

f

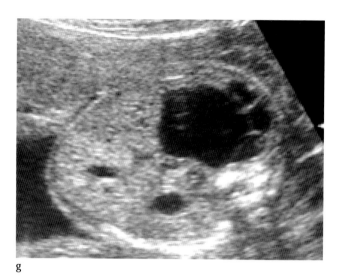

g

Figure 8.13 continued
Duplex systems. A duplex with a dilated upper pole and cystic lower pole in shown in the axial view (f) and sagittal plane (g).

Absent bladder[10]

Failure to identify a fetal bladder situated within the abdomen has a number of etiologies (Table 8.4). If the kidneys are normal and there is no anterior abdominal wall defect, the etiology is likely to lie outside the renal tract. Generalized poor fetal growth in association with oligohydramnios may indicate intrauterine growth retardation, when uterine and fetal Doppler assessment may help confirm the diagnosis.

Bladder exstrophy

Bladder exstrophy is caused by incomplete closure of the inferior part of the anterior fetal abdominal wall and, in its complete form, is often associated with abnormal development of surrounding structures such that it may be possible to observe separation of pubic bones and a low-set umbilicus. The diagnosis should be suspected when the fetal bladder is not visualized in the pelvis in the presence of normal amniotic fluid. Close examination of the abdominal wall may reveal a soft tissue mass distorting the lower abdominal wall (Figure 8.14). Genital abnormalities are frequently observed in males, where micropenis or separation of the halves of the scrotum have been described. It is important to stress that a normal amount of amniotic fluid is always reported. The differential diagnosis includes all the defects of the anterior abdominal wall, omphalocele, gastroschisis and cloacal exstrophy. In the first two, a normally filled bladder should be seen within the extruded sac or associated with herniated bowel.

Cloacal exstrophy[20] (Figure 8.15)

Cloacal exstrophy is a rare, complex abnormality comprising an omphalocele with an everted bladder together with abnormalities of the bowel and genitalia. This defect is often referred to as the OEIS complex (Omphalocele, Exstrophy of the bladder, Imperforate anus and Spinal anomalies). The major sonographic findings are non-visualization of the fetal bladder within the abdomen associated with an anterior abdominal wall defect in 90% of cases. However, a large range of anomalies may be observed, including renal abnormalities (renal agenesis, hydronephrosis, multicystic kidney, hydroureter and ureteric atresia), spinal defects (spina bifida and kyphoscoliosis), abnormalities of the lower limbs and a single umbilical artery.

Enlarged bladder/megacystis[21]

The fetal bladder empties and fills regularly throughout pregnancy. Megacystis can only be diagnosed if the bladder is seen to be persistently enlarged over a period of time of scanning. The underlying pathology is either obstruction to urine outflow, or a deficiency in the muscular wall or innervation of the bladder (Table 8.4). Megacystis may also occur in the presence of polyhydramnios, presumably due to the effect of increased swallowing, when the prognosis will depend upon the underlying etiology. In a review of 79 cases with megacystis seen in the Fetal Medicine Unit at UCLH, the etiologies were as follows: posterior urethral

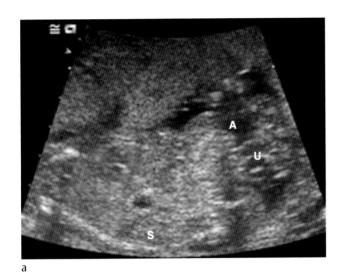

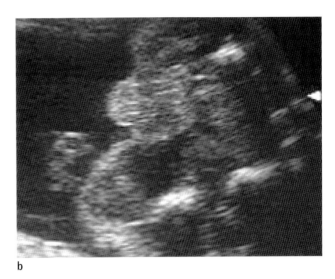

a

b

Figure 8.14
Bladder exstrophy. A fetus with bladder exstrophy is shown in the sagittal plane (a) with the bulge in the anterior abdominal wall (A) seen clearly above the low cord insertion (U) with the spine (S) lying posterior. A view through the pelvis (b) shows the short phallus.

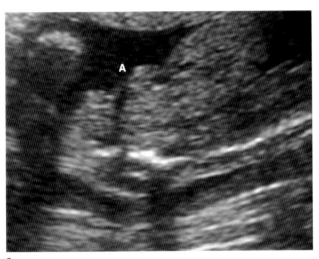

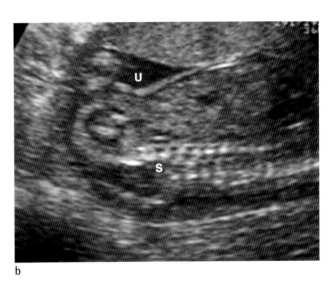

a

b

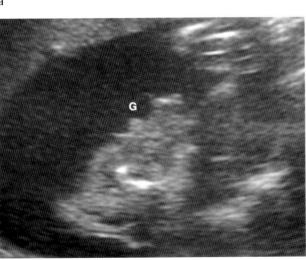

c

Figure 8.15
Cloacal exstrophy. A fetus with cloacal exstrophy scanned at 20 weeks in the sagittal plane (a) showing the abnormal anterior abdominal wall (A), and the short spine (S) in (b) with the axial view (c) demonstrating the splaying of the pelvis with abnormal genitalia (G).

Table 8.5 *Sonographic signs in conditions associated with megacystis*

Diagnosis	Sonographic findings				
	Bladder	Kidneys	Ureters	Liquor volume	Other findings
Urethral atresia	Distended Thin walled	Small Echogenic		Reduced or absent	
Posterior urethral valves	Distended Thick walled	Hydronephrosis +/– echogenic cortex +/– cystic cortex	Dilated	Normal, reduced or absent	Male Dilated posterior urethra
Primary reflux	Distended bladder Thin walled or normal	Hydronephrosis	Dilated (or normal)	Normal	Male or female
Persistent cloaca	Distended Normal or thick walled	Hydronephrosis	Dilated	Normal or reduced	Dilated bowel, dilated vagina, +/– spinal anomalies Usually female
Megacystis microcolon	Distended	Normal	Normal	Normal or increased	

valves (39), reflux (17), complex renal anomalies (7), cloacal anomalies (3), urethral stenosis (4), syndromes (9, megacystis microcolon, oculo-dental-digital, VATER, caudal regression, hollow visceral myopathy).[22] Table 8.5 lists useful sonographic aids to defining the underlying abnormality.

Posterior urethral valves

Posterior urethral valves (PUV) are characterized by redundant folds of mucosa in the posterior wall of the urethra, which result in bladder outflow obstruction. This may be partial or complete and occurs exclusively in males,

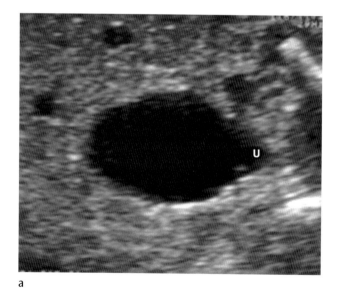

a

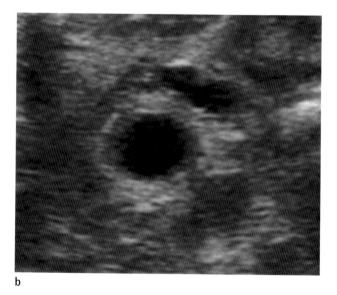

b

Figure 8.16
Posterior urethral valves. A fetus with a thick-walled bladder secondary to posterior urethral valves showing the dilatation with slightly dilated posterior urethra (U) in (a) and incomplete emptying (b) where the thickness of the bladder wall is more evident.

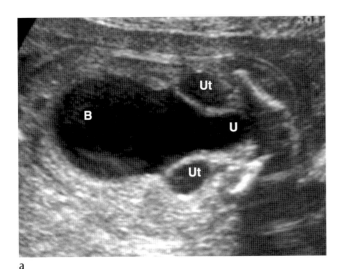

a

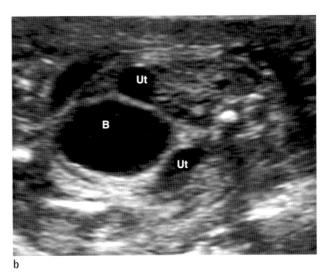

b

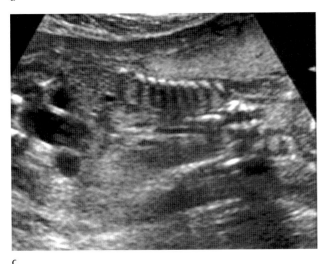

c

Figure 8.17

Posterior urethral valves. A fetus with early and severe presentation of posterior urethral valves showing the classical fusiform shape of the bladder (a) with a dilated posterior urethra (U) and bilaterally dilated ureters (Ut). Another view (b) shows the thin bladder wall and the coronal view (c) shows the very small chest. Note the absence of liquor in all images here taken at 20 weeks' gestation.

where it is the main cause of bladder outflow obstruction. The cardinal sonographic signs of PUV include persistent dilatation of the bladder and proximal urethra with a thickened bladder wall (Figure 8.16), signs of upper tract dilatation and varying degrees of oligohydramnios. The bladder classically has a fusiform or pear-shaped appearance, resulting from the dilated proximal urethra (Figure 8.17). In severe cases, PUV will present in the late first or early second trimester of pregnancy (Figure 8.17). However, the more common presentation is of mild upper tract dilatation with a bladder which may be thick walled and does not empty completely (Figure 8.16b). The fusiform shape may not initially be evident. Serial scanning will show progression of the renal lesion, with increasing dilatation of the renal pelvises and ureters. In some cases liquor volume will reduce over time as the dilatation of the renal tract progresses with increasing bladder distension and thinning of the wall. Renal echogenicity and cystic change may be seen with the development of renal damage secondary to obstruction (Figure 8.18). In other cases

liquor volume can be conserved throughout pregnancy. Spontaneous decompression of the urinary tract may cause extravasation of urine resulting in urinary ascites or a paranephric urinoma.

In the first trimester in severe cases, a large bladder and hyperechogenic kidneys with dilated renal pelvises can be seen (Figure 8.19). Liquor volume is often preserved as amniotic fluid and is not primarily of renal origin prior to 16 weeks of pregnancy. Occasionally, a completely obstructed, hugely dilated bladder will assume a spherical shape and appear to occupy the entire abdomen; alternatively, the bladder will have an irregular outline. In a few cases resolution appears to occur in utero and in others the bladder appears to empty (although complete emptying may not be observed), the wall remains thickened, upper tract dilatation resolves and liquor volume is preserved.

Prenatal management includes a detailed examination of the fetal anatomy to exclude the presence of other genitourinary or extrarenal abnormalities, although oligohydramnios may impair visualization. Karyotyping should

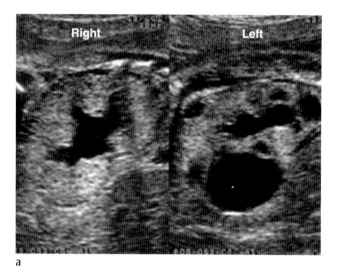

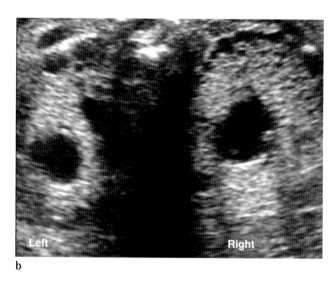

a

b

Figure 8.18

Posterior urethral valves. A fetus with posterior urethral valves demonstrating the variety of cystic change seen at 29 weeks' gestation. Both kidneys are demonstrated in the sagittal plane (a) and axial plane (b). Both kidneys are echogenic; the right is developing small cortical cysts with larger cysts seen in the left kidney.

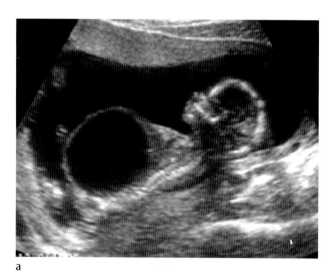

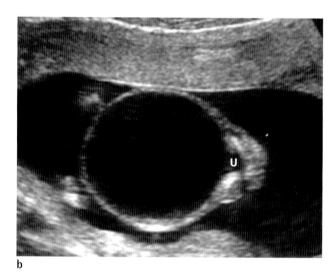

a

b

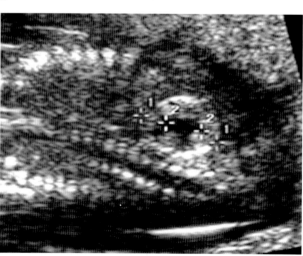

c

Figure 8.19

Posterior urethral valves. Ultrasound scan at 12 weeks' gestation showing a hugely dilated bladder in the sagittal plane (a); the axial plane (b) demonstrates the dilated posterior urethra (U), and the echogenic kidneys with dilated pelvises are also demonstrated (c).

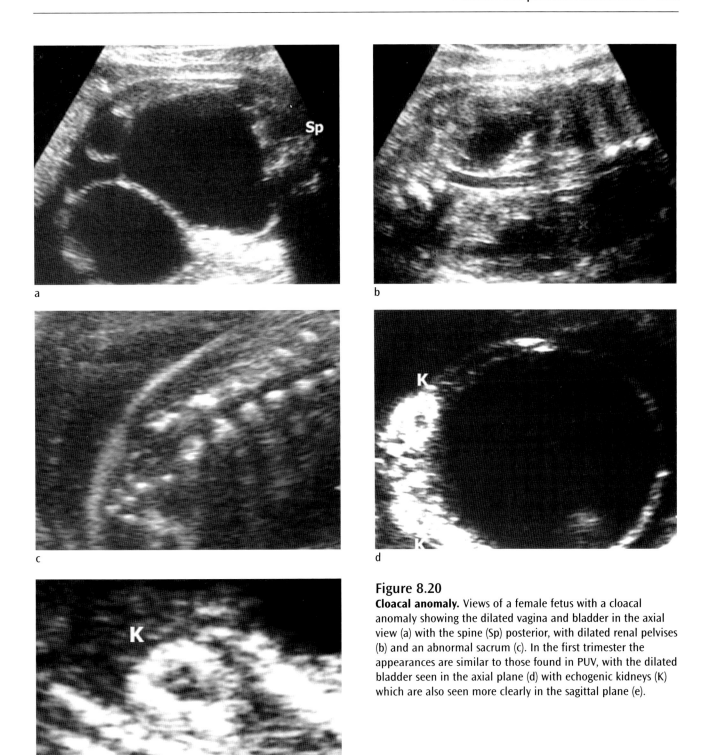

a

b

c

d

e

Figure 8.20
Cloacal anomaly. Views of a female fetus with a cloacal anomaly showing the dilated vagina and bladder in the axial view (a) with the spine (Sp) posterior, with dilated renal pelvises (b) and an abnormal sacrum (c). In the first trimester the appearances are similar to those found in PUV, with the dilated bladder seen in the axial plane (d) with echogenic kidneys (K) which are also seen more clearly in the sagittal plane (e).

be discussed, as aneuploidy may be associated with PUV, particularly when other risk factors are present. Poor prognostic signs include presentation prior to 24 weeks' gestation, oligohydramnios, loss of corticomedullary differentiation, renal cortical cysts and increased cortical echogenicity (Figure 8.18). Renal size and degree of pelvic and ureteric dilatation do not seem to correlate well with outcome, as dysplastic kidneys secondary to obstruction may be large or small. Fetal urinalysis may have some place in evaluating prognosis, as the composition of fetal urine depends only on fetal renal function.[23] The composition of the urine changes with gestational age and normal values have been established, although the normal ranges are quite wide at 20 weeks. The use of urinalysis in clinical practice remains controversial, as long-term follow-up data are largely lacking and renal failure may ensue during childhood, resulting in long-term morbidity. A urinary calcium concentration of >8 mg/dl or sodium concentration of >100 mEq/L and high levels of urinary beta 2 microglobulin (> 4 mg/L) are generally considered to be the most sensitive prognostic indicators.

The prognosis in severe cases is often relatively easy to predict: if the bladder is dilated with obviously dysplastic kidneys and oligohydramnios (see Figure 8.17), perinatal death will ensue secondary to pulmonary hypoplasia and renal failure. However, when the obstruction is partial outcome is more variable, with renal failure occurring in around 30–50% at some time in childhood, but perinatal death is rare. Once the prognosis has been determined as accurately as possible, various options should be discussed, including in-utero follow-up with planned postnatal investigations, termination of pregnancy and, very occasionally, in-utero therapy using a vesicoamniotic shunt to bypass the obstruction.[24]

Reflux or megacystis/megaureter

Reflux or megacystis/megaureter should be suspected if a large, thin-walled bladder is found together with dilated ureters, bilateral hydronephrosis, but normal renal parenchyma and amniotic fluid volume.[25] The differential diagnosis includes other forms of megacystis, and definitive diagnosis usually has to await results of postnatal investigations.

Persistent cloaca

Persistent cloaca is a rare anomaly. The typical ultrasound findings include the presence of two or more cystic structures within the pelvis, often associated with upper renal tract abnormalities (Figure 8.20b), resulting from intestinal, vaginal (hydrometrocolpus) and bladder obstruction.[20] In the first trimester the finding of an enlarged bladder and abnormal kidneys (Figure 8.20d,e) in a female fetus are suggestive of a cloacal anomaly. Even when suspected prenatally, accurate definition of the extent of the abnormalities is difficult, as the involvement of structures in cloacal malformations is varied and serial examinations should be performed as the sonographic abnormalities evolve over time. Abnormalities of the spine are particularly common (Figure 8.20a,c). The differential diagnosis includes ovarian cysts, intestinal duplication, Hirschsprung's disease, colic dilatation, hydrometrocolpus resulting from an imperforate hymen and megacystis microcolon syndrome. A potentially useful sonographic sign in cloacal anomalies is the variation in size of the cystic structures with bladder emptying and filling.

Genital anomalies

A range of genital anomalies can be detected prenatally, including hydroceles (Figure 8.21), which are common and usually benign, varying degrees of hypospadias and micropenis (Figure 8.22) and cliteromegaly (Figure 8.23). These conditions may be isolated or found in association with other anomalies or metabolic or endocrine disorders.[26]

PEDIATRIC IMAGING

This section will be specifically concerned with those conditions found in the postnatal and pediatric age group and will highlight the differences found in children and adults.

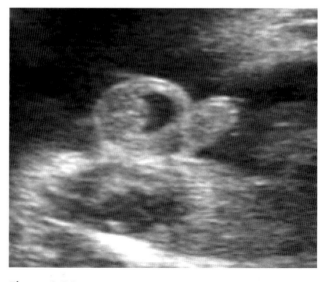

Figure 8.21
A fetus seen at 26 weeks' gestation with hydroceles.

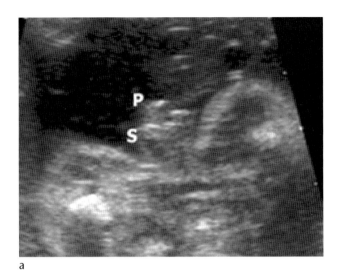
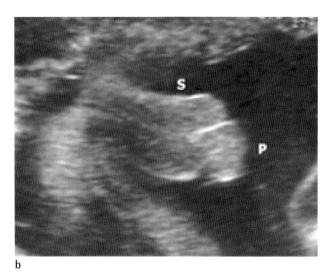

a   b

Figure 8.22
Hypospadias. A fetus with a severe hypospadias seen at 24 weeks (a) and again at 30 weeks (b). The normal scrotum (S) is seen with the micropenis (P).

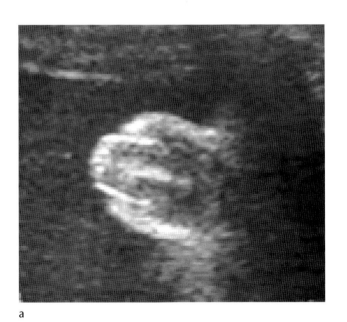
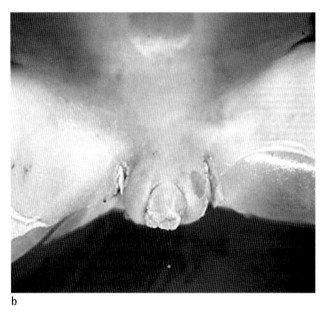

a   b

Figure 8.23
Cliteromegaly. Enlarged clitoris seen at 28 weeks' gestation (a). Other abnormalities were present and a stillbirth occurred a few weeks later (b).

Ultrasound and nuclear medicine are ideally complementary techniques by which the kidneys and bladder can be imaged both anatomically and functionally. Consequently, reference to isotope studies will be regularly made. It is possible that in the future other modalities such as magnetic resonance imaging (MRI) will provide functional imaging information (Table 8.6).

Ultrasound technique

Nowadays, most mothers have had experience of an ultrasound examination during pregnancy and have explained this and reassured their child prior to the examination. A peaceful, warm, soothing environment with musical toys and mobiles on the ceiling providing distraction is an

Table 8.6 *The different imaging modalities used in children and their indications*

Investigation	Description	Indications
Micturating cystourethrogram (MCUG)	Requires bladder catheterization and instillation of radiographic contrast medium. Demonstrates bladder size and shape. VUR if present. Only test which will show urethral abnormalities in boys	Suspected PUV. Thick-walled bladder. Ureteric dilation. UTI in boys <1 year. Antenatal diagnosis of bilateral renal tract dilatation
Direct isotope cystogram (DIC)	Bladder catheterization and isotope contrast	First investigation in girls and for follow-up in toddlers who are not potty-trained. Lower radiation dose than IRC
Voiding urosonography	Bladder catheterization and ultrasound contrast	Similar to DIC. Not universally accepted. Contrast medium not licenced for use in children. Urethra not shown
Indirect radioisotope cystogram (IRC)	Dynamic renogram followed by voiding to look for VUR	Follow-up of VUR in older continent children. Gives additional functional information about kidneys
Dimercaptosuccinic acid (Tc99m DMSA)	Isotope gets fixed in the kidney	To look for scars in the kidney following UTI. To search for functioning renal tissue not seen on US. To assess differential renal function
Diethylenetriamine pentaacetate (Tc99m DTPA) Mercaptoacetyltriglycine (Tc99m MAG3)	Dynamic renogram. Isotope taken up by kidney and passed in urine. After 30 minutes micturition, views to look for VUR (indirect radioisotope cystogram) IRC	Assess differential renal function and drainage. Postoperative evaluation of the collecting system. Indirect cystography following renal transplantation. Renography with captopril stimulation for renovascular hypertension
Intravenous urogram (IVU)	Radiographic contrast injected intravenously. Series of views of the kidneys and bladder as the contrast passes through the system	To demonstrate calyceal anatomy In the work-up of calculi To demonstrate ureteric anatomy Difficult duplex systems

PUV, posterior urethral valves; UTI, urinary tract infection; VUR, vesicoureteric reflux; US, ultrasound.

important contributor towards a successful examination. Warming the gel is essential if children are not to be frightened in the first few minutes. Restraining devices are never used and, once reassured that they are not going to be hurt, most children will settle. Sedation is rarely, if ever, employed, but timing the examination for after food in a neonate will produce both a sleepy infant and a full bladder. A cache of dummies (soothers) is essential. There is no specific preparation, but all children are requested, potty-training permitting, to have a full bladder for the examination. Without a full bladder, dilated lower ureters behind the bladder and intravesical pathology will be missed. In this way children are also well hydrated, allowing full distension of the calyces and renal pelves, especially important in suspected PUJO. A successful examination is critically dependent on the skill and experience of the sonographer. Ultrasound examination of the kidneys and bladder in children, although similar to that in adults, has a few important differences in the technique.

Kidney

Use transducers with highest frequency both to produce images of the highest parenchymal detail and to keep insonation to the minimal levels necessary. Phased-array sector probes or (tightly) curved arrays with a small footprint are generally preferred and allow relatively easy visualization on the small abdomen both in the supine and prone positions. The kidney is normally examined in quiet respiration, but if it is obscured by bowel gas, using deep inspiration or expiration (blow up your tummy like a balloon) usually allows complete visualization. Linear probes, while now much smaller in length at the higher frequencies, still do not provide consistently good overall visualization to measure renal lengths, although they may be useful to examine parenchymal detail.

The examination should always start with the child supine. In this way an anxious child can see the gel being applied, the transducer and the television monitor. The sonographer should begin with the full bladder, scanning both longitudinally and transversely. The bladder should then be emptied and, on returning to the couch, the residual volume should be calculated. The kidneys are then examined both longitudinally and transversely using the

liver and spleen as acoustic windows and comparing their reflectivity. In neonates, this is the best position in which to detect dilatation of the ureters within the abdomen.

Once the kidneys and renal vasculature have been fully evaluated supine, the child is routinely turned prone. This

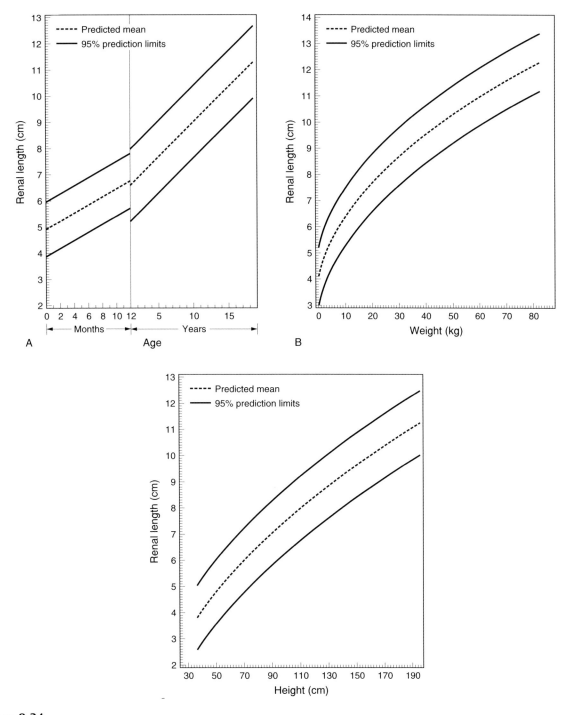

Figure 8.24

Normal renal charts for children. (After Han BK, Babcock DS. Sonographic measurements and appearance of normal kidneys in children. AJR Am J Roentgenol 1985; 145: 611–16.) These charts represent the maximum renal length (A) for age, (B) for weight and (C) for height.

position is ideal in children as the ribs rarely, if ever, obscure the kidneys and, without much body fat or retroperitoneal tissue, the kidneys lie relatively close to the skin surface. Scanning longitudinally and obliquely with the transducer along the long axis of the kidney, the maximum renal length is measured and compared to normal charts. If hydronephrosis or separation of the central sinus echoes is present, the maximum transverse pelvic diameter (either intra- or extrarenal) is measured. This position is used as it can be reliably reproduced when following the degree of central sinus separation at follow-up examinations. Tables of normal renal length compared to height and weight and age are available[27] and this information should form part of the routine examination and report (Figure 8.24).

Supine and prone positions are generally sufficient for a successful examination but rarely, especially in fractious children, one may modify these positions while the child is being held in the mother's arms.

Table 8.7 *Use of urethrograms*	
Year	Number of contrast micturating cystourethrograms
93/94	462
94/95	370
95/96	399
96/97	327
97/98	282
98/99	251
99/2000	225
00/01	213
01/02	180
02/03	173

Bladder

The bladder is an important part of the examination in children and as far as possible should be examined full and first. In this way dilated lower ureters will not be missed and intravesical pathology such as ureteroceles and masses will not be overlooked. The bladder wall must be measured in all boys with suspected outflow obstruction, bladder instability and neuropathic disorders. This is best done away from the trigone. The normal bladder wall measurements are 3 mm and 5 mm full and empty, respectively.[29] In male neonates with bilateral hydronephrosis, the urethra must be examined for posterior urethral valves. This is achieved by using a high-frequency linear probe, scanning the perineum and urethra longitudinally during micturition when the posterior urethra is maximally distended with urine. Post-micturition views of the bladder are routine in all nephro-urologic patients to assess for any residue and to calculate the residual volume (according to a prolate ellipse). A volume of over 30 ml is generally considered pathologic.

Of particular interest in recent years has been the use of ultrasound contrast media in order to perform urosonography. The bladder is catheterized in the conventional way and then ultrasound contrast media instilled. The presence of the echogenic microbubbles in the bladder can be easily seen, and if reflux is present the microbubbles can be seen in the ureters and renal pelves. Clearly, however, no voiding views of the urethra can be obtained in males.

While the use of ultrasound to detect vesicoureteric reflux (VUR) is extremely attractive in children, this technique has not gained widespread acceptance for a number of reasons. Pediatric radiologists are trying to move away from tech-

niques requiring bladder catheterization, as it is invasive and sometimes even introduces infection. The numbers of cystograms performed in pediatric practice have markedly decreased over the years (Table 8.7). It is almost never used in the older child and is almost exclusively used in the infants with an antenatal diagnosis, suspected PUV, complicated duplex systems and neuropathic bladders.

Ultrasound contrast media is expensive, is not universally licensed for use in children and a major drawback is that the urethra is not visualized. The bladder still has to be catheterized. There is potentially only a small group of children in whom this method can be justifiably used: i.e. follow-up cystography in infants with VUR who are not yet potty-trained.

Doppler examination

The technique of Doppler ultrasound examination in children is identical to that used in adult practice and the use of Doppler ultrasound should form part of the normal routine examination as well as the more complex examinations for hypertension. The major difficulty in children is the prolonged period of immobility, as examinations are often long and time consuming.

Doppler is integral to examining the kidneys, in particular in the following instances:

1. To clarify the position of the renal hilar vasculature and renal pelvis.

2. To define the nature and vascularity of any cystic renal lesions.
3. After renal transplantation.
4. Following a renal biopsy and bleeding.
5. For suspected renovascular hypertension.
6. Trauma.

There are a number of patterns of Doppler flow that are peculiar to children:

- reversal of flow in the renal artery may be due to a patent ductus arteriosus in the neonate
- normal neonates may have a markedly low or absent diastolic renal artery flow
- the relatively high heart rate in infants produces low resistance index values and this is exacerbated by a tachycardia.

In practice, however, the resistive index is of very little value in pediatric patients as it has not been shown to be discriminatory.

Anatomical considerations

The appearance of the kidney and related structures is identical in children to that in thin adults with one important exception, the neonate.

The normal neonatal kidney has distinct differences and these must be recognized if the sonographer is not to over-diagnose pathology. The cortical echogenicity is iso- or hyperechoic, as compared to the liver and the cortex, and thinner in relation to the rest of the kidney as compared to an adult kidney. The hyperechoic cortical echogenicity can persist as a normal physiologic appearance for up to 6 months of life and is thought to be related to the cortical position and packing of the neonatal glomeruli. The medullae are echo-poor as compared to the cortex, triangular in shape, with the base of the triangle on the cortex and regularly arranged around the central collecting system. In the past they were often mistaken for cysts due to the echo-poor appearance. They can be distinguished from cysts by the bright 'dot' of the arcuate artery on the triangle base. The central sinus complex appears as an echogenic cluster of echoes in the center of the kidney and little or no sinus fat is present. The renal capsule is thin and poorly differentiated from the rest of the cortex (Figure 8.25).

Most infant kidneys have a smooth outline, very few displaying fetal lobulation.

As in the adult, separation of the central sinus is observed normally with hydration and with a full bladder. Most pediatric sonographers take the somewhat arbitrary figure of 10 mm separation as the upper limit of normal.

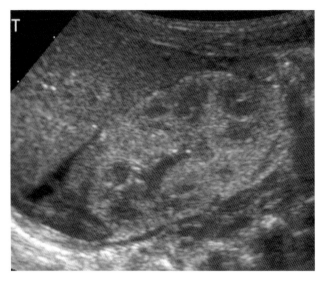

Figure 8.25
Longitudinal sonogram of the normal right kidney in a neonate. The medullary pyramids are echo free, triangular in shape and regularly arranged around the echogenic central collecting system echoes. The renal cortex is relatively thin as compared to the adult kidney. Very little sinus fat is present in children.

However, unlike in adult practice, detection of children with vesicoureteric reflux is important and may only be reflected by minor separation of the central sinus echoes without renal scarring. It is generally considered that if a ureter can be seen it is abnormal.

Postnatal imaging of infants with antenatally detected nephrourological disorders

The antenatal detection of urologic abnormalities has made an enormous impact on postnatal imaging of neonates over the last 10–15 years. In the early years all the neonates had a full nephrologic work-up, but protocols have been better refined over the years so that now, on the whole, the maximum amount of information is obtained using the minimum number of investigations.

Postnatal ultrasound is optimally performed when the infants are well hydrated: i.e. when the mother's milk has come on and generally after 48–72 hours after birth. The role of the initial ultrasound is to confirm the antenatal diagnosis and detect any obstructive uropathy that will require urgent treatment such as duplex systems and posterior urethral valves. The initial postnatal ultrasound will also direct any appropriate further imaging.[29] Table 8.8 lists the abnormalities which can be either unilateral or bilateral.

Table 8.8 *The differential diagnosis of prenatal hydronephrosis*

Unilateral	Bilateral
• RPD • VUR • Megaureter (± VUR) • MCDK (simple) • Complicated duplex kidney, i.e. obstructed upper moiety with ureterocele and/or refluxing lower moiety	• RPD • VUR • Megaureters (± VUR) • MCDK (complicated) cystic dysplastic or dilated (PUJ) kidney on the opposite side • Bilateral complicated duplex kidneys • Bladder or outlet pathology, e.g. neurogenic bladder or PUV with bilateral upper tract dilatation

RPD, renal pelvic dilatation; VUR, vesicoureteric reflux; MCK, multicystic dysplastic kidney; PUJ, pelviureteric junction; PUV, posterior urethral valves.

Unilateral and bilateral renal pelvic dilatation

Unilateral RPD is the commonest abnormality to be detected antenatally and in the majority this appears to be a relatively benign condition. Currently, ultrasound alone is used for a renal pelvic diameter measuring 15 mm or less. It is important for the sonographer to clearly state whether there is calyceal dilatation, as the prognosis for the kidney is considered to be worse. These are manifest as in the adult, as fluid-containing structures separating the renal sinus and connecting with the renal pelvis (Table 8.9).

Table 8.9 *The imaging protocol for renal pelvic dilatation (RPD)*

Unilateral	Bilateral
• Postnatal ultrasound after 2–3 days • MAG3 renogram after 2–3 months if RPD >15 mm • No MCUG if no dilated ureter	• Same as unilateral, but add MCUG

For abbreviations, see Table 8.6.

Megaureter

The term megaureter simply applies to a dilated ureter. Most megaureters are associated with obstruction but they may also be associated with vesicoureteric reflux. Megaureters may be unilateral or bilateral. If detected antenatally, then a micturating cystourethrogram should be performed at the same time as the initial imaging. The dilated ureter is visualized alongside the aorta or inferior vena cava (IVC), perhaps using gentle compression. Ureteric dilatation may be accompanied by marked tortuosity if the dilatation is marked. If there is no reflux, then the infant can be followed as for bilateral RPD.

Multicystic kidney (multicystic dysplastic kidney)

Before the routine use of antenatal scanning, the multicystic kidney (MCK) was reportedly the commonest cause of an abdominal mass in a neonate. The hallmark of the multicystic kidney is an atretic ureter: classically, they are non-

functioning. The multicystic kidney may involve the whole or part of a kidney and, if bilateral, is incompatible with life. Common ultrasound findings are those of a large cyst with multiple smaller cysts peripherally and no normal renal parenchyma (Figure 8.26). It has become increasingly apparent that this condition has a wide spectrum of appearances, with a small cystic kidney at the one end and a large multicystic kidney at the other. Some may even involute in utero. The importance of diagnosing this entity is the high incidence (30%) of associated anomalies in the contralateral kidney; these are termed 'complicated MCK', which is important for the long-term prognosis of the child. Abnormalities seen in the contralateral kidney include pelviureteric abnormalities and ureteral narrowing. There is an increase of vesicoureteric reflux and ureteroceles on the ipsilateral side of the multicystic kidney. It is for this reason that all these neonates must be investigated further.

After the initial detection, the role of ultrasound lies in monitoring the size of the multicystic kidney. The associations with hypertension and malignancy are not used as

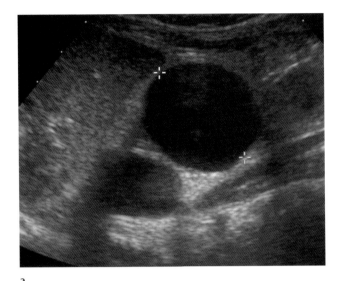

a

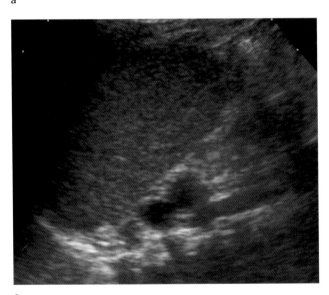

c

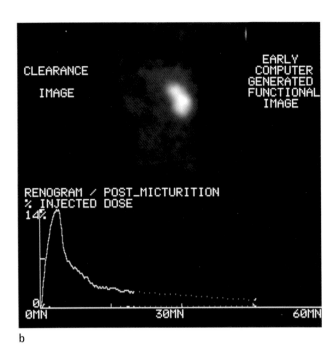

b

Figure 8.26

Multicystic kidney. (a) Longitudinal sonogram of a left multicystic kidney (MCK). There are only two large cysts with no renal parenchyma. This MCK is relatively large, but there is a wide spectrum of appearances and sizes in those detected antenatally. (b) MAG 3 renogram. There is no function in the multicystic kidney. (c) After 1 year, the MCK had involuted, which is the natural history in the majority of these kidneys.

indications for removal of the multicystic kidney (Table 8.10).

Posterior urethral valves

Many male infants with PUV are detected antenatally with a thick-walled bladder (see antenatal diagnosis). However, the clinical presentation is very variable, with the most obstructed systems detected antenatally and the less severely affected in early infancy. There are other causes of a thick-walled bladder such as a neuropathic bladder, a prolapsed ureterocele obstructing the urethra, a syringocele and, more rarely, an anterior urethral diverticulum: i.e. any cause that may obstruct the urethra.

Posterior urethral valves are simply described as a flap of mucosa that obstructs the urethra. The appearances seen on ultrasound are related to hypertrophy of the bladder wall as it tries to overcome the outflow obstruction. The kidney changes depend on the time of onset of the obstruction in intrauterine life: the earlier the onset, the higher the risk of severe consequences to the kidneys such as dysplasia; the later the onset, the more likely the kidneys will be simply hydronephrotic or in older boys may even be normal. Urinomas or collections of urine around the kidney may develop from calyceal rupture due to the high pressure in the system.

Infants detected antenatally need urgent postnatal imaging in order to make the diagnosis and allow early relief of the bladder outflow obstruction. These infants have a high risk of developing a urinary tract infection, which could further compromise the kidneys.

Table 8.10 *Imaging protocol for multicystic kidney (MCK)*

Simple	*Complicated*
• Postnatal ultrasound after 2–3 days to confirm the antenatal diagnosis • No need for prophylactic antibiotics • Repeat scan at 6 weeks • DMSA or MAG3 renogram. If any function on these tests, MCK is unlikely. Refer to urologist	Contralateral kidney dilated >15 mm. Exclude obstruction: • MAG3 renogram after 2–3 months • Prophylactic antibiotics Contralateral kidney <15 mm with ureteric dilatation: • MCUG and if VUR; then follow as for VUR. If no VUR, then follow as for simple kidney

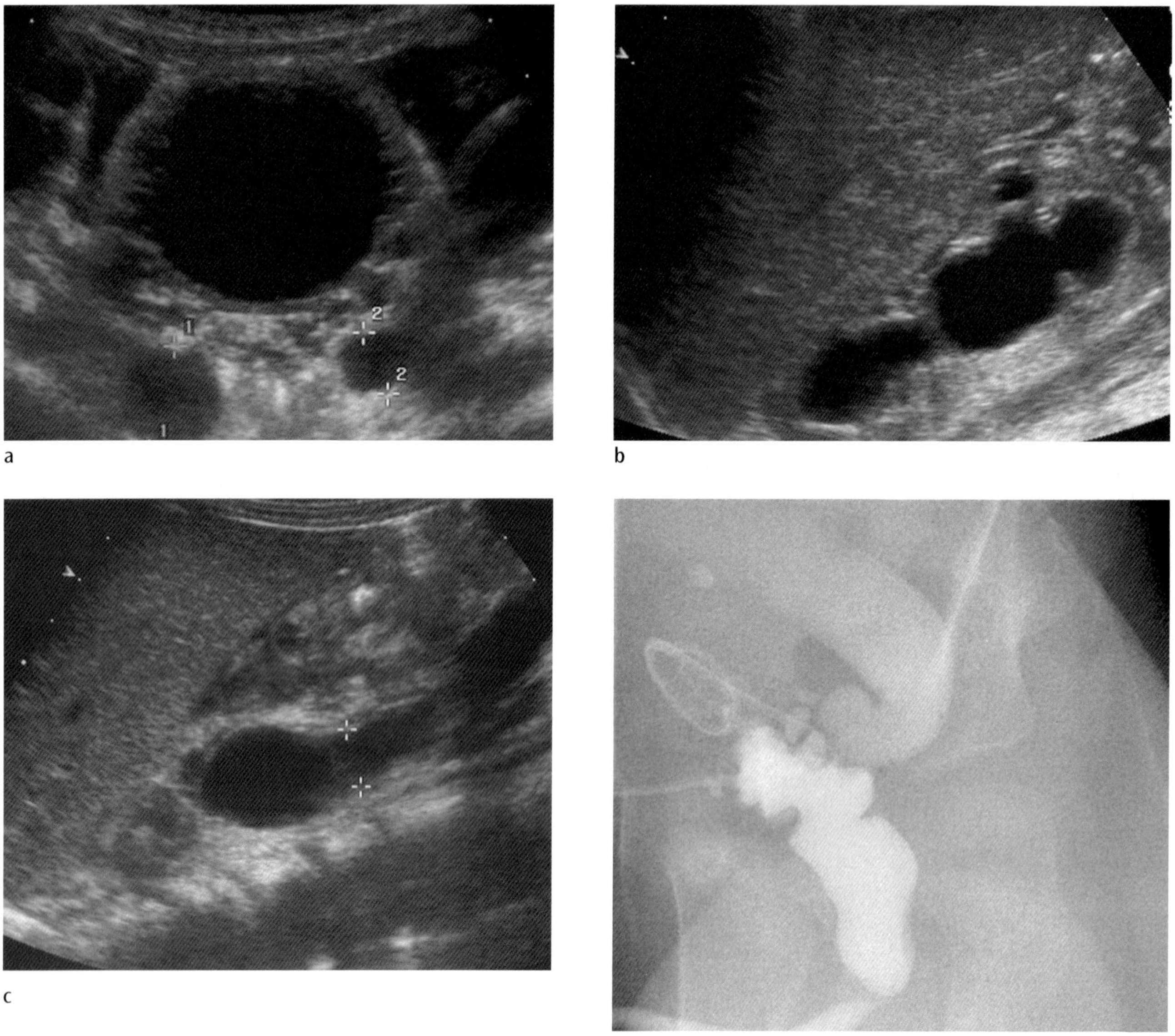

a

b

c

d

Figure 8.27

Posterior urethral valves. (a) Transverse sonogram of the bladder in an 18-month-old boy presenting with a urinary tract infection. Notice both lower ureters are dilated (between calipers) and the bladder wall is irregular and thick. (b,c) Longitudinal sonograms of both kidneys, showing that there is bilateral hydronephrosis and hydroureters. (d) Micturating cystourethrogram via a suprapubic catheter shows a small-volume bladder with a markedly irregular trabeculated wall and thickened bladder neck. The posterior urethra is dilated with a sharp transition to the anterior urethra. There is vesicoureteric reflux into the ureters.

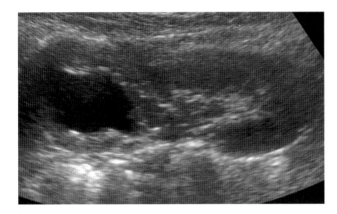

a

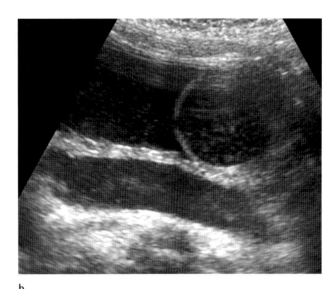

b

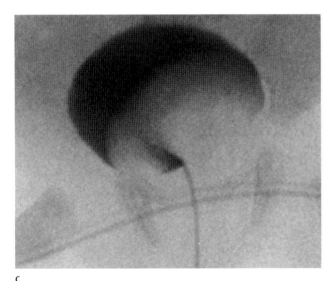

c

Figure 8.28
Duplex kidney. (a) Prone longitudinal scan of the right kidney showing the obstructed upper moiety of a duplex system. (b) Longitudinal sonogram of the bladder showing the thin-walled ureterocele and dilated ureter associated with it. Notice the dilated ureter contains multiple echoes in keeping with an infected system. (c) Micturating cystourethrogram showing the filling defect of the large ureterocele in the bladder.

Postnatal ultrasound findings would include bilateral hydronephrosis and hydroureters, echogenic cystic dysplastic kidneys, a urinoma where the urine has ruptured out of the kidney from a calyx and a thick-walled bladder (Figure 8.27).

In suspected PUV a longitudinal ultrasound examination of the perineum using a high-frequency linear transducer, will be able to demonstrate the thick-walled bladder base and a dilated posterior urethra. This should be done when the infant is voiding so that there is maximal dilatation of the posterior urethra. Dilatation of the posterior urethra measuring more than 7 mm is abnormal.

The infant suspected of having posterior urethral valves should have an urgent micturating cystourethrogram (MCUG).

The duplex kidney

The duplex kidney can be very easy to diagnose but can also be one of the most difficult and complex conditions requiring the use of all imaging modalities. Ultrasound plays an important diagnostic role, with the dilated obstructed systems and ureteroceles primarily detected antenatally (Figure 8.28).

Typically, the upper moiety obstructs and is associated with either a ureterocele in the bladder or ectopic drainage, for instance into the vagina. The upper moiety may have small peripheral cortical cysts and evidence of increased echogenicity and dysplasia. The lower moiety dilates, which is usually vesicoureteric reflux but may be renal pelvic dilatation (PUJ) alone. Duplex kidneys are often bilateral.

On functional imaging, there may be equal function between upper and lower moiety. In some cases, the upper moiety function may be reduced due to dysplasia or obstruction. Lower moiety function may also be reduced due to scarring from the VUR.

Cystograms must be performed in order to document any suspected ureteroceles and VUR.

Nuclear medicine studies such as DMSA (dimercaptosuccinic acid) and MAG3 (mercaptoacetyltriglycerine) are performed to show a differential function and drainage.

Intravenous urography (IVU) is generally not needed in all duplex systems. However, when the ultrasound and nuclear medicine studies do not entirely complement each other, the situation may then necessitate a carefully performed IVU.

Renal anomalies in association with other congenital anomalies

Renal anomalies are known to be associated with other congenital anomalies. All neonates with esophageal atresia, rectal atresia and VATER association should have screening ultrasound of the renal tract. In addition, these children should have routine screening spinal ultrasound examinations. Single kidneys and crossed fused ectopia are the commonest associated abnormalities. There is also a high incidence of renal anomalies in congenital heart disease, especially cyanotic congenital heart disease.

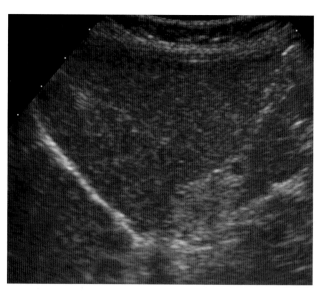

Figure 8.29
Longitudinal sonogram of a dysplastic kidney. Notice the kidney is small and echogenic with no corticomedullary differentiation and a small cyst in the lower pole.

Cystic renal disease

Cystic renal disease of the kidney in children is not an uncommon finding. The more commonly found cystic conditions, the possible pitfalls and potential differential diagnoses are now considered.

Renal dysplasia

Renal dysplasia is diagnosed when the kidney appears small and highly reflective with loss of the normal corticomedullary differentiation. Dilatation of the renal pelvis may be present. Occasionally, small 1–2 mm parenchymal or cortical retention cysts may be visible, in which case they are termed 'cystic dysplastic'. Dysplastic kidneys are known to be associated with obstruction of the ureters or bladder outflow, as in posterior urethral valves. Their association with VUR is less clear. With antenatal detection, there is clearly a spectrum of 'cystic' dysplasia, with the multicystic kidney at one end and cystic dysplasia at the other (Figure 8.29).

Simple cysts

Simple cysts, although relatively infrequent in pediatric compared with adult practice, do occur. Care should be taken when diagnosing a simple renal cyst in the upper pole of the kidney, as this may reflect the obstructed upper moiety of a duplex system. The sonographer should

actively search for a dilated ureter or the ureterocele in the bladder. An old adrenal hemorrhage which has central liquefaction may also appear as a cyst related to the upper pole of a kidney. All children with a simple renal cyst should have an IVU in case this is a calyceal diverticulum, which is prone to calculus formation and infection. Also, they should be followed into adulthood in case this is the first cyst of adult polycystic renal disease.

Polycystic renal disease

This collective term refers to both autosomal recessive polycystic kidney disease and autosomal dominant polycystic kidney disease.

Autosomal recessive polycystic kidney disease

This condition is inherited as an autosomal recessive trait, and pathologically is a disorder resulting from the cystic dilatation of the collecting ducts. The liver is always involved, with hepatic fibrosis and bile duct proliferation. ARPKD is a spectrum of disease, with involvement of these two organs being inversely proportional. Younger children with severe renal impairment have minimal hepatic disease, but in older children the hepatic fibrosis may lead to portal hypertension and varices.

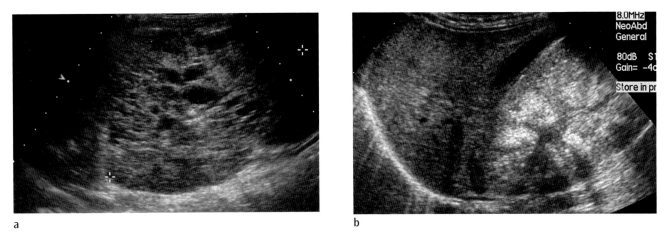

Figure 8.30

(a,b) Longitudinal sonograms of the kidney in two different children with ARPKD. The kidneys are markedly enlarged, hyperechoeic and contain multiple small cysts, giving the posterior acoustic enhancement. (b) The medullae are predominantly affected.

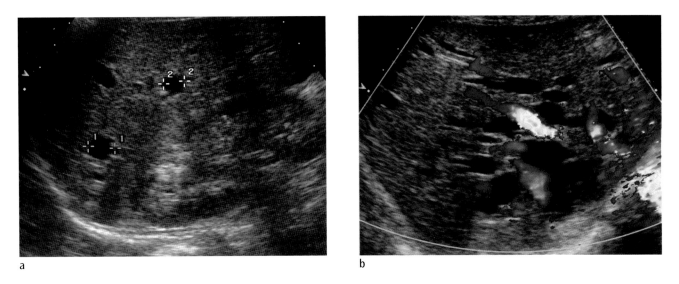

Figure 8.31

(a,b) Longitudinal sonograms of the liver in a child with ARPKD. The liver contains multiple 'cystic' areas which are not vascular when Doppler is used. These are multiple cystic dilatations of the biliary tree. This is associated with hepatic fibrosis and ultimately portal hypertension.

In the neonatal period in an infant with predominantly renal disease, ultrasound will reveal bilateral symmetrical enlargement of the kidneys. The kidneys are filled with tiny cysts, causing the kidneys to appear globally hyperechoic – often this is predominantly medullary.

Small cysts, 1–2 mm in diameter, may be visible in the cortex and medullae. These may enlarge and become multiple as the child grows older (Figure 8.30).

The liver may appear normal or with hyperechoic portal tracts or with cystic dilatation of the bile ducts.

A hepatobiliary iminodiacetic acid (HIDA) scan may demonstrate pooling of isotope in the liver if cystic dilatation of the biliary tree is present.

In an older child with predominantly hepatic manifestations, the kidneys may be normal in size with hyperechoic medullae reflecting the tubular ectasia. Hepatic cysts reflect the bile duct ectasia (Figure 8.31).

In portal hypertension the spleen is enlarged. Esophageal and perisplenic varices may be seen with reverse flow on Doppler studies.

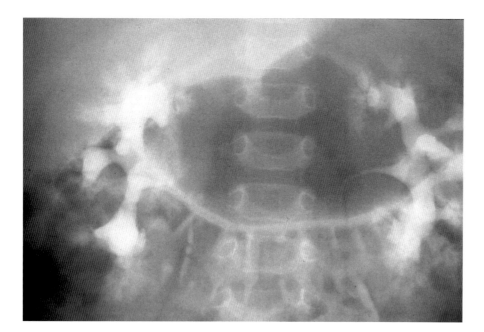

Figure 8.32
IVU in a child with ARPKD. Notice the streaky radiating pattern of contrast excretion that is typical of this condition.

The intravenous urogram is mandatory to confirm the diagnosis of ARPKD, and demonstrates enlarged kidneys with radiating streaks of contrast as it passes through the ectatic tubules. This is best demonstrated on delayed 24-hour images and is optimally performed after 3 months of age (Figure 8.32).

Often, echogenic ('bright') kidneys detected antenatally are erroneously labeled ARPKD, with all the implications for the family concerning genetic counseling. As increasing reports in the literature indicate, the detection of 'bright' kidneys occurs in a heterogeneous group of conditions (see above), and it is for this reason that the intravenous urogram is mandatory for diagnosis in the infant.

Autosomal dominant polycystic kidney disease

ADPKD is inherited as an autosomal dominant trait and classically presents in the fourth and fifth decades of life.[31] The ultrasound appearances are well described elsewhere in the text. It rarely presents de novo in the neonate or child but is seen in our practice particularly in families with ADPKD1 who want to know if the children are affected. Cysts are found in the kidneys of 64% of children with PKD1 under 10 and in 90% under 19 years of age.

Infants are most often detected antenatally with echogenic 'bright' kidneys. The diagnosis of ADPKD in a child with multiple renal cysts relies very heavily on a positive family history.

In the neonate, ultrasound appearances similar to those of ARPKD have been reported and a definitive diagnosis may only be possible with a family history or normal liver biopsy. Visible cysts develop early in these children.

In the older child, the appearances of the kidneys are identical to those seen in adults.

In children, it is important to be aware that tuberous sclerosis may present with cystic kidneys very similar in appearance to those in ADPKD before any other manifestations of this condition are seen, and this alternative diagnosis should always be considered in a child presenting de novo with bilateral cystic kidneys (Figure 8.33). In the infant with tuberous sclerosis there is a high incidence of cardiac rhabdomyomas, and a cardiac echo should be included in the initial work-up in these children together with a brain MRI. The renal manifestations are secondary only to those in the brain and, as well as cysts, the kidneys may contain small echogenic angiomyolipomas.

Syndromes associated with cystic kidneys

Although rare, there are many syndromes associated with cystic renal disease. In practice, the renal cysts are usually diagnosed when infants suspected of having the syndrome are screened. Cysts may be visible in both kidneys and they do not conform to any specific pattern. The commonest syndromes are tuberous sclerosis, asphyxiating thoracic dystrophy, Meckel–Gruber syndrome and Zellweger syndrome.

Cysts in von Hippel–Lindau disease are frequently quoted in the pediatric literature, although this condition is rarely if ever seen in children.

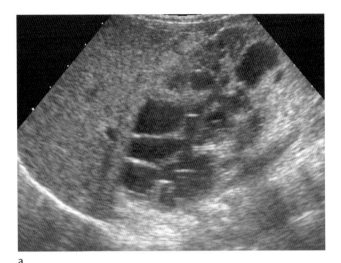

a

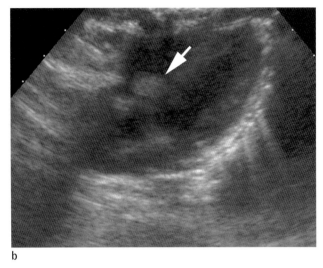

b

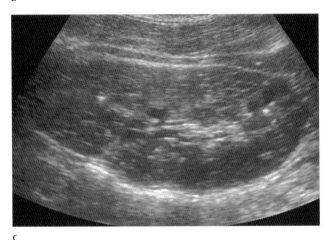

c

Figure 8.33
(a) **Longitudinal sonogram of the right kidney in a baby presenting with fits.** The kidney is completely filled with multiple cysts of varying sizes. Both kidneys looked like this. There was no family history of cystic kidneys. These appearances are identical to ADPKD. (b) **Longitudinal sonogram of the heart in the same baby showing a small ventricular rhabdomyoma (arrow).** (c) **Longitudinal sonogram in an older child with tuberous sclerosis, demonstrating the mixed appearance when cysts and angiomyolipomas are present.**

Medical renal disease

In children, the assessment of the kidneys in medical conditions covers a number of parameters. A kidney is termed 'bright' when the echogenicity is equal to or more echogenic than the liver or spleen.

It is essential to know something about:

- the size of the kidney
- what the corticomedullary differentiation looks like and whether cysts are present or not
- age of the child
- clinical presentation.

An increase in the cortical echogenicity, while sensitive, is a relatively non-specific finding in children and may occur in a number of medical conditions. In neonates and infants up to 6 months of age, this is usually a normal physiologic finding.

In acute tubular necrosis in the neonate from whatever cause, such as diarrhea and vomiting, the kidneys are equally enlarged, with a variable increase in the parenchymal echogenicity and preservation of corticomedullary differentiation. Clinically, the kidneys recover rapidly.

The infant with renal vein thrombosis is typically the child of a diabetic mother, but any condition causing hemoconcentration, e.g. dehydration, may result in renal vein thrombosis. In the early phase the kidney shows increased echogenicity and is enlarged. Later, echogenic interlobular vessels become apparent, with a patchy echonephrogram (Figure 8.34). In most instances there is unequal renal involvement. Clot is sometimes seen extending into the IVC and there is a known association with adrenal hemorrhage, especially on the left. Doppler studies of the renal artery will produce the typical reversal in diastole from the swollen kidney, obstructing the forward flow of blood into the kidney in diastole (see Chapter 1).

Ultrasound cannot differentiate medullary necrosis from these conditions, and any infant suspected of having medullary necrosis should have an intravenous urogram to document the calyceal anatomy and changes 3 months after the acute event.

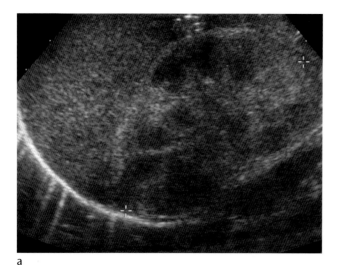

a

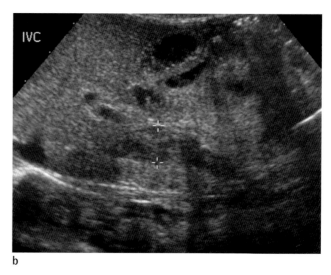

b

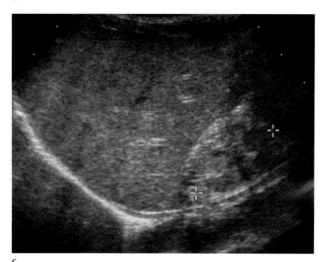

c

Figure 8.34

Renal disease. (a) Longitudinal sonogram of the right kidney in a newborn presenting with hematuria. The kidney measures over 6.5 cm in length and appears swollen with a patchy increase in echogenicity. (b) Longitudinal sonogram of the inferior vena cava (IVC), showing a large clot (between calipers) obstructing the IVC. (c) Longitudinal sonogram of the right kidney after 6 weeks. The kidney has shrunken in size and contains fine echogenic vessels where the thrombus has calcified.

The commonest conditions in the pediatric population resulting in an increased parenchymal echogenicity are glomerular disease, the nephrotic syndrome and glomerulonephritis, but it may also be seen in infection, polycystic kidney disease, oxalosis, renal dysplasia, renal scarring, storage disorders and end-stage renal disease of any pathogenesis.

Isolated increase in the medullary echogenicity invariably indicates nephrocalcinosis.[31] The earliest calcium deposits appear as an echogenic rim around the periphery of the medullae, with a preserved echolucent center. As the deposition progresses, the medullae 'fill in' and become densely hyperechoic. These appearances may be detected ultrasonically before there is evidence of nephrocalcinosis on plain abdominal radiographs. Once acoustic shadowing is detected ultrasonically, there will be plain film evidence of nephrocalcinosis (Figure 8.35). Nephrocalcinosis is

known to occur in premature infants treated with long-term furosemide for bronchopulmonary dysplasia.

If the diagnosis of nephrocalcinosis has been excluded, a large differential remains. In children, this would include medullary tubular ectasia, urate deposition, vascular congestion, renal infection and intrarenal reflux. Transient increase in the medullary echogenicity has been reported in the newborn.

Urinary tract infection

Urinary tract infection (UTI) is common in the under 5 year olds. Boys are more susceptible before the age of 3 months; thereafter, the incidence is substantially higher in girls. The aim of management is the prompt diagnosis and

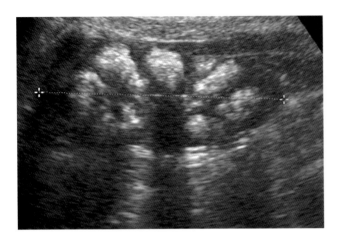

Figure 8.35
Prone longitudinal scan of a kidney with severe nephrocalcinosis. There is marked increase in echogenicity of the medullae and acoustic shadowing in keeping with nephrocalcinosis. Ultrasound is the best imaging modality to use in order to diagnose nephrocalcinosis.

treatment and the detection of an underlying cause. All children presenting with a proven UTI should be investigated. With the introduction of new imaging techniques, antenatal diagnosis and a better understanding of the natural history of VUR, the protocols for investigating children with UTI are constantly under review and changing. The drive in imaging these children is to perform the least-invasive imaging with the highest diagnostic yield, always mindful of the radiation burden.

No child should have an invasive investigation of the renal tract before an ultrasound examination has been performed, and it will be best able to rule out a hydronephrosis, abscess or calculus together with a renal malformation such as a duplex kidney.

Imaging first-proven urinary tract infection

The protocol for imaging first urinary tract infections depends on the age of the child. The reason for this is that the natural history of VUR is to resolve and disappear in the older child, so that cystography is likely to be negative in an older child. Also, the progression of renal damage from VUR is extremely rare in the older child.

Over 5 years of age, only an ultrasound is required. No further imaging should be done if this is normal.

Under 5 years of age the initial investigation is an ultrasound examination, with a DMSA 3–6 months after the UTI. The rationale behind this is that a normal DMSA excludes significant reflux.

If the DMSA is abnormal, some form of cystography is required, and this will depend on the child's age and sex.

In children who are not yet potty-trained, males require a conventional contrast cystogram (MCUG) in order to demonstrate the urethra. Females can have a direct isotope cystogram (DIC), as there is no pathology of the urethra and the radiation burden is less with a DIC. It is in this small group of girls that urosonography can potentially be used, but in many centers it has been tried and abandoned in favor of the DIC.

In older potty-trained children, a MAG3 and indirect radioisotope cystogram (IRC) are sufficient to show differential function of the kidneys, drainage and VUR.

The intravenous urogram is no longer routinely performed but is reserved for those instances when precise calyceal or ureteric anatomy is sought or when all is not clear on other imaging.

It is well recognized that the kidney is most vulnerable to renal scarring and damage in the first year of life. Even with antenatal detection, some infants still present in the first year of life with a UTI. All infants should undergo a micturating cystourethrogram. If VUR is present, then a DMSA should be performed to detect the presence and extent of renal damage (Figure 8.36).

In children, calculi are frequently associated with UTI, in particular a *Proteus* sp. infection, and a plain abdominal radiograph should be included in the initial imaging, to look for calculi and spinal abnormalities which may result in bladder instability or a neuropathic bladder.

Focal bacterial nephritis, renal abscess, lobar nephronia and renal carbuncle occur in children of all ages and have similar appearances to those in the adult. They are often misdiagnosed as a Wilms' tumor.

Of particular note, and worthy of further mention in pediatric practice, is renal candidiasis. Immunocompromised premature neonates, usually on long-term antibiotic therapy, and children with immune deficiency states are particularly likely to develop this. Ultrasonically, the kidneys may have diffuse or focal parenchymal changes and obstruction due to mycetoma formation, and fungal balls in the dilated pelvicalyceal system may also be seen (Figure 8.37).

Renal tumors

Wilms' tumor is the commonest malignancy in childhood and mesoblastic nephroma is the commonest solid renal tumor in the first 6 months of life.[32] Most children present with an abdominal mass, but other signs such as hypertension and hematuria may also present, although this is rare in the neonate.

Ultrasound is the examination of choice in a child presenting with an abdominal mass. Solid masses are easily distinguished from cystic masses, which will then direct further imaging.[33] Solid masses are rarely benign.

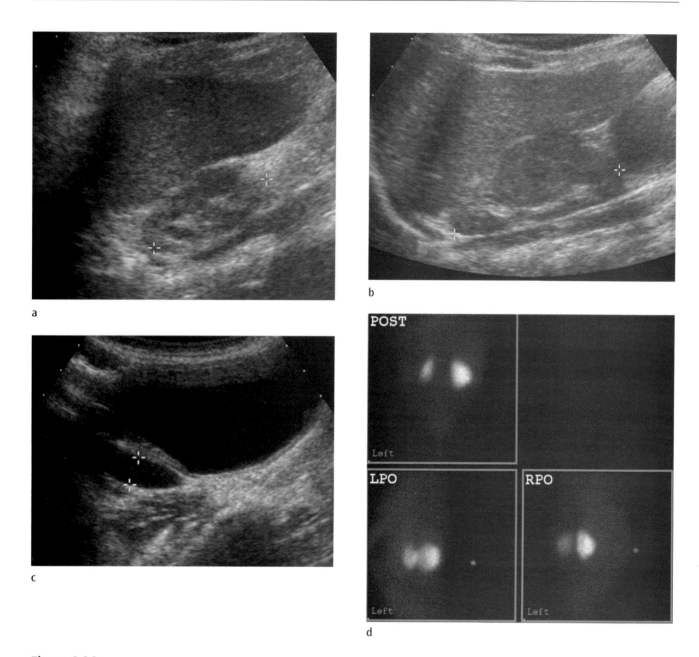

Figure 8.36
This child presented with recurrent urinary tract infections. (a) Longitudinal sonogram of the left kidney. The left kidney is small and scarred with global cortical thinning. (b) Longitudinal sonogram of the right kidney showing a larger kidney but with an irregular cortex with varying thickness of the cortex. (c) Transverse sonogram of the bladder in the same child showing a dilated left lower ureter. (d) DMSA scan showing the smaller scarred left kidney and an irregular outline of the right kidney. This child had bilateral scarred kidneys.

Wilms' tumor (nephroblastoma)

Nephroblastomas were first classified in 1899. The favorable types include multilocular cysts, congenital mesoblastic nephroma and nephroblastomatosis. The unfavorable types, accounting for over 60% of deaths, are anaplastic, rhabdoid and clear cell sarcoma. The clear cells are of particular interest, as they may metastasize to bone.

The classic ultrasound appearance of a Wilms' tumor is of a solid intrarenal mass, often containing hypoechoic lakes or localized areas of necrosis, replacing all or part of a kidney (Figure 8.38). Areas of increased echogenicity

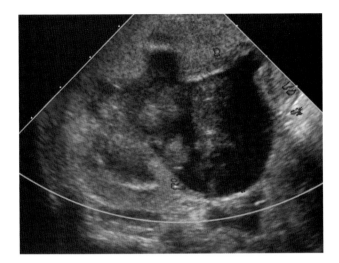

Figure 8.37
This was an immunocompromised neonate who had candida cultured from the urine. The right kidney is echogenic and hydronephrotic. The dilated collecting contains clumps of debris typical of fungal balls.

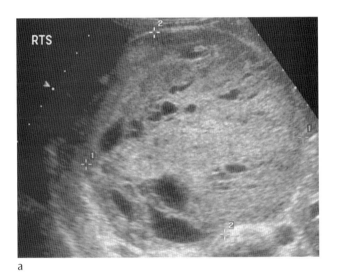

a

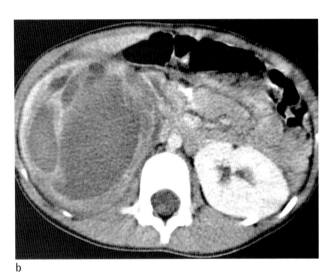

b

Figure 8.38
Wilms' tumor. (a) Longitudinal sonogram of the right flank showing a large predominantly solid mass with cystic areas almost completely filling the right renal bed. Normal renal tissue is difficult to clearly define. (b) CT scan at the level of the right kidney, showing the large mass in the renal fossa with just a thin sliver of enhancing kidney laterally. This was a Wilms' tumor on biopsy. These tumors can often appear very cystic.

may also be present if there has been recent hemorrhage. Obstructed and displaced calyces can be identified if the tumor has not replaced the whole kidney. The contralateral kidney should be carefully examined, as a significant number (10%) are bilateral. The IVC must also be evaluated for secondary spread and, if containing tumor, the IVC (in our experience) has always been expanded. Most commonly, however, it is displaced or compressed by the tumor mass (Figure 8.39). Lymphadenopathy, although present on histology, is rarely appreciable on ultrasound.

Rarely, pedunculated tumors may appear entirely extrarenal.

The staging of Wilms' tumor is dependent on degree of spread: Stage 1 is confined to the kidney and completely resected; in Stage 4 hematogenous spread is present; and Stage 5 is bilateral renal involvement. Generally, however, the outcome for this tumor has improved in recent years.

Nephroblastomatosis is the persistence of primitive embryologic blastema and may occur normally in the

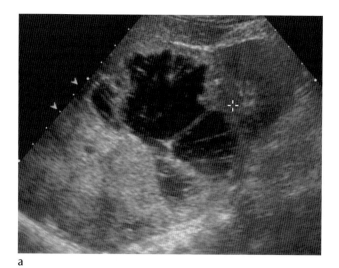

a

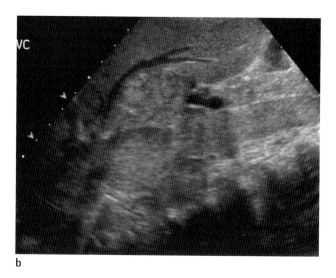

b

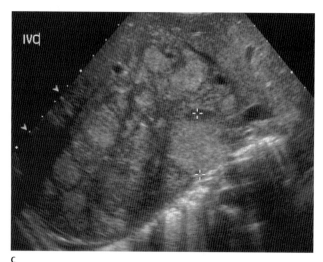

c

Figure 8.39
(a) This child presented with a very large renal tumor and liver secondaries. This longitudinal view of the renal mass shows a small portion of normal kidney inferiorly and a large solid and cystic mass. (b,c) Longitudinal and transverse views of the IVC. The IVC is filled with echogenic tumor thrombus which is expanding the IVC. Ultrasound is the best imaging modality to delineate the IVC and it should always be carefully examined in renal tumors in children.

neonate. Usually it matures without any associated consequence. However, it is known to be premalignant and associated with the development of Wilms' tumors. The ultrasound appearances are of a solidly enlarged kidney(s) with hyper/hypo- or isoechoic masses. If the masses are small, discrete and isoechoic, they may be difficult to identify on ultrasound. It is for this reason that all children with a suspected Wilms' tumor of one kidney should have an abdominal enhanced computed tomography (CT) examination or MRI.

Mesoblastic nephroma is a benign condition, in that complete surgical removal with no spillage results in complete cure. The attempt to distinguish between Wilms' tumor and mesoblastic nephroma on ultrasound may be difficult, although the mesoblastic nephroma is reportedly more uniformly solid.

Doppler studies of Wilms' tumors will produce abnormal Doppler traces ('tumor signals') at the margins of the renal mass.

Certain more common conditions are known to be associated with the development of Wilms' tumors: aniridia, hemihypertrophy and the Beckwith–Wiedemann syndrome.

Bladder

Children should always, as far as possible, be examined with a full bladder.

Neurogenic bladder

In childhood, neurogenic bladder is most commonly seen in association with meningomyeloceles and spinal pathology. The role of ultrasound is to monitor the kidneys for hydronephrosis, to assess the bladder capacity and post-

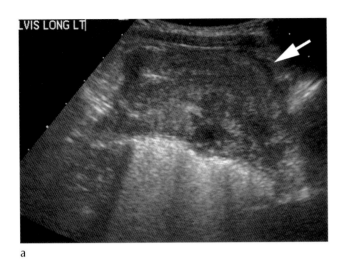
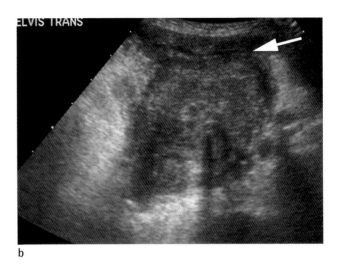

a   b

Figure 8.40
Rhabdomyosarcoma. (a, b) Longitudinal and transverse sonogram of the pelvis in a child presenting with a pelvic mass. The solid well-defined mass is intimately related to and lying behind the bladder, which is squashed anteriorly (arrow). The diagnosis was made on a biopsy.

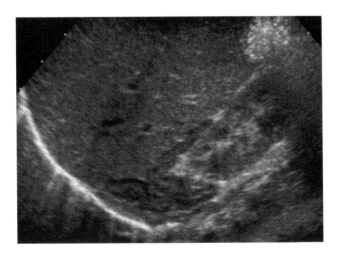
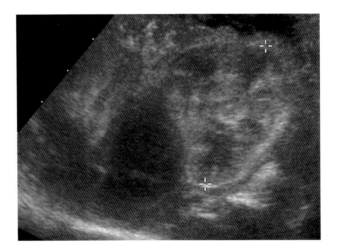

Figure 8.41
Longitudinal sonogram of the normal neonatal adrenal.
They are often surprisingly large in appearance with a hypoechoic cortex and hyperechoeic medulla.

Figure 8.42
Longitudinal sonogram of the left kidney in an infant presenting with a palpable mass. The left kidney (between calipers) is pushed inferiorly by a predominantly cystic adrenal mass. This is the typical appearance of an adrenal hemorrhage of at least a week's duration. Liquefaction and involution occur quite rapidly.

drainage residue and to detect the development of calculi from stasis of urine.

Exstrophy of the bladder

Exstrophy of the bladder refers to an abnormal embryologic development where the abdominal wall below the umbilicus is open, exposing the posterior wall of the bladder, the symphysis pubis is split and the male and female genitalia are incomplete and separated. There are a number of associated anomalies, e.g. spina bifida, imperforate anus, absence of the vagina and small uterus. Renal anomalies are rarely associated.

Imaging the neonate and child with exstrophy is directed towards monitoring renal function, a deterioration of

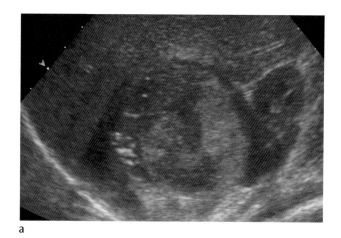

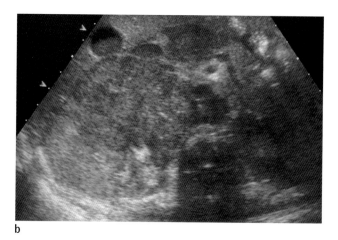

a

b

Figure 8.43
Two examples of the differing appearances of neuroblastoma. (a) Longitudinal sonogram of the right kidney and adrenal. There is a well-defined solid adrenal mass with fine echogenic areas of calcification in keeping with a neuroblastoma. This is a Stage 1 tumor and is confined to the adrenal gland. (b) Transverse sonogram of the upper abdomen in a child with a more advanced adrenal tumor. The mass is solid, crossing the midline and undermining the major vessels, elevating the pancreas and mesenteric vessels to the left. Echogenic calcification is seen posteriorly in the mass and there is sludge in the gallbladder.

which may be a direct consequence of the type of treatment employed. Later, imaging is directed towards bladder continence.

Bladder outflow obstruction

Bladder outflow obstruction is most commonly seen in boys due to posterior urethral valves but may also occur in anterior urethral valves, urethral polyps, a prolapsing ureterocele in a duplex system or a bladder tumor. All these conditions require conventional contrast cystography to demonstrate the urethra.

Tumors

Tumors of the bladder are rare in children, the commonest being the rhabdomyosarcoma.[34] The child may present in acute retention, with a pelvic/abdominal mass or hematuria.

Rhabdomyosarcomas usually arise in the region around the bladder base, the trigone or prostate and may be intra- or extravesical. Typically, if intravesical, rhabdomyosarcomas infiltrate the bladder wall and mucosa and produce a polypoidal mass (Figure 8.40). If extravesical, they may

arise from the fundus of the bladder and appear uniformly solid.

Cystitis

Inflammation of the bladder may be caused by a heterogeneous group of disorders. It is most commonly due to eosinophilic cystitis but can be due to viral, parasitic or bacterial infection or may occur after cytotoxic drug administration. It has been reported specifically occurring in children with chronic granulomatous disease.

Ultrasonically, cystitis may appear very similar to a rhabdomyosarcoma and is sometimes termed 'pseudo-tumoral cystitis'. It may be localized or diffuse and even obstruct the ureteric orifices, producing hydronephrosis.

Conclusion

Ultrasound is the prime imaging modality of the renal tract in children and accounts for over half the workload in most departments. The more widespread use of routine antenatal diagnosis has profoundly changed urologic practice and referral patterns over the last decade. The sonologist must perform a meticulous examination, with careful attention to measuring renal size and cortical thickness. The use of Doppler ultrasound in children should be standard and routine.

RETROPERITONEUM AND ADRENALS

Introduction

Ultrasound is the imaging modality of choice for evaluating the adrenal gland in neonates. In the child presenting with an abdominal mass or with a suspected adrenal tumor, ultrasound is used for first-line imaging, but CT or MRI is the preferred method of evaluating the entire retroperitoneum and extent of disease. Radioisotope MIBG (*m*-iodobenzylguanidine) scans are used in patients with biochemically suspected pheochromocytoma.

Technique

With modern real-time equipment, the adrenals can be reliably detected at birth, but in the child over 1 year old the reliability approximates that of adult adrenal sonography.

The right adrenal gland is most easily visualized using the anterolateral approach, using the liver as an acoustic window. By scanning longitudinally over the IVC and then obliqueing the transducer and scan plane to include the upper pole of the right kidney, the triangle where the adrenal gland lies is reliably shown. Similarly, on the left, the spleen and, in addition, a fluid-filled stomach can be used as an acoustic window.

As in the adult, demonstrating the adrenal gland in children over 1 year of age is time-consuming and requires considerable skill.

Anatomy

Evaluation of the adrenal gland in neonates and children relies primarily on appreciating the age-related changes that occur. At birth the adrenal appears large, with the outer hypoechoic cortex and the linear hyperechoic medulla separately identifiable (Figure 8.41).[35] By 2 months of age, the cortex has involuted and is thinner and by 6 months this differentiation has almost been lost. After 1 year the gland appears similar to that of an adult. Due to this rapid cortical involution, standards for the normal changes in size and appearance are available but are really of very little use in routine clinical practice.

Adrenal hemorrhage

Adrenal hemorrhage most commonly occurs in the neonatal period, and there is a well-recognized association with renal vein thrombosis, particularly on the left due to the drainage of the adrenal vein into the left renal vein. Conditions resulting in hemoconcentration – e.g. dehydration, polycythemia, sepsis and maternal diabetes – are known predisposing factors.

Ultrasonically, the appearances depend on the age of the hemorrhage. Early on, the hemorrhage appears as an echogenic suprarenal mass. As the hemorrhage liquefies, the echogenic mass gradually becomes more cystic (Figure 8.42). Finally, it shrinks down and commonly becomes calcified within weeks or months. The hemorrhage may be indistinguishable ultrasonically from a neuroblastoma, particularly in the early echogenic phase, and if any clinical suspicion exists of the latter, follow-up sonograms and urinary vanillylmandelic acid (VMA) estimations must be performed.

Adrenal hemorrhage may complicate disseminated intravascular coagulation, a well-recognized complication of meningococcemia, the Friderichsen–Waterhouse syndrome.

Adrenal abscess is seen as a complication of adrenal hemorrhage.

Neuroblastoma

Neuroblastoma is the most common extracranial tumor of childhood.[36] The tumor originates in neural crest cells of the sympathetic system. Sixty percent of neuroblastomas arise in the abdomen, most commonly the adrenal gland. At presentation, only about one-fifth of children present with local or regional disease, the majority having distant metastases.

The role of ultrasound is in the first-line imaging of a child with an abdominal mass. Frequently, the diagnosis is made using ultrasound alone, but other imaging modalities are employed to accurately define the extent of disease. Various imaging modalities are used in the diagnosis of neuroblastoma, but MRI, CT and MIBG are particularly useful. The role of imaging is to make the diagnosis, to document the extent of disease at presentation and to assess the response to treatment. Ultrasound may be used to guide percutaneous needle biopsy.

Ultrasonically, neuroblastoma appears as a solid extrarenal tumor (Figure 8.43). Approximately 40% calcify on plain radiography (up to 85% on CT), and this can also be detected ultrasonically. In contrast to Wilms' tumor, neuroblastoma undermines and surrounds the great vessels with tumor. The kidney is usually displaced by the mass, but rarely invaded. Lymphadenopathy is frequently associated. Liver metastases, if present, classically have a 'bull's-eye' appearance. Spinal extension may occur. In the older child this is usually imaged on CT or MRI, but in the younger child ultrasound may be used.

4S neuroblastoma, the neonatal good-prognosis form, has specific ultrasound features. The primary tumor is small – usually Stage I or II. The liver is enormously enlarged and has a 'pepperpot' appearance.

Adrenocortical tumors

These tumors are extremely rare in children, accounting for less than 1% of childhood tumors.[37] The majority present with clinical signs and symptoms of hormonal activity such as Cushing's syndrome and virilism in females. The differentiation between adenomas and carcinomas is made on size: less than 6 cm is classified as an adenoma and over 6 cm a carcinoma. Ultrasonically, they are generally solid, well-defined adrenal masses and cannot be differentiated on imaging. The larger masses may show evidence of necrosis and areas of hypoechogenicity.

Vascular invasion such as tumor growth into the adrenal vein and IVC must be looked for and may be identified with ultrasound.

Pheochromocytoma

Pheochromocytomas are rare in children. If suspected clinically, and if there is biochemical evidence to support this, a radioisotope MIBG scan is performed. Only if this is positive does one proceed to further imaging. Once the MIBG has been performed and is positive, further imaging can be tailored. CT or, if available, MRI is the preferred method of imaging these tumors, as in children they are often bilateral, extra-adrenal and multiple. Ultrasonically, there is little to differentiate them from other adrenal tumors.

Conclusion

The adrenal gland when involved with a pathologic process either presents as an abdominal mass or hormonal disturbances. Ultrasound is the first-line investigation upon which further imaging is directed.

References

1. Winter RM, Baraitser M. The London dysmorphology database. Oxford: Oxford University Press. Electronic Publishing Division; 2000.
2. Wellesley D, Howe DT. Fetal renal anomalies and genetic syndromes. Prenat Diag 2001; 21: 992–1003.
3. Levi S, Schaaps JP, De HP, et al. End-result of routine ultrasound screening for congenital anomalies: the Belgian Multicentric Study 1984–92. Ultrasound Obst Gynecol 1995; 5: 366–71.
4. Levi S, Hyjazi Y. Sensitivity of routine ultrasonographic screening for congenital anomalies during the last 5 years. J Ultrasound Med 1992; 11: 188.
5. Chitty LS, Hunt GH, Moore J, et al. Effectiveness of routine ultrasonography in detecting fetal structural abnormalities in a low risk population. BMJ 1991; 303: 1165–9.
6. Crane JP, LeFevre ML, Winborn RC, et al. A randomized trial of prenatal ultrasonographic screening: impact on the detection, management, and outcome of anomalous fetuses. The RADIUS Study Group. Am J Obstet Gynecol 1994; 171: 392–9.
7. Smith NC, Hau C. A six year study of the antenatal detection of fetal abnormality in six Scottish health boards. Br J Obstet Gynaecol 1999; 106: 206–12.
8. Chitty LS, Altman DG. Charts of fetal size: kidney and renal pelvis measurements. Prenat Diagn 2003; 23(11): 891–7.
9. Efrat Z, Akinfenwa OO, Nicolaides KH. First trimester determination of fetal gender by ultrasound. Ultrasound Obstet Gynecol 1999; 13: 305–7.
10. Wilcox DT, Chitty LS. Non-visualisation of the fetal bladder: aetiology and management. Prenat Diagn 2001; 21: 977–83.
11. Winyard P, Chitty LS. Dysplastic and polycystic kidneys: diagnosis, associations and management. Prenat Diagn 2001; 21: 924–35.
12. Roy S, Dillon MJ, Trompeter RS, et al. Autosomal recessive polycystic kidney disease: long-term outcome of neonatal survivors [published erratum appears in Pediatr Nephrol 1997; 11(5): 664]. Pediatr Nephrol 1997; 11: 302–6.
13. MacDermot KD, Saggar-Malik AK, Economides DL, Jeffery S. Prenatal diagnosis of autosomal dominant polycystic kidney disease (PKD1) presenting in utero and prognosis for very early onset disease. J Med Genet 1998; 35: 13–16.
14. Chitty LS, Griffin DR, Johnson P, Neales K. The differential diagnosis of enlarged hyperechogenic kidneys with normal or increased liquor volume: report of 5 cases and review of the literature. Ultrasound Obstet Gynecol 1991; 1: 115–21.
15. Elliott M, Maher ER. Beckwith–Wiedemann syndrome. J Med Genet 1994; 31: 560–4.
16. Chitty LS, Clark T, Maxwell D. Perlman syndrome: a cause of large hyperechoic kidneys. Prenat Diagn 1998; 18: 1163–8.
17. Chudleigh T. Mild pyelectasis. Prenat Diagn 2001; 21: 936–41.
18. Mouriquand PDE, Whitten M, Pracros JP. Pathophysiology, diagnosis and management of prenatal upper tract dilatation. Prenat Diagn 2001; 21: 942–51.
19. Whitten M, McHoney M, Wilcox DT, New S, Chitty LS. Accuracy of antenatal fetal ultrasound in the diagnosis of duplex kidneys. Ultrasound Obstet Gynecol 2003; 21: 342–6.
20. Warne S, Chitty LS, Wilcox DT. Prenat diagnosis of cloacal anomalies. Br J Urol Int 2002; 89: 78–81.
21. McHugo J, Whittle M. Enlarged fetal bladders: aetiology, management and outcome. Prenat Diagn 2001; 21: 958–63.
22. Whitten SM, Smeulders N, Wilcox DT, Chitty LS. Outcome of prenatally diagnosed bladder dilation. Ultrasound Obstet Gynecol 2003; 22(Suppl 1): 17.
23. Nicolini U, Spelzini F. Invasive assessment of fetal renal abnormalities: urinalysis, fetal blood sampling and biopsy. Prenat Diagn 2001; 21: 964–9.
24. Agarwal SK, Fisk NM. In utero therapy for lower urinary tract obstruction. Prenat Diagn 2001; 21: 970–6.
25. Mandell J, Lebowitz RL, Peters CA, et al. Prenatal diagnosis of the megacystis–megaureter association. J Urol 1992; 148(5): 1487–9.
26. Pajkrt E, Chitty LS. Prenatal gender determination and the diagnosis of ambiguous genitalia. Br J Urol Int 2004; 93 (Suppl 3): 12–19.
27. Rosenbaum DM, Korngold E, Teele RL. Sonographic assessment of renal length in normal children. AJR Am J Roentgenol 1984; 142: 467–9.
28. Jequier S, Rousseau O. Sonographic measurements of the normal bladder wall in children. AJR Am J Roentgenol 1987; 149: 563–6.

29. Tibballs JM, De Bruyn R. Primary vesicoureteric reflux – how useful is postnatal ultrasound? Arch Dis Child 1996; 75: 444–7.

30. Bear JC, Parfrey PS, Morgan JM, et al. Autosomal dominant polycystic kidney disease: new information for genetic counselling. Am J Med Genet 1992; 43: 548–53.

31. Alon US. Nephrocalcinosis. Pediatrics 1997; 9: 160–5.

32. Strouse PJ. Pediatric renal neoplasms. Radiol Clin North Am 1996; 34: 1081–100.

33. Goske MJ, Mitchell C, Reslan WA. Imaging of patients with Wilms' tumor. Semin Urol Oncol 1999; 17: 11–20.

34. McHugh K, Boothroyd AE. The role of radiology in childhood rhabdomyosarcoma. Clin Radiol 1999; 54: 2–10.

35. Oppenheimer D, Carroll B, Vousem S. Sonography of the normal neonatal adrenal gland. Radiology 1983; 146: 157–60.

36. Lonergan GJ, Schwab CM, Suarez ES, et al. Neuroblastoma, ganglioneuroblastoma and ganglioneuroma: radiologic-pathologic correlation. Radiographics 2002; 22: 911–34.

37. Abramson SJ. Adrenal neoplasms in children. Radiol Clin North Am 1997; 35: 1415–53.

Further reading

Carty H, Brunelle F, Shaw D, Kendall B. Imaging children. Edinburgh: Churchill Livingstone; 1994 .

De Bruyn R. Pediatric ultrasound. How, why and when. Edinburgh: Elsevier; 2005.

Dewbury K, Meire H, Cosgrove D, et al. Clinical ultrasound a comprehensive text, 2nd edn. Edinburgh: Churchill Livingstone; 2001.

Te Haar G, Duck FA. The safe use of ultrasound in medical diagnosis. BMUS. 2000

9

The renal transplant

Simon J Freeman

GENERAL CONSIDERATIONS

Introduction

Following the first successful renal transplant operation, performed in the USA in 1954, renal transplantation has emerged as the optimal treatment for almost all patients with end-stage renal disease. Not only does transplantation improve quality of life and end dependence on dialysis, it also appears to confer a significant survival benefit. One study showed that recipients of cadaveric kidney transplants benefited from an increase in predicted life expectancy of 10 years compared with similar patients remaining on the transplant waiting list. Renal transplantation is also cost-effective, providing a much less expensive alternative to long-term dialysis. This procedure has become so successful that, in the UK a year after surgery, 94% of living donor transplants and 87% of cadaveric transplants are still functioning well, these figures falling to approximately 70% and 60%, respectively, at 10 years.

Significant improvements in short- and medium-term graft survival have been achieved over the last decade, mainly through better and more intensive immunosuppressive regimens, but also through refinements in surgical technique, advances in preoperative tissue typing and in postoperative medical care. Early success rates are now so good that increasingly attention is being directed towards addressing the problems occurring late after transplantation. These problems include premature death (predominantly attributable to high rates of cardiovascular disease) and also the long-term effects of immunosuppression that result in increased susceptibility to infection and certain types of cancer. Chronic allograft nephropathy (chronic rejection) is a complex process whose incidence has remained relatively unchanged over the past 10 years and continues to be a major cause of long-term graft failure. Recurrence of the original disease in the transplant is now seen more frequently as graft survival improves.

Lack of donor organs remains the major factor limiting transplantation. Despite relatively static transplant activity, the number of patients with end-stage renal disease suit-

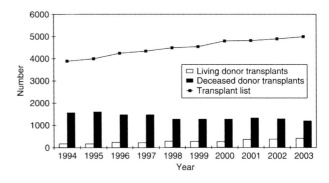

Figure 9.1
UK transplant activity and waiting list 1994–2003. (Redrawn with permission of UK Transplant: website accessed December 2004.)

able for transplantation is steadily increasing, mainly due to an aging population, and therefore the number of patients on waiting lists for transplantation continues to rise (Figure 9.1). To address this issue, several measures have been adopted to improve the supply of donor organs. Most notably, the number of living organ donors is steadily rising; in the UK, living organ donation now accounts for more than one in four kidney transplants. An advantage of living organ donation is that these grafts show consistently higher survival rates than cadaveric transplant kidneys. Living donor morbidity has been significantly reduced in recent years with the more widespread adoption of laparoscopic surgical nephrectomy. Other strategies employed to increase the number of donor organs include the use of suboptimal or marginal kidneys that would previously have been regarded as unsuitable for transplantation and kidneys from non-heart-beating donors. In some countries the rate of organ donation has increased by appointing specialized transplant coordination staff at each hospital and in other countries a system of 'presumed consent to donation' has increased the supply of transplant organs. Research continues into the use of xenotransplantation, but overcoming rejection and concerns regarding the transmission of disease make this unlikely to provide a solution in the short term.

Although the incidence of early and medium-term complications of transplantation is falling, complications do still occur. There are now more than 16 000 patients with a functioning cadaveric transplant and more than 3000 patients with a functioning living donor transplant in the UK. It is therefore likely that these patients will present periodically to most hospitals, not just to transplant centers, for assessment and treatment when problems arise. Ultrasound is the most valuable initial imaging investigation employed in this setting, and it is important that the expertise for sonographic evaluation of a transplant kidney is widely available. Clinical features of graft failure are often lacking or non-specific and unhelpful in differentiating between the different causes of graft dysfunction. Pain, fever, focal swelling and tenderness are all features that may be seen in a number of different pathologies. Ultrasound imaging can contribute to a diagnosis in many of the causes of transplant dysfunction and may also aid in the follow-up and subsequent management of such complications. In addition, it is frequently employed to delineate graft anatomy prior to intervention, including biopsy, antegrade pyelography and drainage procedures. Frequent and repeated ultrasound examinations are usually required, particularly when graft function is suboptimal. For this reason it is important that the examinations are reproducible by the same and different operators. Careful attention to examination technique and to the normal morphologic appearances as well as the normal appearances of the color and spectral Doppler patterns obtained from the main and branch renal arteries is essential, not only for initial diagnosis but also for accurate graft follow-up.

Surgical technique

A basic understanding of surgical technique is helpful for performing and interpreting ultrasound examinations of the renal transplant. Although several surgical approaches have been described, the most commonly used technique places the transplant kidney in a retroperitoneal position in the iliac fossa. The right side is preferred, as the external iliac vein is more easily mobilized. The left iliac fossa is used for second transplants or in situations where vascular disease is present on the right. The rectus muscle is divided, inferior epigastric vessels ligated and the retroperitoneal space and iliac vessels exposed. The renal vein is first anastomosed end-to-side to the external iliac vein. The arterial anastomosis is then performed either end-to-side (usually in cadaveric kidneys with an aortic patch) with the external iliac artery or end-to-end (usually in living donor organs that do not have an arterial patch) with the internal iliac artery. Before the vessels are unclamped, the patient receives a bolus of intravenous fluid and often furosemide and mannitol to maximize renal perfusion. The transplant ureter is then attached to the recipient's bladder by extravesical ureteroneocystostomy in which the posterolateral aspect of the bladder is incised, the donor ureter anastomosed to the bladder mucosa and the detrusor muscle closed over the distal ureter to create an intramuscular tunnel; a ureteric stent may or may not be placed. In patients who have had several prior transplants or with severe atheromatous or venous disease, a lower abdominal transplant or orthotopic (lumbar) transplant may be performed.

A number of other techniques are occasionally adopted to overcome a variety of different surgical problems; in cases where the procedure differs from standard technique, this information must be made available to the ultrasound practitioner performing postoperative evaluation of the transplant. Illustrations of the surgical procedure in the patient's record can prove invaluable in this setting, particularly when there are multiple vascular anastomoses.

Technique of examination

Before embarking on an ultrasound study of a renal transplant it is important for sonologists to familiarize themselves with certain key points in the patient's history. Of particular importance is the vascular anatomy of the transplant being studied. Other information that may be of value is:

- cause and duration of renal failure
- previous history, including length and method of dialysis and outcome of any previous transplants
- quality of the donor kidney
- cold and warm ischemia times.

Comprehensive ultrasound evaluation of the renal transplant requires the use of equipment with high-quality gray-scale and Doppler imaging capabilities. The superficial location of most grafts frequently allows the use of high-frequency transducers (5–7.5 MHz), with the result that images of high resolution can usually be achieved. Occasionally in obese patients, where there is induration of the wound, or in the presence of large peritransplant fluid collections, the use of lower-frequency transducers may be necessary. The examination can be performed within the first 24 hours after surgery, if care is taken over the operative site. No patient preparation is required. A full bladder may occasionally be helpful in demonstration of pelvic anatomy and in the delineation of an obstructed distal ureter. However, in any patient with transplant pelvicalyceal dilatation, the examination should be repeated after the bladder has been emptied to exclude backpressure as the cause of the collecting system dilatation. Ultrasound evaluation may be, and frequently is, performed at the patient's bedside.

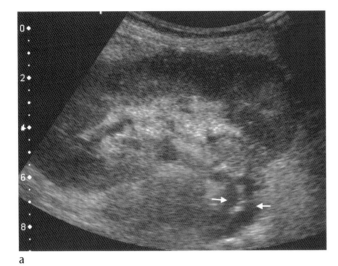

a

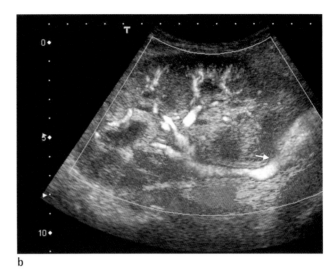

b

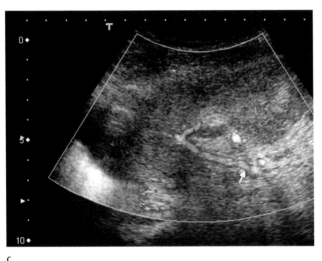

c

Figure 9.2
Normal transplant vessels. (a) The main vessels are sometimes visible on gray-scale imaging (arrows) but the addition of color Doppler facilitates identification of the renal vein (b) and artery (c) and usually allows their courses to be traced back to the vascular anastomoses (arrows).

The examination begins with a careful gray-scale assessment. The transplant can usually be evaluated with the patient lying supine, although it is occasionally necessary to move the patient into the oblique position to obtain adequate views. The axis of the kidney is variable, and therefore a standard approach to establish the axis and orientation of the kidney, ureter and renal vessels is not possible. The transducer is placed in either the right or left iliac fossa, depending on graft site, in a plane running from the anterior superior iliac spine to the pubic tubercle. This is frequently the axis in which the graft comes to lie but the transducer position is then altered to achieve a true long axis of the kidney. Occasionally the transplant may lie in a transverse or almost anteroposterior orientation, particularly in obese patients. Scans are performed in longitudinal and transverse axes and the transducer position is then modified to achieve a coronal plane through the kidney, which allows better demonstration of pelvicalyceal anatomy as well as the vascular supply and drainage. It is impor-

tant also to assess the superficial soft tissues and the perirenal areas as well as the lower pelvis, bladder and retrovesical space in order to detect fluid collections and the presence of dilatation of the ureter.

Measurements are made of the maximum length of the kidney. Transplant volume can be estimated by use of the modified ellipsoid formula:

$$V = 0.612 \times L \times W \times APD$$

where V = renal volume, L = renal length, W = renal width and APD = anteroposterior diameter. However, volume assessment is subject to significant inter- and intra-observer error. Furthermore, changes in renal volume are a normal feature in the period following transplantation. It is now thought to be of limited value and is not therefore performed in many institutions. An assessment is made of the relative reflectivity of the renal cortex, medulla and renal sinus, although this is rather more difficult in the absence of adjacent comparative organs such as are used for the native kidney, i.e. the liver and spleen.

Doppler examination of the renal transplant begins with a color Doppler survey, using a large sample volume, to confirm that all areas of the transplant are perfused. Power Doppler has the advantage of sensitivity to low-velocity flow and relative angle independence and can be a useful additional technique, particularly when perfusion is poor and in evaluation of the smaller vessels in the periphery of the transplant. It does not, however, provide directional information and is more prone to motion artifact. The sample volume can then be reduced and appropriate intrarenal arteries identified for spectral Doppler interrogation. Spectral Doppler traces should be taken from interlobar arteries (identified by their color signal at the borders of the medullary pyramids) or arcuate arteries (identified at the corticomedullary junction). Routine spectral Doppler analysis of the smaller more peripheral vessels, such as the interlobular arteries, is not recommended. Inter- and intra-observer error is greater when analyzing these small vessels; normal resistance index measurements appear to be lower than in the interlobar and arcuate arteries and are less extensively studied. A minimum of three spectral Doppler traces should be obtained, one each from the upper-polar, inter-polar and lower-polar regions.

The examination should then evaluate the main transplant vessels, which are sometimes visible on gray-scale imaging, although they are much more easily identified with color and power Doppler (Figure 9.2). The transplant artery can usually be traced from the renal hilum to the vascular anastomosis, although it will often follow a tortuous path and requires skill and patience on the part of the examiner to demonstrate its entire course. The main renal vessels are more readily demonstrated in the established renal transplant; in the immediate postoperative period wound dressings, induration, edema, pain and tenderness may limit visualization, except at the renal hilum. Spectral Doppler traces are taken from the arterial anastomosis and at any points along the course of the artery where disturbed flow is demonstrated as aliasing of the color Doppler signal. Patency of the main transplant vein should be confirmed with color and spectral Doppler. Finally, it is sometimes necessary to evaluate the iliac artery to identify evidence of iliac stenosis, which is an unusual cause of transplant dysfunction.

As with all Doppler examinations, careful attention to technique is critical and the angle of incidence of the ultrasound beam should be optimized to less than 60°. The color signal is often poor at the polar regions of the kidney due to the unfavorable Doppler angle (Figure 9.3). 'Heel-toe' transducer pressure at this site will often improve the angle and confirm satisfactory perfusion. The pulse repetition frequency (Doppler scale) and Doppler gain controls should be appropriately set to allow identification of low-velocity flow and then altered if aliasing or color noise

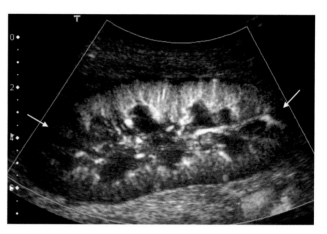

Figure 9.3
Dynamic Flow color Doppler survey of a normal transplant.
Note that the polar regions of the kidney appear not to be perfused (arrows) due to the unfavorable Doppler angle, despite excellent perfusion of the remainder of the transplant.

occur. Doppler filtration should be reduced when areas of low-velocity flow are being examined, because low-level diastolic flow in particular can be masked. Excessive transducer pressure on the transplant should be avoided, as this can result in artifactual reduction of diastolic flow in the intrarenal arteries and so invalidate spectral Doppler measurements.

NORMAL APPEARANCES

Normal gray-scale appearances

The sonographic features of the renal transplant are very similar to those of the native kidney. The superficial location of the graft, however, permits the use of high-frequency transducers and allows definition of the renal parenchyma with much greater clarity. Resolution of cortex and medulla is seen in almost all cases, except where there is obesity, a large peritransplant fluid collection or wound induration. The renal cortex returns mid-range echoes, whereas the medullary pyramids are seen as echo-poor oval or triangular structures with the apex directed towards the renal sinus (Figure 9.4). The cortex forms a substantial rim of the parenchyma not only in the outermost portion of the kidney but also between the pyramids, extending towards the sinus and forming the columns of Bertin. The renal sinus is highly reflective and of variable thickness, depending upon the degree of renal sinus fat. Calyces are frequently visualized in the normal transplant kidney, particularly in the immediate postoperative period when there

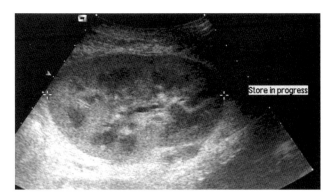

Figure 9.4
Normal renal transplant. The superficial location of the transplant allows the use of a high transducer frequency (6 MHz), accentuating corticomedullary differentiation.

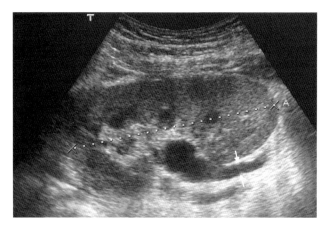

Figure 9.6
Visualization of the proximal transplant ureter. Note that despite good demonstration of the renal pelvis and proximal ureter (arrows), there is no calyceal dilatation in this normally functioning transplant.

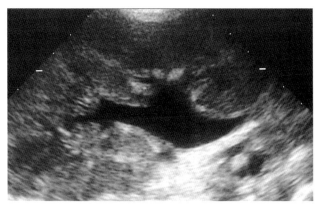

Figure 9.5
Separation of the renal sinus echoes by mild pelvicalyceal dilatation. The renal pelvis is distended and there is mild dilatation of the calyces, although normal calyceal cupping is maintained. This is a frequent 'normal' finding, particularly in the immediate postoperative period.

is edema at the vesicoureteric anastomosis; however, normal calyceal cupping should be maintained (Figure 9.5). The renal pelvis can usually be seen on gray-scale imaging, but the ureter is only occasionally identified for 1–2 cm distal to this (Figure 9.6) and the non-obstructed ureterovesical anastomosis is not demonstrated.

Normal measurements of renal size

Ultrasound is an accurate tool for the measurement of renal size. Studies comparing the correlation between various different methods and the size of the kidney measured

at the time of removal and transplantation indicate that ultrasound provides the closest approximation to the true renal length. Variation in normal size is similar to that of native adult kidneys: length varies between 9 and 11 cm, width between 4 and 6 cm and depth between 4 and 5 cm. Volume measurements vary from 90 ml to 180 ml. The importance of renal measurements, however, lies not in the absolute size of the kidney but in the change in size that may be demonstrated. There is a gradual increase in all renal dimensions after renal transplantation, with an increase of up to 25% by the end of the second week and up to 32% by the end of the third week. Graft size appears to stabilize at around 6 months, although it may increase in situations such as pregnancy or the onset of diabetes mellitus following transplantation or if a pediatric donor has been used. Similarly, forced diuresis may produce an increase in volume of up to 10%. Measurements of the parenchymal internal anatomical structures have been suggested, including measurements of cortical thickness and size of the medullary pyramids; however, the value of these measurements in establishing the cause of transplant dysfunction appears to be limited and they are no longer in widespread use.

Normal transplant Doppler

Color and power Doppler usually permit easy identification of the normal intrarenal arteries and veins (Figure 9.7). Color flow is usually demonstrable to the level of the arcuate vessels and frequently into interlobular and cortical branches, particularly if power Doppler imaging is employed (Figure 9.8).

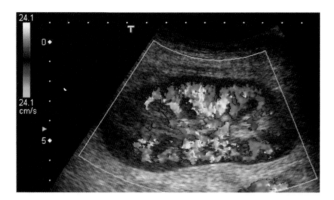

Figure 9.7
Color Doppler in a normal transplant. Good global perfusion of the transplant is well demonstrated; however, note that color flow clearly overestimates vessel size.

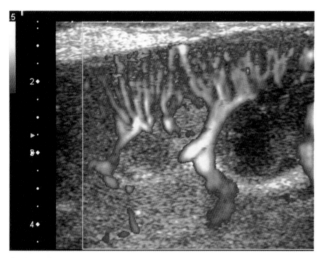

Figure 9.8
Power Doppler in a normal transplant. High-resolution image obtained with a linear array transducer demonstrates small interlobular and cortical branches almost to the capsule of the kidney.

The spectral Doppler trace is a graphical representation of the Doppler frequency shift within the vessels related to time. Angle correction is not required for analysis of the intrarenal arterial waveform but should be applied when evaluating the main transplant vessels, so that frequency shifts can be converted to velocity measurements. The normal transplant arterial Doppler spectrum is almost identical to that of the native kidney showing a 'low resistance' pattern with forward flow throughout the cardiac cycle. There is a rapid upstroke to peak velocity in systole, followed by a gradual decay, with normal diastolic flow velocity being between one-third to one-half of peak systolic

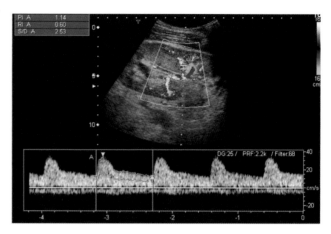

Figure 9.9
Intrarenal arterial spectral Doppler trace from a normal transplant. A low-resistance flow pattern is present, with forward flow throughout the cardiac cycle and a relatively high ratio of diastolic to systolic flow.

flow. The pattern obtained is often described as having a 'ski-slope' appearance (Figure 9.9). The role of spectral Doppler in identifying transplant parenchymal pathology depends upon the presumption that such pathology will alter, and usually increase, resistance to blood flow, reducing diastolic flow to a greater degree than systolic flow. Although it is possible to recognize visually a change in diastolic flow velocities, a number of attempts have been made to quantify such changes so that progress of graft function might be followed. Many different indices quantifying aspects of the spectral Doppler trace have been devised but the indices that have found greatest application in renal transplant ultrasound are the resistance index (RI), pulsatility index (PI) and acceleration time (AT).

The main transplant artery shows a low-resistance Doppler spectral pattern similar to the trace obtained from the intrarenal interlobar arteries. Flow velocities in the main transplant artery are usually in the order of 60–100 cm/s; values of greater than 200–250 cm/s are considered to be abnormal. Flow in the main transplant vein usually shows some variation in velocity with cardiac activity (Figure 9.10).

Doppler indices

Both the *resistance index* and *pulsatility index* are parameters quantifying the ratio of diastolic to systolic flow (Figure 9.11).

The resistance index has been most extensively researched and its value appears to be dependent on changes in both intrarenal vascular compliance and

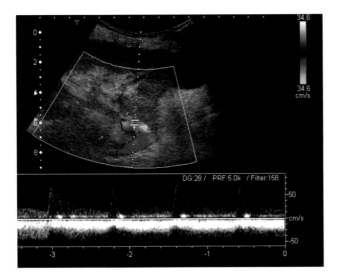

Figure 9.10
Normal spectral Doppler trace from the main transplant vein. Note that there is variation in flow with cardiac activity (periodicity). Flow velocity is reduced just before systole (the arterial trace can be seen faintly above the line).

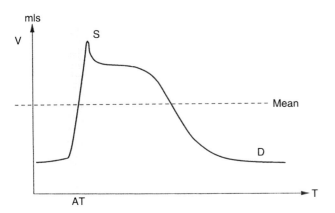

Figure 9.11
The normal Doppler sonogram indicating the methods for calculating the various Doppler indices. S = peak systole; D = minimum diastole; T = time; V = velocity (m/s); AT = acceleration time.

resistance. The normal value for RI is approximately 0.60, with the upper limit of normal being 0.70. The normal range of values for PI in various studies in the literature is 0.63–1.5, without close agreement about a mean. A PI value of greater than 1.8 is often regarded as being significantly abnormal.

The *acceleration time* (or the *time to maximum systole*) is the interval between the onset of systole and the early systolic peak. An AT value of greater than 70 ms is considered to be abnormal in native kidneys, although this index has

been less extensively studied in transplant kidneys and so it is uncertain whether the same cut-off value should be employed. Some authorities consider that an AT value above 90 ms should be regarded as abnormal in transplants; this index reflects upstream disease and is used in assessment of disease in the main transplant artery and the anastomosis.

COMPLICATIONS OF RENAL TRANSPLANTATION

Complications of renal transplantation can be artificially grouped into those that most commonly occur in the early period following transplantation (within the first 3 months) and those that occur later. Although there is some overlap between the two groups, it provides a useful framework to assist with interpretation of an ultrasound study in a patient with a failing transplant. Complications can be further divided into those that are mainly surgical (anatomical) and those that are medical (functional).

Unfortunately, symptoms of transplant dysfunction are non-specific; patients presenting with any combination of diminished urine output, deteriorating renal function, graft swelling and tenderness, fever or leukocytosis may have any one of a number of medical or surgical complications. Early diagnosis of the complications of transplantation is, however, vital to ensure optimal management and survival of the transplant. Ultrasound occupies a central role in early detection of complications, particularly those in the surgical group, and even when it does not allow a definitive diagnosis of the cause of transplant dysfunction can help in determining the optimal time for transplant biopsy and can then guide biopsy or other percutaneous procedures.

EARLY COMPLICATIONS

Delayed graft function (DGF) is a common occurrence following transplantation and is often defined as the need for postoperative dialysis. DGF is often due to acute tubular necrosis, but other medical and surgical causes such as acute rejection and vascular and urologic complications need to be excluded.

Early medical complications

Acute tubular necrosis (ATN) is a significant complicating factor in approximately 20% of cadaveric renal transplants,

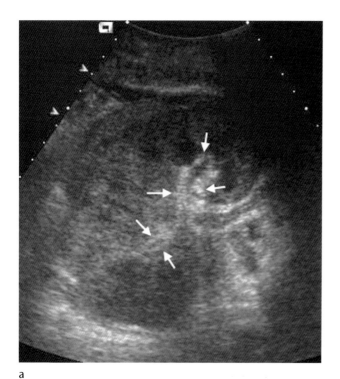

a

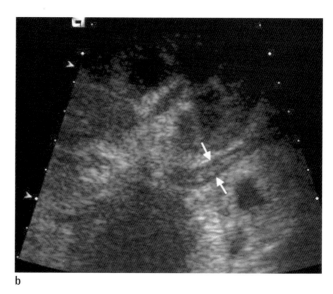

b

Figure 9.12
Gray-scale appearances of severe acute rejection. (a) The transplant is swollen and rounded, with compression of the renal sinus (arrows). (b) Urothelial edema best seen in the magnified view of the ureter (arrows).

with a particularly high incidence in non-heart-beating donor kidneys. It is rarely seen in living donor transplants. The causes of ATN are complex, although it appears to be caused by a combination of ischemia and reperfusion injuries, resulting in the production of reactive oxygen species that cause tissue injury. Many factors predispose to ATN, but prolonged warm and cold ischemic times are particularly implicated. Although ATN will usually recover in 1–2 weeks, it does carry an increased risk of acute rejection, and the combination of ATN and acute rejection appears to carry a particularly poor prognosis.

The incidence of *acute rejection* following renal transplantation has fallen significantly over the past 10 years, but it remains one of the most important causes of early graft dysfunction, usually occurring within the first 6 months after surgery. Improvements in preoperative cross-matching, combined with the introduction of new immunosuppressive agents – notably, tacrolimus, mycophenolate mofetil and sirolimus – have decreased acute rejection rates to approximately 20%. Although effective treatment for acute rejection is now available, a single episode of acute rejection is a major adverse prognostic factor for long-term graft survival. One study showed that the predicted half-life of a graft without an episode of rejection was almost double that of one that had undergone one or more episodes of acute rejection.

Evaluation of DGF is further complicated by the fact that several of the immunosuppressive drugs used to prevent and treat rejection may of themselves be nephrotoxic;

this applies particularly to the calcineurin inhibitors (cyclosporine and tacrolimus). It can be very difficult to distinguish between transplant dysfunction due to acute rejection and that due to drug toxicity, but clearly this is of great importance, as the appropriate management of these two complications will be completely different.

Ultrasound of early medical complications

Clinical differentiation between ATN, acute rejection and drug toxicity is a frequent dilemma in a patient with early transplant dysfunction. Serial ultrasound examinations are commonly employed in this setting. Several early reports indicated that altered gray-scale appearances of the transplant correlated with acute rejection. Graft swelling was thought to be a useful indicator of rejection but, as has been discussed above, an increase in volume is a normal feature post-transplantation. Additionally, graft swelling also occurs in ATN and is therefore an unhelpful feature in establishing the cause of DGF. Severe graft swelling, however, is most commonly due to acute rejection. Other features that were initially considered to be useful in diagnosing acute rejection were alterations in renal cortical echogenicity (increased or decreased), thickening of the renal cortex, decreasing renal sinus area, decreased echogenicity of the renal sinus fat, loss of corticomedullary

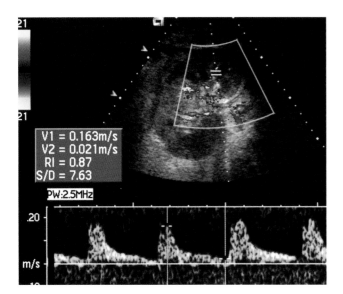

Figure 9.13
Acute rejection. The spectral Doppler trace obtained from an interlobar artery shows a relative reduction in diastolic flow, resulting in an elevation of the resistance index (RI).

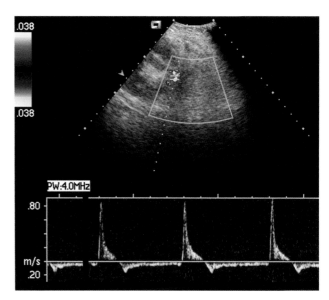

Figure 9.14
Acute rejection. In this example, intrarenal pressures are elevated sufficiently to cause a reversal of diastolic flow. In this situation, it is essential to exclude renal vein thrombosis, which may also produce diastolic flow reversal.

differentiation, prominence and splaying of the renal pyramids and thickening of the collecting system urothelium (Figure 9.12). More recent studies, however, have found these features are both insensitive and non-specific in the diagnosis of acute rejection and occur relatively late. For these reasons, the morphologic changes of early transplant failure are of limited use and acute rejection is not excluded by a normal gray-scale ultrasound examination.

Doppler ultrasound was also initially thought to provide a sensitive and specific non-invasive test for acute rejection. Increased intrarenal pressures due to rejection reduce diastolic flow to a greater extent than systolic flow, leading to an elevation of the RI (or PI) values in the intrarenal arteries (Figure 9.13). More recent work, however, has shown that elevation of the RI is a non-specific finding. In addition to acute rejection, an elevated RI may be seen in cases of ureteric obstruction, external graft compression and renal vein obstruction. Although these conditions will usually be accompanied by other abnormal ultrasound findings, severe ATN and pyelonephritis, which may also result in an elevated RI, may not. A significantly elevated RI (>0.8) is thus best regarded as a non-specific sign of renal transplant dysfunction and can be used to help monitor progress of the transplant. The combination of Doppler ultrasound and a clinical 'rejection score' was shown in one study to achieve a sensitivity of 96% and specificity of 66% for prediction of acute rejection. Doppler ultrasound can thus help guide clinical decisions regarding the need for biopsy. The Doppler spectrum is probably not significant-

ly affected by mild or early acute rejection, and thus many centers advocate the use of protocol-driven routine transplant biopsy in the early stages following surgery to allow prompt identification and treatment of rejection episodes before clinical or sonographic abnormalities are evident. Severe acute rejection may produce such high intrarenal pressures that intrarenal diastolic flow is abolished or even reversed (Figure 9.14). In this situation, careful Doppler examination of the main transplant vein is needed to exclude venous thrombosis, which may produce similar appearances, and where there is doubt surgical exploration may be justified. Although the use of postoperative Doppler spectral analysis is limited in its ability to differentiate between the medical causes of early transplant dysfunction, perioperative Doppler may be a more specific technique. One study showed that the use of ultrasound could accurately predict which patients would develop ATN. An RI value of greater than 0.7 at 30 minutes after unclamping the renal artery correctly identified the transplant kidneys most at risk of developing ATN.

More recently, there have been several studies evaluating qualitative and quantitative analysis of power Doppler (PD) images of the transplant kidney, mainly in the setting of suspected acute rejection. PD is superior to conventional color Doppler in demonstrating flow in the small peripheral vessels, and it has been suggested that reduced flow in these small vessels due to the inflammation and microvascular thrombosis that occur in acute rejection might be detected with PD. Reduced cortical perfusion and

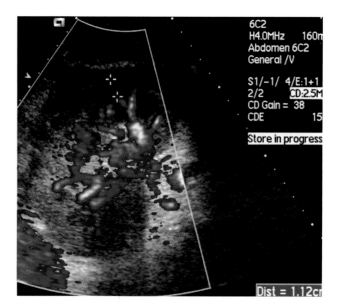

Figure 9.15
Acute rejection. This power Doppler image shows a loss of cortical perfusion despite adequate perfusion of the larger vessels in the more central areas of the transplant.

vascular pruning can be identified in some cases of acute rejection with PD (Figure 9.15). Unfortunately, these appearances have also been reported in chronic allograft nephropathy, ATN, calcineurin inhibitor nephrotoxicity and cytomegalovirus infection and are therefore a non-specific finding of transplant dysfunction. Additionally, this work has not been reproducible and, at present, there is insufficient evidence to recommend its use in replacing biopsy for identifying episodes of acute rejection.

The use of ultrasound contrast agents in identifying early medical complications of renal transplantation is at an early stage, but a recent report has demonstrated changes in contrast medium time–intensity curves in patients with acute rejection compared with normal controls. This may provide a basis for earlier and more accurate sonographic identification of acute rejection in the future, although further studies are necessary before this becomes established as a routine clinical tool.

Doppler ultrasound is unhelpful in diagnosing nephrotoxicity caused by the calcineurin inhibitors cyclosporine and tacrolimus as they do not produce a consistent effect on the intrarenal Doppler spectral trace.

Ultrasound guided-biopsy is frequently required in response to suboptimal graft function, particularly when accompanied by an abnormal Doppler ultrasound study, or as part of a post-transplant management protocol. It has been shown to be a safe and effective procedure; complication rates of 5–30% are quoted, although these are usually insignificant perirenal hematomas or self-limiting episodes of hematuria. One study of 210 renal transplant biopsies

reported an 8% rate of macroscopic hematuria following biopsy, with no graft losses; this study used 14G needles, and it might be expected that the 18G biopsy needles now in routine use would result in a lower complication rate. In order to minimize the risks in biopsy, however, it is important to pay careful attention to technique to maximize diagnostic yield and minimize complication rates. The position of the needle tip must be positively identified before the biopsy is taken. Complications are more frequent in deep biopsies, in the region of the medulla, and therefore biopsy should be targeted as superficially as possible, with the angle between needle and transplant optimized to ensure a long core of cortex and minimal transgression into the medulla.

Early surgical complications

Peritransplant fluid collections

Small fluid collections around a transplanted kidney are a common finding in the first few weeks following surgery and are seen in approximately a third of cases. Small crescentic collections in an asymptomatic patient that do not compress the graft and do not increase in size on serial ultrasound examinations are unlikely to be significant and do not usually require further investigation (Figure 9.16). Larger collections, however, may directly compromise the function of the graft due to pressure on the vessels or ureter. Some collections, such as urinoma, provide indirect

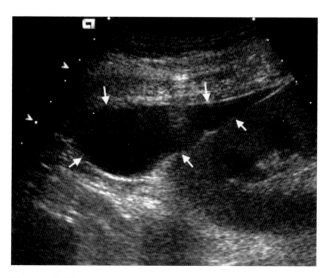

Figure 9.16
Small postoperative fluid collection. This small collection above the upper pole of the transplant (arrows) is not causing compression and is unlikely to be significant.

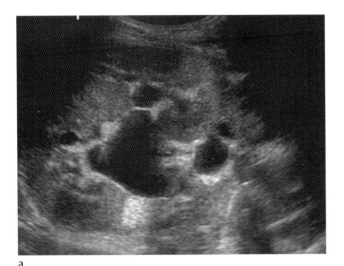

a

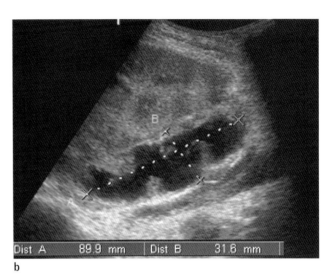

b

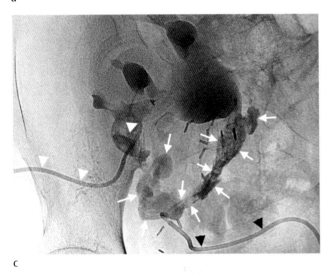

c

Figure 9.17

Urinoma. The transplant is hydronephrotic (a) and there is a fluid collection deep to the transplant (b) aspiration confirmed this to be an infected urinoma. Following nephrostomy drainage, a nephrostogram (c) shows extravasation of contrast from the renal pelvis (arrows) to fill the peritransplant collection. There is a lower pole nephrostomy tube (white arrowheads) and pigtail catheter in the infected urinoma (black arrowheads). At surgery, the transplant ureter was found to be completely necrotic.

evidence of another cause of transplant dysfunction. Ultrasound cannot usually differentiate between the different types of peritransplant collection but can be used to detect and monitor fluid collections and, where necessary, guide diagnostic aspiration to establish the nature of a collection, proceeding to formal drainage if necessary.

Urinoma (Figure 9.17)

Urinoma is an unusual complication, seen in 1–6% of transplants, and is suggested by fever, pain, deteriorating graft function and falling urine output. If not recognized at an early stage it can be a sinister development, particularly if sepsis occurs, which may then necessitate withdrawal of immunosuppression and probable loss of the transplant. Urinomas usually occur as a result of either a leak at the bladder anastomosis or ureteric necrosis due to ischemia of the distal ureter. Bladder leaks are now uncommon, with the use of extravesical anastomosis techniques. The

appearances of a urinoma are usually those of an echo-free collection, although there may be septa, which are usually fine. The diagnosis can be confirmed by biochemical analysis of an ultrasound-guided aspiration of the collection. Isotope renography may also be helpful in diagnosing this complication, demonstrating extravasation of the radiopharmaceutical around the transplant. It is then often necessary to proceed to antegrade contrast pyelography to demonstrate the location of the leak. Early transplant nephrostomy is advised to minimize morbidity and sepsis and to maintain graft function. Many patients will then require surgical exploration and repair.

Lymphocele (Figure 9.18)

Collections of lymphatic fluid derive from division of either donor or recipient lymphatics. Lymphocele incidence is as high as 20% overall and is more common in obese patients, following episodes of acute rejection and with certain

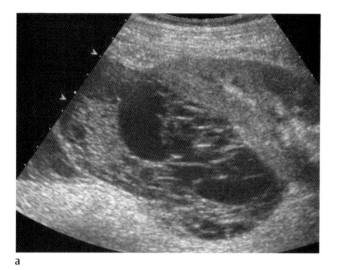

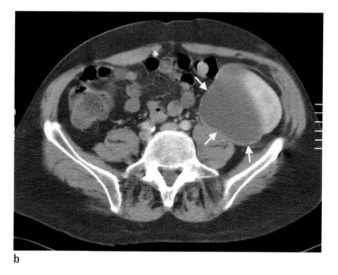

a

b

Figure 9.18
Lymphocele. Ultrasound (a) and CT (b) images showing a large multiseptated fluid collection deep to the transplant typical of a lymphocele (arrows).

immunosuppressive regimens. While most commonly located inferomedial to the graft, lymphoceles may occur at any site. They are usually echo-free but may contain numerous internal fine septa, and in this respect they most closely mimic urinomas. As management of these two complications is completely different, differentiation between these two possibilities by radionuclide scintigraphy or by ultrasound-guided aspiration should be performed at an early stage if there is any suggestion of graft dysfunction. In patients with features of infection, aspiration is also particularly important to identify an infected lymphocele. Lymphoceles will frequently persist, and if producing symptoms related to a mechanical effect such as ureteric obstruction then ultrasound-guided percutaneous drainage may be used as a short-term measure to resolve these symptoms. However, lymphoceles so drained frequently recur and will then usually require formal surgical treatment. Laparoscopic marsupialization to the peritoneum has been shown to be an effective procedure to treat sterile lymphoceles with minimal morbidity. As lymphoceles may be difficult to identify laparoscopically, both intraoperative ultrasound and preoperative ultrasound-guided guidewire or catheter placement into the lymphocele have been successfully used to guide laparoscopic surgery. If the lymphocele is infected on the first aspiration attempt, internal marsupialization becomes no longer appropriate and in these cases long-term catheter drainage may be necessary.

Hematoma (Figure 9.19)

Hematomas are common, particularly in the immediate postoperative period. They may occur subcutaneously or

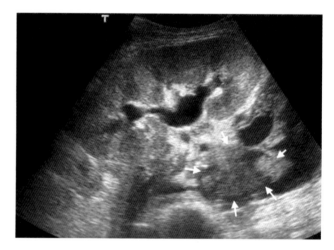

Figure 9.19
Hematoma. A large complex collection deep to the transplant (arrows) represents a hematoma. Note the associated hydronephrosis secondary to extrinsic ureteric compression.

immediately related to the transplant. The ultrasound characteristics of the hematoma depend upon its age and the extent to which coagulation has occurred. Thus, hematomas may be echo-free or contain clumps of echoes, both within the fluid and adherent to the wall of the lesion as a result of clot aggregation. They usually resolve spontaneously and, indeed, overzealous needling may increase the risk of super-added infection. However, needle aspiration and drainage may be necessary, either if the clinical symptoms suggest that infection is present, if the diagnosis is in doubt or if ureteric or vascular compromise is suspected.

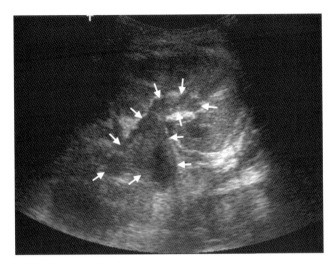

Figure 9.20
Collecting system obstruction by hematoma. Following a percutaneous procedure in this patient, there was a profound reduction in urine output and hematuria. Ultrasound shows that the collecting system is dilated and filled with mid-range echoes representing hematoma (arrows).

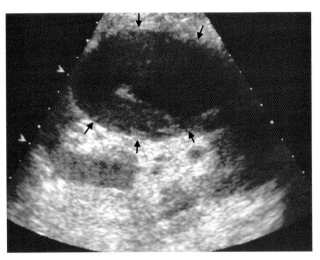

Figure 9.21
Peritransplant abscess. A complex fluid collection superficial to the transplant (arrows). Despite there being no clinical indication of infection, ultrasound-guided needle aspiration produced thick pus.

The regular use of renal biopsy to monitor the progress of renal transplant function is a further potential cause for the development of a hematoma, although the use of smaller-gauge needles (18G) and spring-loaded automatic biopsy devices as well as ultrasound guidance has improved the safety of renal transplant biopsy. Occasionally, postbiopsy hemorrhage can be catastrophic and result in the loss of the graft or cause bleeding into the pelvicalyceal system and ureteric obstruction with clot (Figure 9.20).

Abscess formation (Figure 9.21)

Any of the perirenal fluid collections may become infected. There are no specific features on ultrasound that reveal that a hematoma, urinoma or lymphocele has become infected. Furthermore, the clinical features of infection are often masked by immunosuppression. Although the classical features of an abscess are those of a fluid collection whose contents are of fine echogenic fluid with finely irregular margins, these features are seen in only a small percentage of abscesses. A high index of suspicion for the development of an abscess needs to be held and diagnostic aspiration performed in any fluid collection where the condition of the patient gives cause for concern. Most abscesses can be diagnosed by a combination of ultrasound imaging and ultrasound-guided needle aspiration. Many can also be treated by a combination of antibiotic therapy and percutaneous catheter drainage, although fungal infections

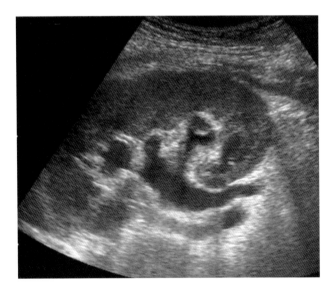

Figure 9.22
Mild transplant hydronephrosis and hydroureter. This examination, performed in the early postoperative period, shows mild hydronephrosis secondary to edema of the ureteric anastomosis. The extent of hydronephrosis did not progress on subsequent studies and the graft maintained good function throughout.

respond poorly to catheter drainage and it is perhaps worthwhile considering an initial aspiration of the abscess with microscopic analysis prior to the insertion of a percutaneous drain.

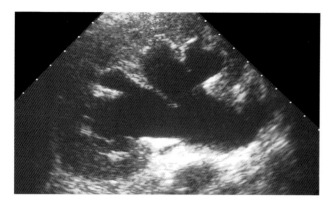

Figure 9.23
High-grade transplant hydronephrosis with marked calyceal clubbing secondary to ureteric obstruction.

Hydronephrosis

Mild, transient, hydronephrosis is a common finding in the first few days following transplantation and usually reflects edema of the ureterovesical anastomosis (Figure 9.22). Other causes of early transplant hydronephrosis are clot in the transplant ureter or bladder or non-obstructive causes such as bladder distension combined with the effects of denervation of the transplant kidney collecting system. In patients with hydronephrosis and a full bladder, the examination should always be repeated after voiding to exclude bladder distension as the cause.

Ultrasound is very accurate in demonstrating transplant hydronephrosis, and the absence of collecting system dilatation makes ureteric obstruction very unlikely. However, interpretation of hydronephrosis in the early period following transplantation is more difficult and, as in the native kidney, the presence of pelvicalyceal dilatation does not always indicate that ureteric obstruction is present. In a patient with mild stable pelvicalyceal dilatation and a well-functioning transplant, further investigation is probably unnecessary. A transplant showing progressive hydronephrosis on serial ultrasound studies, where there is high-grade hydronephrosis (Figure 9.23), a peritransplant collection that may be compressing the ureter (see Figure 9.19) or where the transplant is functioning suboptimally, may indicate ureteric obstruction. It has been suggested that Doppler ultrasound may be helpful in distinguishing obstructive from non-obstructive hydronephrosis in a similar manner to native kidneys. In a hydronephrotic transplant where the intrarenal arterial RI is less than 0.75, and where there is no urine leak, obstruction is unlikely. This may help improve the specificity of ultrasound in identifying obstruction, although clearly elevation of the RI is not limited to obstruction and can be due to many other causes of transplant dysfunction. Given the difficulty of interpreting transplant pelvicalyceal dilatation in a patient with a failing transplant, it is often necessary to proceed to further imaging studies such as computed tomography (CT) and, if doubt remains, ultrasound-guided antegrade pyelography, a Whittaker test or trial of percutaneous nephrostomy may be required.

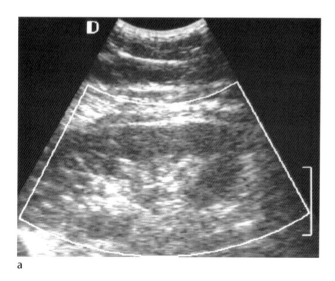

a

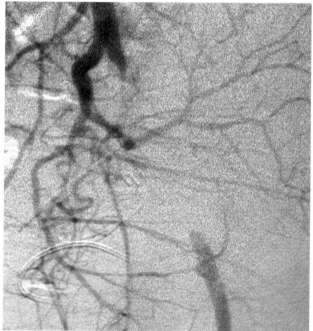

b

Figure 9.24
Transplant artery thrombosis. (a) Ultrasound, performed on the first postoperative day, shows absence of color signal throughout the kidney, indicating absence of perfusion. A subtraction angiogram (b) confirms that both the transplant and external iliac arteries are occluded.

Vascular complications

Fortunately, early occlusive vascular complications of transplantation are now rare but when they do occur they usually result in loss of the transplant and carry significant risk to the patient. Doppler ultrasound is the cornerstone of early identification of these complications. For an adequate ultrasound study, it is vital to be aware of the surgical anatomy, particularly the number of transplant vessels and the site of their anastomoses. As with all vascular Doppler studies, careful attention must be directed to selection of pulse repetition frequency (scale), Doppler gain and wall filter settings appropriate to the vessels being examined.

Renal arterial thrombosis

Renal artery thrombosis occurs in 0.5–3.5% of renal transplants and almost always within the first month after surgery. Risk factors for development of this complication include acute rejection, multiple renal vessels, hypotension, atherosclerosis of the donor or recipient vessels, perfusion injury, vascular kinking, diabetic nephropathy, prolonged ischemic times and extremes of donor age. It may be discovered on routine postoperative ultrasound before there is clinical evidence of graft failure.

Doppler examination will show complete absence of color signal in the transplant and main renal vessels (Figure 9.24). Spectral Doppler examination at the arterial anastomosis will occasionally demonstrate a short systolic peak of low velocity with no diastolic flow. When identified, this complication almost always leads to graft nephrectomy, although there are reports of successful graft fibrinolysis.

In a transplant with multiple renal arteries, thrombosis of one vessel will result in segmental infarction. Gray-scale ultrasound may demonstrate a swollen echo-poor area of infarction and color or power Doppler will show absent perfusion of this area (Figure 9.25). Subsequently, the infarcted segment reduces in volume, and becomes increased in reflectivity, forming first an echogenic wedge and finally a linear echogenic focus with a cortical scar unless the infarct is large enough to remain as a wedge-shaped area of increased reflectivity. Lower-pole infarcts may compromise the blood supply to the ureter.

Renal vein thrombosis

Although this is an unusual complication, it is more common than arterial thrombosis and is seen in up to 5% of transplants, usually in the first postoperative week. It is a more common occurrence in children, presumably due to the smaller size of the renal vessels. Renal vein thrombosis

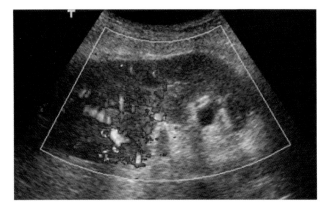

Figure 9.25
Segmental infarction. There were three arteries supplying this transplant kidney. Color Doppler ultrasound obtained on the first postoperative day shows no perfusion of the lower part of the transplant, indicating thrombosis of the lower polar artery.

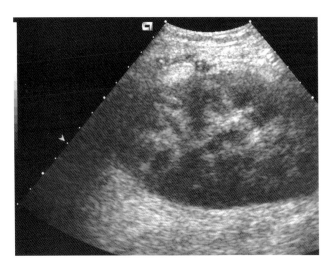

Figure 9.26
Renal vein thrombosis. Gray-scale image showing that the transplant is swollen with compression of the renal sinus. These appearances are non-specific and could also be seen in severe acute rejection.

usually presents as sudden oliguria, graft swelling and tenderness. The gray-scale appearances are non-specific but graft enlargement and decreased corticomedullary differentiation may be seen (Figure 9.26). Color Doppler imaging usually shows flow only during systole in the intrarenal vessels but may occasionally demonstrate a 'to and fro' pattern of alternating red and blue. Spectral Doppler examination of the intrarenal arteries, however, often shows a striking reversal of diastolic flow (Figure 9.27), sometimes with a 'reversed M' appearance. This spectral pattern is highly suggestive of renal vein thrombosis and, although reversed

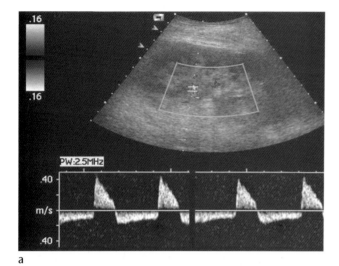

a

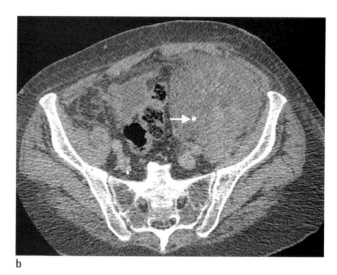

b

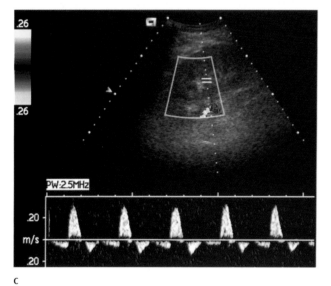

c

Figure 9.27
Renal vein thrombosis. (a) Intrarenal arterial Doppler spectral trace showing that diastolic flow is reversed. (b) Venous phase contrast-enhanced CT performed 6 hours later reveals a swollen non-perfused transplant consistent with venous infarction (there is a ureteric stent in situ – arrow). (c) Another case of renal vein thrombosis, showing the 'reverse M' appearance of diastolic flow.

diastolic flow is occasionally seen in cases of severe rejection, absence of venous signal at the renal hilum and in the transplant itself in combination with this spectral pattern is virtually pathognomonic for renal vein thrombosis. It is occasionally possible to directly visualize the thrombus within a dilated main transplant vein (Figure 9.28). Incomplete renal vein thrombosis will produce less marked Doppler abnormality with reduced diastolic flow. Incomplete luminal obstruction may be visible on color or power Doppler examination. There is a report of two cases of early renal vein thrombosis where a spectral pattern of a low systolic peak with maintained diastolic flow was seen in the intrarenal arteries resembling the 'parvus and tardus' pattern seen in renal artery stenosis.

Although most cases of renal vein thrombosis will result in the need for graft nephrectomy, early detection may allow graft salvage through surgical thrombectomy or radiologic catheter clot aspiration. Thus, a high level of suspicion should be maintained for this complication in early postoperative ultrasound.

Patients suffering vascular occlusion (arterial or venous) after transplantation in the absence of an obvious technical cause should be screened for a thrombophilic disorder and, if present, should be treated with thrombosis prophylaxis at the time of retransplantation.

Arteriovenous fistulae and pseudoaneurysms

These complications are usually the result of transplant biopsy. In spite of attempts to use non-invasive methods to monitor the progress of the transplant, biopsy remains the mainstay of graft monitoring for detection of medical causes of graft failure. Biopsy under direct ultrasound vision is a safe and well-tolerated procedure, but arteriovenous fistulae remain very frequent and may complicate as many as

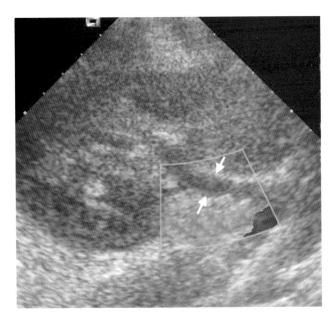

Figure 9.28
Renal vein thrombosis. No color flow can be seen in the main transplant vein (arrows).

17% of transplants undergoing biopsy. As a general rule, these fistulae are small, clinically insignificant and 75% will occlude spontaneously within 4 weeks. Occasionally, however, the fistulae have a very high flow volume and may have significant pathologic sequelae. They may, for instance, cause hematuria, peritransplant hematoma, hypertension, poor function (due to an intrarenal vascular steal) or precipitate cardiac failure. In these cases, coil embolization may be indicated, although this will inevitably lead to loss of a variable amount of functioning renal tissue. Occasionally arteriovenous fistulae may result in graft loss.

Doppler features of arteriovenous fistulae are characteristic. High-velocity flow is demonstrated by aliasing of the color signal at the fistula site. The fistula may then be more elegantly demonstrated by reducing overall color sensitivity and increasing the pulse repetition frequency (scale). In this way, demonstrable flow within the other vessels in the kidney is lost, while the feeding artery, nidus and draining vein are usually clearly seen (Figure 9.29). Spectral Doppler examination of the fistula nidus will show a characteristic disturbed high-velocity, low-resistance pattern (Figure 9.30). If flow through the fistula is particularly disordered, then tissue vibration around the fistula will produce a 'tissue bruit', being seen as a diffuse area of high-velocity color signals (Figure 9.31). While volume flow in a large number of these fistulae is relatively low compared to overall flow to the graft, in the larger and clinically significant fistulae shunting may be sufficient to alter the blood flow characteristics within the main renal artery and renal vein. Characteristically, the renal artery demonstrates increased

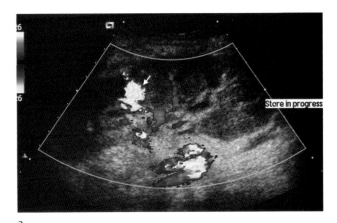

a

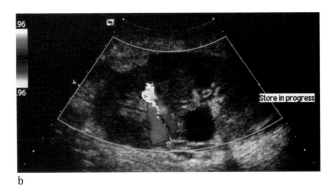

b

Figure 9.29
Transplant arteriovenous fistula. (a) Color Doppler examination shows a focal area of high velocity with aliasing of the color signal (arrow). (b) After increasing the pulse repetition frequency (PRF), color flow in the kidney is largely abolished, but the fistula is now well seen with the feeding artery, draining vein and nidus clearly visible.

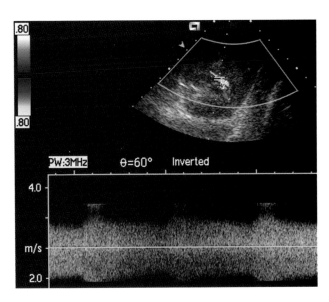

Figure 9.30
Transplant arteriovenous fistula. A spectral Doppler trace shows the typical high-velocity, low-resistance flow pattern.

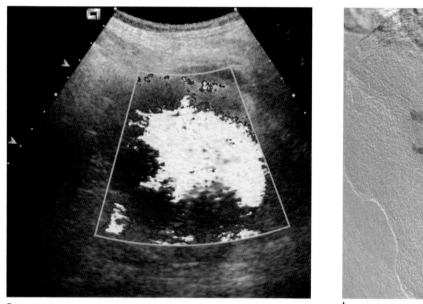

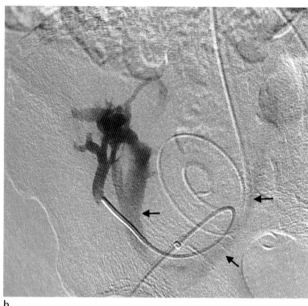

a

b

Figure 9.31

Large post-biopsy transplant arteriovenous fistula. (a) Color Doppler examination shows that the entire renal sinus is filled with color signal representing the tissue bruit from a high-flow fistula. (b) A subtraction arteriogram shows a large central fistula with early venous filling (arrows) and no significant cortical perfusion. Unfortunately, it was not technically possible to occlude the fistula and the transplant eventually failed.

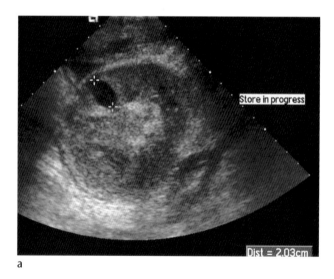

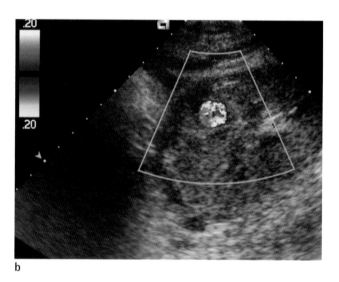

a

b

Figure 9.32

Post-biopsy transplant pseudoaneurysm. The gray-scale image (a) shows a small cystic structure in the renal parenchyma that fills with color on the corresponding color Doppler image (b).

blood flow velocities with reduction in the peripheral resistance to blood flow (low PI and RI). In the renal vein the signal may resemble that in the renal artery, i.e. an arterialization of venous blood flow with an increased PI related to the arteriovenous shunting within the large arteriovenous fistula. It is important to remember that a large AV fistula may result in a reduction of the RI value in the main renal artery and in the larger segmental branches supplying the affected area of the kidney. In a transplant that has otherwise increased vascular resistance, e.g. due to rejection or ATN, any elevation of RI in these vessels may be masked by the hemodynamic effects of the fistula.

Intrarenal pseudoaneurysms are also usually the result of biopsy and often coexist with arteriovenous fistulae. The incidence of pseudoaneurysm formation following biopsy is approximately 6%. They appear as cystic structures that fill with color on color or power Doppler examination (Figure 9.32) and show a 'to and fro' pattern at the aneurysm neck on spectral Doppler examination. Like arteriovenous fistulae, intrarenal pseudoaneurysms are likely to resolve spontaneously. Extrarenal pseudoaneurysms are fortunately rare; they are most frequently seen at the anastomosis site and are often the result of infection. They usually result in the need for graft nephrectomy.

LATE COMPLICATIONS

Long-term renal transplant survival continues to improve such that the principal cause of graft loss following the first year of transplantation is patient death with a functioning graft. Cardiovascular disease is the leading cause of death in transplant patients and aggressive treatment of the risk factors for cardiovascular disease, such as hypertension, anemia and dyslipidemia, is important post-transplantation. Renal transplantation also carries an increased risk for the development of cancer; this is thought to be primarily due to the use of immunosuppression, permitting proliferation of oncogenic viruses and inhibiting normal tumor surveillance. This increased risk applies to most cancers, but is particularly high for lymphomas and skin cancer. Management consists of reducing immunosuppression to minimum levels acceptable to prevent rejection and providing general advice on lifestyle factors known to reduce cancer, particularly avoiding excessive exposure to sunlight. Post-transplant lymphoproliferative disease (PTLD) has an incidence of 1–2% in renal transplant recipients and most commonly occurs 3–4 years after transplantation (Figure 9.33). The majority are B-cell non-Hodgkin's lymphomas associated with Epstein–Barr virus (EBV). The liver is the most commonly involved organ and extranodal disease is more common than in lymphoma in non-immunocompromised patients. The transplant itself may be involved either as focal masses or diffuse infiltration. In approximately half the cases disease is present outside the abdomen. The prognosis for PTLD is relatively poor with a 5-year mortality of 40–50%. Treatment consists of reduction or cessation of immunosuppression, antiviral therapy, radiotherapy, chemotherapy and surgery. Transplant patients are also at increased risk of infection; risks are greatest in the period between 1 and 6 months post-transplantation, particularly for EBV, cytomegalovirus and *Pneumocystis carinii*, and

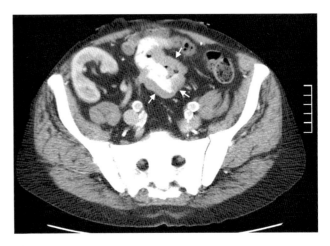

Figure 9.33
Post-transplant lymphoproliferative disease. CT image demonstrating an area of focal small bowel wall thickening (arrows), representing small bowel lymphoma adjacent to the transplant.

routine anti-infective chemotherapy is usually given in this period. The risk of infection decreases in the long term, but remains high in patients with poor graft function and those on high doses of immunosuppression.

Disease recurrence in the transplant is of increasing clinical importance as graft survival improves; this may involve either primary glomerulonephritis or systemic disease that

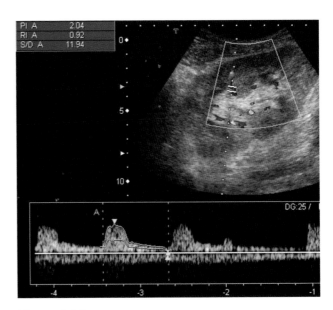

Figure 9.34
Recurrent diabetic nephrosclerosis in a transplant. This patient's transplant had functioned well for 19 years but started to fail. Gray-scale appearances were normal, but the intrarenal Doppler spectrum shows reduced diastolic flow (raised RI). Biopsy confirmed recurrent diabetic nephropathy.

involves the kidneys. The overall incidence of graft failure from disease recurrence is usually thought to be in the order of only 2%, but this figure is likely to be an underestimate, mainly due to difficulties in differentiating the histologic changes of rejection from those of transplant glomerulonephritis. Disease recurrence usually manifests as deteriorating graft function with proteinuria. The probability of recurrent disease varies according to the disease process involved: e.g. almost all patients with type 1 diabetes will develop changes of diabetic nephropathy in the transplant (Figure 9.34), but this is very unlikely to lead to transplant failure in the first 10 years. Disease recurrence is, however, particularly problematic in patients with oxalosis (primary hyperoxaluria type 1), and this condition may be a relative contraindication to transplantation. Systemic diseases that involve the kidney do not usually represent an absolute contraindication to transplantation but in certain conditions, such as Henoch–Schönlein purpura, systemic lupus erythematosus (SLE) and Wegener's granulomatosis, transplantation should be delayed until the disease is quiescent to minimize the risk of disease recurrence.

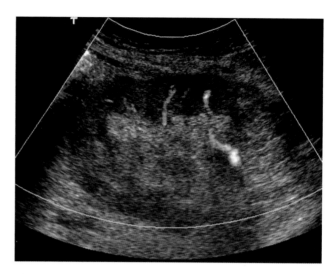

Figure 9.35
Chronic allograft nephropathy. This color Doppler image shows a reduced number of 'straightened' vessels.

Chronic allograft nephropathy (chronic rejection)

Acute rejection is an unusual occurrence in the late period following transplantation and, if present, may indicate lack of compliance with immunosuppressive treatment. An episode of acute rejection is, however, the most important factor in predicting which patients will develop chronic allograft nephropathy (CAN). The incidence of CAN has remained relatively unchanged and, after death with a functioning transplant, is now the most important cause of long-term graft loss. CAN usually develops more than 6 months after transplantation and presents as deteriorating graft function, proteinuria and hypertension. Histologically, there are features of interstitial fibrosis, tubular atrophy, glomerulosclerosis and vascular intimal thickening.

A number of ultrasound features of CAN have been described, including a reduction in graft size, increased parenchymal echogenicity, reduced numbers of intrarenal vessels and straightening of the vessels (Figure 9.35). However, these features are subjective and unreliable, and the role of ultrasound has traditionally been to exclude other causes of graft dysfunction and guide biopsy. Measurement of RI in the transplant arteries is not of value in identifying CAN, as it frequently does not show any alteration. Recent reports suggest that new ultrasound techniques may be of value in detecting CAN. One study analyzed color Doppler images from renal transplants and found that renal cortical hypoperfusion was present in patients with CAN (but also in patients with calcineurin inhibitor toxicity) and suggested that this technique could

be used to select patients that require needle biopsy. In another approach comparing ultrasound strain imaging in a single transplant with CAN and a normal control, a threefold difference in cortical strain was seen between the two grafts. Although of interest for the future, these approaches need to be validated in larger studies before their use can be recommended in routine practice. Unfortunately, there is no effective treatment for CAN and patients progress to renal failure but are often suitable for retransplantation.

Although intrarenal Doppler measurements are not helpful in identifying CAN, an RI of 0.80 or higher 3 months or more after transplantation appears to be an adverse prognostic factor predicting both transplant failure and patient death with a functioning graft.

Late surgical complications

Vascular: transplant artery stenosis

Transplant artery stenosis is the most common vascular complication following transplantation and is seen in 3–15% of cases. It most often occurs between the first and third year post-transplantation and usually presents as hypertension and deteriorating graft function, particularly when precipitated by treatment with an angiotensin-converting enzyme inhibitor drug. Stenosis may occur at any site along the length of the transplant artery, but is most commonly at, or close to, the vascular anastomosis. Unlike

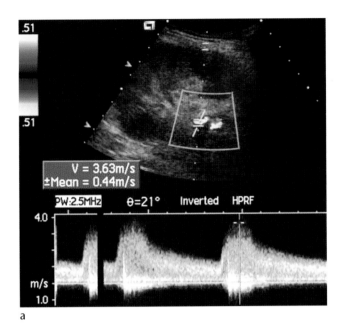

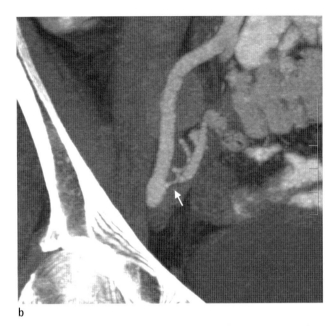

Figure 9.36

Transplant artery stenosis. The spectral Doppler trace (a) from the transplant artery adjacent to the anastomosis shows high peak systolic velocity (363 cm/s) consistent with high-grade stenosis. A coronal oblique maximum intensity projection reconstructed image from CT angiography (b) confirms high-grade proximal stenosis (arrow).

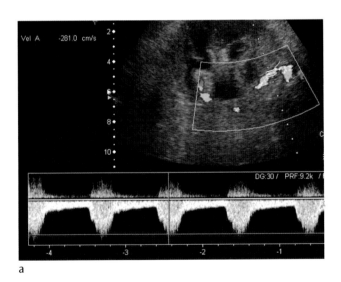

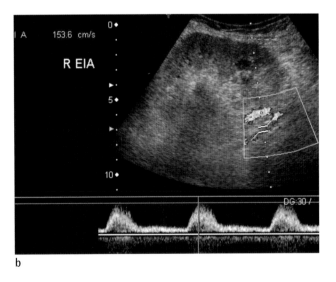

Figure 9.37

(a,b) Transplant artery stenosis. In this case, there is color aliasing in the transplant artery. Both the main renal artery PSV (281 cm/s) and transplant artery/external iliac artery PSV ratio (1.83) show a borderline increase consistent with hemodynamically significant transplant artery stenosis. (Figure reproduced with permission from Freeman S. Ultrasound investigation of suspected renal artery stenosis. Ultrasound 2004; 12(2): 69–74, published by Maney Publishing on behalf of the British Medical Ultrasound Society.)

the native renal artery, the transplant artery is usually readily identified using color Doppler imaging, making ultrasound an ideal non-invasive test for identification of transplant artery stenosis. The transplant artery is examined from the anastomosis to the renal hilum with spectral Doppler tracings at regular intervals along the course of the artery and particularly at any sites of aliasing of the color Doppler signal. The transplant artery may follow a very tortuous course, and care must be taken to ensure accurate angle correction. Power Doppler may be helpful

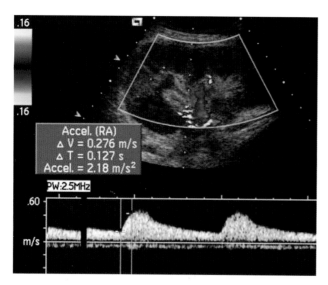

Figure 9.38
Transplant artery stenosis. Intrarenal arterial spectral Doppler trace showing a parvus and tardus pattern with a prolonged systolic acceleration time (127 ms).

in demonstrating the course of a tortuous artery but should not be used in isolation, as it lacks the ability of color Doppler to identify disturbed flow and does not provide directional information. An increase in peak systolic velocity (PSV) in the main transplant artery to above 200–250 cm/s is an indication of hemodynamically significant stenosis and is reported to give sensitivity of 90–100% and specificity of 87.5–95% in identifying this condition (Figure 9.36). Significant stenosis can also be diagnosed by a raised PSV ratio between the transplant artery and external iliac artery; if the ratio is greater than 1.8, a significant stenosis is also deemed to be present (Figure 9.37). A positive ultrasound study is sufficient to recommend formal catheter or CT angiography proceeding to angioplasty if stenosis is confirmed.

As in the native kidney, the 'parvus and tardus' spectral Doppler pattern is also described in the intrarenal arteries in patients with high-grade main artery stenosis. This pattern describes a spectral trace that shows a prolonged systolic upstroke and reduced systolic peak (Figure 9.38). Identification of this pattern may be helpful to raise

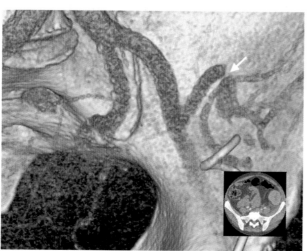

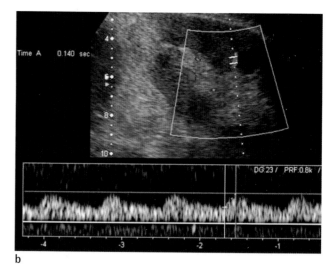

Figure 9.39
Transplant artery kink. (a) The color Doppler image shows a color tissue bruit at the renal hilum. (b) Intrarenal arterial spectral Doppler trace shows a parvus and tardus arterial flow pattern. (c) A volume-rendered CT image confirms an arterial kink at the renal hilum (arrow). As the transplant was functioning poorly, it was explored and the redundant artery excised, following which, function improved.

a

b

c

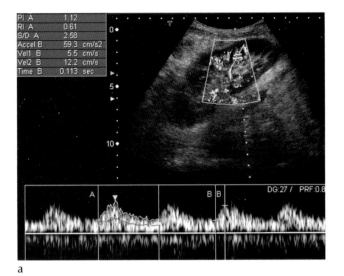

a

Figure 9.40
Transplant artery fibromuscular hyperplasia. (a) The intrarenal arterial Doppler spectrum shows a parvus and tardus pattern, but no focal stenosis was demonstrated on Doppler examination of the main transplant artery. (b) A coronal maximum intensity projection reconstruction from a CT angiogram shows the typical beaded appearance of fibromuscular hyperplasia in the main transplant artery.

b

suspicion that a stenosis is present. An acceleration time of greater than 90 ms is an objective measure of the tardus element of the parvus and tardus pattern. Intrarenal spectral Doppler patterns in renal artery stenosis are, however, less extensively studied in transplant kidneys than in native kidneys and there is conflicting literature on whether it is a valuable sign in its own right. As the main transplant artery can usually be directly identified, assessment of the intrarenal spectral Doppler trace is not of critical importance. Routine ultrasound surveillance of the renal artery in low-risk patients following transplantation is not proven to be of value, although it has been suggested that, in this patient population, a higher cut-off PSV of 300 cm/s may be more appropriate to indicate a positive study. Branch artery stenosis can occur in transplant kidneys but is usually difficult to demonstrate sonographically.

The Doppler ultrasound features of stenosis can be mimicked by arterial kinking, particularly where there is a long and redundant transplant artery. Although not a true stenosis, a major arterial kink may compromise blood supply to the kidney and thus be clinically significant. It can be demonstrated as an area of color aliasing and disturbed flow at the site of the kink, often with the parvus and tardus pattern present in the downstream arteries (Figure 9.39). Surgical correction may be necessary. Rarely, unrecognized fibromuscular hyperplasia in the donor transplant artery may cause significant arterial stenosis (Figure 9.40).

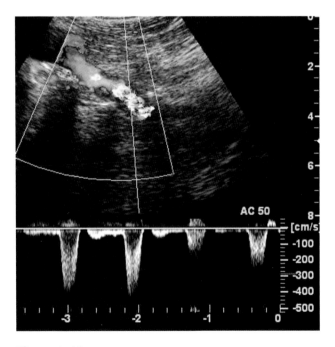

Figure 9.41
Iliac artery stenosis. Color aliasing and high peak systolic velocities are demonstrated at the site of a significant iliac stenosis.

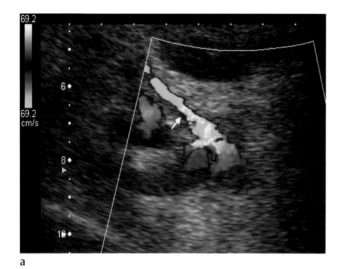

a

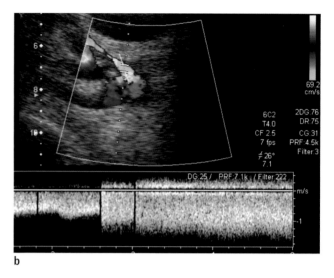

b

Figure 9.42

Transplant vein stenosis. (a) Colur Doppler image showing high-velocity flow with aliasing next to the venous anastomosis (arrow); note the high PRF. (b) A spectral Doppler trace is shown where the sample gate has been moved through the stenosis, demonstrating very high venous flow velocities at the stenosis site with a twofold velocity gradient between the proximal and distal vein.

Perinephric fluid collections may also result in vascular compression occasionally sufficient to produce vascular compromise.

Stenosis of the iliac artery proximal to the transplant renal artery is an uncommon cause of transplant dysfunction reported to occur in 1.5–2.4% of transplants; a high index of suspicion should be present in a patient who has known peripheral vascular or coronary artery disease or in patients with a 'parvus and tardus' pattern of intrarenal arterial blood flow and no ultrasound evidence of transplant artery stenosis or kinking. A high-velocity jet (>200 cm/s) may be seen at the site of the stenosis itself (Figure 9.41), alternatively, a proximal stenosis can be inferred by the normal external iliac triphasic waveform distal to the transplant artery anastomosis being replaced by a monophasic flow profile. A monophasic iliac waveform proximal to the arterial anastomosis is not necessarily abnormal due to flow modification by the low vascular resistance of the transplant itself. Identification of iliac stenosis is critical because radiologic or surgical correction of the iliac stenosis will usually result in improvement of graft function.

Venous stenosis

Occasionally, venous rather than the arterial stenosis may occur. Narrowing of the lumen of the renal vein can occur anywhere along the course of the vessel, usually as a result of perivascular fibrosis, trauma during surgery or perinephric fluid collections. Color Doppler will show an area of color aliasing and the spectral pattern demonstrates increased flow velocities (Figure 9.42). No absolute velocity measurements are described to indicate a stenosis, but a focal increase of venous velocity of greater than two- to threefold is usually taken to indicate a hemodynamically significant lesion.

Urologic: ureteric stricture

Ureteric stricture occurs in between 1 and 5% of all transplants and is usually due to ischemia, although surgical technique and rejection may also play a role. Blood supply to the proximal third of the ureter is derived from the main transplant artery and can therefore be preserved by careful harvesting of the transplant. The blood supply to the mid and distal donor ureter is, however, always lost during graft harvesting, and therefore the distal transplant ureter is at risk of ischemia and subsequent fibrosis and is the most common site of stricture formation. For this reason, the transplant ureter is usually fashioned as short as possible. This complication is more common in living donor transplantation, probably due to greater surgical dissection around the ureter with loss of the periureteral vasculature. Occasionally, obstruction may occur at the pelviureteric junction either due to undiagnosed pelviureteric junction obstruction in the donor kidney, extrinsic compression by a peritransplant collection or trauma during graft harvesting. Other causes of ureteric obstruction such as renal calculi, papillary necrosis or fungal balls are also occasionally encountered.

Ultrasound will demonstrate progressive hydronephrosis, usually accompanied by deteriorating graft function. Spectral Doppler will often show an elevated RI. Ultrasound may be able to demonstrate the level of the obstruction but further evaluation with spiral CT, antegrade pyelography and, when available, a Whittaker test may be needed to define its cause and significance. Initial management is with percutaneous nephrostomy and an antegrade ureteric stent can be placed as a temporizing procedure. Definitive treatment may be achieved with balloon dilatation for short ureterovesical strictures, particularly if occurring in the first 3 months after surgery, but surgical correction is usually required for other cases. Occasionally, long-term ureteric stenting may be selected for high-risk surgical patients.

Miscellaneous conditions

Miscellaneous cardiovascular abnormalities may cause alteration in the spectral Doppler pattern. Abnormalities of heart rate and rhythm will produce unusual appearances in the arterial spectrum, and high-output cardiac failure with functional tricuspid incompetence may be reflected in an unusual, highly pulsatile flow within the transplant renal vein. Torsion of an intraperitoneal renal transplant around its vascular pedicle is a rare complication but one where early recognition can lead to surgical graft salvage. Clinical features are non-specific, and diagnosis is dependent upon the ultrasound demonstration of a change in the axis of the transplant relative to a baseline scan, which may be accompanied by a variety of vascular changes, including reversed arterial diastolic flow or absence of flow in the transplant artery or vein.

SUMMARY

Renal transplantation is the optimal treatment for almost all patients with severe chronic renal failure; its success is tempered by a shortage of donor kidneys. Recent improvements in management, and particularly the introduction of new immunosuppressive regimens, have significantly reduced the incidence of early graft failure and 1-year graft survival rates are now in the region of 90%. Attention is now being increasingly directed towards preventing the long-term complications of transplantation, particularly premature cardiovascular disease and immunosuppression-associated malignancy. Chronic allograft nephropathy

remains a major cause of long-term graft loss that, at present, has no effective treatment.

Complications of transplantation do, however, still frequently occur and serial ultrasound is pivotal in their timely detection. Ultrasound remains central to identification of the vascular and urologic complications of transplantation but currently lacks the ability to reliably differentiate between the different medical complications of transplantation. Demonstration of abnormal intrarenal blood flow is a non-specific indicator of transplant dysfunction and, in combination with clinical findings, should help influence the decision-making process for graft biopsy.

Ultrasound has also made transplant biopsy a safe and reliable technique and is frequently used to guide other interventional therapeutic maneuvers.

Further reading

General

Andrews PA. Renal transplantation: recent developments. BMJ 2002; 324: 530–4.

Baxter GM. Ultrasound of renal transplantation. Clin Radiol 2001; 56: 802–18.

Baxter GM. Imaging in renal transplantation. Ultrasound Q 2003; 19: 123–38.

Benedetti E, Hakim NS, Perez EM, Matas AJ. Current topics in medicine: renal transplantation. Acad Radiol 1995; 2: 159–66.

Solvig J, Ekberg H, Hansen F, Brunkvall J, Länne T. Accuracy of noninvasive ultrasonic volume measurements on human kidney transplants: presentation of a new formula. Nephron 1998; 80: 188–93.

Hariharan S, Johnson CP, Bresnahan BA, et al. Improved graft survival after renal transplantation in the United States, 1988 to 1996. N Engl J Med 2000; 342: 605–12.

Khauli RB. Surgical aspects of renal transplantation: new approaches. Urol Clin North Am 1994; 21: 321–41.

Magee CC, Pascual M. Update in renal transplantation. Arch Intern Med 2004; 164: 1373–88.

Martinoli C, Bertolotto M, Crespi G, et al. Duplex Doppler analysis of interlobular arteries in transplanted kidneys. Eur Radiol 1998; 8: 765–9.

Mathew TH. Recurrent disease after renal transplantation. Transplant Rev 1991; 5: 31–45.

Pozniak MA. Doppler ultrasound evaluation of renal transplantation. In: Allan PL, Dubbins PA, Pozniak MA, McDicken WN, eds., Clinical doppler ultrasound. Edinburgh: Churchill Livingstone; 2000.

Radermacher J, Mengel M, Ellis S, et al. The renal arterial resistance index and renal allograft survival. N Engl J Med 2003; 349: 115–24.

Sandhu C, Patel U. Renal transplant dysfunction: the role of interventional radiology. Clin Radiol 2002; 57: 772–83.

Scarsbrook AF, Warakaulle DR, Dattani M, Traill Z. Post-transplantation lymphoproliferative disorder: the spectrum of imaging appearances. Clin Radiol 2005; 60: 47–55.

Vincenti F. A decade of progress in kidney transplantation. Transplantation 2004: 77: S52–S61.

Wolfe RA, Ashby VB, Milford EL, et al. Comparison of mortality in all patients on dialysis, patients on dialysis awaiting transplantation, and recipients of a first cadaveric transplant. N Engl J Med 1999; 341: 1725–30.

Rejection

Allen KS, Jorkasky DK, Arger PH, et al. Renal allografts: prospective analysis of Doppler sonography. Radiology 1988; 169: 371–6.

Beckingham IJ, Nicholson ML, Bell RPF. Analysis of factors associated with complications following renal transplant needle core biopsy. Br J Urol 1994; 73: 13–15.

Chow L, Sommer FG, Huang J, Li KCP. Power Doppler imaging and resistance index measurement in the evaluation of acute renal transplant rejection. J Clin Ultrasound 2001; 29: 483–90.

Fischer T, Mühler M, Kröncke TJ, et al. Early postoperative ultrasound of kidney transplants: evaluation of contrast medium dynamics using time–intensity curves. Fortschr Röntgenstr 2004; 176: 472–7.

Griffin JF, McNicholas MMJ. Morphological appearance of renal allografts in transplant failure. J Clin Ultrasound 1992; 20: 529–37.

Jindal RM, Hariharan S. Chronic rejection in kidney transplants. Nephron 1999; 83: 13–24.

Lu M, Yin X, Wan G, Xie X. Quantitative assessment of power Doppler mapping in the detection of renal allograft complications. J Clin Ultrasound 1999; 27: 319–23.

Nankivell BJ, Chapman JR, Gruenewald SM. Detection of chronic allograft nephropathy by quantitative Doppler imaging. Transplantation 2002; 74: 90–6.

Perrella RR, Duerinckx ÁJ, Tessler FN, et al. Evaluation of renal transplant dysfunction by duplex Doppler sonography: a prospective study and review of the literature. Am J Kidney Dis 1990; 15: 544–50.

Salgado O, García R, Gutiérrez H, et al. Accuracy and predictive value of ultrasound in acute rejection. Transplant Proc 1994; 26: 335–6.

Shoskes DA, Shahed AR, Kim S. Delayed graft function: influence on outcome and strategies for prevention. Urol Clin North Am 2001; 28: 721–31.

Sidhu MK, Gambhir S, Jeffrey RB Jr, et al. Power Doppler imaging of acute renal transplant rejection. J Clin Ultrasound 1999; 27: 171–5.

Tranquart F, Lebranchu Y, Haillot O, et al. The use of perioperative Doppler ultrasound as a screening test for acute tubular necrosis. Transpl Int 1993; 6: 14–17.

Venz S, Kahl A, Hierhlozer J, et al. Contribution of color and power Doppler sonography to the differential diagnosis of acute and chronic rejection, and tacrolimus nephrotoxicity in renal allografts. Transpl Int 1999; 12: 127–34.

Warshauer DM, Taylor KJW, Bia MJ, et al. Unusual causes of increased vascular impedance in renal transplants: duplex Doppler evaluation. Radiology 1988; 169: 367–70.

Weitzel WF, Kim K, Rubin JM, et al. Feasibility of applying ultrasound strain imaging to detect renal transplant chronic allograft nephropathy. Kidney Int 2004; 65: 733–6.

Wollenberg K, Waibel B, Pisarski P, et al. Careful clinical monitoring in comparison to sequential Doppler sonography for the detection of acute rejection in the early phase after renal transplantation. Transpl Int 2000; 13(S1): S45–S51.

Urologic

El-Mekresh M, Osman Y, Ali-El-Dien B, et al. Urological complications after living-donor renal transplantation. BJU Int 2001; 87: 295–306.

Lojanapiwat B, Mital D, Fallon L, et al. Management of ureteral stenosis after renal transplantation. J Am Coll Surg 1994; 179: 21–4.

Platt JF, Ellis JH, Rubin JM. Renal transplant pyelocaliectasis: role of duplex Doppler US in evaluation. Radiology 1991; 179: 425–8.

Vascular

Baxter GM, Ireland H, Moss JG, et al. Colour Doppler ultrasound in renal transplant artery stenosis: which Doppler index? Clin Radiol 1995; 50: 618–22.

Brandenburg VM, Frank RD, Riehl J. Color-coded duplex sonography study of arteriovenous fistulae and pseudoaneurysms complicating percutaneous renal allograft biopsy. Clin Nephrol 2002; 58: 398–404.

de Morais RH, Muglia VF, Mamere AE, et al. Duplex Doppler sonography of transplant renal artery stenosis. J Clin Ultrasound 2003; 31: 135–41.

Humar A, Key N, Ramcharan T, et al. Kidney retransplants after initial graft loss to vascular thrombosis. Clin Transplant 2001; 15: 6–10.

MacLennan AC, Baxter GM, Harden P, Rowe PA. Renal transplant vein occlusion: an early diagnostic sign? Clin Radiol 1995; 50: 251–3.

Patel U, Khaw KK, Hughes NC. Doppler ultrasound for detection of renal transplant artery stenosis – threshold peak systolic velocity needs to be higher in a low-risk or surveillance population. Clin Radiol 2003; 58: 772–7.

Rerolle JP, Antoine C, Raynaud A, et al. Successful endoluminal thrombo-aspiration of renal graft venous thrombosis. Transpl Int 2000; 13: 82–6.

Rouvière O, Berger P, Béziat C, et al. Acute thrombosis of renal transplant artery: graft salvage by means of intra-arterial fibrinolysis. Transplantation 2002; 73: 403–9.

Voiculescu A, Hollenbeck M, Plum J, et al. Iliac artery stenosis proximal to a kidney transplant: clinical findings, duplex-sonographic criteria, treatment and outcome. Transplantation 2003; 76: 332–9.

Wong-You-Cheong JJ, Grumbach K, Krebs TL et al. Torsion of intra-peritoneal renal transplants: imaging appearances. AJR Am J Roentgenol 1998; 171: 1355–9.

10

Combined renal and pancreatic transplantation

Dennis Ll Cochlin

Although pancreatic transplantation could be carried out for diabetes alone, current medical opinion suggests that the hazards and effects of immunosuppression outweigh the advantages. In patients receiving renal transplants for renal failure caused by diabetic nephropathy, immunosuppression will be given to protect the renal allograft and the same regimen will protect the pancreatic allograft. At present, therefore, pancreatic transplantation is combined with renal transplantation in these patients and both organs are monitored ultrasonically in similar ways. It is therefore appropriate to discuss pancreatic transplantation in this text.

Pancreatic transplantation is an operation that endeavors to correct the metabolic abnormalities associated with diabetes mellitus. The transplanted pancreas behaves like a normal pancreas and responds to elevated glucose levels by secreting insulin into the circulation. The pancreas has an exocrine secretion of enzymes and these usually need to be drained in some manner. A common operation is that depicted in Figure 10.1. The whole pancreas is transplanted to the right side of the abdomen, where the feeding arteries are anastomosed to the common iliac artery, and the splenic vein joined to the common iliac vein.

The exocrine secretion passes into a segment of the second part of the duodenum which is connected to the recipient's bladder (Figure 10.1). In this way the enzymes are lost from the body in the urine. These urinary enzymes, particularly the amylase, can be easily measured and this provides an indication as to how well the pancreas is functioning. Another operative technique is to anastomose the duodenal segment to part of the recipient's small intestine; although under these circumstances the enzyme secretion by the pancreas is less easy to measure, this is still possible. A further technique is to occlude the pancreatic duct so as to prevent all exocrine secretion. Although the pancreas atrophies, the islets are preserved and insulin secretion can be remarkably normal. Transplantation of the pancreatic islets alone is an attractive proposition but clinical studies to date have not been universally successful.

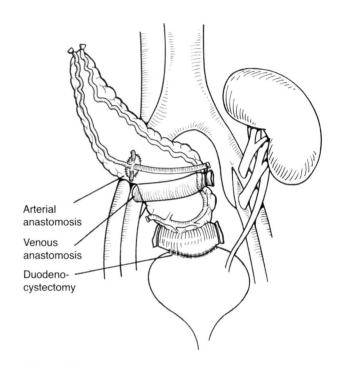

Arterial anastomosis

Venous anastomosis

Duodeno-cystectomy

Figure 10.1
Surgical technique of combined renal and pancreatic transplantation.

Patients selected for pancreatic transplantation are usually diabetic individuals who have already developed renal failure as a consequence of their disease. They receive a pancreas and a kidney from the same donor, these being accommodated in the left and right iliac fossae (see Figure 10.1). The patients receive immunosuppression from the time of transplantation, and should rejection occur it usually takes place in both organs at the same time. Treatment is usually successful and the survival rate for a pancreas transplant is 60–70% at 1 year. With a successful pancreatic transplant a patient no longer requires insulin injections and there is usually a great improvement in the quality of life. Established diabetic complications such as poor vision are not usually reversed, however.

Early complications

As with any surgical procedure, there may be early complications. These include hematoma, urinoma caused by a leak from the bladder, lymphocele caused by damage to the lymphatic channels when dissecting out the iliac vessels, and leakage of pancreatic enzymes due to the surgical insult or damage to the pancreas. It appears, however, that such complications are unusual, and we have seen few in our center. A small amount of fluid around the pancreas is common in the immediate postoperative period, and this disappears during the first 7 days. It represents serous fluid formed as a reaction to the tissue insult of the surgery, and some leakage from the pancreas (pancreatic weeping). Only if the amount of fluid is excessive or increases should aspiration be carried out. An excessive or increasing fluid collection may be due to a sterile serous collection, a pancreatic leak, abscess, urinoma, lymphocele or hematoma. Percutaneous needle aspiration is the only certain way of distinguishing between these.

Venous thrombosis

One possible common early complication is venous thrombosis. This is more common than in the transplanted kidney. Venous blood flow is slower in the transplanted pancreas than in the transplanted kidney and, because of the way the venous drainage is constructed, there are necessarily large changes in the caliber of the veins draining the pancreas, causing flow disturbance. Both these factors contribute to the incidence of venous thrombosis.

Rejection

Rejection is the other major complication. The original method of detecting rejection is by monitoring blood sugar. A rise in the blood sugar, however, occurs late in the rejection process, and is therefore of limited value. Allowing the pancreatic duct to drain into the bladder enables the amylase level in the urine to be measured. The urinary amylase in such patients drops earlier in rejection and is a more useful test than blood sugar estimation. Another approach is to assume that rejection episodes in the transplanted pancreas and kidney are concomitant. If this is so, the kidney may be monitored in the usual way, and rejection episodes treated. Such treatment will also treat the concomitant pancreatic rejection. Unfortunately, however, the pancreas may sometimes reject without obvious rejection signs in the kidney. Percutaneous biopsy, often used to detect renal transplant rejection, is more hazardous in the transplanted pancreas, although it is used in

some centers. Doppler ultrasound monitoring of pancreatic transplant rejection is relatively new, but sufficient work has been done to document the changes that take place. Large series have not been carried out, however, so the sensitivity and specificity of the test are not established. Changes in the gray-scale ultrasound scan also take place in rejection but these occur relatively late in rejection and are non-specific. They are far less useful than the Doppler study.

Ultrasonic scanning technique

The patient is best studied with a full bladder, if this is possible, as the pancreatic head and the loop of duodenum, whether anastomosed to the bladder or the jejunum, may be more easily identified when the full bladder displaces adjacent bowel.

An oblique plane best demonstrates the head of the pancreas lying anteriomedial to the iliac vessels, although various changes of angulation or turning the patient into a 45° oblique position may be necessary to avoid overlying bowel loops. With this approach, color Doppler reveals the arteries in the head of the pancreas which may be interrogated by spectral analysis to give a resistance index (RI) value (Figure 10.2). The body and tail of the pancreas may be shown lying in the paracolic gutter on a scan taken in a longitudinal plane through the anterior abdominal wall or flank. In this view, the portal vein is seen lying posterior to the body of the pancreas (Figure 10.3). Sufficient angulation may usually be obtained to permit a color flow image

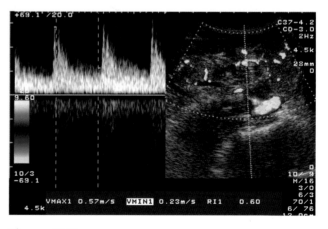

Figure 10.2
Artery in the head of the pancreas. A branch artery in the head of the pancreas has been interrogated by spectral Doppler. This shows a normal pattern with a resistance index of 0.6.

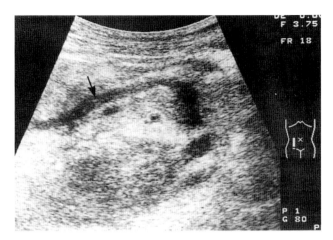

Figure 10.3
Portal vein. The long portal-splenic vein (arrow) is seen lying posterior to the pancreatic body and tail (see also Figure 10.8). In an alternative surgical technique, a short segment of vein is anastomosed to the iliac vein.

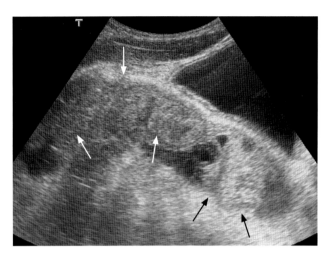

Figure 10.4
Normal pancreatic transplant. The pancreas is seen, with the bladder to the right. The pancreas is marked with white arrows, the duodeno-jejunal anastomosis by black arrows.

and a diagnostically useful spectral Doppler signal. The arteries in the body and tail are more difficult to find. The main artery lies parallel to the duct, and may usually be seen, but it is relatively small, and the disadvantageous angle to the Doppler beam make it difficult to get good Doppler signals. Branches of the main artery are very small, but may sometimes be seen in slim subjects, using high-frequency Doppler transducers. Sometimes the main artery has a kink in it, producing a short length of artery with an advantageous angle for Doppler.

Doppler studies are often requested in the early postoperative period, to exclude venous thrombosis. Studies are difficult at this time, as dressings and drains hinder access, there is often overlying bowel gas, accentuated by a partial ileus, and the wound area is edematous and tender. Any dressings that are obstructing access must be removed. The surgeons at our center use an adhesive clear plastic dressing (OpSite), taking care to exclude air bubbles. The scan may be performed through this dressing, which only slightly degrades the ultrasound image.

Normal ultrasound appearances[1]

The normal transplanted pancreas has an appearance similar to that of the native pancreas (Figure 10.4). It gives the impression of being larger, presumably because it is more superficial, although measurements reveal that, after the initial postoperative edema has subsided, the transplanted pancreas is the same size as the native pancreas. The length of portal vein used for venous drainage to the iliac veins is

clearly seen lying posterior to the body of the pancreas (Figures 10.3–10.5) and the loop of duodenum anastomosed to the bladder or ileum may also be seen (Figure 10.6). This is difficult to identify as duodenum, and often appears as a nondescript, sometimes fluid-filled structure, which should not be confused with a pathologic fluid collection.

In the immediate postoperative period, the pancreas is often somewhat enlarged due to edema, and there is often a collection of serous fluid around the head, body and tail. The picture is essentially that of pancreatitis caused by the transplantation procedure (Figure 10.7). This returns to a normal appearance after about a week. Fluid collections should not increase in size after the first 48 hours, and, if they do so, a pathologic cause should be considered. It must be remembered, however, that patients who continue on peritoneal dialysis because of delayed renal function may have dialysis fluid in this region. The duodenal loop produces mucus, which, when anastomosed to the bladder may be seen as fronds extending into the bladder (see Figure 10.6).

Normal Doppler appearances[2]

The venous flow in the portal vein is turbulent, with a variable degree of phasic swing and a velocity of about 0.2 m/s. It has no special characteristics (Figure 10.8) and the only importance of its study is in suspected venous thrombosis.

Arterial flow has the typical low-resistance spectral pattern shown in all the solid organs of the body, with a shallow systolic descent and continuing diastolic flow.

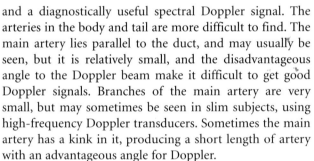

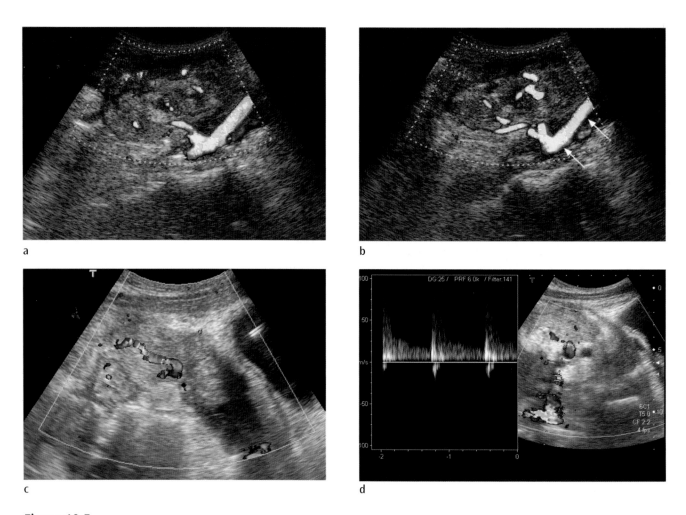

a

b

c

d

Figure 10.5

Vascular anatomy. (a) The porto-splenic vein is seen anastomosed to the iliac vein. The main arterial trunk is shown below it. (b) A portion of the portal vein is shown posterior to the body of the pancreas (arrow). Multiple arteries and veins are seen in the pancreatic head. (c) A portion of the arterial trunk is shown. (d) The artery is seen passing along the pancreatic body.

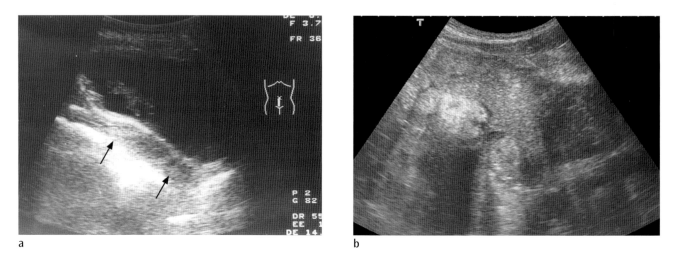

a

b

Figure 10.6

Duodenal anastomosis. (a) The loop of duodenum (arrow) is anastomosed to the bladder. Mucus strands project into the bladder. This is occasionally seen and is not abnormal. (b) Duodeno-jejunal anastomosis.

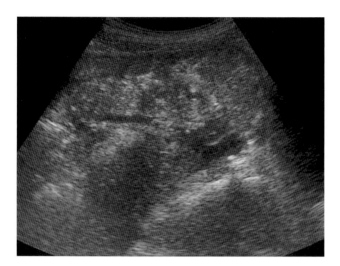

Figure 10.7
Fluid around the pancreatic body. This quantity of fluid is normal in the first postoperative week. Compare the case of rejection shown in Figure 10.12.

Diastolic flow is higher than in the kidney, with RI in the range 0.35–0.75. Values are similar in the head and the body and, provided that intrapancreatic arteries are studied, it does not seem to matter which are used. Peak systolic velocities are in the range 0.2–0.8 m/s (Figure 10.9).

Venous thrombosis[2-4]

Venous thrombosis of the pancreatic and portal vein is a common early complication of pancreatic transplantation. It produces some swelling of the pancreas, with a heterogeneous echo pattern and a small amount of peripancreatic fluid (Figure 10.10). These signs are, however, non-specific and some swelling and peripancreatic fluid may be normal in the early postoperative period. A heterogeneous echo pattern is abnormal, but this may be a difficult feature to be certain about, and may also occur in rejection. Thrombus in the portosplenic vein is not usually demonstrated on the gray-scale image, probably because of the relatively poor visualization of these structures.

Doppler studies show a portal vein with severely reduced or absent Doppler flow (Figure 10.10b). Arterial flow may be difficult to detect in cases of venous thrombosis, but a few vessels may usually be found in or around the pancreatic head. These show a high systolic peak, and reversed diastolic flow, similar to that seen in the kidney with renal vein thrombosis (Figure 10.10c). Because of the reversed diastolic flow, the real-time color Doppler image shows the arteries flashing red and blue, although spectral Doppler is necessary to confirm the flow pattern.

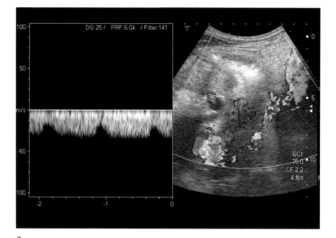

a

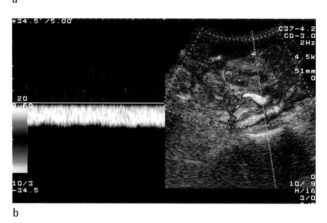

b

Figure 10.8
Portal vein flow. (a) The section of portal vein draining the transplanted pancreas shows a gently undulating Doppler flow pattern. (b) A more continuous pattern, with a fairly typical velocity of about 0.2 m/s. The normal range of velocities has not been established.

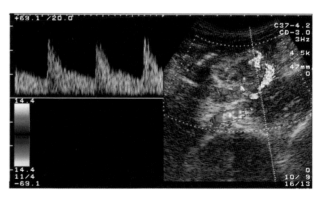

Figure 10.9
Normal arterial flow pattern. This is the normal spectral pattern in the arteries supplying a pancreatic allograft. There is a smooth curve from systole to diastole, with continuing diastolic flow; resistance index (RI) = 0.6. This is the main pancreatic artery, seen between the duodenal loop and the head of the pancreas.

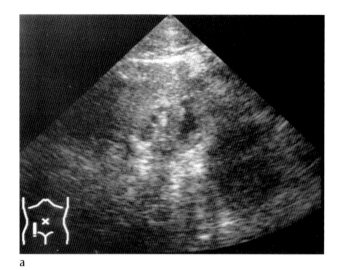

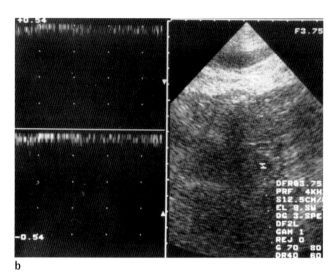

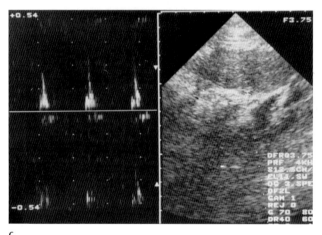

Figure 10.10
Pancreatic/portal vein thrombosis. (a) A swollen, inhomogeneous pancreatic head. (b) There is very reduced flow in the portal vein (measured at less than 0.1 m/s). (c) Arterial flow was difficult to find but a few arteries were shown at the pancreatic head with reversed diastolic flow. The steep descent from peak systole to maximal reversed flow seems to be typical of venous thrombosis.

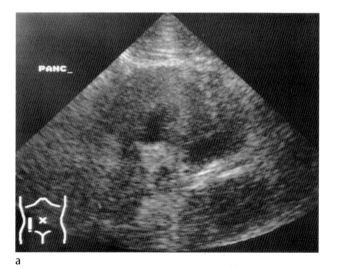

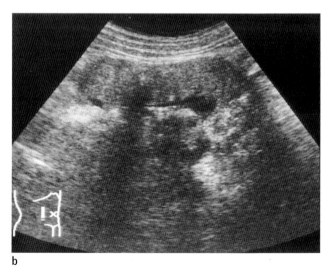

Figure 10.11
Early rejection. (a) The head of the pancreas is swollen with a heterogeneous echo pattern. (b) The body is swollen but with a homogeneous echo pattern.

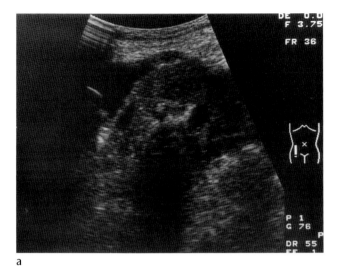
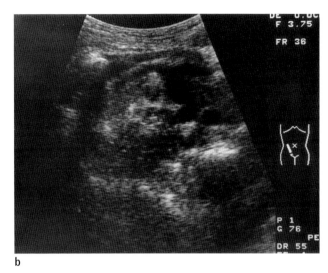

a   b

Figure 10.12
Rejection: peripancreatic fluid. The pancreatic head has a very inhomogeneous echo pattern. The fluid seen around the pancreatic body is too large in volume to be normal in the third postoperative week. This proved to be rejection.

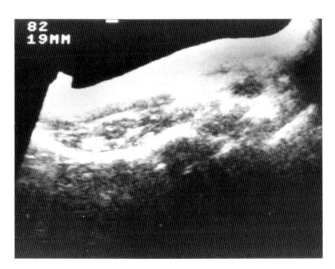

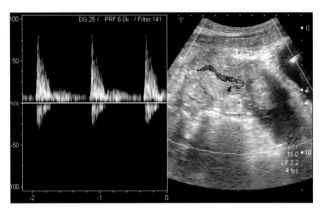

Figure 10.14
Rejection. The end-diastolic flow is low, the resistance index (RI) is 0.9 and there is an early diastolic notch. As in the kidney, an early diastolic notch is a sign of increased vascular resistance.

Figure 10.13
Rejection. In this case of severe rejection the pancreas is very heterogeneous and difficult to distinguish from surrounding bowel and other tissues.

Isotope studies have also been used in the attempted diagnosis of venous thrombosis. Non-visualization of the pancreas with Tc-DTPA suggests venous thrombosis, but the normal transplanted pancreas shows relatively little uptake compared with the kidney, and non-visualization has been found in normal pancreatic transplants. Indium-labeled platelets may produce more specific results, but Doppler with color flow is probably superior to isotope studies. Some centers prefer to confirm venous thrombosis suspected on Doppler or isotope by the 'gold standard' of arteriography, or MR angiography before transplantectomy.

Rejection[5,6]

Pancreatic rejection may give normal appearances on the gray-scale (non-Doppler) scan, or it may produce enlargement of the pancreas with a heterogeneous echo pattern (Figure 10.11). After 24–48 hours, there may be peripancreatic fluid (Figure 10.12), and later the pancreas may become very heterogeneous and difficult to distinguish from the surrounding tissues and bowel loops (Figure 10.13). As in the kidney, rejection causes increased arteriolar resistance, characterized by reduced, absent or

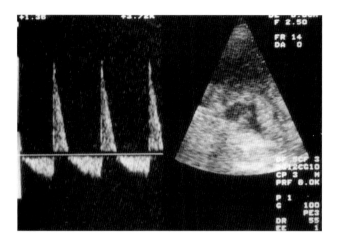

Figure 10.15
Rejection. There is reversed diastolic flow. Note that there is a shallow curve from the point of reversal to maximum reversed flow, unlike the pattern in venous thrombosis (Figure 10.10), where there is a sharp descent from end diastole to maximum reversed flow.

Figure 10.16
Established rejection. The rejection episode has been present for about a week despite treatment with increased immunosuppression. A large quantity of fluid is seen around the pancreatic head. Note that the Doppler flow shows reversed diastolic flow and also reduced systolic flow. The reduction in systolic velocity probably indicates that the rejection episode is severe.

reversed diastolic flow in the arteries (Figures 10.14–10.16). The mechanism for this increased resistance is, however, clearly different from that in the transplanted kidney, and its etiology is unknown. Unlike the kidney, there is no equivalent to acute tubular necrosis, the pancreas having normal or possibly slightly increased diastolic flow immediately following transplantation. Cyclosporine toxicity does not appear to affect the pancreas, so reduction

in diastolic flow seems to be specific for rejection. Published series are, however, few and of small numbers, so that a high specificity, although likely, is not definitely established, nor is the sensitivity. The value of RI at which rejection should be diagnosed has also not been established. In our center we use a figure of above 0.8 as giving a high probability of rejection, and between 0.7 and 0.8 as indeterminate. We regard an RI of less than 0.7 as being

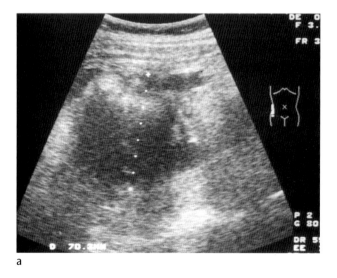

a

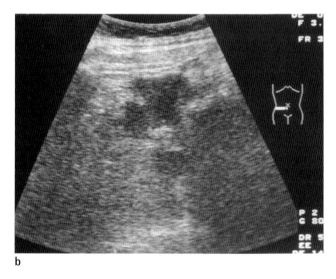

b

Figure 10.17
Abscess. (a,b) An irregular fluid-filled cavity is seen related to the pancreatic head. This is unlike 'normal' peripancreatic fluid because of its shape. Needling produced coliform pus. Percutaneous drainage was carried out but was followed by open surgical drainage 2 days later. The pancreatic graft survived, although this is unusual in these circumstances.

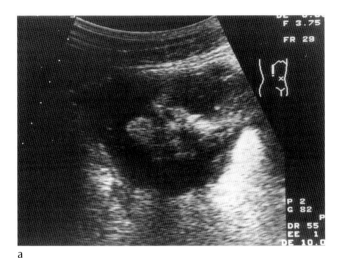
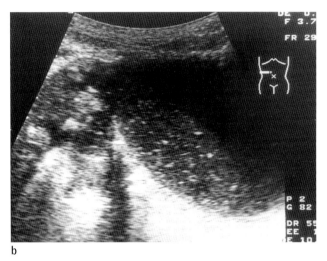

a
b

Figure 10.18
Abscess. (a) In this case, there is a large amount of fluid around the pancreatic tail, which is very irregular. (b) The abscess extends towards the central abdomen.

normal. Successful treatment of rejection results in an early return to a normal RI value.

Peripenacreatic fluid collections²

As with most surgical procedures, a small amount of serous fluid at the operation site is normal for the first week or so.

In the case of the pancreas, this is more likely, as operative damage to the pancreas causes some leakage of pancreatic enzymes from the surface of the pancreas. This is sometimes referred to as 'pancreatic weeping' (see Figure 10.7). Such collections are of little concern, but may be aspirated if excessive, or if the patient shows symptoms and signs suggestive of sepsis.

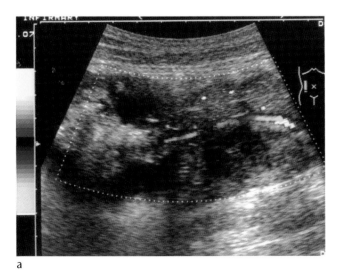
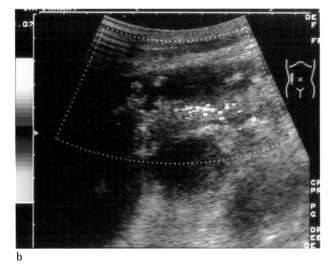

a
b

Figure 10.19
Abscess. The pancreas is very irregular with a large amount of fluid around it. The actual outline of the pancreas is difficult to define. The pancreas is hyperemic and, in this case, the color image helps to identify the body of the pancreas, showing the portal vein (a) and the pancreatic arteries (b).

Both venous thrombosis and rejection cause increased peripancreatic fluid, although the amount is not large unless the process persists for some days, by which time the diagnosis is usually established (see Figure 10.16).

Excessive or persistent pancreatic leaks may occur due to damage to the pancreas, usually during removal from the cadaveric donor. These collections may be larger than the usual postoperative peripancreatic fluid collections, but are otherwise indistinguishable. Unlike the 'normal' postoperative collections, however, they do not resolve. Aspiration produces fluid with very high amylase levels.

Peripancreatic abscesses, like abdominal abscesses in general, have appearances ranging from echo-free collections indistinguishable from other peripancreatic collections to typical thick-walled abscess cavities with medium or mixed echodensity fluid (Figures 10.17–10.19). The diagnosis is established by percutaneous aspiration, but percutaneous drainage has been found to be ineffective in most cases, surgical drainage being preferable. Despite surgical drainage and antibiotic therapy, however, most cases ultimately require removal of the pancreas.

Urinomas, lymphoceles and hematomas may also occur. Their appearances when they occur as a complication of pancreatic transplantation are similar to those when they occur at other sites. Their appearances are discussed in Chapter 9. The true nature of such collections may, however, only be ascertained with certainty by percutaneous aspiration.

Conclusion

Pancreatic transplantation is an established procedure, although still only a relatively small number are performed. It is a procedure that carries a reasonably high graft survival rate and, in successful cases, provides marked patient benefit. The procedure is therefore likely to increase in importance.

Ultrasound is clearly the first-line investigation for imaging postoperative problems, and is usually the only imaging procedure necessary. Interpretation is, however, sometimes difficult and the ultrasound image may need to be supplemented by CT or MRI images.

Doppler studies are definitive in the diagnosis of venous thrombosis, and are clearly very valuable in showing perfusion of the pancreas and investigating suspected rejection. Larger series are, however, necessary to determine the sensitivity and specificity of Doppler studies in rejection.

References

1. Freund MC, Steurer W, Gassner EM, et al. Spectrum of imaging findings after pancreas transplantation with enteric exocrine drainage: Part 1, posttransplantation anatomy. AJR Am J Roentgenol 2004; 182(4): 911–7.
2. Gilabert R, Fernandez-Cruz L, Bru C, Sans A, Andrew J. Duplex-Doppler ultrasonography in monitoring clinical pancreas transplantation. Transplant Int 1988; 1: 172–7.
3. Freund MC, Steurer W, Gassner EM, et al. Spectrum of imaging findings after pancreas transplantation with enteric exocrine drainage: Part 2, posttransplantation complications. AJR Am J Roentgenol 2004; 182(4): 919–25.
4. Letourneau JG, Maile CW, Sutherland DER, Feinberg SB. Ultrasound and computed tomography in the evaluation of pancreatic transplantation. Radiol Clin North Am 1987; 25: 345–55.
5. Patel B, Markivee C, Mahanta B, et al. Pancreatic transplantation: scintigraphy, US and CT. Radiology 1988; 167: 685–7.
6. Patel B, Wolverson MK, Mahanta B. Pancreatic transplant rejection: assessment with duplex US. Radiology 1989; 173: 131–5.

11

Renal dialysis

Dennis Ll Cochlin

GENERAL CONSIDERATIONS

Renal dialysis is a long-established treatment for acute and chronic renal failure: peritoneal dialysis was first used by Ganter in 1923, whereas hemodialysis, although introduced for the treatment of acute renal failure by Kolff in 1949, only became a practical treatment for chronic renal failure with the introduction of the Quinton–Scribner arteriovenous shunt in 1960. The use of double-lumen central venous dialysis cannulae is more recent.

Renal dialysis may be achieved by a number of methods, depending on clinical circumstances. The major division is into peritoneal dialysis and hemodialysis. Peritoneal dialysis is achieved by placing a cannula through the anterior abdominal wall into the peritoneal space, with the coiled tip ideally lying in the pelvis. Dialysis fluid is alternately run into and out of the peritoneal cavity, the dialysis exchange being achieved across the peritoneum, which acts as a dialysis membrane. Peritoneal dialysis may be used in acute or chronic renal failure. Fluid exchange may be carried out while patients undergo their normal daily activities (continuous ambulatory peritoneal dialysis, CAPD).

Hemodialysis involves the passage of the patient's blood across the semipermeable membrane of a dialysis machine. This requires access to a site on the patient that will provide a high blood flow and is amenable to repeated access procedures in the case of chronic renal failure.

Temporary access may be achieved by insertion of a double-lumen cannula into a central vein, usually the superior vena cava via the subclavian or jugular veins, whereas long-term access is achieved by the surgical construction of an arteriovenous fistula. This causes the draining veins to become enlarged, and the wall to thicken (arteriolization). The thickened vein wall allows safe repeated venepuncture, and the high blood flow necessary for dialysis is also achieved.

It is important to consider the subject of dialysis in this text for several reasons. First, dialysis, particularly peritoneal dialysis, may alter the ultrasound image. Secondly, ultrasound may be used to assist in the placement of peritoneal and intravenous dialyses access cannulae, and for the preoperative assessment of vessels prior to construction of arteriovenous dialysis fistulae. Thirdly, ultrasound has a role in the investigation of some of the complications of renal dialysis.

PERITONEAL DIALYSIS

Preoperative assessment[1,2]

A cannula, usually a Tenckhoff cannula, is introduced percutaneously into the peritoneal cavity. Ideally, the tip should lie in the pelvic cavity. The only preliminary investigations usually considered necessary are a clinical examination of the abdomen and a plain abdominal X-ray to ensure that there are no abdominal masses or aneurysms. If either of these investigations produces any doubt, ultrasound examination should be performed. Some centers routinely perform an abdominal ultrasound scan as well as a plain X-ray on all patients for prospective peritoneal cannula insertion, but this is probably unnecessary.

A large bladder may be emptied by catheterization, and a large liver may be avoided by a low insertion, possibly under ultrasound control, but other abdominal masses may be a contraindication to cannula insertion. Even with careful assessment, misplacement does sometimes occur (Figure 11.1).

A history of previous abdominal sepsis or surgery raises the possibility of adhesions. Differential motion of the intraperitoneal structures and retroperitoneal tissues may be reduced in the presence of adhesions and this feature may be studied by ultrasound (visceral slide). The ultrasound study is, however, of limited value, barium follow-through examination with screening being the more appropriate investigation.

When peritoneal dialysis is established, on subsequent scans it is important to recognize that the patient is on dialysis and not suffering from ascites or other pathologic fluid

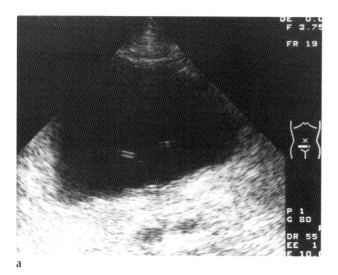

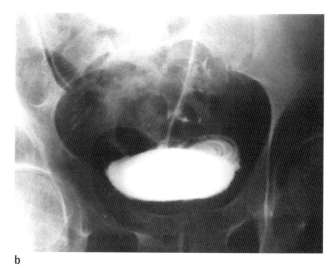

a

b

Figure 11.1
Misplaced Tenkhoff cannula. The cannula lies with its tip in the bladder. When peritoneal dialysis commenced, the patient miraculously started to pass 'urine'! A good clinical examination followed by an abdominal ultrasound scan would have detected the enlarged bladder and prevented the misplacement of the cannula. (a) Cannula lying in the bladder on an ultrasound scan. (b) Contrast injected through the cannula confirming the situation.

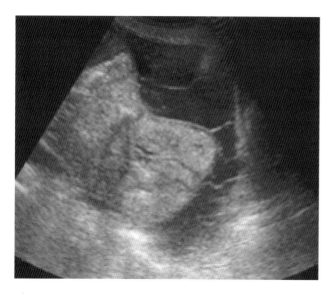

Figure 11.2
Residual dialysis fluid. A small collection of fluid remains in the subhepatic area 4 weeks after peritoneal dialysis was discontinued. This is not unusual.

collections. Even after drainage, some fluid usually remains (Figure 11.2). Although the presence of a peritoneal dialysis cannula should be obvious, in ill patients with multiple lines and drains the presence of a peritoneal dialysis cannula may be missed leading to a mis-diagnosis of a pathological collection.

Complications of peritoneal dialysis[3]

Poor dialysis

Failure to dialyse may be due to a blocked, kinked, poorly placed or 'migrated' cannula or omental 'wrapping' of the catheter tip. Although the cannula may sometimes be seen on ultrasound (Figure 11.3), this is not the appropriate investigation for occlusion, kinking or poor placement. Contrast injected through the cannula under screening control is far superior.

Failure to drain adequately is also usually due to poor placement. Ultrasound may provide a subjective assessment of the residual fluid remaining after drainage, but the position of the cannula tip should be checked with X-ray, with or without contrast injected through the cannula.

Infection or peritonitis

Infection of the peritoneal fluid is suspected when the returned fluid is cloudy or contains fibrinous strands and is confirmed by bacteriologic culture. Negative culture suggests 'mechanical' or aseptic peritonitis. Ultrasound may be used to detect abscess cavities or loculated collections and guide their drainage.

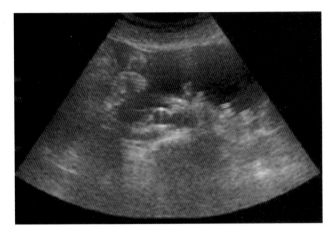

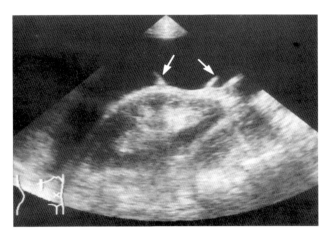

Figure 11.3
Cannula tip. Several sections of the curled cannula tip are seen within dialysis fluid in the pelvis. They appear as short parallel lines.

Figure 11.4
Peritoneal dialysis fluid: normal appearances. The fluid is anechoic. Fine strands are often seen crossing the fluid. These are generally of no significance. In symptomatic patients, however, they may be the first sign of sclerosing peritonitis. The fluid surrounds full bowel loops and the peritoneal membrane is seen.

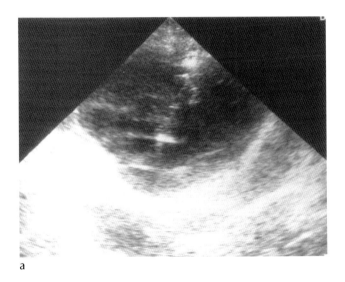

a

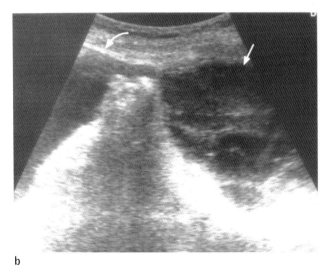

b

Figure 11.5
Abdominal abscess complicating peritoneal dialysis. A well-circumscribed lesion of mixed echodensity such as this is almost certain to be an abscess. This was confirmed in this case by percutaneous aspiration. (a) A transverse section of the abscess. (b) An oblique section showing the abscess (straight arrow) and non-infected dialysis fluid (curved arrow).

Interpretation may be a problem, as varying amounts of fluid normally remain after drainage of peritoneal dialysate. A thick wall around a fluid collection may indicate abscess formation, or the appearance of the fluid itself may suggest pus. Peritoneal dialysis fluid is anechoic, whereas pus is often echogenic, with small mobile echogenic foci within it. These 'speckles' may be seen to move with respiration or transducer pressure. Very fine particles also move away from the transducer due to the mechanical force of the ultrasound beam (Figures 11.5–11.7).

In the absence of these signs, loculated collections or abscess cannot be excluded by ultrasound. In these circumstances, a computed tomography (CT) scan after the injection of dilute contrast through the peritoneal dialysis (PD) cannula is the investigation of choice.[4] After injection of contrast, the patient walks around for a short time. The contrast diffuses throughout the peritoneal cavity and any fluid collections not opacified are assumed to be loculated and possibly infected. Infection is then confirmed or excluded by percutaneous aspiration under CT control.

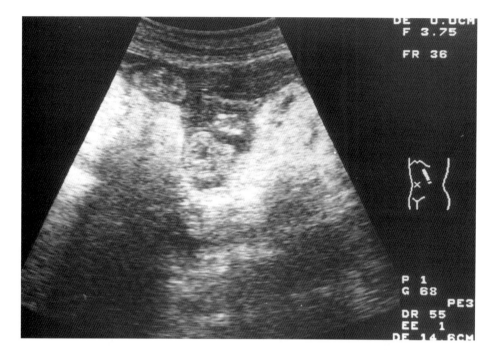

Figure 11.6
Intra-abdominal abscess. Turbid fluid of medium echodensity surrounds loops of small bowel. This infected fluid was of higher echodensity than the rest of the dialysis fluid and did not drain with the normal fluid. Both these features strongly suggest loculated infected fluid.

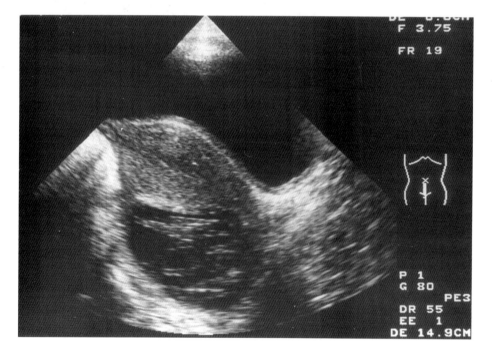

Figure 11.7
Pelvic abscess. There is an abscess in the pouch of Douglas with multiple echoes within the abscess fluid.

Sclerosing peritonitis[5–7]

This is a serious, often fatal complication of peritoneal dialysis, presenting with abdominal pain, progressive loss of ultrafiltration and, in the later stages, intestinal obstruction. This is a different disease from infective peritonitis. The cause is unknown, but substances such as acetate and chlorhexidine introduced in or with the dialysis fluid have been implicated. It is probable that there is no single cause that accounts for all cases.

The disease produces a thick fibrous membrane on the peritoneum which encapsulates the small bowel and causes thickening and contraction of the mesentery. This leads to acute or subacute small bowel obstruction. Surgery for this condition is very difficult and death from the disease or complications of the surgery are common.

There is no evidence that discontinuation of peritoneal dialysis prevents progress of the disease, but it has been noted that in some patients who receive renal transplants, the disease is arrested. This is thought to be due to the immunosuppression.

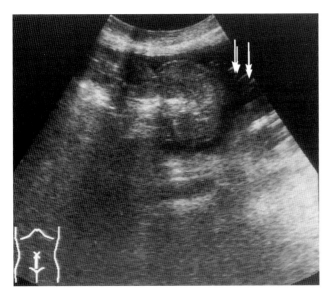

Figure 11.8
Sclerosing peritonitis. Fine strands cross the peritoneal cavity (arrows). These are a feature of the disease, especially when associated with tethering of the bowel and hypoperistalsis. This is minimal change, and fine echogenic strands similar to these may also be seen in peritoneal dialysis patients without the disease.

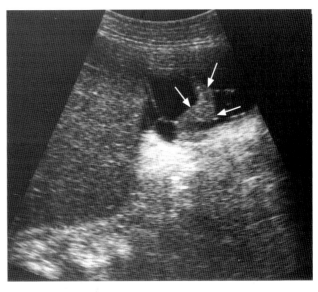

Figure 11.9
Sclerosing peritonitis. In this case a thick fibrous band crosses the dialysis fluid (arrows), from which finer strands project.

Imaging

Reports on imaging in sclerosing peritonitis are few, but ultrasound, carried out with peritoneal dialysis fluid in the abdomen, seems to be the imaging method of choice. In our experience ultrasound gives more diagnostic information than CT or magnetic resonance imaging (MRI). A barium small bowel study is complementary to the ultrasound study but inferior to ultrasound if used on its own.

The characteristic ultrasound appearances comprise tethering of bowel loops to the posterior abdomen and covering of bowel loops with a thick previsceral membrane. The bowel loops may be drawn into a short mesentery and some bowel loops may be hypoperistaltic or aperistaltic. Fine echogenic strands often cross the peritoneal cavity through the dialysis fluid but although these are a prominent feature of the disease they may also be seen in some patients who do not have the disease.

The thickened membrane is the most diagnostic feature but is only seen as a late feature in advanced disease. Early disease may show only subtle changes such as echogenic strands, minimal posterior tethering of bowel loops and perhaps a change in the peristaltic pattern of some bowel loops. In patients on peritoneal dialysis who develop colicky abdominal pain, the diagnosis of sclerosing peritonitis should be considered and the early ultrasonic signs should be diligently sought (Figures 11.8–11.13).

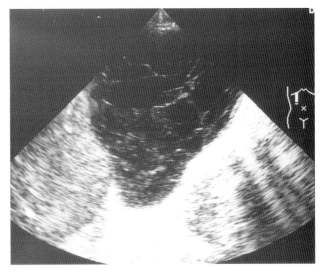

Figure 11.10
Sclerosing peritonitis. In this advanced case, with symptoms of bowel obstruction, there are very extensive fibrous bands. This degree of change is never seen in normal patients.

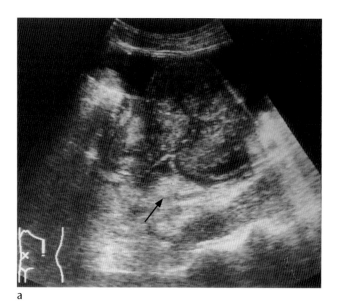

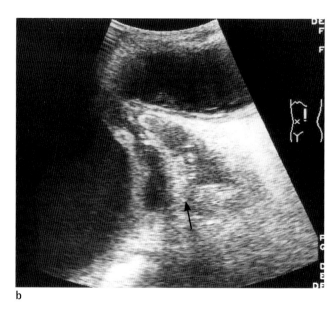

a

b

Figure 11.11
Sclerosing peritonitis. (a,b) The bowel is drawn into a thickened mesentery (arrow). On real time the bowel was hypoperistaltic.

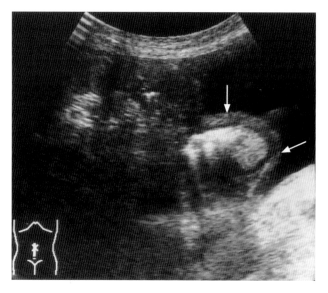

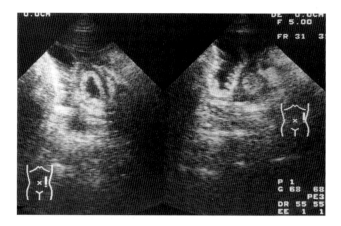

Figure 11.13
Sclerosing peritonitis. There is thickened membrane and aperistaltic loops of small bowel.

Figure 11.12
Sclerosing peritonitis. The thickened peritoneal membrane (arrows) is the most characteristic feature of the disease but is only seen in advanced cases.

required. If isotope enters the scrotom, the diagnosis is confirmed (Figure 11.14).

Hydrocele

Hydroceles may complicate peritoneal dialysis due to a patent processus vaginalis. Ultrasound will confirm a hydrocele, but will not distinguish a patent processus vaginalis from other causes of hydrocele. For this distinction, introduction of isotope into the peritoneal dialysis fluid is

Pleural fluid

Pleural fluid may accumulate due to small defects in the diaphragm. These may also be demonstrated by ultrasound, but are indistinguishable from pleural effusions (Figure 11.15). As with scrotal fluid, an isotope peritoneogram will differentiate between the two.

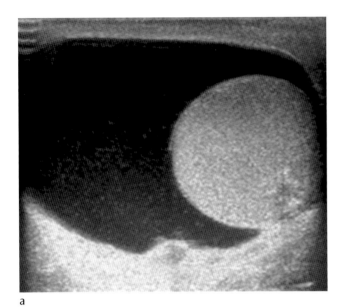

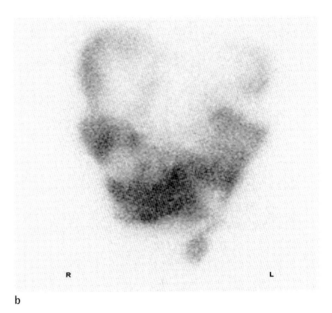

a

b

Figure 11.14

Hydrocele due to patent processus vaginalis. (a) These hydroceles are indistinguishable from other forms of hydroceles. However, an isotope peritoneogram (b) reveals a communication with the peritoneal cavity.

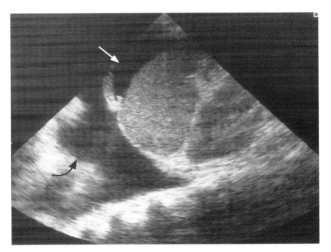

Figure 11.15

Pleural effusion complicating peritoneal dialysis. There is dialysis fluid around the spleen (straight arrow) and a left pleural effusion (curved arrow). An isotope peritoneogram showed a communication between the peritoneal and pleural spaces.

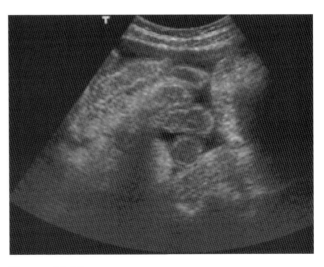

Figure 11.16

Ascites. In this patient a greater quantity of dialysis fluid was being drained than was introduced. Peritoneal dialysis was discontinued in favor of hemodialysis but the ascites continued, necessitating repeated drainage. No cause was found and the ascites subsided some months later. It was presumably caused by the peritoneal dialysis.

Ascites[8]

Ascites is an occasional complication of peritoneal dialysis, and is presumably due to peritoneal irritation by the hypertonic dialysis solution. Abdominal ultrasound cannot distinguish between dialysis fluid and ascites. The diagnosis of ascites is usually made clinically, more fluid being returned than run into the abdomen. Sometimes, however, the ascites only becomes obvious when peritoneal dialysis is discontinued in favor of hemodialysis or transplantation. In these cases, abdominal ultrasound will reveal the ascites, which is identical to ascites from other causes (Figure 11.16).

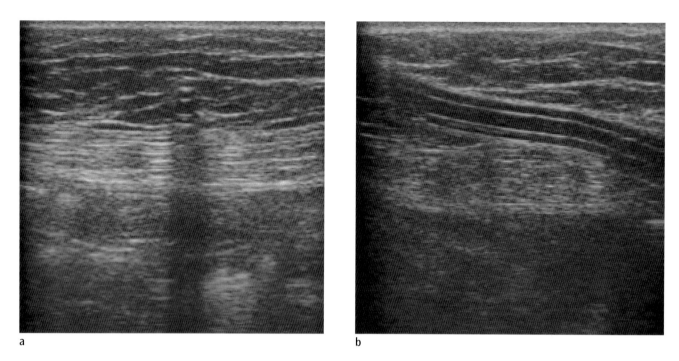

a   b

Figure 11.17
Tenckhoff cannula. (a) Transverse and (b) longitudinal sections of the cannula passing through the oblique tunnel in the abdominal wall and into the peritoneal cavity.

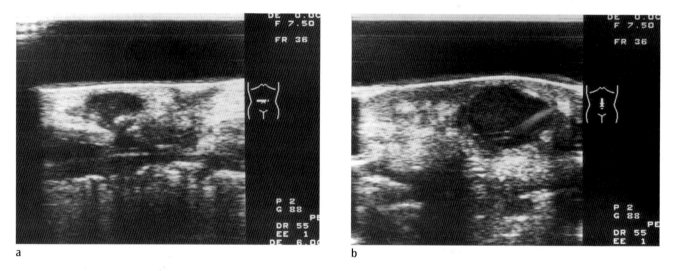

a   b

Figure 11.18
Tenckhoff track abscess. (a,b) There is an abscess cavity at the point where the cannula passes into the abdomen. Tramline echoes representing the cannula are seen running through the abscess.

Tunnel infection[9]

Infection around that portion of the catheter that lies in the subcutaneous tunnel usually necessitates removal of the cannula. It sometimes presents as a discharge at the exit site, swelling, tenderness or pain along the subcutaneous track and fever. Often, however, tunnel infections are asymptomatic and eventually present with peritonitis that does not resolve with antibiotic therapy. Diagnosis is thus usually made on clinical symptoms and signs. Ultrasound may, however, aid in the diagnostic process. The cannula may be clearly seen passing obliquely through the

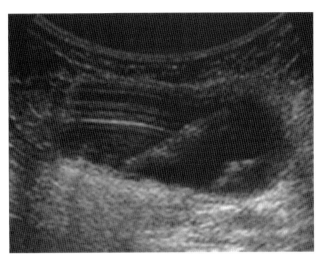

Figure 11.19
Tenckhoff cannula tunnel infection. In this case, there is a small track which led to a tiny discharging sinus on the skin. The tramline echoes representing the cannula are shown (arrows).

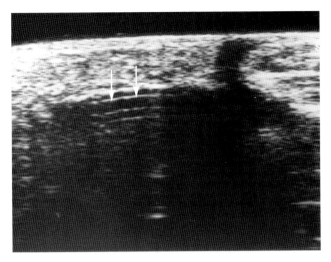

Figure 11.20
Collection of dialysis fluid in the cannula tunnel. An anechoic collection with fine septa is seen around the Tenckhoff cannula in the abdominal wall tunnel. Aspiration revealed non-infected fluid.

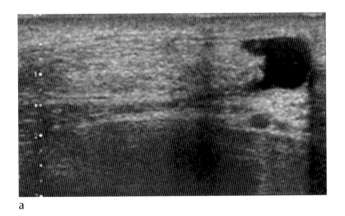

a

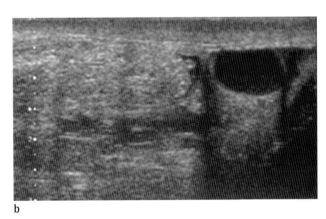

b

Figure 11.21
Femoral hernia complicating peritoneal dialysis. (a,b) Omentum and dialysis fluid are seen in the femoral canal. The hernia only became apparent after the commencement of peritoneal dialysis.

abdominal wall into the peritoneal cavity (Figure 11.17). Occasionally, however, initial presentation is as a swelling over the tunnel track and ultrasound may be used to confirm abscess formation (Figures 11.18 and 11.19). Sometimes a swelling around the cannula may be due to leak of dialysis fluid from the peritoneal cavity (Figure 11.20). These patients present with a swelling at the cannula track, discomfort and sometimes discharge. In the absence of infection they are apyrexial. If there is doubt, the fluid may be aspirated percutaneously and sent for bacteriologic analysis.

Hernias

Hernias at all the common sites are more common in peritoneal dialysis patients. Also, previous asymptomatic hernias may become obvious during dialysis. Diagnosis is usually made on clinical grounds. Incisional hernias after removal of a cannula may, however, cause diagnostic difficulty if a loop of bowel is trapped, presenting as obstruction. Such hernias are well demonstrated by ultrasound (Figures 11.21–11.23).

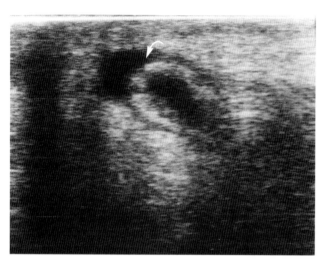

Figure 11.22
Incisional hernia complicating peritoneal dialysis. Dialysis fluid is seen in the hernia (straight arrow) together with a loop of small bowel (curved arrow).

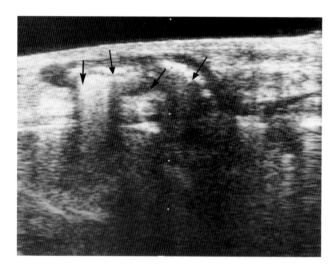

Figur 11.23
Incisional hernia. In a different case, a loop of small bowel (arrows) passes through the defect in the abdominal wall caused by insertion of the Tenckhoff cannula.

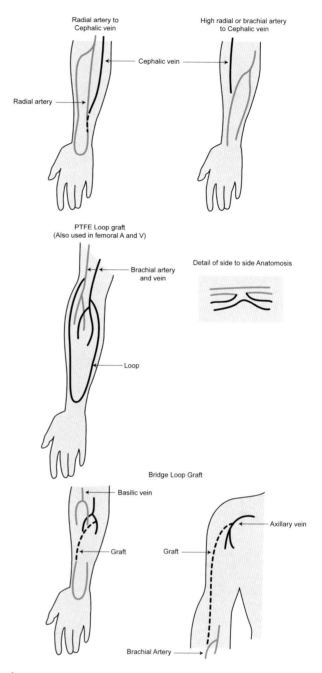

Figure 11.24
Common fistula sites.

HEMODIALYSIS

Permanent vascular access for hemodialysis is now achieved almost exclusively by means of surgically constructed arteriovenous fistulae where this is possible. These fistulae, described by Breschia and Cimino, are constructed at radio-cephalic, ulnar–ulnar or brachial–basilic sites. Biologic or synthetic arteriovenous shunts are occasionally used where suitable adjacent arteries and veins are not available. The most common sites are shown in Figure 11.24. When good arteries and veins are scarce, they may be constructed at other sites, including the legs. External arteriovenous shunts are now rarely used. Long-term access may also be achieved by inserting a double-lumen cannula (such as Permacath) into a subclavian vein, usually via a subcutaneous tunnel.

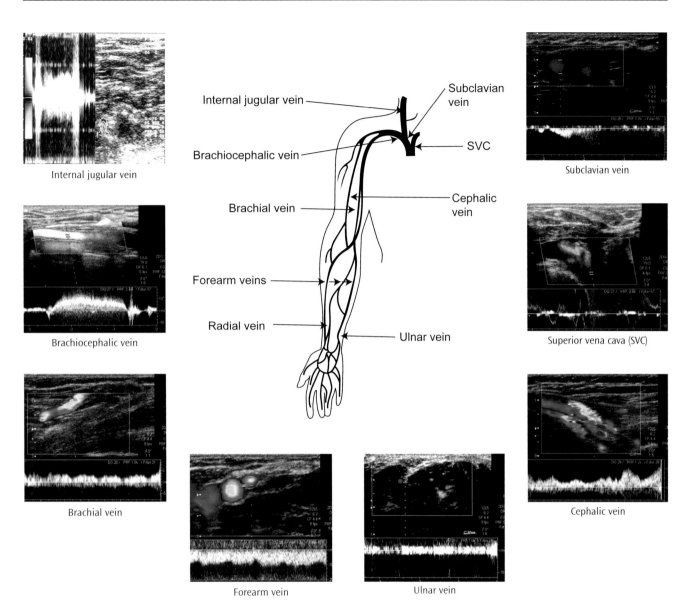

Figure 11.25
Normal Doppler patterns in arm veins.

Short-term vascular access for reversible renal failure or while waiting for an arteriovenous fistula to be constructed, or to mature, is achieved by insertion of a double-lumen cannula with its tip in a large central vein. Subclavian or jugular veins are the preferred introduction sites, with the tip lying in the superior vena cava, although a femoral vein may be used with the cannula tip lying in the inferior vena cava.

Ultrasound may play a role in planning hemodialysis by investigating the state of vessels and blood flow prior to a vascular access procedure, as an aid to the actual access procedure, and more often in the investigation of vascular complications of the procedure. This requires a combina-tion of ultrasound imaging and venous and arterial Doppler studies.

Doppler venography of the arm

Contrast venography has been the traditional 'gold stan-dard' for studying the arm veins, but venous access may be difficult in the swollen limb, resulting in an uncomfortable, painful or unsuccessful procedure. The jugular vein is not demonstrated by contrast venography.

Color Doppler studies are a viable non-invasive alterna-tive investigation which also demonstrate the jugular vein

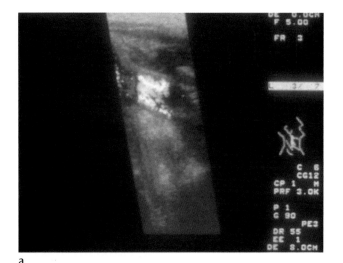

a

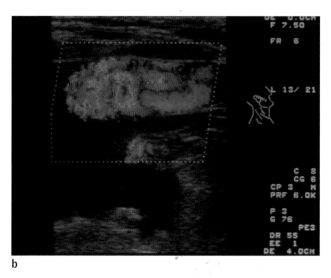

b

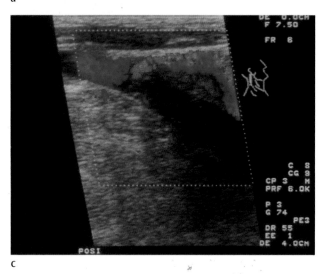

c

Figure 11.26
Jugular vein thrombosis. (a) Thrombus occluding the jugular vein. (b) This case is more chronic; the thrombus is not seen but the vein is occluded with reversal of flow seen on the color Doppler image at the occlusion. (c) Marked distension of the jugular vein by thrombus with recannulation and flow through the thrombus. All three cases were caused by central venous lines.

(Figure 11.25), but do not demonstrate the superior vena cava because of lack of an adequate window. The patency of the superior vena cava may, however, be inferred from a study of the waveform pattern in the subclavian veins (see below). In the investigations of thrombosis there is a 100% correlation with venography, although in the investigation of stenosis, the sensitivity compared with venography is only about 90%, partly because of blind areas such as the retroclavicular portion of the subclavian vein.

In cases where interpretation of the color Doppler image is difficult, however, usually because of multiple collateral vein formation, contrast venography should be performed.

Technique

The examination requires the use of color Doppler imaging, a short linear array with near focusing and the ability

to offset the beam. Imaging frequency should be in the 6–10 MHz range on current machines.

The examination may be performed with the patient lying supine with the arm in the neutral position but slightly abducted or with the patient seated on the opposite side of the couch from the operator with the arm across the examination couch. The subclavian and axillary veins are identified via the infraclavicular fossa, either directly or by their relationship to the artery, followed by longitudinal scans to the clavicle. The subclavian vein is then scanned via the supraclavicular fossa, and followed into the brachiocephalic vein. The axillary, brachial basilic and, if necessary, the cephalic veins may now be studied, as may the forearm veins (Figure 11.25). The variability of the venous anatomy in the arm is such that it is sometimes not possible to map the exact anatomy as well as with contrast venography. Such detail is not, however, necessary in most cases. In a minority of cases where previous fistulas have failed and the patient is running out of suitable vessels, the

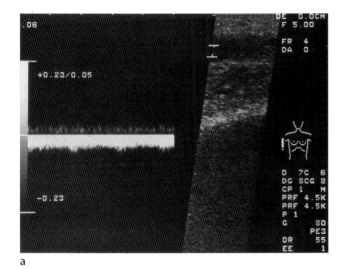

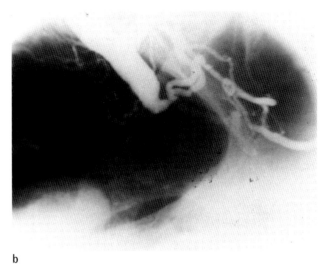

a

b

Figure 11.27
Occlusion of the axillary vein. (a) The vein is distended with slightly hyperechoic thrombus. The Doppler signal upstream to the thrombus shows continuous flow with loss of the normal phasic swing. This is typical of flow into collateral veins. (b) The venogram confirms total occlusion with collateral formation.

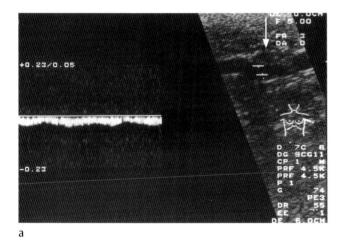

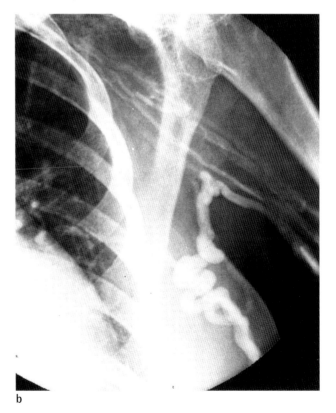

a

Figure 11.28
Axillary vein occlusion. (a) There is echoic thrombus within the vein (arrow). Doppler flow upstream to the occlusion shows total lack of the normal phasic swing. This loss is typical of veins draining via a collateral circulation. (b) Confirmation by contrast venography.

b

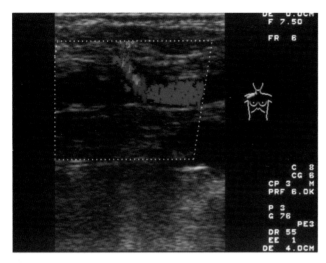

Figure 11.29
Axillary vein thrombosis. The distended thrombosed segment of vein is seen to have no color flow, while there is filling of the downstream vein via a collateral.

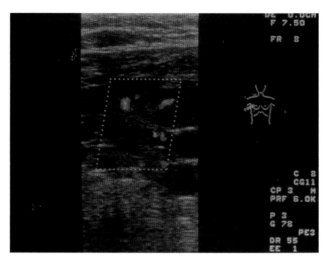

Figure 11.30
Collateral veins bypassing an axillary vein occlusion.

detail afforded by contrast venography is necessary. The internal jugular vein is easily scanned in the neck, and followed to its junction with the subclavian vein. Passive flow is readily seen in all veins and flow can be increased by utilizing the Valsalva maneuver. Sniffing has a similar effect, but neither maneuver is usually needed.

Venous thrombosis

Venous thrombosis results in a segment of vein that is totally or partially occluded by thrombus. The thrombus itself is usually slightly more echoic than flowing blood, but may be isoechoic. The echodensity of thrombus changes with chronicity, but the pattern of change is variable. Acute thrombus distends the segment of vein in which it occurs, and this is perhaps the most valuable gray-scale finding.

Color Doppler imaging is necessary since compression cannot be used. Color flow may be seen up to the occluding thrombus, and distal to it (due to collateral flow), but there is no flow in the thrombus. In the case of non-occluding thrombus, color flow may be seen past the thrombus, but this is clearly different from normal flow. Spectral analysis of flow may also be helpful. The central veins show phasic swing, due to changing pressure in the right atrium during the cardiac cycle and changes in the intrathoracic pressure with respiration. Flow through collateral veins abolishes this swing in the veins distal (anatomically) to the thrombosis (Figures 11.26–11.28).

This may be the first clue to a thrombosis, and may also be the only sign of a thrombosis in ultrasonically 'blind' areas such as the subclavicular area and the superior vena cava.

Collateral veins dilate quite quickly following thrombosis, and these may be shown on the color Doppler image (Figures 11.29 and 11.30).

Venous stenosis

Venous stenosis may occur at the site of previous venous cannulae, or may occur secondary to a surgically constructed arteriovenous fistula. Such stenoses are usually situated within a few centimeters of the anastomosis, but may also occur at areas of physiologic compression of the vein, where the axillary vein is compressed by the pectoralis minor muscle or where the subclavian vein passes between the clavicle and the first rib. They are caused by turbulence in these areas resulting in platelet deposition, leading to intimal hyperplasia or valvular hypertrophy.

Stenoses are seen on the ultrasound image as areas of narrowing, and on Doppler study by increased velocity. The velocity value at which significant stenosis is diagnosed is arbitrary, but a value of three or more times the value in a normal section of the vein is commonly used. Turbulence occurs distal to the stenosis, but turbulence in venous flow is less easy to detect than in arterial flow – particularly if the venous flow is high as in a vein draining a

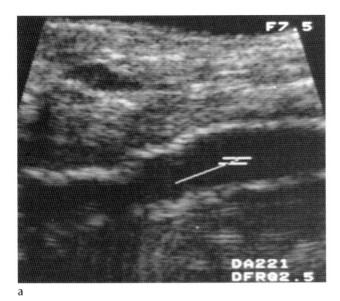
a

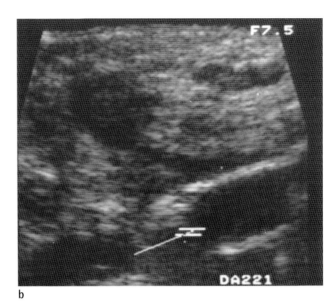
b

Figure 11.31
Minor stenosis of a fistula vein. (a) This degree of stenosis causes no problems but may progress in time to a significant stenosis as shown in (b) taken 6 months later.

fistula, where a degree of turbulence is always present. Where the paths of veins change their angles relative to the transducer, the use of angle correction when estimating velocities is mandatory. Increased velocity normally occurs with a greater than 50% stenosis. Veins in arms without fistulae have relatively low flow. Stenoses may be seen as areas of narrowing on the gray-scale image, but increased flow across the stenosis is difficult to appreciate, although a color change may be seen on color Doppler imaging, particularly in augmented flow. Venography is usually employed to confirm a stenosis suspected on Doppler, often preangioplasty, although with increasing confidence confirmation by contrast venography may not be required. Doppler ultrasound is usually employed as the follow-up procedure after angioplasty (Figures 11.31–11.33).

Arterial Doppler studies in the arm

Doppler studies give poor anatomical information in the arm when compared with an angiogram. The brachial artery may be followed to the bifurcation at the elbow, and the radial and ulnar arteries may be studied at the wrist, but it is not possible to follow the radial and ulnar arteries down the forearm. Doppler imaging does, however, give invaluable physiologic information in the form of flow pattern, response to exercise, velocity and volume flows.[10] For the purpose of hemodialysis assessment, therefore,

Doppler studies are superior to contrast arteriography (Figure 11.34).

Technique

The patient sits on a chair placed on the opposite side of the couch from the examiner. The couch is adjusted to a suitable height, and the patient places his or her arm across the couch. Foam pads are used if necessary to support the arm so that there is no muscle tension, and the arm is comfortable and at rest. The brachial artery is identified at the antecubital fossa, using color flow if available, although color is not essential. A portion of the artery is chosen above the bifurcation into radial and ulnar arteries, the Doppler beam is adjusted by electronic adjustment or transducer angulation so that there is a Doppler angle of 60° or less to the arterial flow and a spectral Doppler trace is obtained. This should be the typical triphasic signal of a musculoskeletal artery supplying a limb at rest. Evidence of arterial disease gives the same changes to the signal as shown in any musculoskeletal artery. It must be remembered, however, that cardiac disease and hypertension may also cause changes in the spectral Doppler pattern. The radial and ulnar arteries are visible at the wrist and lower forearm, and at the antecubital fossa, although they cannot be followed through the mid-forearm. The brachial and subclavian arteries may be imaged throughout their length, apart from the portion beneath the clavicle, by scanning up

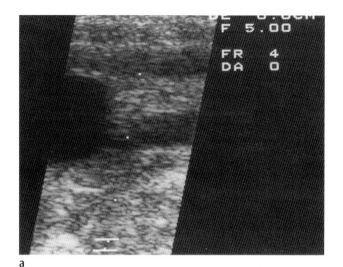

a

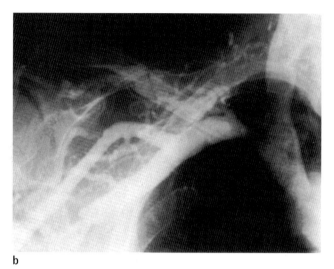

b

Figure 11.32
Subclavian vein stenosis. (a) A supraclavicular scan shows a dilated proximal (upstream) vein and a stenotic area. (b) The venogram confirms the findings. **Axillary vein stenosis.** (c) The color flow image shows the stenosis and aliasing beyond it due to a high-velocity jet.

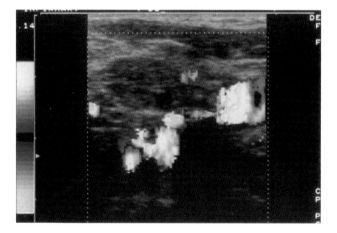

c

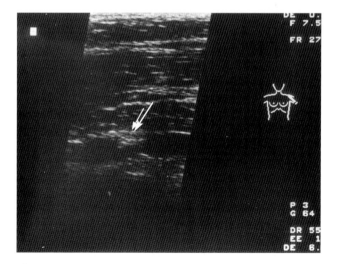

Figure 11.33
Valvular hyperplasia in the axillary vein. The enlarged valve is shown (arrow).

the arm, below and above the clavicle, using a similar technique to that used to follow the veins.

Volume flow estimation

From the spectral trace, a time-averaged velocity may be estimated. If the cross-sectional area of the artery is then measured, a volume flow estimation is possible. It is important to realize that this estimation is subject to several errors that are cumulative. The angle estimation is imprecise. The way that the time-averaged velocity is calculated makes a number of assumptions, and the method varies between different machines. The cross-sectional area of small vessels is difficult to measure with any accuracy. Volume flow estimation is therefore intrinsically inaccurate. In a medium-sized artery, such as the brachial, the error may be as high as ±50%. Nevertheless, the measure-

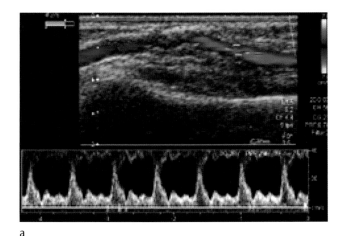

a

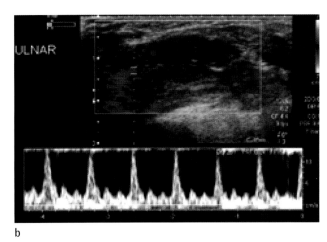

b

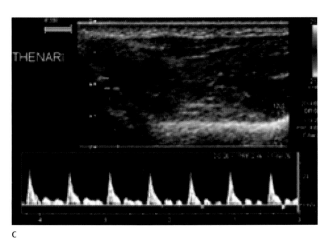

c

Figure 11.34
Arterial studies. Typical Doppler studies of healthy arm arteries at rest are shown: (a) brachial artery, (b) ulnar artery and (c) radial artery at the thenar eminence.

ment is sufficiently accurate for clinical purposes in dialysis fistulae.

Brachial artery volume flow estimation

The cross-sectional area of the artery is measured at the site of the Doppler gate, the time-averaged velocity measured from the spectral trace and volume flow calculated as described earlier. As the brachial artery is relatively large and superficial, sufficiently accurate estimations for clinical use may be obtained, subject to the limitations of the technique (Figure 11.35).

Radial and ulnar artery flow

Radial and ulnar flow are assessed in a similar way. The radial artery is identified at the wrist, in the position where it is normally palpated. The ulnar artery is located on the ulnar side of the wrist. A rather more proximal position than used in the radial artery is usually best. These arteries are very superficial and a stand-off gel pad may be required (Figures 11.36 and 11.37).

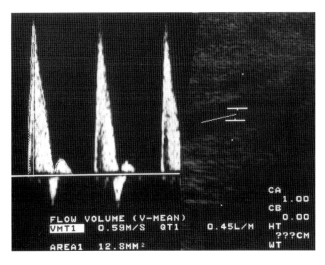

Figure 11.35
Volume flow estimation in a normal brachial artery. The waveform is typical of the triphasic pattern of an artery supplying muscles at rest. The volume flow has been estimated by first measuring the cross-sectional area of the artery and then tracing around the maximum velocity envelope, after correcting for Doppler angle. The machine software then estimates volume flow.

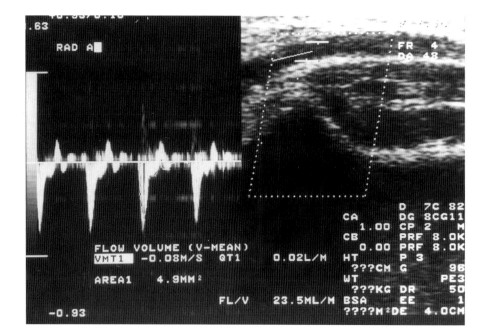

Figure 11.36
Normal radial artery flow. The technique is similar to that used in the brachial artery and the flow pattern is similar. The radial artery is best seen at the wrist.

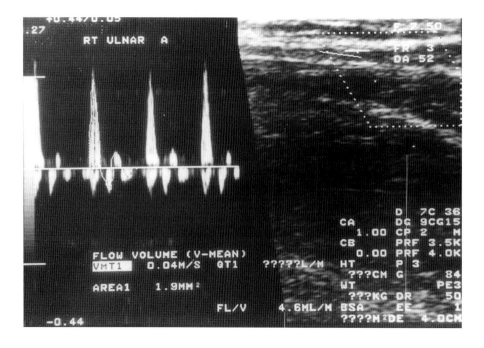

Figure 11.37
Normal ulnar artery flow. The technique is similar to that used in the brachial artery and the flow pattern is also similar. The ulnar artery is best seen slightly higher in the forearm than the radial artery.

The spectral pattern is similar to that of the brachial artery, being a typical triphasic pattern. Change to a low-resistance pattern occurs with exercise, but may also occur if the hand is hot or if there is muscle tension. The arm should therefore be relaxed and cool during the examination. Arterial disease at this level is more common than in the brachial artery, particularly in diabetics. Atheroma plaques may sometimes be visualized, despite the small size of the arteries, but more often the Doppler signs of atheromatous disease are seen. Loss of diastolic flow indi-

cates proximal stenosis or occlusion, although this feature is variable. Increased systolic velocity and turbulence indicates a stenosis at or near the Doppler site. The radial artery may also be identified at the thenar eminence. Here, a reversed direction of flow may occur after fistula construction. Volume flow may be measured at the radial and ulnar artery, but it must be realized that, because of the relatively small size of the arteries, cross-sectional area estimation and hence volume flow estimations in these arteries are very inaccurate.

Central venous dialysis cannulae

Insertion of jugular and subclavian venous cannulae

Jugular or subclavian central venous cannulae for temporary dialysis have traditionally been inserted 'blind' using body surface landmarks and palpation only, and their position is subsequently checked by a chest X-ray (the landmark method). There is rarely any major problem with this method of insertion. In 2002, however, the UK National Institute for Clinical Excellence (NICE) reviewed current evidence. They reported that, while the landmark method works well for experienced operators, overall the complications of arterial puncture – arteriovenous fistula, pneumothorax and nerve injury – are unacceptably high. Multiple unsuccessful attempts are also common. They found that these complications are less common when ultrasound guidance is used. They therefore recommended that ultrasound guidance should be used in all elective cases and in emergency situations when available. In any case, if insertion fails, or there is reason to believe that the veins may not be patent, then color Doppler imaging or contrast venography should be used.

The technique is straightforward and similar to any other ultrasound-guided needle puncture. The veins are so superficial that a needle guide is not necessary. The position of the vein may be marked by ultrasound, and the needle placed according to the mark, but full real-time guidance is best, where the needle tip may be guided under direct ultrasound vision into the venous lumen.[11]

Early complications of venous cannulation

Perhaps the most common early complication of subclavian or jugular venous cannulation is pneumothorax or hemothorax, due to inadvertent puncture of the apical pleura. These complications are revealed by a chest X-ray, and ultrasound has no part to play. Hematomas are usually clinically obvious, and ultrasound only confirms their presence. Doppler ultrasound may, however, be used to exclude arterial damage or venous compression by the hematoma. Intimal dissection may also occur, although in veins this is not normally a serious complication (Figure 11.38). Its detection, however, precludes further attempts at cannulating that vein until the appearances return to normal. Arteriovenous fistulae are uncommon complications. Doppler study shows increased diastolic flow (low resistance index) in the artery, and high-velocity flow in the vein with a similar flow pattern to the artery.

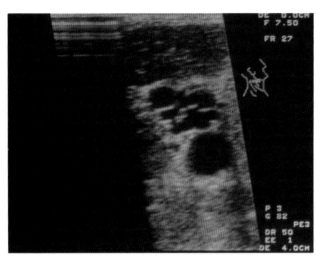

Figure 11.38
Intimal dissection. The jugular vein shows extensive intimal dissection following attempted cannulation. Venous intimal dissection is not a serious complication but precludes further attempts to cannulate that vein until appearances return to normal.

Late complications of venous cannulation

Thrombosis and stenosis are the main late complications of venous cannulation – particularly if the cannula remains in situ for a long period of time, as is usually the case with dialysis cannulae. Occlusions or stenoses may cause acute edema, or may remain asymptomatic until a permanent arteriovenous dialysis fistula is subsequently constructed. The increased venous flow so produced may then cause chronic edema of the arm. Stenosis or thrombosis from previous dialysis or other central venous cannulae may hinder the subsequent insertion of a dialysis cannula.

Arteriovenous dialysis fistulae[12]

Dialysis access fistulae are surgically constructed arteriovenous fistulae at the wrist, between radial or ulnar arteries and accompanying cephalic and ulnar veins or at the antecubital fossa between the brachial artery and the accompanying basilic vein. These result in enlargement of the vein, with high flow and thickening of the vein wall (arteriolization). The thickened wall enables repeated punctures to be performed with safety, thus providing suitable percutaneous access for hemodialysis.

The surgery is relatively straightforward given healthy vessels, and in these cases no preoperative imaging is

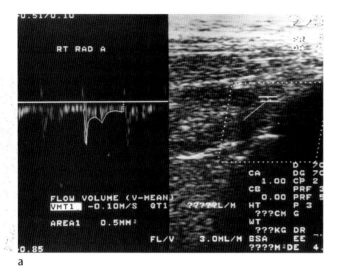
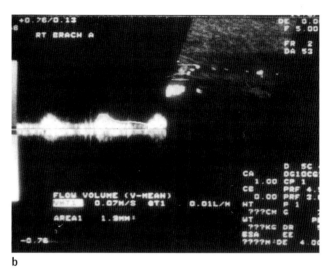

a

b

Figure 11.39
Poor radial artery flow. (a) The artery was detected with difficulty and showed little color flow. Velocity is low (0.1 m/s) and there is loss of reversed diastolic flow. These are signs of severe arterial disease. In the radial and ulnar arteries the flow pattern is often more valuable than volume estimation. **Large vessel disease.** (b) The brachial artery flow is severely reduced and damped, indicating severe proximal disease.

usually necessary. Imaging is, however, necessary in patients in whom there is an increased risk of arterial disease, such as arteriopaths, diabetics or elderly patients, and also in patients who have had multiple venous cannulae or previous complications of venous cannulation, as these have an increased chance of venous stenoses or occlusion.

Arterial flow assessment prior to arteriovenous fistula construction[13]

The traditional method of arterial assessment is firstly to palpate the arterial pulse, and then to carry out a modified Allen test. The patient induces blanching of the hand by tightly clenching the fist. The examiner occludes the radial and ulnar arteries by digital pressure while the patient's fist is clenched. The patient opens the fist, and the examiner releases either the radial or the ulnar artery. The color of the palm should return within 5 seconds. Failure of this response in either artery indicates arterial insufficiency. The test is entirely adequate in most cases. In cases of doubt, however, Doppler ultrasound offers a more sensitive method of arterial flow assessment.

Flow in the brachial artery may be assessed easily by Doppler ultrasound. Estimation of volume flow by Doppler is inherently inaccurate, but in a relatively large superficial artery like the brachial, meaningful estimates may be obtained (see Figure 11.35).

Table 11.1 *Volume flow in forearm arteries (ml/min)*[a]

Brachial artery	60–280	Mean 170
Combined radial and ulnar flow	20–60	Mean 40

[a]Taken from a small survey of healthy volunteers. $n = 40$; 20 male, 20 female, age 20–51 years

Volume flow may also be measured in the radial and ulnar arteries by the same method (see Figures 11.36 and 11.37). In these vessels, the relatively small diameter makes errors in estimating the cross-sectional area far greater. This results in accuracy of perhaps less than ±50%. In practice, however, volume flow estimation taken with the shape of the waveform is sufficient for clinical purposes (Figure 11.39). Normal values for flow in these vessels have been established (Table 11.1), and flow values less than 50% of these are a contraindication to arteriovenous fistula construction. Poor flow or absent flow in the radial or ulnar artery due to a previous failed fistula procedure is not a contraindication, provided there is compensatory increased flow in the other artery. If the radial or ulnar artery is occluded by digital pressure, then flow in the other artery should increase. Failure of this augmentation is a contraindication to arteriovenous fistula construction.

Another way of assessing flow is to compare flow in the brachial artery, and combined flow in radial and ulnar arteries at the wrist. Normally, flow at the wrist is about

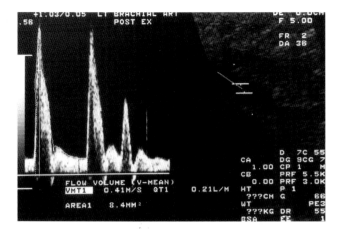

Figure 11.40
Brachial artery flow following exercise. Systolic velocity increases after exercise and rapidly decreases on ceasing the exercise. Diastolic flow also decreases with loss of the reversed component. This response indicates a healthy arterial tree.

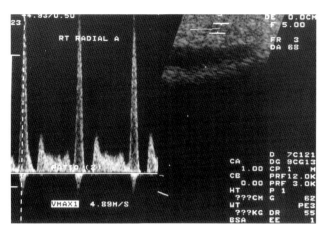

Figure 11.41
Radial artery stenosis. A high systolic velocity is shown at the stenosis.

20% of brachial flow. We arbitrarily use a value of less than 10% as a contraindication to arteriovenous fistula construction.

Exercise testing

An alternative or complementary approach is to study flow before and after exercise. Exercise of the hand may be achieved by compressing a soft ball, and of the forearm by repeated flexion of the elbow while holding a weight. Exercise in the normal subject more than doubles resting flow and changes the triphasic waveform found in the resting state to a low-resistance biphasic waveform. This is caused by dilatation of the muscle arterioles in response to the exercise. This response lasts for several minutes after exercise (Figure 11.40), allowing time to measure Doppler flow. Conversion of triphasic flow to low-resistance flow, but diminished increase in volume flow, occurs in atheroma of the larger arteries, while failure to fully convert to a low-resistance signal indicates small vessel disease, although both patterns frequently coexist in severe disease of either sort. Such failure of response is also regarded as a contraindication to arteriovenous fistula construction.

These are all, at present, empirical rules and no large-scale studies have been performed.

Atheroma may be demonstrated as relatively echogenic homogeneous or inhomogeneous plaques, although the small size of the radial and ulnar arteries makes adequate visualization very difficult. Arterial stenoses, as elsewhere, show increased velocity at the stenosis, turbulence immediately distal, and, in severe cases, damping of the far distal

waveform. A systolic velocity value of 2.5–3 times that in the normal proximal artery is regarded as signifying a hemodynamically significant stenosis (Figure 11.41).

Venous assessment prior to arteriovenous fistula formation

The absence of edema in the arm preoperatively does not exclude the possibility of postoperative problems. Venous thrombosis or stenosis, particularly of the axillary vein, may be asymptomatic until the increased flow from a fistula reveals relative venous insufficiency and causes edema. Patients who have had previous venous cannulation in that limb for dialysis or other central venous access are at risk, particularly if the cannulae were in situ for a prolonged period. Doppler or contrast venography may be employed preoperatively in such cases. For the technique and findings see the 'Doppler venography of the arm' section.

Complications of dialysis fistulae[14,15]

Repeated graft thrombosis and inadequate dialysis may be due to inadequate arterial inflow or inadequate venous outflow.

Ischemia of the hand may be due to arterial disease or excessive flow through the fistula.

Local complications are aneurysm, pseudoaneurysms, hematomas and abscess. All may be detected by ultrasound.

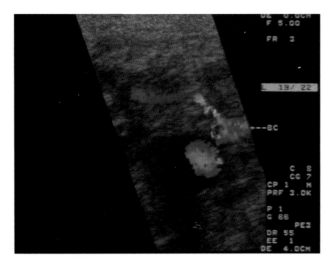

Figure 11.42
Axillary vein thrombosis. The axillary vein is distended, with no flow upstream to the junction with the cephalic vein indicating thrombosis.

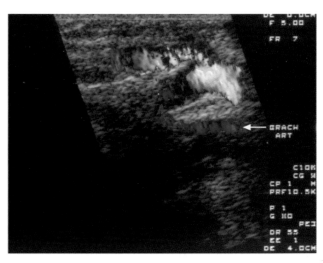

Figure 11.43
Normal brachial fistula. The brachial artery (arrow) is seen supplying a fistula to the brachial vein. Because a high pulse repetition frequency (PRF) is used, the reduced flow in the artery distal to the fistula is not demonstrated.

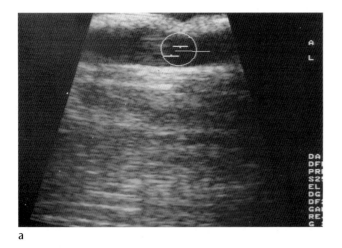

a

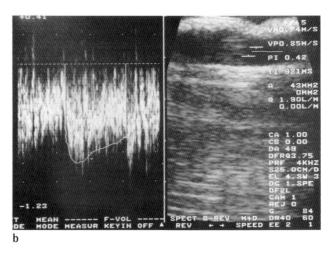

b

Figure 11.44
Forearm fistula: normal flow in the arterialized vein. This degree of turbulence is normal. Volume flow has been estimated by measuring a cross-sectional area of the vessel (a), and then tracing around the maximal velocity envelope for one cardiac cycle (b), after correcting for the angle of insonation. Because of the turbulence the trace is approximate but the estimate of volume flow is sufficiently accurate for clinical use.

Thrombosis

Thrombosis of dialysis fistulae may occur at the venous side of the fistula, in which case the thrombus is usually palpable, although ultrasound may be used as a confirmatory test. Thrombosis of the draining veins at axillary or subclavian level is more insidious and difficult to diagnose. Contrast venography has been the gold standard, but color Doppler ultrasound is now an acceptable alternative (Figure 11.42) (see also the 'Doppler venography of the arm' section).

Arterial steal

Ischemia of the hand may be due to pre-existing subclinical arterial disease that becomes symptomatic when the fistula further reduces flow in the distal arteries. In other cases, it may be due to excessive flow through the fistula. Poor dialysis may be due to insufficient flow. Volume flow through the arterialized fistula vein can usually be assessed sufficiently accurately by Doppler ultrasound, because the vein is large and superficial, cross-sectional area can be

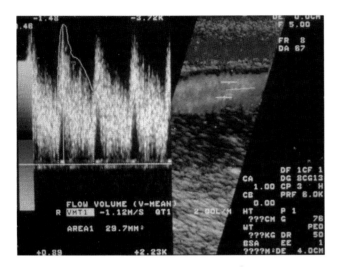

Figure 11.45
Radial fistula: normal radial artery flow. The artery is shown deep to the fistula vein. Note that flow in the artery is greatly increased both by enlargement of the artery and increased flow velocity. The normal triphasic flow seen in the radial artery in the resting limb is replaced by low-resistance flow with very high diastolic flow.

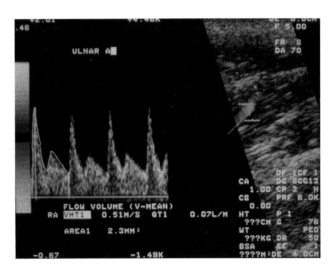

Figure 11.46
Normal ulnar artery flow with radial fistula. The ulnar flow is increased and the normal triphasic flow seen at rest is replaced by a low-resistance flow pattern with continuing high diastolic flow.

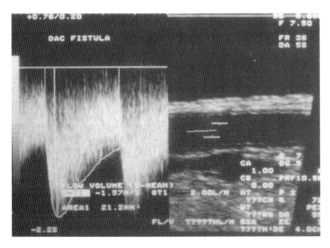

Figure 11.47
Flow in a synthetic shunt. The even echogenic walls of the Dacron shunt are seen with a typical flow pattern.

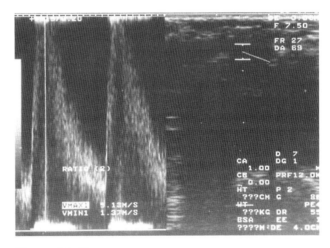

Figure 11.48
Dialysis fistula stenosis. A high-velocity jet of more than 5 m/s is seen at the fistula site, indicating a very narrow stenosed fistula.

accurately assessed. Where the vein is very irregular in size and/or the flow is very turbulent, flow volume estimation is less accurate, but still useful (Figures 11.43–11.48).

Volume flow may be assessed in the feeding artery, and compared with the draining vein.[16] The difference is theoretically the blood supply to the hand. In practice, however, the inaccuracies inherent in the measurements are too great for this method of assessment to be clinically useful.

The radial artery may be identified on color Doppler at the thenar eminence. Retrograde flow at this point indicates arte-

rial steal (Figure 11.49). Retrograde flow, however, occurs in up to 20% of patients with fistulae, and only a small proportion of these will be symptomatic. Moreover, not all symptomatic patients have retrograde radial flow, so the test is of limited value. It has been shown that initially up to one-third of the flow through a radio-cephalic fistula comes from the distal limb of the artery, i.e. retrograde flow from the hand.

In cases of ischemia of the hand, diminished digital artery pulsation may also be demonstrated by Doppler study. This is best achieved with a continuous-wave

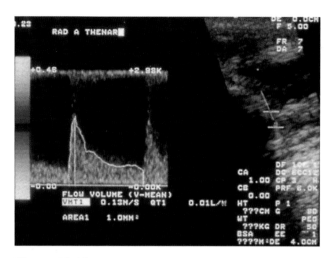

Figure 11.49
Arterial steal causing ischemia of the hand. In this patient with a radial fistula, the radial artery at the thenar eminence shows reversed flow. The patient had ischemia of the hand, explained by the arterial steal. Similar reversal of flow may, however, occur without ischemia and not all patients with ischemia show reversal of flow.

Doppler device. The Doppler study, however, adds little to clinical evaluation.

Local problems and masses at the fistula site

Pseudoaneurysms

A pseudoaneurysm usually occurs as a complication of dialysis venepuncture, usually due to inadequate pressure on the puncture site after removal of the needle. Less commonly, it may be a postoperative complication of arteriovenous fistula construction. A pseudoaneurysm starts with the formation of a blood leak adjacent to the vessel. Such blood collections occasionally maintain a communication with the vessel lumen, allowing blood to flow into the center of a hematoma. The cavity so formed enlarges to produce a pseudoaneurysm. There is no true wall as in the case of a true aneurysm; the solid hematoma forms the wall, and hence the term pseudoaneurysm, or false aneurysm.

Pseudoaneurysms sometimes spontaneously thrombose to form, in effect, hematomas. Other pseudoaneurysms may progressively enlarge and may reach a considerable size if not treated.

Ultrasound imaging and Doppler studies are the appropriate method of investigating masses adjacent to fistula or puncture sites. The ultrasound image will determine whether the center of the mass is solid or liquid. Doppler

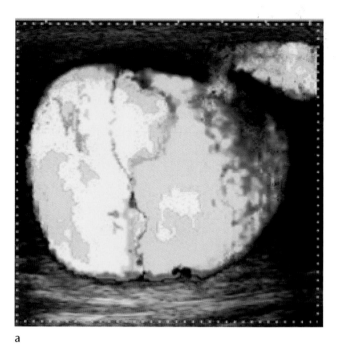

a

b

Figure 11.50
Pseudoaneurysm. (a) There is a large pseudoaneurysm arising from the needling site of the fistula vein. (b) Partial thrombosis following percutaneous thrombin injection. A second injection caused total thrombosis.

will establish whether there is flowing blood in the center, establishing the diagnosis of pseudoaneurysm. The jet at the neck of the aneurysm may be demonstrated. Demonstration of the site of the communication with the

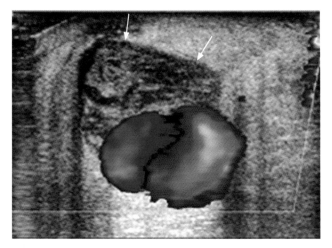

Figure 11.51
Pseudoaneurysm. The typical two-color pattern of the pseudoaneurysm caused by spiral blood flow (yin-yang pattern). There is also a solid hematoma anterior to the dialysis vein (vein arrowed).

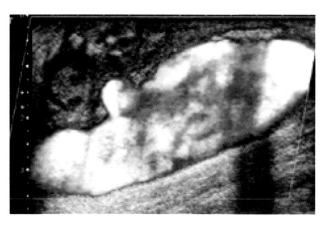

Figure 11.52
Pseudoaneurysm with spontaneous thrombosis: fistula vein aneurysm. Most of the pseudoaneurysm has thrombosed, leaving only a small area of flow in the neck. The fistula vein is also aneurysmal with a fusiform shape.

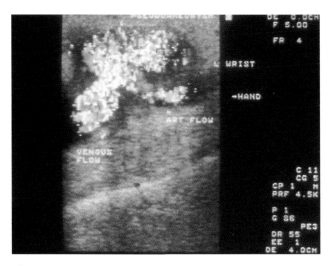

Figure 11.53
Pseudoaneurysm complicating radial fistula. A postoperative pseudoaneurysm is seen at the fistula site. The radial artery and draining vein are shown. Color flow in the pseudoaneurysm gives a mosaic pattern typical of turbulent flow, contrasting with the spiral flow pattern seen in a true aneurysm.

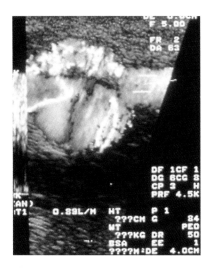

Figure 11.54
Dialysis fistula aneurysm. A saccular aneurysm with typical spiral flow is seen at the needling site of an antecubital fistula vein. At excision this was found to be a true aneurysm rather than a pseudoaneurysm. The nature of the aneurysm on the scan is demonstrated by the clear image of a thin wall. Saccular aneurysms are far rarer than fusiform aneurysms or pseudoaneurysms.

vessel can aid the surgical procedure for closure. On color flow, the pseudoaneurysm may show turbulent flow, or often the characteristic 'two color' pattern more commonly seen in true aneurysms. One half of the aneurysm is shown as blood flowing towards the transducer, the other half flows away, with a clear-cut demarcation between the two. This is due to spiral flow in the pseudoaneurysm lumen.

The 'wall' of a pseudoaneurysm is sometimes thick and irregular, unlike that of a true aneurysm. The 'wall' may, however, thin as the pseudoaneurysm enlarges. Partial clotting of the pseudoaneurysm may result in apparently two

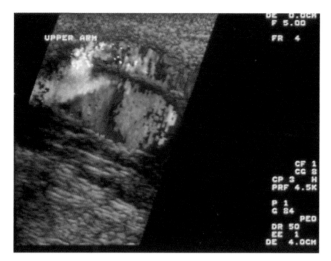

Figure 11.55
Possible mycotic aneurysm. There is an aneurysm in the arterialized axillary vein of a patient with a radial fistula. Such aneurysms occurring at sites remote from the fistula are thought to be mycotic, although their nature is not known with certainty. Typical spiral flow is shown in the lumen.

or more lumenae, although these in fact communicate. Chronic pseudoaneurysms may give a bizarre appearance, as parts of them fibrose or calcify. If the lumen thromboses, they become indistinguishable from chronic hematomas, except for the history of gradual enlargement (Figures 11.50–11.53).

Pseudoaneurysms may be treated by applying pressure to the pseudoaneurysm neck, under Doppler control, until flow ceases. Pressure is continued for 5 minutes or more and reapplied if necessary until the neck thromboses and flow ceases, leaving in effect a hematoma. Another method is direct injection of thrombin into the pseudoaneurysm. This acts almost instantaneously. The injection is guided and the thrombosis is observed by real-time ultrasound (see Figure 11.50).

Aneurysms

The 'arterialized' vein draining a dialysis fistula normally enlarges, sometimes markedly. Such dilatation, particularly if localized, may be termed aneurysmal. It is of little significance. Doppler ultrasound demonstrates that flow in such areas is turbulent, but, unlike true arterial aneurysms, mural thrombus does not form, and rupture does not occur (Figures 11.52 and 11.54).

We have seen several cases of small saccular aneurysms in veins distal to arteriovenous fistulae. The etiology of these is uncertain, although they may be mycotic aneurysms related to previous asymptomatic infections. The cases we have seen have been asymptomatic and have not progressed (Figure 11.55).

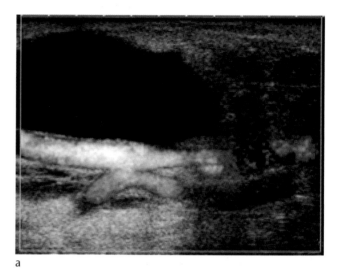

a

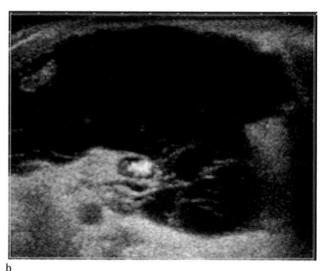

b

Figure 11.56
Hematoma. (a) Longitudinal and (b) transverse sections of a large, mostly liquefied postoperative hematoma anterior to a brachial fistula. The side-to-side anastomosis of the fistula is clearly seen.

Hematomas

The management of vascular dialysis sites is aimed at preventing the formation of hematomas by the use of prolonged pressure over the needle site following removal of the needle, and also good needle insertion technique. Despite this, even in the most careful hands, hematomas do occur. These are often small and asymptomatic and are only seen if ultrasound is carried out for some other reason, such as a clinical study. Occasionally, a hematoma of a palpable size occurs. In these cases, the purpose of ultrasound is to exclude pseudoaneurysm. Pseudoaneurysms

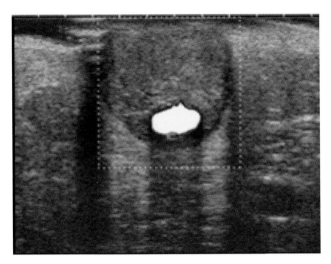

Figure 11.57
Hematoma. There is an echogenic solid hematoma at the needling site of a brachial fistula vein. Transverse view.

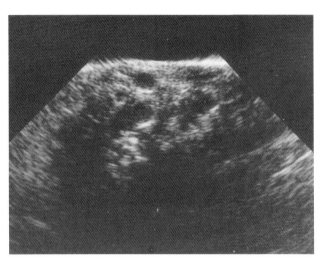

Figure 11.58
Calcified perifistula mass. This complex mass in the antecubital fossa is thought to have started as a hematoma, modified in time to form a calcified mass. Vessels, including the fistula vein, are seen passing through the lesion.

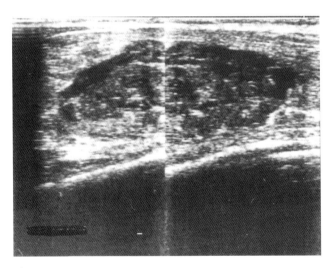

Figure 11.59
Infected hematoma. This large hematoma was clinically infected. This was confirmed by percutaneous aspiration.

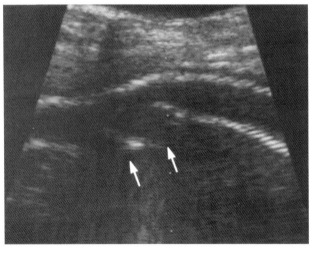

Figure 11.60
Intimal dissection. There is a Goretex fistula graft in the forearm showing the typical wall texture of a synthetic graft. There is a dissection of the vein wall at the anastomosis with the graft (arrows).

need to be treated by occlusion by pressure or prothrombin injection, or surgically excised, particularly if they are enlarging, while hematomas are treated conservatively, unless of a size that causes clinical discomfort or compression of an adjacent vessel. They do not normally cause significant vascular compression of the arterialized fistula vein, but may cause compression of the other veins, resulting in edema of the limb distal to them (see Figures 11.52 and 11.56–11.58).

Abscess

Peregraft abscesses have an ultrasonic appearance similar to that of hematomas. They appear as masses of variable low or mixed echodensity adjacent to the vessel. The clinical situation, however, with fever, high white cell count with local tenderness and erythema usually points to the diagnosis, which is confirmed by percutaneous aspiration (Figure 11.59).

Intimal dissection

This is an unusual complication. It may occur as a complication of the surgical procedure or, rarely, due to poor needling technique (Figure 11.60).

GENERAL DIALYSIS COMPLICATIONS

Congestive cardiac failure

The increased flow in a fistula may precipitate cardiac failure. Doppler ultrasound may be employed to assess whether the fistula flow is excessive.

Acquired cystic disease of the kidneys

About 90% of patients on hemodialysis or peritoneal dialysis develop multiple small renal cysts which have a malignant potential. These are described in Chapter 1.

References

1. Ash SR. Peritoneal dialysis in acute renal failure of adults: the under-utilized modality. Contrib Nephrol 2004; 144: 239–54.
2. Gokal R, Mallick NP. Peritoneal dialysis. Lancet 1999; 353(9155): 823–8.
3. Rottembourg J, Gahl GM, Poignet JL, et al. Severe abdominal complications in patients undergoing continuous ambulatory peritoneal dialysis. Proc Eur Dial Transplant Assoc 1983; 20: 236–42.
4. Twardowski ZJ, Tully RJ, Ersoy FF, Dedhia NM, Computerised tomography with and without intraperitoneal contrast for determination of intraabdominal fluid distribution and diagnosis of complications in peritoneal dialysis patients. ASAIO Trans 1990; 36: 95–103.
5. Kawaguchi Y, Kawanishi H, Mujais S, Topley N, Oreopoulos DG. Encapsulating peritoneal sclerosis: definition, etiology, diagnosis, and treatment. International Society for Peritoneal Dialysis Ad Hoc Committee on Ultrafiltration Management in Peritoneal Dialysis. Perit Dial Int 2000; 20(Suppl 4): S43–55.
6. Holland P. Sclerosing encapsulating peritonitis in chronic ambulatory peritoneal dialysis. Clin Radiol 1990; 41: 19–23.
7. Hollman AS, McMillan MA, Briggs JD, Junor BJ, Morley P. Ultrasound changes in sclerosing peritonitis following continuous ambulatory peritoneal dialysis. Clin Radiol 1991; 48: 176–9.
8. Rodriguez HJ, Walls J, Slatopolsky E, Klahr S. Recurrent ascites following peritoneal dialysis. A new syndrome? Ann Intern Med 1974; 134: 283–7.
9. Holley JG, Foulks CJ, Moss AH, Willard D. Ultrasound as a tool in the diagnosis and management of exit-site infections in patients undergoing continuous ambulatory peritoneal dialysis. Am J Kidney Dis 1989; 14: 211–16.
10. Baxter BT, Blackburn D, Payne K, et al, Noninvasive evaluation of the upper extremity. Surg Clin North Am 1990; 70: 87–97.
11. Sands JJ, Ferrell LM, Perry MA. The role of color flow Doppler ultrasound in dialysis access. Semin Nephrol 2002; 22(3): 195–201.
12. Weiswasser JM, Kellicut D, Arora S, Sidawy AN. Strategies of arteriovenous dialysis access. Semin Vasc Surg 2004; 17(1): 10–18.
13. Lemson MS, Leunissen KM, Tordoir JH. Does pre-operative duplex examination improve patency rates of Brescia-Cimino fistulas? Nephrol Dial Transplant 1998; 13(6): 1360–1.
14. Blankestijn PJ, Smits JH. How to identify the hemodialysis access at risk of thrombosis? Are flow measurements the answer? Nephrol Dial Transplant 1999; 14(5): 1068–71.
15. Haruguchi H, Teraoka S. Intimal hyperplasia and hemodynamic factors in arterial bypass and arteriovenous grafts: a review. J Artif Organs 2003; 6(4): 227–35.
16. Krpan D, Damarin V, Prot F, et al, Measurement of blood flow through AV-fistulae by means of Doppler sonography in regularly hemodialysed patients. Int J Artif Organs 1991; 14: 78.

12

Interventional ultrasound

Dennis Ll Cochlin

GENERAL CONSIDERATIONS

Ultrasound is, in many ways, the ideal method of guidance for placing a needle in the body, as progress of the needle may be followed under direct ultrasound vision in real time, without the use of large obstructing apparatus and without the worry of radiation exposure.

There are, however, disadvantages. The needle and its tip are often not easy to see, and keeping the needle image in the ultrasound beam requires some skill and practice. Even then, various maneuvers may be necessary to visualize the needle. Bowel loops in the proposed needle track may be a problem.

Thin needles (18 gauge or smaller) may be safely passed through the bowel to biopsy deep lesions. Introducing a needle through the colon into a fluid collection, however, introduces a great risk of infecting the collection and should be avoided. Drainage catheters may not be placed across the bowel. It is difficult to accurately place a needle between bowel loops with ultrasound guidance. Unless, therefore, a route clearly free of intervening bowel loops can be found on ultrasound, computed tomography (CT) guidance, where bowel loops are clearly seen, is preferable in these circumstances.

Large blood vessels should be avoided. Color flow imaging may be employed with advantage to ensure that echo-free areas are not blood vessels, and that structures to be needled are not excessively vascular.

Despite the disadvantages, ultrasound is the method of choice when needling the kidney, prostate and other parts of the genitourinary system. For retroperitoneal structures, ultrasound or CT is chosen as appropriate, the safety of the procedure being the prime deciding factor.

TECHNIQUE OF NEEDLE PLACEMENT

The following statements and discussion apply to any ultrasound-guided needle placement, whether it is for biopsy, drainage, or any other procedure.

Patient preparation

Full informed consent is obtained from the patient, and an explanation is given of alternative procedures. The patient is best kept starved, in case of nausea.

Sedation and analgesia

Sedation and analgesia is a matter of choice, depending on the individual procedure and patient. Procedures that are likely to be quick and easy may require no sedation or analgesia in a cooperative patient, while a difficult drainage procedure may require both. Entonox is increasingly being used. It is very effective in some patients. Even when it is not used, its availability may be a psychologic advantage to the patient. In cases that are likely to be difficult or prolonged, and in nervous patients, it is best, in any case, to establish intravenous access before the procedure, so that intravenous drugs may be given during the procedure if necessary. If large doses of benzodiazepines and/or opiates need to be used, then a second person is needed to monitor the patient. Monitoring by pulse oximeter is desirable. In such cases, it may be better for an anesthetist to supervise the sedation and analgesia. This situation rarely arises, however, except in the case of children.

The choice of drugs is a matter of individual preference, but a combination of sedative and analgesic seems appropriate. In most cases we use benzodiazepine emulsion and meperidine (pethedine) for adults, and chlorpromazine and meperidine for children.

Seeing and placing the needle

Needle tip and shaft visualization[1–6]

Placement of needles with ultrasound control for biopsy or drainage is now very often achieved under direct real-time

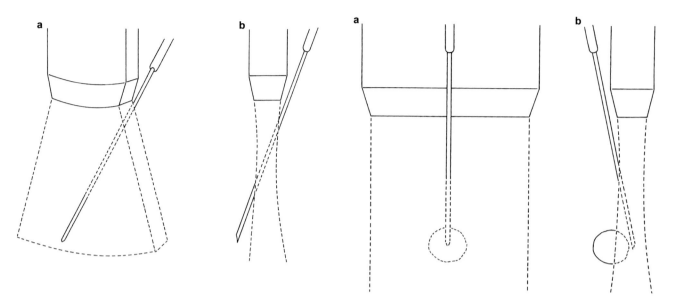

Figure 12.1
Needle straying from the lateral confines of the beam. A small angle discrepancy in the Z-plane will result in part of the needle leaving the beam and not being visible.

Figure 12.2
Effect of a wide beam width. The needle tip lies alongside the lesion. On the ultrasound image, however, as both lesion and needle tip lie within the beam, the needle tip will appear to lie within the lesion. The wider the beam, the more likely is this error to occur.

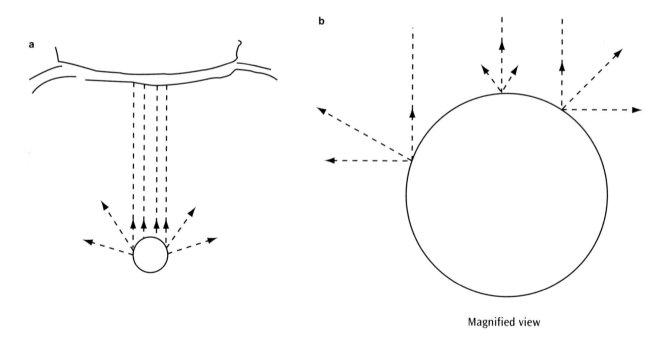

Magnified view

Figure 12.3
Effect of round cross-section of needle on returned echoes. Diagram of transverse section of needle shaft. Apart from the central beam, most of the reflected echoes are directed away from the transducer. The component reflected back to the transducer, which produces the image, is weak.

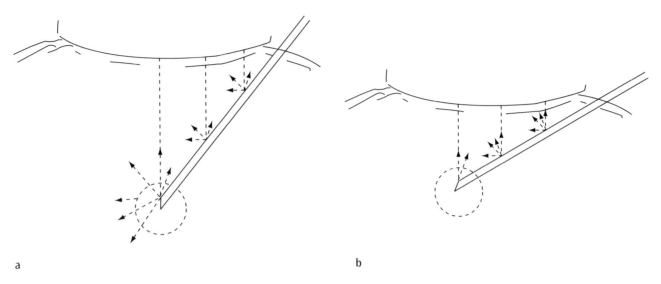

a   b

Figure 12.4

Needle angulation. (a) The needle is placed close to the transducer, making it easier to judge the needle angle and remain within the beam in the Z-plane. The shallow angle to the ultrasound beam, however, makes its visualization poor. (b) The angle to the ultrasound beam is greater and visualization is improved. The needle, however, must enter the skin at some distance from the transducer, making judgment in the X-, Y- and Z-planes more difficult. The effect on the reflection of the beam is shown. This is cumulative to the effect in the other plane shown in Figure 12.3.

ultrasound guidance. This procedure is reliant on the production of good echoes from the tip and shaft of the needle. The most common reason for not seeing the needle echoes is that the needle is not in the lateral (Z) place of the transducer (Figure 12.1). The use of a needle guide helps in this regard, although all needle guides allow some lateral movement and, with fine needles, bending of the needle often occurs. The use of a transducer with a relatively wide beam makes it more likely that the needle will remain in the beam, but with a wide beam the needle can appear to enter the lesion when it is in fact alongside the lesion (Figure 12.2). The ideal beam width is therefore a compromise. The beam width is, in any case, largely a function of the ultrasound system design and may only be changed to a limited extent by altering the focusing controls.

Although a metal needle would intuitively seem likely to be a powerful specular reflector, in practice the smooth rounded surface of the shaft produces a poor echo (Figure 12.3). The shaft often lies at a shallow angle to the transducer beam, which also greatly reduces the echoes.

The bevelled needle tip produces far stronger echoes because of its angular shape, but, because of its angulation, the strength of the echo varies. In a relatively low even-echodensity structure like the liver, needle visualization is rarely a problem. Placing a needle into a kidney for biopsy or antegrade puncture, however, requires visualization of the needle in the lumbar muscles and surrounding tissues. The highly reflective interfaces in this region are of a similar reflectivity to the needle. The inhomogeneous tissues also degrade the ultrasound beam. Visualization of the

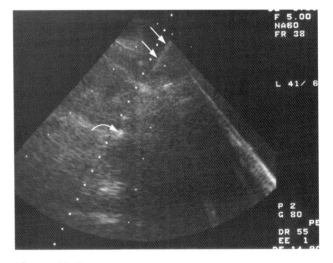

Figure 12.5

Effect of angulation: non-etched needle. Part of the renal biopsy needle shaft is seen (straight arrows). As the needle approaches the central ultrasound beam, the angle that it makes with the ultrasound beam gets smaller and the image of the needle shaft is lost. The needle tip remains visible (curved arrows) because its bevel presents a greater angle to the ultrasound beam.

needle in this area is therefore at best less than ideal and, at worst, the needle is often barely visible. A number of things can, however, be done to improve visualization.

Placing the needle so that its shaft makes a wide angle to the ultrasound beam improves visualization (Figures

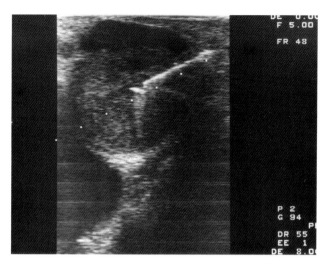

Figure 12.6
Effect of increasing the angle. This image of a prostatic biopsy shows how well the needle is seen when the angle to the ultrasound beam is increased. Such angulation cannot be used for renal biopsy.

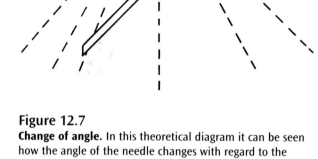

Figure 12.7
Change of angle. In this theoretical diagram it can be seen how the angle of the needle changes with regard to the ultrasound beam as it crosses the image.

12.4–12.7). Such placement, however, may move the puncture site further from the transducer. This makes it more difficult to ensure that the needle stays in a plane that lies within the lateral beam width. It may also make the use of a guide impossible. In the case of the kidney, the position of the kidney, partly beneath the rib cage, limits the options for approach. The angle used is therefore, of necessity, a compromise.

In any ultrasound-guided needle puncture procedure, planning is vital. It is useless having planned an ideal needle track if the transducer cannot be placed in a position that enables monitoring of the progress of the needle. Equally it is no good having an ideal ultrasound image of the target if the needle cannot be placed in that plane because of an obstruction, such as a rib. Time must therefore be taken to choose a route that will allow safe placement of the needle, while also allowing good real-time imaging of the needle passage through the tissues and into the target site. Sometimes in order to achieve this it is necessary to change transducers. A small footprint sector transducer may sometimes be placed in a suitable plane where there in no room for a curved linear.

Method of improving needle visualization[1–6]

Often when the needle lies in mixed echodensity tissue, such as muscle, it is difficult to determine which echoes represent the needle, particularly when the only strong echo from the needle is that from the tip. Moving the needle in and out with a fine movement produces motion

of the needle echoes, often allowing them to be distinguished from those of surrounding tissues. The movement also produces tissue movement around the tip and shaft. This is often a good approximate guide to where the needle lies, although tissues move in a surprisingly wide area around the needle, so that it is not an exact guide. Such movement may identify the needle tip as a small bright area moving rather more than the surrounding tissues.

Withdrawing the needle stylet or injecting a small volume of saline makes the needle tip slightly more echogenic. Because the needle tip echo is generated from the bevel, placement of the needle with the bevel away from the transducer greatly reduces the needle tip echo. The largest echo is produced with the bevel at an indeterminate angle to the transducer. It is best, therefore, to start with the bevel directly facing the transducer and, if difficulty is encountered in seeing the tip echo, to rotate the needle in either direction. The true reason for this is complex, and the image of the needle tip is probably due to the effects of refraction more than reflection.

Manufacturers of needles have attempted to make parts of the needle shaft more echogenic by roughening the surface. Fine etching of the surface produces only marginal improvement, although more deeply etched bands are better (Figure 12.8). It has been observed for some time that needles with side holes produce strong echoes from the margins of the holes. This fact has been utilized by some manufacturers, by placing side holes, or deep circular indentations that do not penetrate the whole thickness of the needle wall. These are far more effective than fine etching.

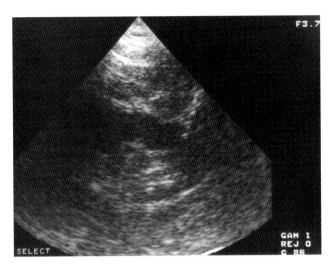

Figure 12.8
Etched needle. This renal biopsy needle has etched marks at 1-cm intervals. They are seen on the ultrasound image as a series of echoes. Such a needle produced echoes from a shaft at a far lower angle to the transducer than a non-etched needle (compare Figure 12.5).

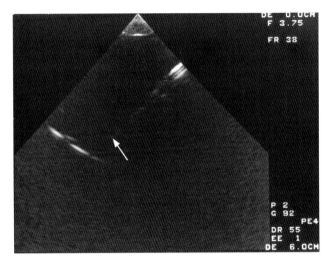

Figure 12.9
False needle tip echo, non-etched needle. A strong echo is produced from the part of the shaft that lies superficially and is nearly at 90° to the transducer beam. As the angle becomes less, the strength of the echo reduces so that the rest of the needle is not seen well. The true needle tip is shown by the arrow. Increasing gain settings helps to reduce this error.

Needles with flexible plastic sheaths are often used for drainage for preliminary puncture prior to insertion of a guide wire. These needles are particularly poor reflectors and so are often difficult to see by ultrasound. A useful technique is to replace the stylet with a flexible guide wire passed to the end of the needle. This usually provides good visualization. Once the position of the needle is known, the wire is replaced by the stylet, and the needle advanced further or repositioned. The maneuver is repeated as often as necessary.

The use of color Doppler imaging has been tried, the color being produced by the movement of the needle. Color gain needs to be set very low; otherwise, a large area of flash artifact is produced. With correct gain settings, however, it is possible to visualize the needle position from the color. It is, however, very difficult to choose ideal settings, and it gives little advantage in most cases.

Transponder needles have a small transducer either at the needle tip, or at the hub of the needle, utilizing the needle itself as a waveguide. The position of the transducer is sensed by the machine, which then places a bright spot on the screen at that point. There may also be an audio signal that changes pitch as the needle tip moves into or strays from the lateral width of the beam. These devices virtually guarantee detection of the needle tip position, but they require special needles and an electronic interface with the machine. A few manufacturers have at various times produced such needles, but the high cost and limited choice of needle size has led to none being commercially successful.

Errors in interpretation of the needle position

A relatively wide transducer beam may produce a 'partial volume' image of the needle tip within a structure, when in fact it lies alongside the structure (see Figure 12.2).

Echoes from part of the shaft of the needle may be interpreted as the tip echo when, in fact, the tip lies deeper. As the needle moves deeper into the tissues, its angle to the transducer becomes less, so that the distal end of the shaft may be less clearly seen than the more superficial part (Figures 12.4, 12.7 and 12.9). In order to minimize the likelihood of making such errors the needle tip echo should be followed on real time as it moves deeper into the tissues. Conversely, when the whole needle is poorly seen, part of the needle may be seen on real time, giving an indication of the needle direction. On moving the needle, tissue movement may be seen deep to the actual needle tip. This may be misinterpreted as the actual needle tip, giving a false impression of the tip depth.

Ideal visualization of the needle therefore depends to some extent on the choice of needle, but far more on the skill and experience of the operator, who will use constant fine transducer movement to keep the needle central in the ultrasound beam, will choose the best compromise of needle angulation, and will use other 'tricks of the trade', such as fine needle movement, to produce tissue movement, and will constantly observe the real-time image, looking for signs like indentation of the renal capsule. There is no 'quick fix' solution, and no substitute, for experience.

Technique of needle placement

As stated earlier, time should be taken to plan the site and angle of needle placement before infiltrating the skin with local anesthetic.

Indirect ultrasound guidance

Large or superficial targets may have their position and depth determined by ultrasound scan. The skin is appropriately marked and, after skin cleansing, local anesthetic is infiltrated and a needle or catheter introduced at the angle and to the depth determined by the ultrasound scan. The position may be checked after insertion by a further scan, if necessary, and the position adjusted. The transducer needs to be rendered sterile by covering it with a suitable condom-like cover.

Freehand direct ultrasound guidance

This involves real-time scanning of the target lesion, while introducing the needle at an angle and position such that the progress of the needle tip is visible on real time throughout its progress.

The target lesion is first scanned, and a transducer position is chosen that will show the target lesion and also permit the needle to be introduced in such a way that it remains in the ultrasound beam throughout its progress, and, in the case of fluid aspiration or catheter insertion, does not traverse bowel. This is not always easy, and as much time as necessary must be spent at this stage. Different transducers, sector curved or linear, may be appropriate for different lesions.

The needle is well seen when it lies at about 60°–90° to the central ultrasound beam (see Figure 12.6). If this technique is chosen, it is best to check the proposed route of the needle by first scanning along the proposed needle track, marking the puncture site and noting the depth. With this technique, it is not easy to judge the angle of the needle in relation to the transducer, because of the physical distance of the transducer from the puncture site. It is helpful if possible to turn the patient so that the proposed needle track is either horizontal or vertical in one or preferably both planes, as this makes it easier than trying to judge angles. It is essential to see the needle at all times. This often involves introducing the needle in small increments, with constant fine adjustment of the transducer angle. The operator must constantly alternate between looking at the ultrasound screen image and looking at the needle and transducer to check their relative alignment.

Alternatively, the needle may be introduced at a shallow angle to the transducer. This may be achieved by introducing the needle at the end of the transducer, so that it

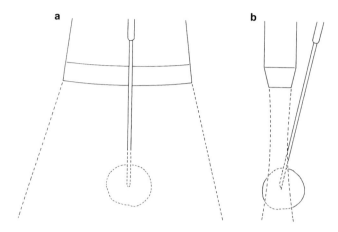

Figure 12.10
Needle placement alongside a linear or curved linear transducer. The needle has been introduced alongside the transducer and angled slightly so that it enters the transducer beam.

enters the beam shortly after introduction and then stays within the beam (see Figure 12.8), or the needle may be introduced alongside the transducer at a slight angle so that it enters the beam (Figure 12.10). In this case, it may be seen that the needle actually traverses obliquely across the width (Z-plane) of the ultrasound beam. Because the beam has finite width, a sufficient length of the needle may be seen for guidance. With the latter method, the angle that the needle makes to the ultrasound beam is necessarily shallow, so the needle is poorly seen. For this reason the former approach is preferred. For some lesions however, because of limited options for needle position and transducer position, the latter approach may be necessary. With either approach it is helpful to turn the patient so that the transducer is vertical (or sometimes horizontal) in at least one plane.

Often, a compromise between these two extreme techniques is used, with an intermediate needle angle. The choice of the angle between the needle and the central beam is a compromise. A shallow angle makes it easier to judge the angle with regard to the transducer in both planes, but the needle is less well seen. A large angle makes the needle echoes stronger, but angles are more difficult to judge. In practice, the options are often limited by the position of the target lesion, overlying ribs, bowel and so on.

An alternative approach is to keep the needle vertical, and angle the transducer (Figure 12.11). This also works well when the position of the lesion permits.

Needle guide technique

Various forms of needle guides are available. These take the form of clip-on guides, which attach to the transducer in

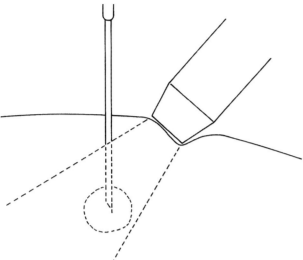

Figure 12.11
Needle placement keeping the needle vertical and angling the transducer.

various ways and have several fixed or continuously variable angles. Most have inserts or adjustments that fit various sizes of needles. All of these systems are used in conjunction with cursor lines on the ultrasound screen, which the needle, when introduced through the guide, theoretically follows (Figure 12.12).

The main advantage of these systems is that they help to keep the needle in the lateral (Z) plane of the transducer beam. They do this with varying success. Although it would seem that the needle must remain in the beam, in practice all systems allow slight lateral movement and, with many clip-on systems, the guide is not truly rigidly attached to the transducer. Although only slight movement is permitted, a very small angulation at the transducer may permit a quite large discrepancy of position of a needle tip in a deep lesion. Also, the needles may bend out of the beam. Nevertheless, needle guides, carefully used, are effective. Angulation in the X–Y plane is also controlled by the guide. In practice, the needle rarely exactly follows the theoretical path displayed on the screen, although the path

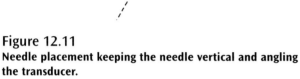

a

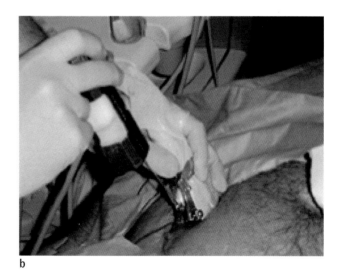

b

Figure 12.12
Use of a needle guide. (a) A clip-on needle guide is shown. (b) A guide in use in a transplant kidney biopsy (see Figure 12.26 for the ultrasound image). (c) An example in a native kidney biopsy. The needle is poorly seen, but can be made out following the theoretical track and touching the renal capsule prior to firing the biopsy gun.

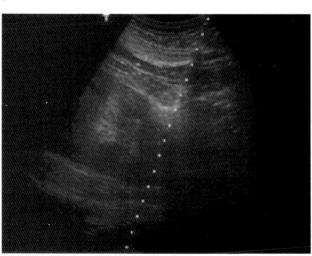

c

is usually close. Variations in this plane are, however, less important, as the needle's progress may be followed on the real-time image and angulation adjusted as necessary.

Many workers have a preference for one or other of the methods outlined above. Different lesions, however, pose different problems, and the technique chosen should be the one most appropriate to the particular circumstance, and to the expertise of the operator and the available equipment.

Needle bending

The use of fine needles is very desirable in many cases, as they have been shown to cause significantly less morbidity than large-diameter needles. The 23-gauge Chiba needle is now commonly used for aspiration biopsy purposes. One problem associated with such needles, however, is bending, causing them to stray from the proposed needle track.

The main reason for bending is differential movement of the tissues during respiration. This mainly occurs in the upper abdomen as the needle passes through the abdominal wall. Provided that the needle tip is monitored throughout its progress, this is not usually a problem. The patient may be instructed to breathe in and out by varying amounts and the needle bending may be controlled to advantageous effect in this way. Another approach used by some is to place a wide-bore 'guide' needle through the abdominal wall, and insert the fine needle through it. This eliminates or reduces bending due to respiration.

There have been reports that the bevel of the needle may cause steering of the needle away from the side of the bevel. Some workers advocate turning the needle as necessary to utilize this effect.

Finally, hard lesions may deflect the needle tip. Occasionally, this may even prevent the tip of a fine needle from entering the lesion. In these cases a stiffer needle must be used.

RENAL BIOPSIES[7–10]

Renal biopsy is an increasingly common method for determining the cause of non-obstructive renal failure in normal-sized kidneys. The patient will have had a thorough clinical history taken and physical examination performed. Biochemical tests are reviewed; prerenal failure is excluded and the degree of renal failure is assessed. An ultrasound study will have excluded obstruction, polycystic kidneys and vascular causes of failure and non-perfusion or renal vein thrombosis. The size of the kidneys is also measured. If the kidneys are found to be small 'end-stage' kidneys, arbitrarily defined as less than 8 cm length, then biopsy is unnecessary, as such kidneys will not recover with treatment, and also biopsy is likely to show fibrous change

with few glomeruli, and will be non-contributory. In kidneys with none of the above features, biopsy is usually performed in order to find the cause of the renal failure and to plan treatment.

Originally, percutaneous biopsy was carried out 'blind', using surface landmarks only. This was largely superseded by fluoroscopic control using intravenous contrast. With this method, however, although the needle is well seen, the nephrogram is short lived, and in cases of renal failure the nephrogram may be absent.

Ultrasound was first used prior to needle placement to determine the position of the kidney. The position of the lower pole was marked on the skin surface, the depth measured and the biopsy needle placed accordingly. This, however, was a halfway measure and now, in most centers, all renal biopsies are carried out under direct ultrasound vision. This has resulted in a marked decrease in morbidity, and an increase in diagnostically useful biopsy samples.

Technique of ultrasound-guided renal biopsy

On the previous day, informed consent is obtained from the patient, and a full coagulation screen is performed. If coagulation is compromised, it is, if possible, corrected. Children are all sedated, whereas adults are only sedated if necessary; Entonox is a useful alternative to sedation. The patient lies prone on the ultrasound couch. Sandbags placed under the abdomen may reduce the amount of kidney that lies beneath the ribs and prevent anterior movement of the kidney during the procedure. The kidneys are carefully examined ultrasonically from the posterior approach. A decision is made as to which kidney will be biopsied. If there are no other considerations, the one that is technically easier is chosen. Even though the kidneys will have been previously scanned, a double check is performed now that there are two normal-sized kidneys. Biopsy of a solitary kidney is not totally contraindicated, but should only be performed after considering that a complication could lead to complete renal failure.

The kidneys lie in a difficult position for biopsy: their upper poles lie within the rib cage. The bowel lies anteriorly. The kidneys are very vascular organs, and, therefore, hemorrhage is a significant risk. A retroperitoneal puncture is preferable, as any perinephric hematoma will tamponade. Also, bowel will not be punctured. A posterolateral approach is usual.

The site of the biopsy is chosen. The aim is to biopsy the lower pole of the kidney tangentially (Figure 12.13). A scan plane is selected, ideally with the transducer vertical, the lower pole of the kidney clearly seen and, if a needle guide is used, the needle track marks on the screen crossing the lower pole. It is useful to do this in quiet respiration, so that

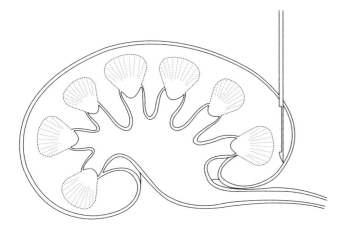

Figure 12.13
Diagram of ideal needle placement. The biopsy is taken across the renal pole, missing the renal pyramid, so that a full biopsy length of cortex is obtained.

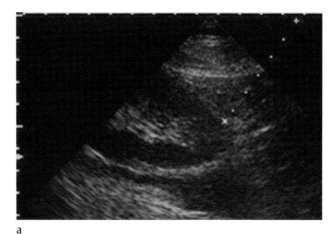

a

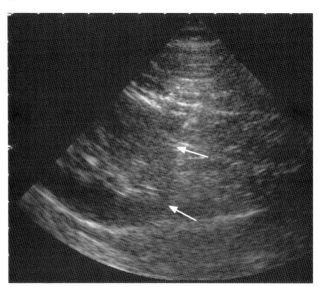

b

Figure 12.14
Ideal renal biopsy. (a) A mark has been placed on the screen to indicate the ideal needle track and to mark the depth. (b) Image taken immediately after firing the needle. A freehand technique was used. The biopsy (position arrowed) was ideally placed tangentially across the renal pole, missing the pyramid.

one may use inspiration or expiration as a further maneuver. If the needle tip is high or low as it approaches the kidney, inspiration or expiration can be used to move the kidney into the correct position for the biopsy. In patients with a high kidney, however, full inspiration may be necessary. The transducer site may be marked, and the skin cleaned and dried. The transducer is covered by a sterile cover and, from then on, asepsis is observed.

A site is selected about 1 cm caudad of the lower end of the transducer and the skin infiltrated with local anesthetic. Further local anesthetic is injected down to the renal capsule using a spinal needle. This may be done blind, but it is useful to use direct ultrasound vision, as this part of the procedure may be used as a 'trial run' for the biopsy needle placement. If the local anesthetic needle is too high or too low, more local anesthetic is injected at a more suitable site or angle. If the local anesthetic needle is not well seen, however, it is not worth struggling to see it at this stage. Ironically, infiltrating the tissue around the lower pole of the kidney may degrade the image, presumably because microbubbles are introduced with the local anesthetic. The depth of the kidney surface may be measured. Even though the biopsy will be performed under real-time ultrasound guidance, the needle is often poorly seen, and the depth may serve as an extra guide.

The skin is now punctured with a scalpel and an automated biopsy needle introduced under direct ultrasound vision, either using a needle guide or freehand, depending on preference. The technique is described in the previous section. The needle is advanced until the tip is seen to indent or just penetrate the renal capsule, and the biopsy is taken. As the needle tip approaches the kidney, inspiration or expiration may be used as a fine adjustment to move the kidney

into an ideal position. If the needle is well placed, it is fired in quiet respiration. The movements of respiration do not damage the kidney with the needle tip in the kidney, and the needle may be fired and removed very rapidly so that suspended respiration is not necessary (Figures 12.14–12.18).

An ideally placed biopsy achieves maximum cortex in the biopsy and also avoids the larger central blood vessels. In practice, this is not always achieved. Placing the needle too low results in skirting the lower pole and only perinephric fat is obtained. This causes no harm, but the biopsy has to be repeated. Biopsying too high often results in part cortex part medulla. There may not be enough glomeruli for interpretation and the biopsy has to be

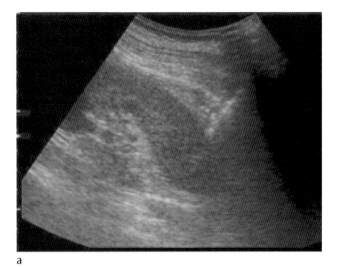
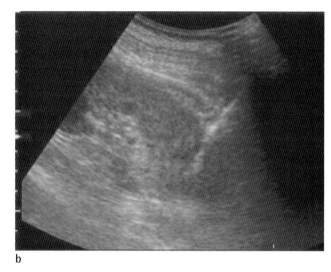

a

b

Figure 12.15
Slightly high biopsy. (a) The needle tip is touching the renal surface prior to firing. (b) Image taken immediately after firing. This is a safe position for a biopsy, being away from the large central vessels. Because it is slightly high, however, half the core was renal medulla. Another core had to be taken to get enough cortex for histologic analysis.

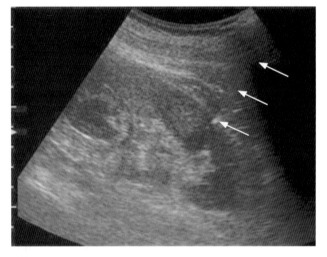

Figure 12.16
Biopsy needle too high. The needle tip is touching the kidney (tip and shaft arrowed). This is dangerously high. The needle was repositioned lower for the biopsy.

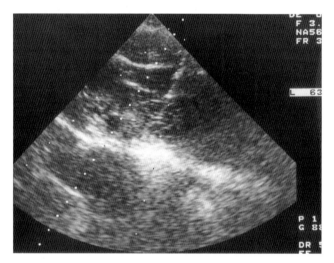

Figure 12.17
Biopsy of a small kidney. The small irregular kidney, although poorly seen from the back, could nevertheless be biopsied under direct ultrasound vision. The regularly placed echoes from the etched bands on the needle are clearly seen.

repeated. More importantly, the risk of significant hemorrhage is increased. A biopsy obtained with the needle insufficiently advanced or advanced too far will obtain renal tissue in only part of the core, which may be insufficient for analysis. In practice, several attempts are often necessary, and more than one core is often needed for sufficient tissue. It is good practice to have an experienced pathology technician to study the cores under low-power microscopy at the time of biopsy. The technician may then assess when sufficient renal tissue has been obtained.

Some have advocated the use of color Doppler to avoid puncturing blood vessels. This is not logical, as the kidney is such a vascular organ that vessel puncture is unavoidable. We have lost one kidney following a well-placed

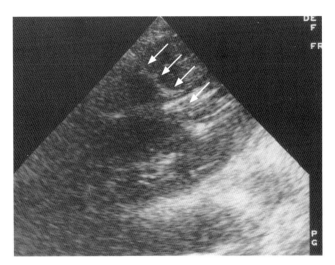

Figure 12.18
Reversed angulation. The patient was large and the kidney could only be well visualized from a low angle. The needle was placed cephalad to the transducer and angled caudad towards the lower pole. This reverse approach, although not often necessary, is sometimes helpful.

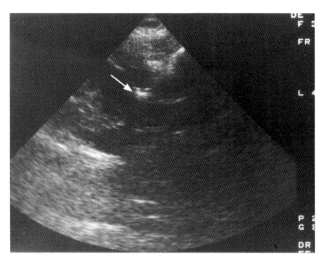

Figure 12.19
Image after firing the biopsy needle. The rapid firing of the highly echogenic needle stylet produces a strong image. Recording this image on a cineloop may be worthwhile, as the image may be reviewed if the biopsy fails. This can give valuable information for resiting the needle. In this case the needle tip (arrow) is only just within the kidney after firing and only a very short core of renal tissue was obtained, most of the core being perinephric fat. Using this information the needle was inserted deeper on the next pass and a good core was obtained.

biopsy, because of puncture of a large branch of an accessory lower pole artery. Accessory lower pole arteries are, however, common and this is an unusual complication. In any case, accessory renal arteries are rarely detected on color Doppler imaging.

Imaging the kidney at the end of the procedure is worthwhile. The needle track is sometimes seen, probably due to hematoma and small air bubbles (Figure 12.19). The kidney should otherwise look normal. A bleed may be seen as an increasing collection of fluid around the renal pole. A perinephric bleed is also suspected if the lower pole of the kidney is originally seen and then becomes difficult to see (Figure 12.20).

The position of the biopsy track should be carefully noted. At further passes, it is important not to misinterpret the previous track as the present needle position (Figure 12.21).

Complications of renal biopsy

It is not a routine practice to perform follow-up imaging after renal biopsy. If patients complain of excessive pain, experience hematuria, become shocked or drop their hemoglobin levels, ultrasound imaging is indicated. These scans may show intrarenal hematomas (Figure 12.22), subcapsular hematomas (Figure 12.23) and/or perinephric retroperitoneal hematomas (Figure 12.24). These are

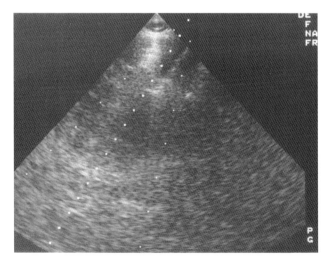

Figure 12.20
Postrenal biopsy intrarenal hemorrhage. This image taken a few minutes after a biopsy shows the needle track, but the lower pole of the kidney, previously well seen, is extremely ill defined. This is a sign of severe hemorrhage. Although this does not change the immediate management, it alerts the renal physician to the situation.

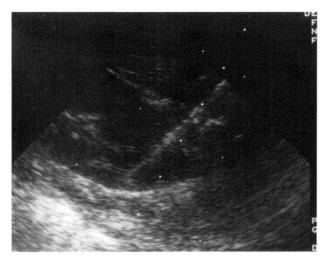

Figure 12.21
Needle track. This image was obtained after a renal biopsy
had been taken and the needle withdrawn. The echogenic track
is probably due to track hemorrhage and bubbles. If a further
pass is made, it is important to distinguish between the old
track and the new needle image.

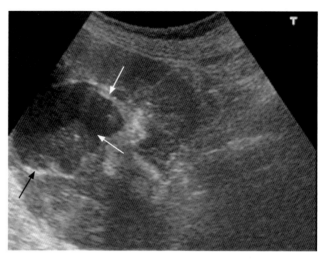

Figure 12.22
Intrarenal hematoma. The patient had excessive pain after
biopsy. Four hours post biopsy there is a mostly liquid
intrarenal hematoma (arrowed). The patient settled on
conservative treatment.

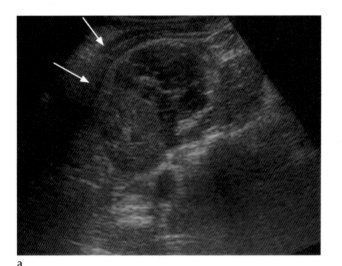

a

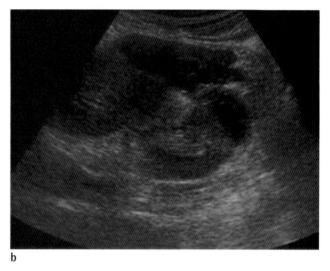

b

Figure 12.23
Subcapsular hematoma. (a) On post-biopsy scanning, as well as an intrarenal bleed, a shallow subcapsular hematoma was seen
(arrows). Such small hematomas are of little significance, but the patient should be carefully monitored and rescanned later to ensure
that the hematoma is not enlarging. (b) This patient with pain 2 hours following a biopsy had a larger subcapsular hematoma.
Hematomas of this size are more worrying. The patient, however, recovered on conservative treatment.

uncommon, although not rare with this method of biopsy.
If they are found, management is initially conservative. CT
will show smaller perinephric hematomas than ultrasound,
but small hematomas are of no clinical significance and so
ultrasound is the appropriate examination. The amount of
hematuria and clinical assessment of rapidity and

chronicity of bleeding are the factors that influence the
decision for surgical or angiographic intervention. If later
follow-up scans are performed, they will show arteriovenous fistulae in 5–10% of patients. In the native kidney,
however, only a very small minority of these will be associated with a large intracalyceal or perinephric bleed

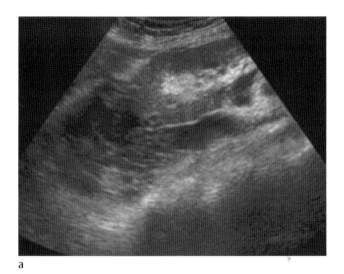
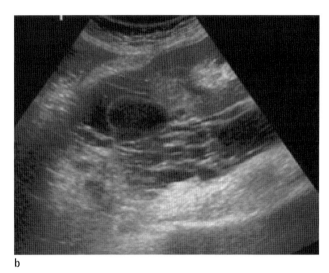

a   b

Figure 12.24
Perinephric (retroperitoneal) hematoma. (a) One hour following a biopsy there is a moderate-sized perinephric hematoma. (b) Two hours later it is slightly larger. It stabilized at this size.

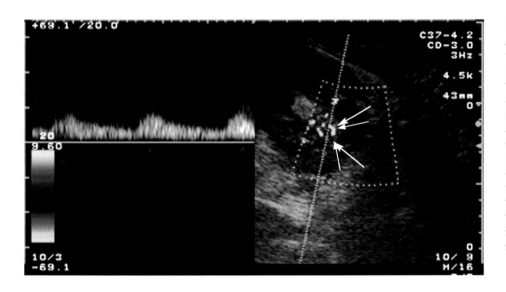

Figure 12.25
Arteriovenous fistula. Twenty-four hours following biopsy the patient had severe hematuria and was shocked. Ultrasound reveals an area of tissue vibration (arrows), indicating an arteriovenous fistula. A vessel is seen flowing into a perinephric hematoma. Angiography confirmed an arteriovenous fistula. The vessel seen was a vein with arterial flow. Bleeding into the calyceal system was also shown. The bleeding vessel was successfully embolized.

requiring intervention (Figure 12.25). The majority are asymptomatic and close spontaneously. There is little point, therefore, in routinely searching for them. Their appearances are listed below in the Renal transplant biopsy section and in Chapter 9 on renal transplants.

Choice of biopsy needle system

Renal biopsies for parenchymal disease require a relatively large core of cortex so that a sufficiently large number of glomeruli are obtained for histologic interpretation. This requires a cut core of about 14 gauge (2 mm). Traditionally, a 'Tru cut'-type needle was used, in which a needle stylet is introduced until its tip lies just through the renal capsule, and then the stylet, which contains a long notch, is advanced. The sheath, which has a cutting edge, is then advanced over the stylet to cut a core of tissue. Stylet and sheath are then withdrawn in this position. There are several spring-loaded devices available that achieve the same procedure automatically. They have the advantage of obtaining more reliable cores, partly because the

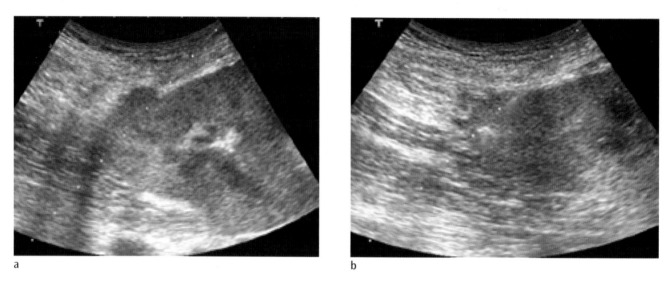

a
b

Figure 12.26

Renal transplant biopsy. A biopsy guide has been used. (a) The needle is seen indenting the kidney prior to biopsy. A shallow angle has been chosen. (b) After firing, the needle is seen to have biopsied tangentially across the anterior context of the uppermost pole.

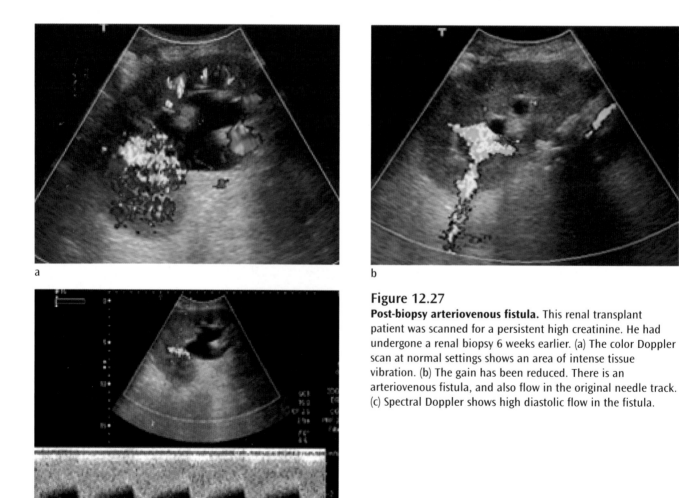

a
b

c

Figure 12.27

Post-biopsy arteriovenous fistula. This renal transplant patient was scanned for a persistent high creatinine. He had undergone a renal biopsy 6 weeks earlier. (a) The color Doppler scan at normal settings shows an area of intense tissue vibration. (b) The gain has been reduced. There is an arteriovenous fistula, and also flow in the original needle track. (c) Spectral Doppler shows high diastolic flow in the fistula.

automated technique is less operator dependent, and partly because the speed of operation gives the tissue less time to move away. They may also be 'fired' with one hand, leaving the other hand free to hold the transducer, if the procedure is done single-handed. Some of the devices available, however, have weaker springs than others and are less reliable at obtaining a good biopsy core.

Non-etched and etched needles are available, the etched needles being etched at the tip or in bands at 1 cm intervals along the shaft. Each gives a different image, and the choice is largely personal, although I prefer those etched in bands. For young children, we use a smaller 18-gauge (1.35 mm) needle. We feel that although the core is not as easy to interpret histologically, the risks of a large needle in a small child's kidney outweigh the advantages of the large core. This is, however, a purely intuitive response, and we have no real proof that the use of a larger needle is contraindicated in children.

RENAL TRANSPLANT BIOPSY[11]

Renal transplant biopsies are extensively used in the investigation of transplant dysfunction (see Chapter 9). The kidney is usually easily palpated, and biopsy may be carried out guided only by palpation. It seems logical, however, to do these also under direct ultrasound vision, and most centers use this method.

Because of the position of the kidney, a different approach has to be used from that in the native kidney. Either pole may be biopsied. The cephalad pole is usually chosen as the easier approach. An anterolateral approach is used in order to prevent the needle crossing peritoneum or bowel. As with the native kidney, a tangential line close to the surface of the kidney is best. A more shallow angle may be employed because of the superficial position of the kidney (Figure 12.26).

For the study of transplant dysfunction, histology does not require large numbers of glomeruli. Large biopsy cores are therefore not needed and 18-gauge (1.35 mm) biopsies are adequate. Some centers take two cores, as rejection may be patchy, affecting some parts of the kidney more than others. Some centers advocate aspiration biopsies from both poles and tangentially from the central kidney. In this case, guidance does not need to be as accurate, as needling the central part of the kidney with a fine aspiration needle is not hazardous, and the peritoneal cavity may be traversed with impunity.

With cut biopsies, arteriovenous fistulae may occur. The majority, as in the native kidney, close spontaneously, but a few enlarge to cause a steal phenomenon or hypertension. The tendency of transplant biopsies to do this may be related to immunosuppression, particularly by cyclosporine, and may be exacerbated by hypertension, which is common in transplant patients. Continuing enlargement of a fistula is much more likely to occur in a more centrally placed biopsy. The Doppler hallmarks of an arteriovenous fistula are increased velocities and decreased resistance in the feeding arteries, increased pulsatility in the draining veins and tissue vibration around the fistula (Figure 12.27). In different patients, different features may predominate (see Chapter 9).

BIOPSIES OF OTHER SITES

Renal tumors[12–16]

Percutaneous biopsy of renal tumors is rarely necessary. A renal tumor proven on imaging is normally treated by nephrectomy without further investigations, unless thought to be an angiomyolipoma or other benign tumor, in which case the diagnosis may be confirmed on CT. Occasionally, however, the nature of a renal mass may be in doubt, and histology may be required before or instead of surgery. Such circumstances include suspected lymphoma of the kidney, which may be treated by radiotherapy, suspected secondary deposits, suspected oncocytomas or xanthogranulomas.

Percutaneous biopsy of any tumor introduces the risk of spread along the needle track. Dissemination of malignant cells along the needle track has been shown to occur commonly, but clinical tumor along the needle track is rare, presumably because the body's defense mechanisms destroy them. A few cases of such spread have been reported in renal tumors, but the risk seems to be small. Hemorrhage is the other risk. The risk is significant, although acceptable with cut biopsy, and there is virtually no risk with fine-needle aspiration biopsy. For this reason, aspiration biopsy is sometimes preferred, using a fine-gauge needle such as a Chiba, with three to six passes, preferably near the periphery of the lesion to avoid any necrotic center (Figure 12.28). The interpretation of aspiration cytology specimens requires a pathologist experienced in the technique. Even with skill and experience, interpretation may be difficult, and a second-cut biopsy may be required for a definitive diagnosis. For this reason, some centers prefer to carry out a cut biopsy de novo, feeling that the small added risk of hemorrhage is acceptable for the higher diagnostic yield. Some workers obtain a cut biopsy specimen, but also roll the needle onto a slide, thus obtaining cytology and histology.

Percutaneous biopsy of renal masses, therefore, has a small but important, place in the investigation of these lesions. Ultrasound guidance follows the same general

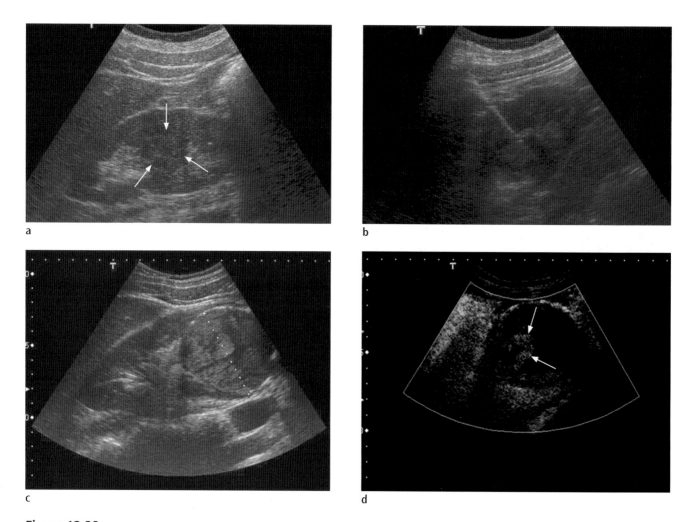

Figure 12.28
Renal tumor biopsy: ultrasound guidance and contrasted ultrasound guidance. (a) This patient had had a left partial nephrectomy for a papillary renal cell carcinoma. Under surveillance he developed a mass in the right kidney. He wanted proof of the diagnosis before agreeing to nephrectomy. (b) The biopsy revealed another papillary renal cell carcinoma. (c) Another patient. This patient had one small end-stage kidney and a mass in the other. Because of the effective single kidney, biopsy, proof was thought necessary. An ultrasound-guided biopsy, however, yielded necrotic tissue only. (d) A contrasted ultrasound scan was therefore performed (Sonovue). This showed a predominantly necrotic tumor. The viable nodule (arrow) was biopsied and showed a renal cell cancer.

principles as discussed earlier. A further guide is the 'feel' of the needle. Renal tumors are usually harder than the surrounding renal tissue, and slightly increased resistance may be felt as the needle enters the lesion. The prime guidance, however, must remain visual guidance, whether by ultrasound or CT control.

Prostate biopsy

The prostate may be biopsied via a transrectal approach, guided by a palpating finger, or may be directly guided under real-time ultrasound. This has been achieved by a transperineal approach, but is now almost exclusively achieved by a guided transrectal route, the needle passing through a biopsy guide clipped onto the transducer.

Because the needle guidance track is long compared with the length of needle in the tissue, the needle stays in the ultrasound beam and follows the indicated path with little problem. The needle track makes a shallow angle to the transducer, and relatively high frequencies are used. All these factors are beneficial, so that there is no problem in visualizing the needle really well in this procedure (Figure 12.29). A cut biopsy 18-gauge needle is used, and an automated needle-firing device is desirable.

Coagulation studies are not necessary unless there is a known reason for coagulation problems. If patients are anticoagulated, it is usual to stop the anticoagulants until the INR (international normalized ratio) is less than 1.5.

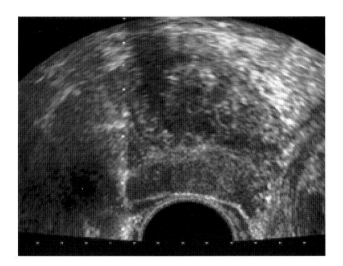

Figure 12.29
Prostate biopsy. The needle (blurred echoes) is seen closely following the predicted path.

immunocompromised patients take ciprofloxacine 500 mg twice daily and metronidazole 400 mg three times daily for a further 5 days. Those with artificial heart valves or other such devices that pose infection risk have, in addition, intravenous ampicillin and gentamicin.

With any antibiotic regimen, there remains a risk of septicemia: 1 or 2% of patients are affected. Patients are warned of this and told to seek medical advice if they develop a fever. The biopsy is performed on a day-case basis. The patient stays in the hospital for 1 hour after the biopsy.

A sample of urine is collected and if there is no blood or moderate blood visible to the naked eye, and the patient has no symptoms, he is sent home, with a document informing him of who to ring if he gets subsequent severe hematuria or symptoms of infection. If the urine is heavily bloodstained, another sample is collected after a further hour. If clear, or clearing, the patient is sent home. If there is continuing heavy hematuria or urinary retention, which is rare, the patient is admitted.

Patients at high risk of stopping anticoagulation are admitted and converted to heparin, which, being short acting, may be briefly stopped for the procedure. Some centers do not stop anticoagulants and there is evidence that this does not lead to an increased risk of hemorrhage, although study numbers are relatively small. Low-dose aspirin is a small risk factor. Some centers stop aspirin for the procedure, some do not. The patient is covered by broad-spectrum antibiotics such as ciprofloxacin and metronidazole. A common regimen is ciprofloxacin 750 mg, metronidazole 400 mg orally 2 hours before the procedure, and repeated 6 and 12 hours after. In addition, diabetic or other

Brachytherapy for prostate cancer

With brachytherapy treatment, radioactive seeds are placed within the prostate in a regular pattern. The pattern is planned from CT images, but placement is achieved by transperineal puncture, under transrectal ultrasound guidance. A guide template attached to the shaft of the transducer ensures accurate placement in a grid pattern. Depth is controlled by real-time ultrasound guidance (Figure 12.30). More detail is outside the scope of this book.

Figure 12.30
Prostate brachytherapy. A diagram of the method of inserting seeds for brachytherapy.

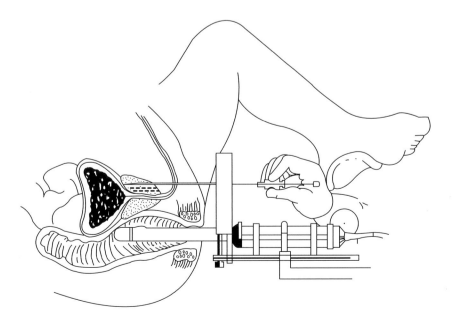

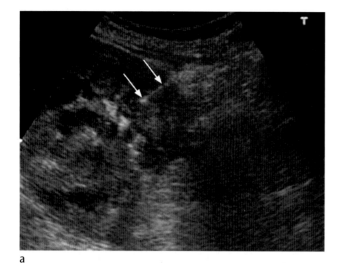

a

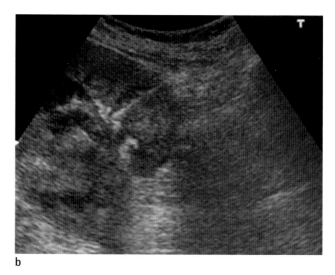

b

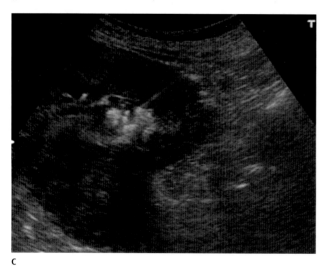

c

Figure 12.31

Antegrade calyceal puncture. (a) The needle (arrow) has entered the kidney and appears to be heading for the chosen calyceal puncture site. (b) The needle has advanced further and is indenting the calyx. (c) The needle has been advanced into the calyceal system. Urine was aspirated. A fine guide wire was introduced through the needle. Some of the echoes in the calyceal system are from the wire, some are from a small volume of air that is often introduced when passing the guide wire.

ANTEGRADE PYELOGRAPHY, DRAINAGE AND STENT INSERTION[17–20]

Antegrade pyelography has traditionally been used to establish the site of obstruction when an intravenous urogram produces insufficient contrast, or the creatinine is raised. This is now almost always achieved by CT. Diagnostic antegrade pyelography is, however, still required in a few cases. More often, antegrade puncture is used for placement of an antegrade nephrostomy drain. A temporary drain may be inserted into an obstructed system until a more permanent drainage procedure is carried out; prior to antegrade stent insertion or prior to percutaneous stone removal (nephrolithotomy).

The antegrade procedure is usually carried out under ultrasound control, although, for percutaneous stone removal from a non-dilated system, a retrograde catheter is often inserted first, the system opacified and dilated and an antegrade drain placed under fluoroscopic control.

Percutaneous puncture of the calyceal system is carried out with the patient prone. The kidney is imaged by ultrasound and a route for the puncture is chosen. Ideally, a calyx should be entered from the periphery of the kidney so as to avoid the larger central vessel (Figures 12.31 and 12.32). This is not always possible and, with a fine needle, the renal pelvis may be entered directly with relative safety (Figure 12.33), although some bleeding into the calyceal system is more likely by this route. Once the route has been chosen, a site must be found at which the transducer may be placed to image the needle entry. Some would advocate placing the transducer so that the ultrasound beam is at an angle of 60–90° to the needle track. This has the advantage that the needle is more echogenic at this angle, but keeping the needle track inside the beam is difficult. It is generally easier to insert the needle via a puncture site near one end

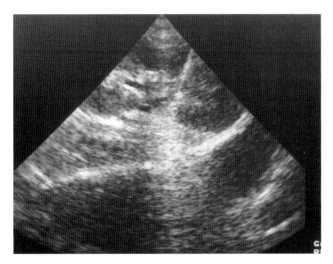

Figure 12.32
Antegrade calyceal puncture of a minimally dilated system.
In this case the needle shaft is well seen. The needle has passed
through the anterior and posterior walls of a minimally dilated
lower pole calyx. The needle was withdrawn slightly while
maintaining suction and the calyx was entered.

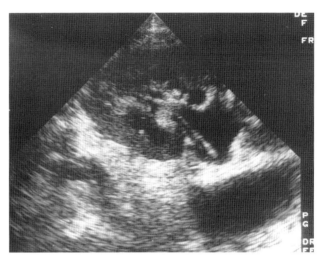

Figure 12.33
Antegrade puncture. In this transplanted kidney the calyces
were difficult to enter, so the renal pelvis was entered directly.
This is acceptable and safe if a fine needle (22 or 23 gauge) is
used.

of the transducer and insert the needle at 30–60° to the
central ultrasound beam, keeping the needle in the ultrasound beam, and hence direct visual control, throughout
its passage (Figure 12.34). The degree of visualization of
the needle varies. Sometimes the whole shaft and tip may
be seen, more often only the tip is seen well, whereas in
other cases only tissue movement on moving the needle is
seen. Fine needles are usually less echogenic than the larger
biopsy needles. All the maneuvers described in the Seeing
and placing the needle section may be needed. It is good
practice to measure the depth of the calyceal system from
the skin surface using the ultrasound image, and to mark
this depth in some way on the needle. On the real-time
image, the needle shaft may be seen, but the tip may be
deeper than it appears. This occurs because the angle that
the needle makes to the ultrasound beam becomes less as
the needle tip approaches and passes the central beam (see
Figure 12.7). Measuring the depth in the needle gives a
second way of assessing the position of the needle tip,
although, in practice, ultrasound measurements tend to
slightly underestimate the depth Fine needles may also
bend out of the ultrasound beam, either because of variations in tissue density, because of differential movement of
superficial and deeper tissues with respiration, or because
of a steering effect caused by the bevel of the needle..

The actual puncture of a dilated calyx may often be seen.
The wall of the calyx bulges as the needle tip indents it, and
then the needle tip is seen entering the calyx. Often, however, the needle passes through the posterior wall of the
calyx. The stylet is withdrawn and gentle aspiration

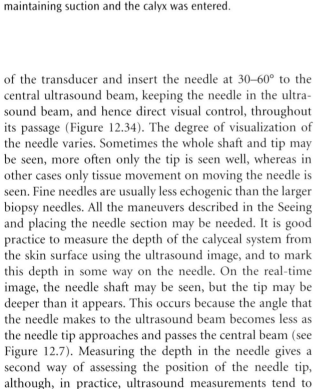

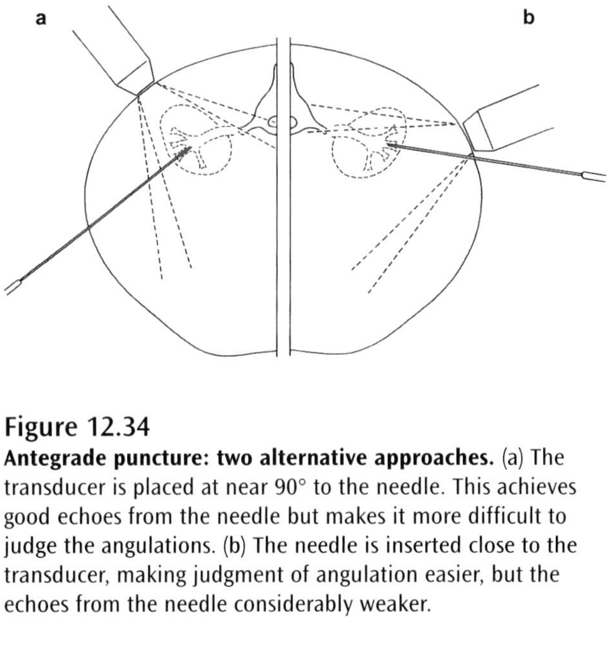

Figure 12.34
Antegrade puncture: two alternative approaches. (a) The
transducer is placed at near 90° to the needle. This achieves
good echoes from the needle but makes it more difficult to
judge the angulations. (b) The needle is inserted close to the
transducer, making judgment of angulation easier, but the
echoes from the needle considerably weaker.

applied. If no urine appears, aspiration is maintained as the
needle is withdrawn.

When the needle has been shown to enter the calyceal
system, contrast is injected under fluoroscopic control to
opacify the system and show the level of obstruction. Care
must be taken not to inject so much contrast that it

extravasates outside the calyceal system, as this will make fluoroscopic control for subsequent drain insertion difficult.

If a percutaneous nephrostomy drain is to be inserted, this may also be done under ultrasound control if the system is sufficiently dilated. For less-dilated systems, however, insertion under fluoroscopic control into the now-opacified system may be performed. If the fine needle is well positioned, then a very fine wire (Neff system) may be passed through the needle into the calyceal system and ideally maneuvered down the ureter, or at least well into the system. The needle is withdrawn over the wire. If the needle is poorly positioned, for instance directly into the renal pelvis, then a second fine needle may be better placed into the opacified system and the wire introduced through this needle. The fine wire is not sufficiently stiff to directly guide the nephrostomy drain. A special dilator is first passed over the wire. This has an outer sheath that allows introduction of a standard guide wire. This is similarly maneuvered into the ureter if possible. The sheath is withdrawn and the nephrostomy drain with a suitable internal stiffener is passed over the wire. The wire and stiffener are withdrawn and the drain is fixed at the skin surface.

This two-stage method is relatively safe, as the initial needle is narrow, and multiple puncture attempts are possible. If the calyceal system is sufficiently dilated, however, experienced operators may be sufficiently confident to directly introduce a larger needle with a sheath that allows introduction of the standard guide wire without the initial use of the fine needle and guide wire.

If the drain is being inserted prior to percutaneous stone removal, then a route must be chosen that will permit easy access to the stone through the subsequent dilated track. If the drain is being inserted prior to stent insertion, a calyx should be chosen that will permit an easy placement of a guide wire down through the renal pelvis and into the ureter.

Once the needle is in place, subsequent maneuvers of wire insertion, drain insertion or stent insertion are usually carried out under fluoroscopic control. Under certain circumstances, such as pregnancy, however, the whole procedure may be carried out under ultrasound control.

Cyst drainage[20]

This procedure is not often necessary, as most renal cysts are asymptomatic. It may be necessary to relieve symptoms in patients who have bled into a cyst. This often occurs in polycystic kidneys, and causes pain by rapidly dilating the cyst. In these cases, drainage relieves the symptoms. Infected cysts and the small minority of cysts where there is a possibility of malignancy may require needling. The procedure of needle placement is the same as previously described. The needle tip is usually clearly seen when it lies within the cyst.

Suprapubic catheter insertion

Insertion of a suprapubic catheter is normally carried out without the need for any ultrasonic guidance. In cases when the bladder is abnormal in some way, however, either from previous surgery or from involvement with tumor, ultrasound guidance may be used. We use a small pigtail catheter, as used for antegrade kidney drainage. This is a perfectly adequate size, unless there is marked hematuria, which may occlude the lumen.

Urinary catheter balloon puncture[21]

Occasionally, the balloon of a urinary catheter will not deflate for removal. This is less common with modern plastic catheters than with the old rubber variety, but still occasionally occurs. A fine needle may easily be inserted under real-time ultrasound control into the balloon via a percutaneous route through the bladder, thus bursting the balloon.

Abscess drainage[22–25]

Abscesses, and other collections associated with the genitourinary system, may be drained percutaneously under ultrasound guidance (Figure 12.35). The principles of needle placement are as described earlier. Small collections may be aspirated to dryness, and this may be curative. There is increasing evidence that the old surgical dictum that all abscesses must be drained is probably not true, and aspiration and antibiotic treatment may be sufficient. For all but the smaller abscesses, however, percutaneous drainage is wise. Drain insertion is usually a catheter over wire technique, as used for antegrade kidney drainage. For larger collections, however, a large-bore sump drain with a rigid metal stylet may be used. If there is any question about traversing bowel, then CT guidance is preferable to ultrasound guidance.

The drain placement is usually straightforward, but success or failure depends on the subsequent management of the drain. Unlike large-bore surgically placed drains, the smaller ultrasonically guided percutaneous drains often need regular flushing with saline and aspiration to be effective. It is good practice to aspirate any collection immediately the drain is inserted, and flush with saline until the returned fluid is clear. This gives the procedure a good start. The drain should subsequently be flushed in a similar way at least 6-hourly until no pus is being returned. Larger collections may have two drains placed one at either end, which will enable saline to be instilled via one, and drained via the other. Some sonologists supervise the drain management themselves, but most lack the time: in this case, the sonologist should leave clear instructions on the ward.

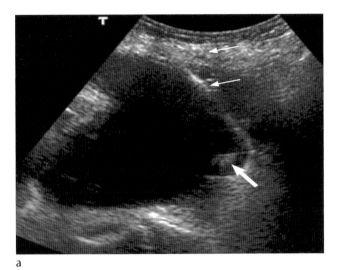 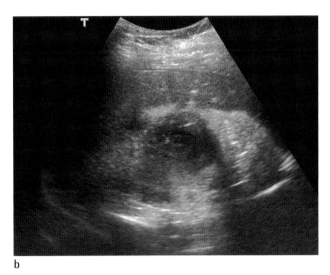

a   b

Figure 12.35

Abscess drainage. (a) The needle is seen entering a perinephric abscess. A wire has been inserted. The narrow arrows point to the needle, the wide arrow to the coiled wire tip. (b) Needle aspirating an intrarenal abscess.

LITHOTRIPSY

General considerations

Lithotripters themselves are ultrasound-guided, but the technique of and indications for lithotripsy are beyond the scope of this text. Early lithotripsy treatment had a number of complications. With more experience, complications are now uncommon. Ultrasound may play a role in the follow-up of patients after lithotripsy and this will be discussed.

Post-lithotripsy appearance[26,27]

Lithotripsy breaks calculi by imparting energy, and in doing so, in effect, causes blunt trauma to the kidney. Early lithotripsy treatment often produced small intrarenal and perinephric hematomas and perinephric urinomas (Figures 12.36–12.38). Such lesions are usually of no consequence and their recognition on a subsequent ultrasound scan should not cause alarm. Some degree of calyceal dilatation as the stone fragments pass is normal (Figure 12.39). Increasing calyceal dilatation, however, may indicate the need for removal of ureteric fragments, particularly if there are also signs of infection. It is this serial scanning for the detection of obstruction that is the main role of ultrasound in the post-lithotripsy patient. Retained stone fragments may be seen (Figure 12.40) but are more usually followed by X-ray, unless non-radiopaque.

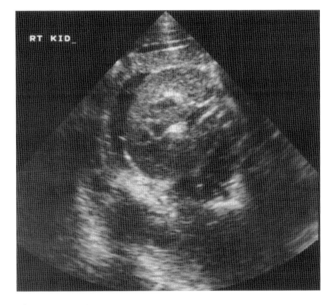

Figure 12.36

Post-lithotripsy perinephric hematoma. Small perinephric hematomas of this size are often seen after lithotripsy and seem to be of little significance.

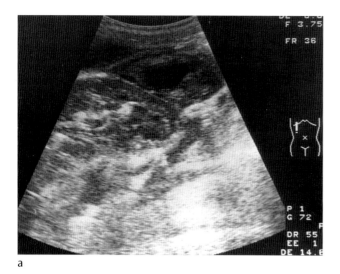

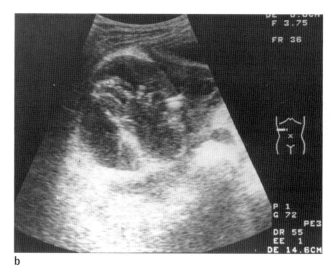

a

b

Figure 12.37
Post-lithotripsy perinephric hematoma. (a,b) A hematoma of this size should not occur and in this case was associated with renal damage as assessed later by isotope renography.

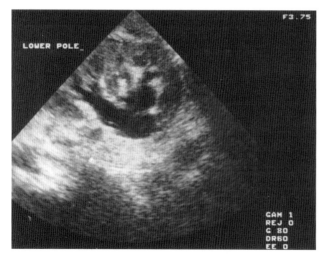

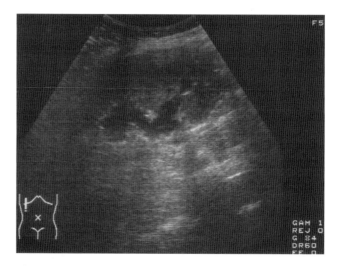

Figure 12.38
Post-lithotripsy urinoma. An anechoic area is seen around the upper pole of the kidney, representing a urinoma. This complication is of no significance.

Figure 12.39
Post-lithotripsy calyceal dilatation. There is dilatation of the calyceal system, particularly the upper pole which previously contained the calculus. Such dilatation is of no significance unless it increases.

References

1. Bondestam S, Kreula J. Needle tip echogenicity. A study with real-time ultrasound. Invest Radiol 1989; 24: 555–60.
2. Aindow JD, Hitchmough MD, Lesner J. The ultrasonic reflectivity of biopsy needles. Hospital Physicists Association 42nd Annual Conference, September 1985, Southampton.
3. Hamper UM, Savader BL, Sheth S. Improved needle tip visualization by color Doppler sonography. AJR Am J Roentgenol 1991; 156: 401–2.
4. Heckemann R, Seidel KJ. The sonographic appearance and contrast enhancement of puncture needles. J Clin Ultrasound 1983; 11: 265–8.
5. Kurohiji T, Sigel B, Justin J, Manchi J. Motion marking in color Doppler ultrasound needle and catheter visualization. J Ultrasound Med 1990; 9: 243–5.

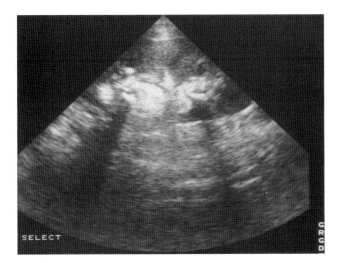

Figure 12.40
Post-lithotripsy renal calculi. These fairly large calculi in the upper and lower poles were treated by lithotripsy. The calculi have broken into small fragments which have a typically blurred outline. Some of the larger fragments failed to pass and a further session of lithotripsy was necessary.

6. McGahan JP. Laboratory assessment of ultrasonic needle and catheter visualization. J Ultrasound Med 1986; 5: 373–7.

7. Eichhorn GL, Berger NA, Butzov JJ, et al. Clinical sonography in urology. Urology 1973; 1(6): 506–22.

8. Nass K, O'Neill WC. Bedside renal biopsy: ultrasound guidance by the nephrologists. Am J Kidney Dis 1999; 34(5): 955–9.

9. Burstein DM, Schwartz MM, Korbet SM. Percutaneous renal biopsy with the use of real-time ultrasound. Am J Nephrol 1991; 11(3): 195–200.

10. Wiseman DA, Hawkins R, Numerow LM, Taub KJ. Percutaneous renal biopsy utilizing real time, ultrasonic guidance and a semiautomated biopsy device. Kidney Int 1990; 38(2): 347–9.

11. Hubsch PJ, Mostbeck G, Barton PP, et al. Evaluation of arteriovenous fistulas and pseudoaneurysms in renal allografts following percutaneous needle biopsy. Color-coded Doppler sonography versus duplex Doppler sonography. J Ultrasound Med 1990; 9(2): 95–100.

12. Helm CW, Burwood RJ, Harrison NW, Melcher DH. Aspiration cytology of solid renal tumors. Br J Urol 1983; 55: 249–53.

13. Juul N, Torp-Pedersen S, Gronvall S, et al. Ultrasonically guided fine needle aspiration biopsy of renal masses. J Urol 1985; 133: 579–81.

14. von Screeb T, Arner O, Skovsted G, Wikstad N. Renal adenocarcinoma. Is there a risk of spreading tumor cells in diagnostic puncture? Scand J Urol Nephrol 1967; 1: 270–6.

15. Wehle MJ, Grabstald H. Contraindications to needle biopsy of a solid renal mass: tumor dissemination by needle aspiration. J Urol 1986; 136: 446–8.

16. Bush WH Jr, Burnett LL, Gibbons RP. Needle tract seeding of renal cell carcinoma. AJR Am J Roentgenol 1977; 129: 725–7.

17. Dyer RB, Regan JD, Kavanagh PV, et al. Percutaneous nephrostomy with extensions of the technique: step by step. Radiographics 2002; 22(3): 503–25.

18. Frede T, Hatzinger M, Rassweiler J. Ultrasound in endourology. J Endourol 2001; 15(1): 3–16.

19. Millward SF. Percutaneous nephrostomy: a practical approach. J Vasc Interv Radiol 2000; 11(8): 955–64.

20. Gross DM. Diagnostic renal cyst puncture and percutaneous nephrostomy. Urol Clin North Am 1979; 6(2): 409–24.

21. Higgins WL, Mace AH. Puncture of a nondeflatable Foley balloon using ultrasound guidance. Radiology 1984; 151: 801.

22. van Sonneberg E, Mueller PR, Ferucci JT Jr. Percutaneous drainage of 250 abdominal abscesses and fluid collections. Part I: Results, failures and complications. Radiology 1984; 151: 337–41.

23. Mueller PR, van Sonneberg E, Ferucci JT Jr. Percutaneous drainage of 250 abdominal abscesses and fluid collections. Part II: Current procedural concepts. Radiology 1984; 151: 343–7.

24. Bernardino ME, Baumgartner BR. Abscess drainage in the genitourinary tract. Radiol Clin North Am 1986; 24: 539–49.

25. Cronan JJ, Amis ES Jr, Dorfman GS. Percutaneous drainage of renal abscesses. AJR Am J Roentgenol 1984; 142: 351–4.

26. Baumgartner BR, Steinberg HV, Ambrose SS, et al. Sonographic evaluation of renal stones treated by shock-wave lithotripsy. AJR Am J Roentgenol 1987; 149: 131–5.

27. Kaude JV, Williams JL, Wright PG, et al. Sonographic evaluation of the kidney following extracorporeal shock wave lithotripsy. J Ultrasound Med 1987; 6: 299–306.

Index

Page numbers in *italics* refer to tables and figures.